BIOMEDICAL APPLICATIONS OF ELECTROSPINNING AND ELECTROSPRAYING

Woodhead Publishing Series in Biomaterials

BIOMEDICAL APPLICATIONS OF ELECTROSPINNING AND ELECTROSPRAYING

Edited by

NARESH KASOJU
HUA YE

ELSEVIER

WP
WOODHEAD PUBLISHING
An imprint of Elsevier

Woodhead Publishing is an imprint of Elsevier
The Officers' Mess Business Centre, Royston Road, Duxford, CB22 4QH, United Kingdom
50 Hampshire Street, 5th Floor, Cambridge, MA 02139, United States
The Boulevard, Langford Lane, Kidlington, OX5 1GB, United Kingdom

Notices
Knowledge and best practice in this field are constantly changing. As new research and experience broaden our understanding, changes in research methods, professional practices, or medical treatment may become necessary.

Practitioners and researchers must always rely on their own experience and knowledge in evaluating and using any information, methods, compounds, or experiments described herein. In using such information or methods they should be mindful of their own safety and the safety of others, including parties for whom they have a professional responsibility.

To the fullest extent of the law, neither the Publisher nor the authors, contributors, or editors, assume any liability for any injury and/or damage to persons or property as a matter of products liability, negligence or otherwise, or from any use or operation of any methods, products, instructions, or ideas contained in the material herein.

Library of Congress Cataloging-in-Publication Data
A catalog record for this book is available from the Library of Congress

British Library Cataloguing-in-Publication Data
A catalogue record for this book is available from the British Library

ISBN: 978-0-12-822476-2

For information on all Woodhead Publishing publications visit our website at https://www.elsevier.com/books-and-journals

Publisher: Matthew Deans
Acquisitions Editor: Sabrina Webber
Editorial Project Manager: Aleksandra Packowska
Production Project Manager: Surya Narayanan Jayachandran
Cover Designer: Christian J. Bilbow

Typeset by TNQ Technologies

Contents

Contributors

Aakriti Aggarwal
Department of Biotechnology, Dr. B. R. Ambedkar National Institute of Technology, Jalandhar, Punjab, India

P.R. Anil Kumar
Division of Tissue Culture, Department of Applied Biology, Biomedical Technology Wing, Sree Chitra Tirunal Institute for Medical Sciences and Technology, Thiruvananthapuram, Kerala, India

Matej Buzgo
InoCure s.r.o., Prague, Czech Republic

Ellen Byrne
Business Development at Spraybase (Biofabrication Division of Avectas), MaynoothWorks, Maynooth, Co. Kildare, Ireland

Andrew J. Carr
Botnar Research Centre, University of Oxford, Oxford, United Kingdom

Chih-Yao Chui
Institute of Biomedical Engineering, Department of Engineering Science, University of Oxford, Oxford, United Kingdom

Duncan Q.M. Craig
UCL School of Pharmacy, London, United Kingdom

Zhanfeng Cui
Institute of Biomedical Engineering, Department of Engineering Science, University of Oxford, Oxford, United Kingdom

Vinod Damodaran
Division of Tissue Culture, Department of Applied Biology, Biomedical Technology Wing, Sree Chitra Tirunal Institute for Medical Sciences and Technology, Thiruvananthapuram, Kerala, India

Pooya Davoodi
Department of Engineering, University of Cambridge, Cambridge, United Kingdom; The Nanoscience Centre, University of Cambridge, Cambridge, United Kingdom

Poornima Dubey
Department of Radiation Oncology, University of Cincinnati College of Medicine Cincinnati, Cincinnati, OH, United States

Rose Ann G. Franco
School of Mechanical, Medical and Process Engineering (MMPE), Science and Engineering Faculty (SEF), Institute of Health and Biomedical Innovation (IHBI), Queensland University of Technology (QUT), Kelvin Grove, QLD, Australia; Translational Research Institute (TRI), Woolloongabba, QLD, Australia

Deepa Garg
Central Scientific Instruments Organization (CSIR-CSIO), Chandigarh, Punjab, India; Academy of Scientific and Innovative Research, CSIR-CSIO, Chandigarh, Punjab, India

Elisabeth L. Gill
Department of Engineering, University of Cambridge, Cambridge, United Kingdom; The Nanoscience Centre, University of Cambridge, Cambridge, United Kingdom

P. Gopinath
Department of Biotechnology, Joint Faculty in Centre for Nanotechnology, Indian Institute of Technology Roorkee, Roorkee, Uttarakhand, India

Naresh Kasoju
Division of Tissue Culture, Department of Applied Biology, Biomedical Technology Wing, Sree Chitra Tirunal Institute for Medical Sciences and Technology, Thiruvananthapuram, Kerala, India

Hae Won Kim
Institute of Tissue Regeneration Engineering (ITREN), Dankook University, Cheonan, Chungcheongnam-do, Republic of Korea; UCL Eastman-Korea Dental Medicine Innovation Centre, Dankook University, Cheonan, Chungcheongnam-do, Republic of Korea

Remya Komeri
Division of Tissue Culture, Department of Applied Biology, Biomedical Technology Wing, Sree Chitra Tirunal Institute for Medical Sciences and Technology, Thiruvananthapuram, Kerala, India

Alok Kumar
Department of Immunology and Genomic Medicine, Graduate School of Medicine, Kyoto University, Yoshida Campus, Yoshida Konoe-cho, Kyoto, Japan

Antonina A. Lach
Botnar Research Centre, University of Oxford, Oxford, United Kingdom

Joana A. Martins
Botnar Research Centre, University of Oxford, Oxford, United Kingdom

Ishita Matai
Central Scientific Instruments Organization (CSIR-CSIO), Chandigarh, Punjab, India; Academy of Scientific and Innovative Research, CSIR-CSIO, Chandigarh, Punjab, India

Deepthy Menon
Amrita Centre for Nanosciences and Molecular Medicine, Amrita Vishwa Vidyapeetham, Kochi, Kerala, India

Manju Misra
Graduate School of Pharmacy, Gujarat Technological University Gandhinagar Campus Nr. Government Polytechnic K-6 Circle, Gandhinagar, Gujarat, India

Jimna Mohamed Ameer
Division of Tissue Culture, Department of Applied Biology, Biomedical Technology Wing, Sree Chitra Tirunal Institute for Medical Sciences and Technology, Thiruvananthapuram, Kerala, India

Hayley L. Morris
Botnar Research Centre, University of Oxford, Oxford, United Kingdom

Pierre–Alexis Mouthuy
Botnar Research Centre, University of Oxford, Oxford, United Kingdom

Shantikumar V. Nair
Amrita Centre for Nanosciences and Molecular Medicine, Amrita Vishwa Vidyapeetham, Kochi, Kerala, India

Chikim Nguyen
Department of Dentistry - Regenerative Biomaterials, Radboud university medical center, Nijmegen, the Netherlands

Linh Nguyen
UCL Eastman-Korea Dental Medicine Innovation Centre, Dankook University, Cheonan, Chungcheongnam-do, Republic of Korea; Division of Biomaterials and Tissue Engineering, Eastman Dental Institute, University College London, Royal Free Hospital, London, United Kingdom

Andrew R. Padalhin
Beckman Laser Institute Korea, College of Medicine, Dankook University, Dankook, Cheonan, Chungcheongnam-do, Republic of Korea

Roopesh Pai (R)
Division of Tissue Culture, Department of Applied Biology, Biomedical Technology Wing, Sree Chitra Tirunal Institute for Medical Sciences and Technology, Thiruvananthapuram, Kerala, India

Geoff J.M. Parker
Centre for Medical Image Computing, Department of Computer Science, University College London, London, United Kingdom; Bioxydyn Limited, Manchester, United Kingdom

Kapil D. Patel
Institute of Tissue Regeneration Engineering (ITREN), Dankook University, Cheonan, Chungcheongnam-do, Republic of Korea; UCL Eastman-Korea Dental Medicine Innovation Centre, Dankook University, Cheonan, Chungcheongnam-do, Republic of Korea

Seeram Ramakrishna
Center for Nanotechnology and Sustainability, Department of Mechanical Engineering, National University of Singapore, Singapore, Republic of Singapore

C.R. Reshmi
Amrita Centre for Nanosciences and Molecular Medicine, Amrita Vishwa Vidyapeetham, Kochi, Kerala, India

Mahesh Kumar Sah
Department of Biotechnology, Dr. B. R. Ambedkar National Institute of Technology, Jalandhar, Punjab, India

Yan Yan Shery Huang
Department of Engineering, University of Cambridge, Cambridge, United Kingdom; The Nanoscience Centre, University of Cambridge, Cambridge, United Kingdom

Aiva Simaite
InoCure s.r.o., Prague, Czech Republic

Vinita Takiar
Department of Radiation Oncology, University of Cincinnati College of Medicine Cincinnati, Cincinnati, OH, United States; Cincinnati Department of Veterans Affairs (VA) Medical Center, Cincinnati, OH, United States

Shreya Thakkar
Department of Pharmaceutics, National Institute of Pharmaceutical Education and Research (NIPER), Ahmedabad, Gujarat, India

Fiona Verisqa
Division of Biomaterials and Tissue Engineering, Eastman Dental Institute, University College London, Royal Free Hospital, London, United Kingdom

Wenyu Wang
Department of Engineering, University of Cambridge, Cambridge, United Kingdom; The Nanoscience Centre, University of Cambridge, Cambridge, United Kingdom

Gang Wei
College of Chemistry and Chemical Engineering, Qingdao University, Qingdao, Shandong Province, PR China

Gareth R. Williams
UCL School of Pharmacy, University College London, London, United Kingdom

Fang Yang
Department of Dentistry - Regenerative Biomaterials, Radboud university medical center, Nijmegen, the Netherlands

Hua Ye
Institute of Biomedical Engineering, Department of Engineering Science, University of Oxford, Oxford, United Kingdom

Deng-Guang Yu
School of Materials Science and Engineering, University of Shanghai for Science and Technology, Shanghai, China

Fenglei Zhou
Centre for Medical Image Computing, Department of Computer Science, University College London, London, United Kingdom; UCL School of Pharmacy, University College London, London, United Kingdom

Foreword

It gives me immense pleasure to write this foreword for the book entitled *Biomedical Applications of Electrospinning and Electrospraying*, edited by my colleagues Dr. Naresh Kasoju and Professor Hua Ye. The editors of this book have several years of diverse, hands-on field experience, and have published seminal works on electrospinning and electrospraying (*abbreviated henceforth as ES for simplicity*), including development of a portable point-of-care ES device. Furthermore, the various chapters are contributed by domain experts from around the world. They are known for their passion and sustained contributions.

I have had a long association with ES technologies throughout my career, and I am happy to see that many more young researchers are venturing into this field in recent times. ES technologies, though introduced in the early 1900s, have gained momentum only in recent times partly due to the acceleration received from the biomaterials field. Given the simplicity of the process, yet extraordinary features of ES products, ES technologies gained much attention and appreciation from many. The field continues to evolve, by not only interacting with other emerging techniques such as 3D printing, but also by finding applications in point-of-care devices. I am happy to see that *Biomedical Applications of Electrospinning and Electrospraying* covers the field from the very basics to the translational aspects.

As I write this foreword, humanity is battling COVID-19 pandemic, thus throwing an unprecedented challenge to the scientific community to come up with ways and means for rapid testing and screening, effective medical treatments, and preventive and protective measures. This has been an opportunity for ES researchers and technologists to come up with an array of ES medical devices, such as ES face masks for preventing aerosol spread and antiviral hospital apparel. Moreover, ES technologies could be further explored in rapid diagnosis, sustained drug delivery, and lung regeneration. Perhaps, the range of innovations to mitigate COVID-19 will see useful technologies from the ES community and be included in future editions of this book.

I congratulate the editors Dr. Naresh Kasoju and Professor Hua Ye and all the expert contributors of this book for their excellent contributions. I am sure this book will provide sound, clear, inspiring guidance to young minds new to the ES technologies, and as a comprehensive state-of-the-art update on R&D innovations and translational affairs to the experts engaged in several ES medical device development programs worldwide.

In a nutshell, if you are looking for a single reference on the ES technologies, with details on (i) basic principles; (ii) technological advances; (iii) applications in tissue engineering, drug delivery, biosensing, and beyond; (iv) combinatorial approaches including 3D printing; (v) practical considerations for setting up ES units; and (vi) regulatory pathway for bringing the ES medical devices from bench to bedside, this timely book *Biomedical Applications of Electrospinning and Electrospraying* is just apt for you.

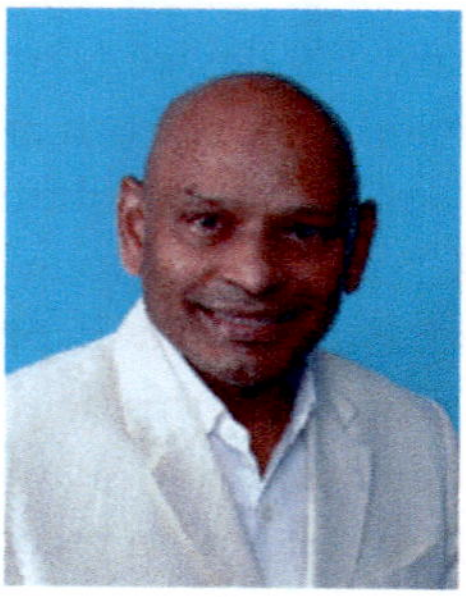

Professor Seeram Ramakrishna, *FREng, Everest Chair*
PhD (Cambridge), TGMP (Harvard), FIES, FIMMM, FIMechE, FAIMBE, FASME, FNAE, FBSE
Director, Center for Nanofibers and Nanotechnology
National University of Singapore, Singapore
WhatsApp +65 90107766
https://blog.nus.edu.sg/seeram/
https://www.linkedin.com/in/seeram-ramakrishna/
https://www.eng.nus.edu.sg/me/staff/ramakrishna-seeram/
https://www.uib.no/en/sdgbergen/141236/members-unesco-expert-group

Preface

Electrospinning and electrospraying techniques have evolved significantly from being methods to prepare fibers and powders to processes of fabricating highly complex and ordered materials. Several innovative approaches have been described in the literature including combinations of electrospinning, electrospraying, and 3D printing. Unfortunately, there is no work so far to cover these similar yet unique techniques, and therefore, this book aims to fill this gap.

We are confident that *Biomedical Applications of Electrospinning and Electrospraying* would appeal to readers, both academic and professionals, who are interested in understanding fundamental concepts on fabrication of micro- and nanoscale materials, state-of-the-art setups in electrospinning and electrospraying, potential applications of these materials in biomedical field, considerations for setting up a facility, and translational path for e-spun/e-spray devices from bench to bedside. This book covers both fundamental and advanced aspects in electrospinning and electrospraying so as to attract the readers at beginner's as well as advanced level.

We greatly acknowledge all the contributors for their wonderful efforts in compiling the best of the dedicated topics in a timely manner. We are also indebted to the reviewers for their precious time and critical suggestions. We take this opportunity to extend our thanks to *Mathew Deans, Sabrina Webber, Aleksandra Packowska, Surya Narayanan Jayachandran, Christian J Bilbow*, and *the entire editorial team* from Elsevier Inc. and Woodhead Publishing Ltd. for their invaluable efforts in the successful publication of this book. We extend our sincere thanks to *Professor Seeram Ramakrishna,* FREng, Everest Chair, Director, Center for Nanofibers and Nanotechnology, National University of Singapore, Singapore, and *World's Most Influential Scientific Minds* (Thomson Reuters) for critically reviewing this book and for offering an encouraging foreword.

Finally, we deeply believe that electrospinning and electrospraying have been and would remain as favorite techniques to prepare nanomaterials for biomedical applications, and this book is an attempt to compile the latest trends in the field. However, we appreciate any constructive comments or suggestions from peers and experts in academics and industries to enhance the quality of the work as well as further expand the scope of the field in the future.

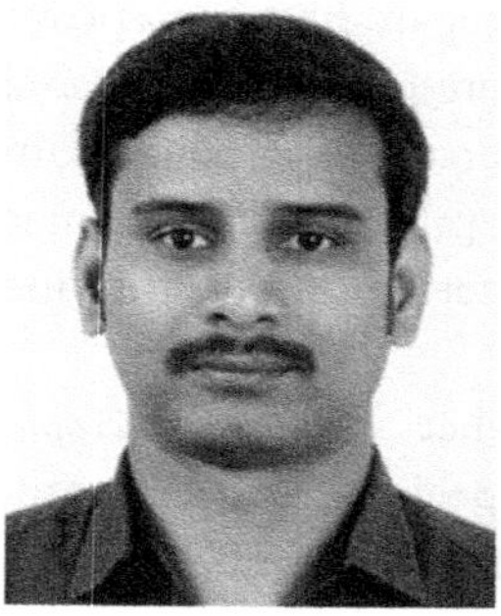

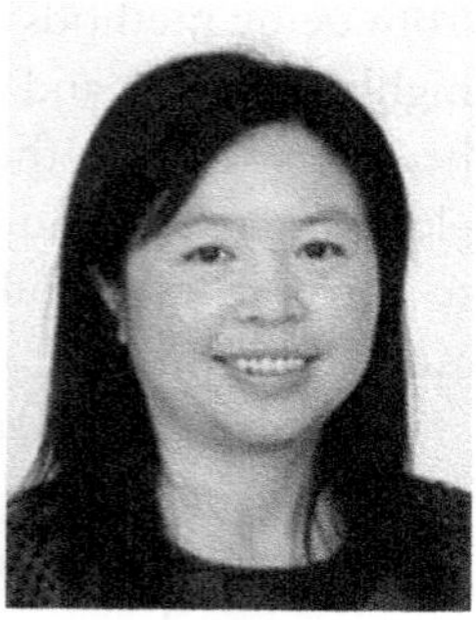

Naresh Kasoju **Hua Ye**

Introduction

Biomedical Applications of Electrospinning and Electrospraying aims to introduce electrospinning and electrospraying concepts; describe the state-of-the-art technological advancements; provide a comprehensive coverage of electrospun/electrospray materials in drug delivery, tissue engineering, and biosensor applications; present details on practical considerations for setting up a unit; and finally offer translational path for electrospun and electrospray medical devices from bench to bedside.

This edited book consists of a total of 15 chapters written by a mix of young scientists as well as well-established experts in the field, including those from the industry. These chapters are categorized into four parts for effective dissemination of the contents to the readers.

Part I deals with "*Electrospinning*" theme, wherein Chapter 1 introduces the basic concepts and fundamental insights in electrospinning, Chapter 2 deals with advances and innovations in electrospinning technology, Chapter 3 details about the electrospun materials as scaffolds in tissue engineering and regenerative medicine, Chapter 4 describes the applications of electrospun fibers in the field of drug delivery, and Chapter 5 provides latest applications of electrospun nanomaterials as biosensors in diagnostics and beyond.

Part II deals with "*Electrospraying*" theme, wherein Chapter 6 describes the fundamental concepts and insights in electrospraying for biomedical applications, Chapter 7 provides latest advances and innovations in electrospraying technology, Chapter 8 reviews the applications of electrospraying materials in tissue engineering and beyond, Chapter 9 details about the applications of electrospray particles as drug delivery systems, and Chapter 10 covers the applications of electrospray systems as biosensors in diagnostics and beyond.

Part III deals with "*Trends in electrospinning and electrospraying*" theme, wherein Chapter 11 describes various state-of-the-art combinational approaches in electrospinning and electrospraying, Chapter 12 covers several combinational approaches in electrospinning/electrospraying and 3D printing, and Chapter 13 offers comprehensive retrospective and prospective analysis on electrospinning and electrospraying for biomedical applications.

Finally, Part IV deals with "*Laboratory and translational aspects in electrospinning and electrospraying*" theme, wherein Chapter 14 describes considerations for setting up e-spin/e-spray setups, and Chapter 15 provides the translational path for electrospun and electrospray medical devices from bench to bedside.

With such an amazing mix of topics, it is anticipated that this book would attract a wide spectrum of readers from different levels across multiple disciplines.

Naresh Kasoju
Hua Ye

PART ONE

Electrospinning

CHAPTER ONE

Basic concepts and fundamental insights into electrospinning

Kapil D. Patel[1,2] Andrew R. Padalhin[3], Rose Ann G. Franco[4,5]
Fiona Verisqa[6], Hae Won Kim[1,2], Linh Nguyen[2,6]
[1]Institute of Tissue Regeneration Engineering (ITREN), Dankook University, Cheonan, Chungcheongnam-do, Republic of Korea
[2]UCL Eastman-Korea Dental Medicine Innovation Centre, Dankook University, Cheonan, Chungcheongnam-do, Republic of Korea
[3]Beckman Laser Institute Korea, College of Medicine, Dankook University, Dankook, Cheonan, Chungcheongnam-do, Republic of Korea
[4]School of Mechanical, Medical and Process Engineering (MMPE), Science and Engineering Faculty (SEF), Institute of Health and Biomedical Innovation (IHBI), Queensland University of Technology (QUT), Kelvin Grove, QLD, Australia
[5]Translational Research Institute (TRI), Woolloongabba, QLD, Australia
[6]Division of Biomaterials and Tissue Engineering, Eastman Dental Institute, University College London, Royal Free Hospital, London, United Kingdom

List of abbreviations

AC Alternating current
ACP Alternating current power
AFM Atomic force microscopy
BCP Biphasic calcium phosphate
BSA Bovine serum albumin
CNTs Carbon nanotubes
DC Direct current
DSC Differential scanning calorimetry
EDS Energy dispersive spectroscopy
FT-IR Fourier transform infrared spectroscopy
HA Hydroxyapatite
HRTEM High-resolution transmission electron microscopy
HVAC High-voltage alternating current
HVDC High-voltage direct current
IR Infrared
mBGNs Mesoporous bioactive glass nanoparticles
MFAES Magnetic field–assisted electrospinning
MNPs Magnetic nanoparticles
MS Mesoporous silica
mZnO Multidrug-loaded mesoporous zinc oxide
NEFS Near-field electrospinning
PAN Polyacrylonitrile

Biomedical Applications of Electrospinning and Electrospraying
ISBN: 978-0-12-822476-2
https://doi.org/10.1016/B978-0-12-822476-2.00010-8

PCL Polycaprolactone
PLA Polylactic acid
PLGA Poly(D,L-lactic-co-glycolic acid)
PLLA Poly (L-lactic acid)
PU Polyurethane
PVP Poly(vinyl pyrrolidone)
SBF Simulated body fluid
SEM Scanning electron microscope
SNFs Silk nanofibers
TEM Transmission electron microscope
XRD X-ray diffraction spectroscopy

1.1 Introduction

Electrospinning is related to the principle of spinning of polymeric solutions or melts at elevated temperatures in a high DC electric field. Most of the synthetic and naturally occurring polymers can be electrospun after dissolving in appropriate solvents. In conventional spinning, shearing, rheological, gravitational, inertia, and aerodynamics forces act on the fibers. However, in electrospinning, only electrostatic forces are used to generate fibers. In electrospinning, the shearing forces are generated by the interaction of an applied electrostatic field with the electrical charges carried by the polymer jet rather than by the spindles utilized in conventional spinning. The mechanism of electrospinning is accumulated of charge at the liquid surface under the electrostatic repulsion which is higher than the surface tension of the liquid meniscus and deformed into a conically shaped structure [1]. Further, the charged liquid jet is ejected toward the collector (flat plates, rotating drums, mandrels, and disks). Depending on the solution viscosity, solid fibers will be formed as the solvent evaporates from the whipping motion that occurs during its flight time from the cone-shaped structure to the collector. The result is a nonwoven fiber mat that is deposited on the collector. Similarly, the polymer concentration in the slurry could either hinder the production of fibers (if too high, due to the high viscosity) or result in the formation of globules of polymer (if too low). The same effect will have a too high flow rate, while if the flow rate is too low, the deposition of the fibers onto the collector will be inconsistent. Electrospun setup parameters such as the needle diameter and the collector speed exhibit a strong influence on the diameter of the fibers as well as their alignment [2,3].

Moreover, the fibers' diameter and orientation (random and alignment) can be controlled by optimizing the polymers viscosity, applied voltage, needle gauge, and rotational speed of the collector, respectively.

Electrospinning is the simplest, straightforward, cost-effective, and most versatile technique to produce a few hundred nanometers to micrometers-sized fibers at room temperature [4]. Although there are many other techniques/methods for producing nano-/microfibers, electrospinning has more advantages over others. The main advantages of electrospinning over other techniques/methods are to produce high surface area, easy handling, high yields, and varying fibers diameters. The fibers produced from electrospinning are more exceptional physical properties particularly mechanical, due to the degree of orientation of fibers compared to random and their bulk-sized fibers. The first man-made fabrics of cotton and wood cellulose fibers were developed by Rayan in 1891 [5]. It was I. V. Petryanov-Sokolov and collaborators who developed the rapid production and industrial facility for electrospun fibrous materials in the 1930s [6]. Nylon was the first synthetic fiber produced commercially by DuPont in 1938 and gained huge public attention [7,8]. The factory production capacity reached to 6.5 kg/h during 1950–60 [9]. Moreover, the first commercial products based on submicrometer fibers were launched by the US Company named Donaldson Co. Inc. in 1989 [6]. Reneker and et al. produced nanoscale and high added value of organic nanomaterials by electrospinning in 1995 and the method is still in use for the production of micro-/nanofibers [10]. Currently, the electrospinning technique has gained huge interests among scientists, researchers, and clinicians because of its easy handling, versatility, and cost-effectiveness for fiber productions. Moreover, electrospinning has relatively fewer steps involved and has very straightforward methods for nanofibers preparation compared to wet spinning, mats-spinning fiber drawing, and extrusion molding methods. Therefore, a number of companies are manufacturing electrospun nanofibers in large volumes and setting industrial production line for commercial products for various applications, including biomedical applications such as drug delivery and tissue engineering.

Although several book chapters, review papers, and research articles have been published to discuss the fundamentals and advancements in electrospinning techniques, however, there is always space to discuss the basics of electrospinning techniques in a specific context. In this chapter, we have summarized the basics of the electrospun technique for the production of micro-/nanofibers for biomedical applications. This chapter begins from Section 1.2 with comprehensive details on the electrospinning apparatus, including different types of nozzles, a variety of collectors, and visual simulation of electric field on an electrospinning setup with a single-charge needle tips or conducting plates. In Section 1.3, we have discussed the effect of processing parameters, including environmental (humidity and temperature), solution (molecular weight, concentration, solvent, conductivity, viscosity, and molecular structure), and electrospinning (tip-collector distance, voltage, flow rate, collectors types, and speed) variables on nanofibers production. Section 1.4 is focused on the selection of materials including polymers (natural, synthetic, semisynthetic), composites (nanoparticles in polymer or on the surface), and ceramics (template method, melt quenching). Sections 1.5 and 1.6 are targeted at the production of different types of fibers morphologies and its morphological, physical, chemical, and mechanical characterization, respectively. Finally, thermal property, electrical conductivity, and cellular behaviors (cellular toxicity, blood compatibility) are discussed.

1.2 Electrospinning apparatus and diversity of various components

The oldest record for the electrospinning process dates back to the early 1900s which was patented for both the method of electrical method of fluid dispersion and the associated equipment [11]. This was then followed by another patent detailing a modified experimental process for producing artificial threads using the same principles supplemented with variable collecting methods [12]. The electrically charged spinning methods were then further popularized during the 1990s up to the early 2000s through models and actual experiments [2,13,14]. As outlined in the previous section, the basic electrospinning setup is composed of at least three main components: a spinneret, an electrical power supply, and a collector (Fig. 1.1).

These basic components are positioned accordingly (either in a vertical or horizontal orientation) to permit the induction of electrical charge into the polymer solution/melt and accommodate the proper formation of a stable Taylor cone during the electrospinning process.

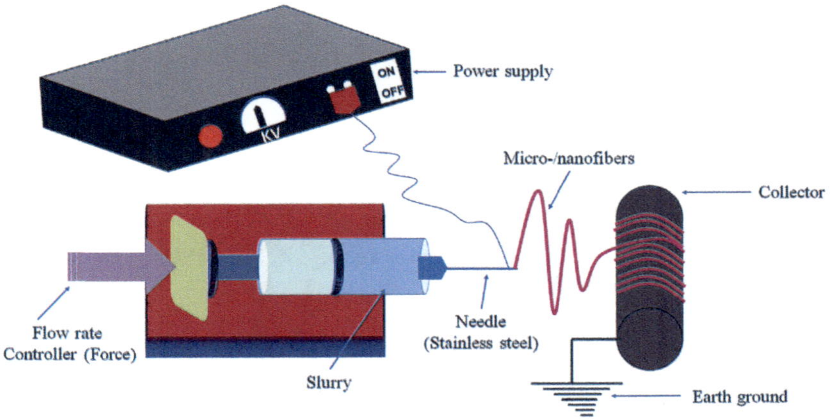

Figure 1.1 Schematic illustration of electrospinning setup, consisting of high-voltage power supply, polymer solution–filled needle with pump, and rotating drum as a collector.

The spinneret consists of a polymer reservoir attached to an adjustable feed system. Depending on the method of processing, the spinneret could either include a syringe pump with an airtight syringe containing the polymer solution or an extruder equipped with adjustable heating elements to fluidize polymer solids. Both types of spinneret could be configured without needles or use single or multiple needles or nozzles. Electrospinning nozzles can be single channeled, multiple channeled, coaxial, or a combination of any of the previous types. For most experimental setups, a single nozzle spinneret is used since this offers the best venue for observation and permits calculated adjustments of the different electrospinning parameters [15]. Multiple needle setups are more common in industry-scale electrospinning because it can provide increased product output necessary for commercialization. Single-channeled nozzles make use of a single polymer feed system, while a multiple-channeled nozzle could either make use of a single feed system for increased production of fibers composed of the same polymer or operate with two or more polymer feeds to fabricate a composite fibrous material [16] (Fig. 1.2a–c). A coaxial nozzle makes use of multiple polymer reservoirs configured with separate feed mechanisms or pumps [17,18]. Coaxial nozzles allow fabrication of a core shell or even multilayered electrospun fiber composed of different polymers (Fig. 1.2d). In addition to the different

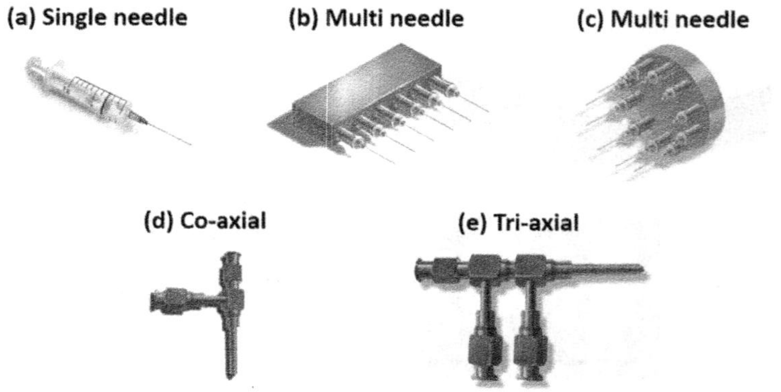

Figure 1.2 Different electrospinning nozzle/needle configurations are used for electrospinning. (a) Single needle; (b) Multi needle; (c) Multi needle; (d) Co-axial and (e) Tri-axial.

polymer feed systems and nozzle types, some advanced electrospinning setups are also equipped with electric motors that allow linear movement of the spinneret allowing shifting deposition of the electrospun fibers on a collector [15,19,20].

The second crucial component for an electrospinning setup is the inclusion of a suitable electrical power supply that can deliver the voltage range, typically 0−50 kV, required to apply electrical charge into polymer solutions or polymer melts. The common electrical power delivery system applies high-voltage direct current (HVDC) unto the electrodes attached to the spinneret [20]. The HVDC power delivery system permits the designation of a positive and negative charge induction on the polymer feed electrode, collector, auxiliary electrode, or all these components. Assigning a specific polarity on a particular electrospinning component facilitates the manipulation of the existing electrical field and could induce targeted attraction or repulsion depending on the configuration. This type of power supply has been the basis for the majority of the research involving electrospinning [21,22]. The lesser-known power delivery system for electrospinning is the high-voltage alternating current (HVAC). This type of power supply provides an electrical charge with switching polarity. Aside from the high-voltage setting, the HVAC power delivery adds frequency as another parameter during electrospinning. This is the rate at which the electrical charge switches between polarities and is common within the range of 60 Hz–1 kHz [23]. Previous researches have indicated that making use of an AC instead of DC power delivery during electrospinning lessens fiber whipping which consequently mitigates the effect of fiber instability. The AC enables the formation of smaller aligned nanofibers through the straightforward accumulation of the developed fibers on the collectors [24]. Both types of electrical power delivery systems induce the presence of a very strong electrical field, which greatly influences the behavior of the fluid polymer making electrospinning possible. In an intensified electric field, once the critical voltage is attained, the surface tension is overwhelmed by the repulsive electrostatic force forming single or multiple fluid jets from the tip of the electrospinning nozzle or needle [2,25–27] (Fig. 1.3).

The third component of an electrospinning setup is the collector, the surface upon which the formed fibers deposit and accumulate. Fibers accumulate and deposit on the surfaces of collectors because of the inherent attraction of electrically charged fibers to electrically grounded materials. Several designs have been implemented to achieve different forms of materials. The most basic collector type is a flat electrically grounded surface such as a metallic plate or a sheet of aluminum foil. This allows the accumulation of randomly oriented electrospun fibers on a large surface area as a sheet type of material [19,28]. Alternatively, a collector composed of an edge profile of flat conductive material can be used to achieve aligned electrospun fibers [29]. A conductive solid drum, rod, wire drum, or disc equipped with a controllable electric motor, to incorporate rotational movement, can also be used as a collector to fabricate several forms of electrospun material [30]. Both the rotating solid drum and wire drum collector allow fabrication of a nonwoven large diameter tubular material which can be crosscut into rings or cut lengthwise to form a large sheet. A rotating rod collector allows the creation of small diameter tubular material ideal for certain applications. On the other hand, using a rotating disc collector results in the formation of a thin ring composed of highly oriented fibers. Adjusting the speed at which these types of collectors rotate can increase or decrease the organization and orientation of the collected electrospun fibers. In addition to solid surface collectors, liquid bath collectors can also be used to gather electrospun fibers. Instead of a static flat surface or a rotating collector, a liquid bath collector makes use of a container with a grounded nonsolvent liquid (commonly water) to collect the fibers. Depending on the composition, the fibers can accumulate within the fluid volume or along the surface. The resulting material can take an amorphous form similar to loose cotton or a stringlike

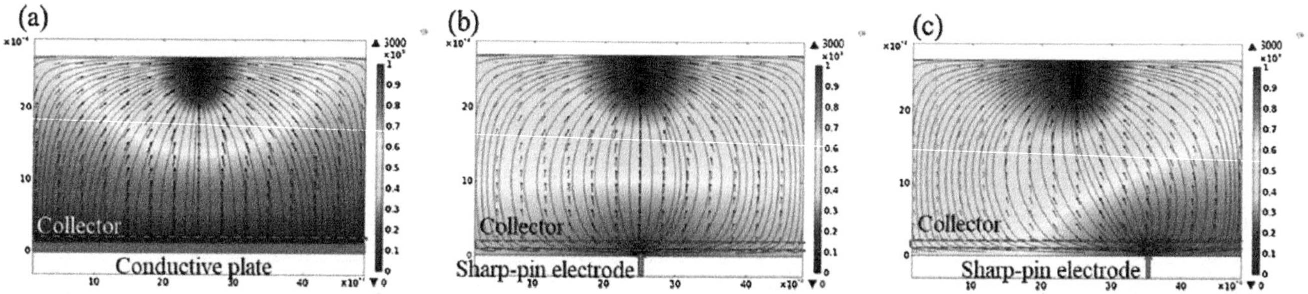

Figure 1.3 Visual simulation of the electric field on an electrospinning setup with a single charged nozzle/needle tip and a conductive plate (a), Sharp-pin (b), or a sharp-pin electrode offset from the nozzle. *Reproduced with permission from Y. Xiangyu, C. Ye, P. Guo, Electric field manipulation for deposition control in near-field electrospinning, J. Manuf. Process. 30 (2017) 431–438. https://doi.org/10.1016/j.jmapro.2017.10.005; © 2017 The Society of Manufacturing Engineers. Published by Elsevier Ltd.*

form reminiscent of yarn if further drawing is applied using a rotating drum. Compared to solid surface collectors, liquid bath collectors make the formation of bulky three-dimensional material with enhanced porosity possible [31,32]. These different collector types and their combinations allow accumulation of nonwoven polymer fibers, aligned fibers, stratified fibers, as a monolithic sheet, multilayer sheet, large and small diameter tube, crimped tube, ring, or porous cottonlike material. In addition to the variable structural forms, electrospinning collectors could also be modified through induction of electrical current, which in turn alter attachment and accumulation behavior of the electrically charged fibers (Fig. 1.4).

1.3 Effects of process parameters on electrospinning

Numerous factors should be considered for conducting electrospinning, particularly when trying to produce high-quality micro- and nanoscale fibers, which require specific morphology to achieve functionality. Electrospinning parameters can be fine-tuned through understanding the governing

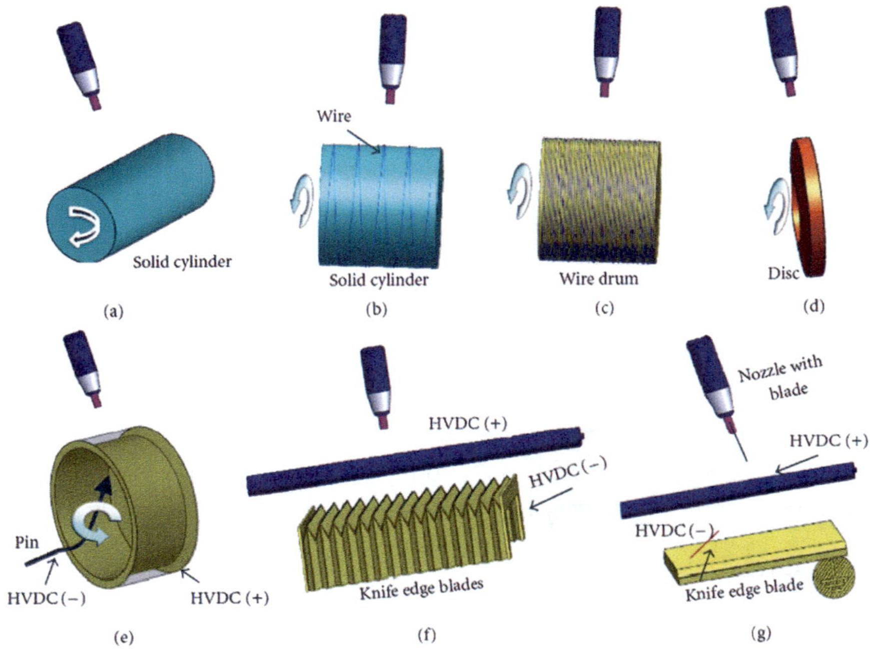

Figure 1.4 Different types of collectors are used in electrospinning polymeric fibers [20]. *HVDC*, high-voltage direct current. *Reproduced with permission from R. Sahay, V. Thavasi, S. Ramakrishna, Design modifications in electrospinning setup for advanced applications, J. Nanomater. 2011 (2011) 17. https://doi.org/10.1155/2011/317673; Copyright © 2011 Rahul Sahay et al.*

principles that affect the spinning process [33]. The polymer solution composition, electrical charge, and the ambient conditions all play a key role in generating electrospun fibers. The formation of a stable Taylor cone during electrospinning relies on balancing the governing principles of the aforementioned factors. In addition to the possibility of generating beads, sputter, or fibers, these parameters also affect the resulting fiber morphology. Widespread studies and exhaustive research have been conducted regarding the numerous parameters and properties that influence fiber diameter and morphology [34] (Fig. 1.5).

1.3.1 Solution properties

Choosing the material for electrospinning provides the initial reference in defining the appropriate settings for electrospinning. Aside from possessing the necessary properties for the intended application, the material dictates the possible processing techniques to achieve its spinnable fluid state. The type of spinneret system to be used directly affects the polymer spinnability. Previous studies have demonstrated that some polymers require additional components for melt electrospinning to reduce fiber diameter, improve processing current and thermal properties, or act as a plasticizer to prevent premature thermal degradation [35]. Just about any polymer/polymer combination can be electrospun within a workable range. Nevertheless, the basis of the workable range, specifically the lower limit of the concentration, remains controversial [3,36,37]. Solvent-based electrospinning can be

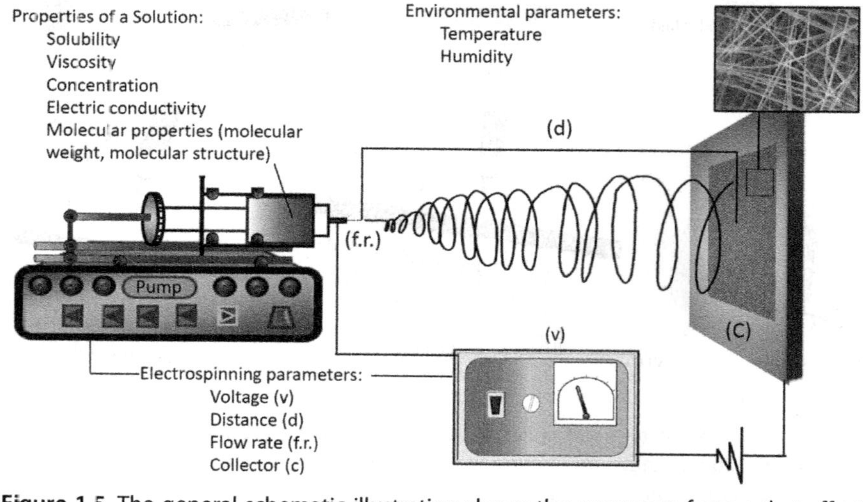

Figure 1.5 The general schematic illustration shows the numerous factors that affect the initiation of the electrospinning process and the morphology of resulting fibers.

considered as more complicated since several aspects should be considered that will be detailed in the subsequent sections.

1.3.1.1 Polymer composition and viscosity

The nature of the chosen polymer/polymer blends (e.g., chemical composition, structure, and molecular weight) and the associated intermolecular interactions within the resulting polymer solution dictate the relationship between the polymer concentration and viscosity. Establishing an all-inclusive formula to determine the suitable polymer—solvent system for an electrospinning process is difficult. Fiber diameter and morphology are commonly modified by adjusting the solution concentration relative to the spinning conditions [38]. Reduced polymer concentration leads to decreased fiber diameter. However, electrospinning a highly dilute polymer solution can lead to particulate matter due to a very low viscoelastic force [15,39]. Highly charged parts of the polymer jet separate into droplets because of surface tension at which point the solvent readily evaporates and forms droplets midair. Elongation of the polymer jet results in the increased surface area aiding the evaporation of the rapid solvent evaporation [40]. The choice of solvent not only determines the dissolution of the chosen polymer but also affects the formation of the solid fibers.

1.3.1.2 Solution surface tension

Since surface tension is determined by the intermolecular attractions within a solution, it follows that the polymer concentration and the nature of the solvent affect the affinity of the solution to maintain minimal surface area [33,41,42]. Earlier studies have attempted to devise a formula to determine the relationship between polymer concentration and surface tension through extrapolated experimental data and factoring in the properties of the solution components [43,44]. The cohesive forces between the molecules of the dissolved polymer and the solvent dictate the intensity of the solution surface tension and the energy required to increase the relative surface area of the solution. A Taylor cone and polymer jet are formed through the deformation of the polymer droplet brought about by the increased influence of the electric field upon reaching the electric charge threshold. Bead formation results from surface tension attempting to shrink the mass unit area of the viscoelastic polymer jet [13,45,46]. Several studies have shown that reduction of surface tension through either solvent substitution or addition of surfactant leads to improved electrospinning ability and uniform fiber formation [47,48]. Nevertheless, a lower polymer solution surface tension does not always equate to improved electrospinning [49,50].

1.3.1.3 Conductivity and solution dielectric properties

Electrical conductivity pertains to the ease of flow of electrical charge across a material. The presence of electrolytes and polyelectrolytes in polymer solutions imparts electrical conductivity. Polyelectrolytes are macromolecules that separate into highly charged molecules once placed in an ionizing solvent. Polyelectrolytes enhance the charge density along the surface of a polymer jet since ionic charges are directly related to electric conductivity. This leads to greater elongation, preventing bead formation during the electrospinning process [51]. Taylor's investigation on the electrohydrodynamics led to the idea of dielectric fluids accumulating charges at the interface between two materials with different conductivity. The same idea was then extended toward applying the same theory with adjusted principles unto "leaky dielectrics" or poorly conducting fluids in which charge accumulates at the interfaces because of varied conductivity between the solution and air [52]. The electrospinning process calls for a minimum electrical conductivity of a polymer solution to function; thus, solutions with very low conductivity would be very difficult to electrospun if not impossible [53]. The accessibility of ionic species increases the conductivity of a polymer solution. These ionic species could come from the dissociated polymer molecules, impurities, and/or additives. Solutions composed of polyelectrolytic polymers have higher conductivity compared to electrically neutral polymers due to their ionic potentials. In this case, increasing the polymer concentration would lead to increased solution conductivity. Nonetheless, in some instances, an increase in polymer concentration could result to a lower conductivity for the resulting polymer solution [54]. Solutions lacking the minimal conductivity required for electrospinning can be modified with the addition of electrolytes such as inorganic salts [55,56] or ionic compounds [54,57]. These additives increase the electrical charge of the resulting polymer by introducing ions upon dissociation, which in turn enhances the influence of the induced electrical field. Several studies have indicated that augmenting the polymer solution conductivity through the addition of salts leads to defect-free [58] and finer fibers [59]. Other investigations revealed that bead formation could be significantly reduced through the increased dielectric constant of the polymer solution. Dielectric constant pertains to the ability of a material to polarize upon exposure to an electric field or its permittivity. Materials with high dielectric constant develop a greater degree of polarization in response to an applied electric field. Solvent polarity is a crucial factor when evaluating solvents to be used for polymer dissociation [60,61].

1.3.2 Voltage and electrical field

The elongation of a polymer solution into a fine continuous filament during electrospinning is governed by the principles of electrohydrodynamics. A stable cone-jet is formed through the leveling effect of a polymer solution's viscosity on the electrical field–induced tangential stress present at the interface of air and the electrically charged polymer solution [62,63]. Hence, understanding the effect of voltage and the formation of the associated electrical field upon application of said voltage is important in operating electrospinning setups.

1.3.2.1 Relation of induced voltage and flow rate

The amount of electrical voltage applied to the polymer solution has a significant effect on the initiation of electrospinning and the resulting fiber morphology. In theory, increased voltage results in decreased fiber diameter due to the strengthened electrical field. Given that all the previous parameters discussed are constant, higher voltage makes it possible to create submicron fibers [64–66]. However, a continuous increase in voltage can ultimately lead to instability at a certain point. Recent studies demonstrate the relationship between applied voltage and polymer solution flow rate. Based on the numerical simulation proposed by Liu [37], which was verified through the accompanying experiment, the application of an ever-increasing voltage in an electrospinning setup results in the evolution of multiple jets. The increased delivery of voltage intensifies the electric field, which easily overcomes the surface tension of the polymer solution readily forming a polymer jet, elongating the polymer solution. Under a constant flow rate, the droplet at the tip of the electrospinning nozzle would eventually drop below the top edge of the electrospinning nozzle. Upon the absence of a droplet volume at the tip of the electrospinning nozzle, the electrical field concentrates along the edge of the nozzle tip, and more than one jet forms. Formation of multiple jets leads to reduced electrical field per jet even at high voltage. This unstable condition results in increased fiber diameter and less uniform fiber diameter distribution [26,62,63,67]. Increasing the applied voltage during electrospinning would typically require adjustment of flow rate to maintain a certain volume of polymer solution at the nozzle tip to avoid the development of multiple jets. However, it should be noted that increasing the flow rate places the polymer solution under pressure, which could lead to undesirable effects such as pressure-induced phase separation. Thus, in most instances, the adjustment in flow rate during electrospinning is less prioritized compared to previously discussed parameters.

1.3.2.2 Presence of auxiliary electrodes

Modifying the electric field is one of the most effective ways to regulate an electrospinning jet. Numerous studies have been conducted in manipulating the electric field to control fiber deposition during electrospinning [27,68]. The addition of electrodes and modification collectors used in electrospinning accommodates the alteration of the electrical field present within the electrospinning setup. In a direct current–powered electrospinning setup, auxiliary electrodes can be configured to repel, attract, and control polymer jets depending on the polarity of the charge applied to it. Previous studies have demonstrated that applying the same polarity results in the repulsion of the polymer jet from the electrode and applying an opposite charge polarity would increase attraction. Blocking out some portions of a conductive electrospinning collector enables the collection of highly oriented fibers [69]. A similar effect can be achieved using the parallel edge of two conductive plates as a collector [70]. One research even demonstrated that adding a ring electrode [71] or parallel plates [72] charged with similar polarity along the path of the polymer jet stream could aid in stabilizing the bending stability of the polymer jet. It is also possible to introduce a nanofibrous pattern into fibrous mats by placing a sharp conductive pin adjacent to a collector drum [73] (Fig. 1.6).

1.3.3 Jet instability and tip-to-collector distance

Maintaining a stable polymer jet stream is imperative when conducting electrospinning. Based on previous experiments and formula derivations, two types of instabilities can be identified during electrospinning [44,67,74]. The classical Rayleigh instability (axisymmetric instability) states that perturbations are introduced into the jet stream due to vibration between the interface of a nozzle and the fluid media. These perturbations exist as smooth radial oscitations (varicosity) along the length of the jet, components of which can degrade or intensify over time [67,75,76]. Intensified axisymmetric instability leads to jet stream breakup producing micro/nanopolymeric spheres. It has been found that in an electrospinning setup, this type of instability can be modulated by the electric field [76].

Another type of instability is described as a nonaxisymmetric instability or bending instability. Uneven distribution of electrical charge along the length of the polymer jet induces Coulombic repulsion, resulting in a radical shift of the polymer axis (bending). This lateral motion in combination leads to the evolution of a whipping cone [40,74,77]. The whipping cone further

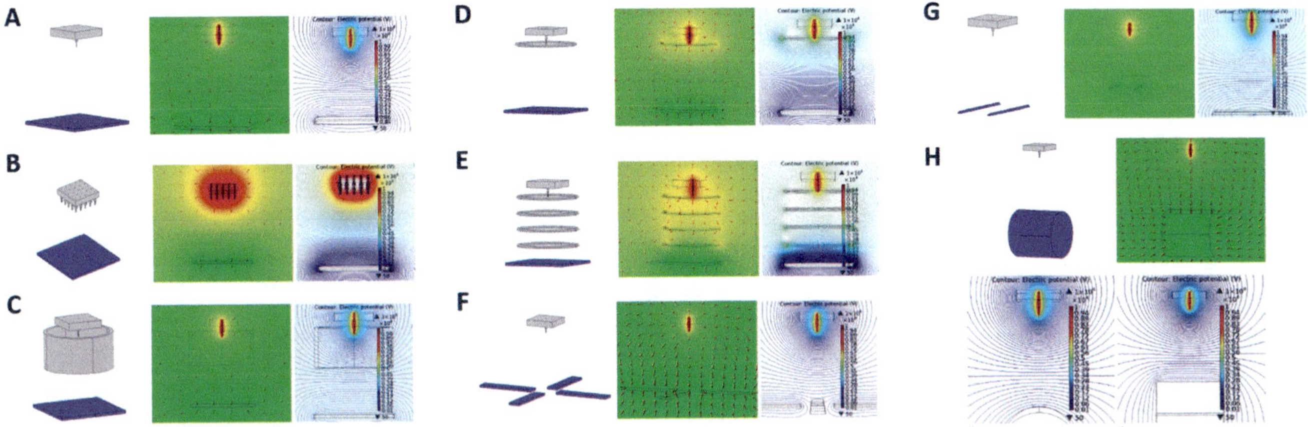

Figure 1.6 Some simulations showing the geometry, electric field behavior (red–green heatmap), and electric potential distribution (linear heatmap) in different electrospinning setups; single needle and plate collector (a); multineedle single plate collector (b); single needle with a cylindrical auxiliary electrode and single plate collector (c); single needle with ring auxiliary electrode and plate collector (d); single needle with multiple ring auxiliary electrode and plate collector (e); single needle and cross-positioned multiple strip collectors (f); single needle and parallel rod collectors (g); and single needle with the cylindrical collector (h). The electrospinning nozzle, collector, and presence of auxiliary electrodes affect the path of the electric field with a commensurate effect on polymer jet stabilization and fiber deposition. *Reproduced with permission from S. Krzysztof, F.-N. Anna, L. Marcin, Three-dimensional computer models of electrospinning systems, Open Phys. 15 (1) (2017) 777–789. https://doi.org/10.1515/phys-2017-0091; © 2017 K. Smółka et al.*

accelerates the polymer jet, which facilitates the reduction of fiber diameter. Bending instability subsequently develops into even smaller coils formed along the path of the previous whipping action [78]. It should be noted that this type of instability is utilized in the electrospinning process to not only decrease the resulting fiber diameter but also create the nonwoven microstructure.

The effects of jet instability become more evident as the distance between the nozzle tip increases. Previous studies indicate that greater tip-to-collector distance permits the development of larger bending/coiling behavior with lower frequency, while a shorter tip-to-collector distance results in a tighter bending/coiling at a higher frequency [79] (Fig. 1.7).

1.3.4 Ambient electrospinning conditions

The formation of the electrospun fibers can also be affected by ambient conditions such as temperature and relative humidity. In general, elevating the ambient temperature of melt electrospinning would aid in maintaining the "fluidity" of the polymer and permit further elongation resulting in the decrease in fiber diameter. Lowered ambient temperature during melt electrospinning will minimize the time needed to consolidate the polymer jet into a solid fiber, which could affect the resulting fiber diameter [18,35,80]. Previous studies have indicated that ambient relative humidity does not influence the formation of fibers in melt electrospinning [81].

The effect of ambient temperature and relative humidity on solvent-based electrospinning is mainly based on the evaporation of the solvent used to create the polymer solution. Higher ambient temperature increases the evaporation rate, while lower temperatures reduce the evaporation rate. Elevated ambient temperature aids in the early formation of fibers [82], while lowered ambient temperature makes the polymer jet receptive to elongation and thinning [82,83]. Increased relative humidity leads to lowered evaporation rate, while lowered relative humidity would lead to increased solvent evaporation affecting the rate of solidification of the polymer jet [81,84,85].

1.4 Choice of materials

The electrospinning technique has been used for the production of fibers from materials such as polymers, ceramic, and composites. Materials in form of either solution or melted in slurry condition can be utilized for

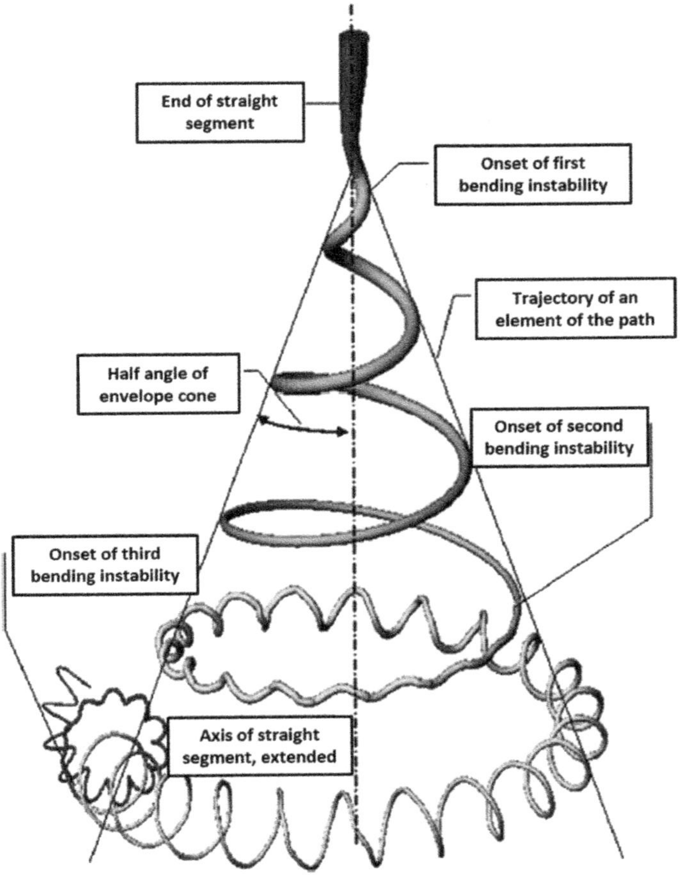

Figure 1.7 Schematic illustration showing the progressing evolution of jet instability during a basic electrospinning setup. It has been observed that subsequent smaller bending instability develops from the primary bending instability from the end of the straight path of the polymer jet. *Reproduced with permission from D.H. Reneker, A.L. Yarin, Electrospinning jets and polymer nanofibers, Polymer 49 (10) (2008) 2387–2425. https://doi.org/10.1016/j.polymer.2008.02.002; Copyright © 2008 Elsevier Ltd.*

electrospinning. Polymers and copolymers are the ideal candidates for electrospinning and easy-to-produce fibers compared to natural polymers as there is a possibility of denaturation and other complications such as limited solubility in an organic solvent to achieve ideal viscosity. A solution made of mixing nanomaterials (nanoparticles, nanotubes, nanosheets) in a polymer can be utilized for electrospinning. Based on materials used in electrospinning, we have categorized in three different choices of materials for electrospinning namely polymers (synthetic and natural), composites, and ceramics.

Polymers (natural, synthetic, semisynthetic) are the most frequently used materials to produce micro-/nanofibers. The blending of natural and synthetic polymers has also been used to produce nanofibers. Until today, hundreds of polymers have been utilized to produce either micro- or nanofibers using electrospinning. The choices made for the production of nanofibers are based on the requirements and tissue specificity. For example, soft tissue such as skin, muscle, and nerve regeneration requires mostly polymer-based micro-/nanofibrous scaffolds. When the polymer nanofibers were incorporated or embedded with micro-/nanoparticles (metals, ceramics), they are called composite fibers. Various strategies have been developed to fabricate composite nanofibers, in straightforward nanoparticles mixed in polymer solution [86,87]. The composite micro-/nanofibers are also produced by molecularly imprinted composite electrospun nanofibers that can be used in biosensing and imaging applications [88]. Generally, the introductions of the nanoparticles such as mesoporous bioactive bioglass or mesoporous silica nanoparticles are used as drug/biomolecules delivery carriers and osteoinduction [89,90]. Another strategy for the preparation of composite polymer nanofibers is first to prepare polymer nanofibers and then modify the fiber surface with a ceramic layer or nanoparticles/nanotubes [91,92]. Tailoring the surface of electrospun membrane/scaffolds is a key strategy to modulate the cellular interactions that are helpful for the tissue healing process as well as for biomolecules and drug loadings. Several strategies have been developed to fabricate composite nanofibers using inorganic nanoparticle modification through chemical or electrostatic/physical reactions. Ceramic-based materials alone are difficult to perform electrospinning and thus not possible to process electrospun nanofibers. However, ceramic materials can melt at high temperatures and can produce ceramic micro-/nanofibers at a high temperature which is also known as melt spinning [13]. The limitation of the melt spinning technique is the produced fibers' diameters in the range of micrometers [93]. Ceramic-based nanofibers can be produced by two different methods: first, fabrication of polymer—ceramic composite nanofibers and then selective thermal treatments, which will help to remove the polymer components and left with ceramic nanofibers. Second, prepare the polymer nanofibers and then coat with ceramics materials and then remove the polymers fiber through thermal treatments. Ceramic micro-/nanofibers can be achieved with high surface area, porous surface, and hollow morphology. The composite and ceramics micro-/nanofibers are commonly used for hard tissue such as bone, osteochondral, and dental repair/regeneration applications.

1.5 Morphology of the electrospun materials

As it has been mentioned previously, the morphology of electrospun fiber is affected by several process parameters such as electrospinning solution, polymer composition and viscosity, solution surface tension, electrical properties, jet instability, tip-to-collector distance, as well as ambient conditions. While the most common shape of fibers produced by electrospinning is in a circular cross-section form that composes a nonwoven structure, changing the parameters could be resulting in a different morphology.

1.5.1 Classical morphologies

1.5.1.1 Nonwoven fibers

Electrospun fibers result from a straight fluid extension that undergoes splitting due to fluid and electrical bending instability and then deposited on the collector [94]. Continuous fibers then are collected on the collector in a nonwoven morphology. Nonwoven morphology itself is an arrangement of fibers without knots or entanglement. The structure is fabricated layer by layer with various arrangements of the fibers, which can be in 1D, 2D, or 3D form. Furthermore, the fibers can create an open mesh nonwoven surface with pores. These irregular pores are made as the fibers are crossing each other during the deposition. Porosity and surface areas that are generated by the multilayered crossing fibers can provide support for cell proliferation in tissue engineering [95]. Electrospun polyamide 6 in formic acid showed different porosity values between circular cross-section nonwoven fibers and ribbon nonwoven fibers, with the former having higher porosity percentage [95]. The result suggested that nonwoven fiber structure and properties can be modified by changing the electrospinning parameter accordingly.

1.5.1.2 Aligned fibers

The alignment of electrospun fibers can be achieved by using rotating collectors or by manipulation of electric or magnetic field or by centrifugal electrospinning that combines centrifugal and electrical forces. Rotating collector such as a wire-framed drum can form axially aligned fibers. The degree of alignment of the fibers is dependent on the velocity of the collector's rotation that should match the spinning rate of the fiber. While slow rotating velocity could not initiate the alignment of the fibers, a very high rotation speed would cause fiber fracture [94]. Rotation speed also affects the fiber diameter. The higher the rotation speed, the smaller the fiber diameter. Crossed fiber alignment can be produced by using two perpendicular rotating collectors as well. To generate highly oriented fiber alignment, applying the supplementary electrical field can be an alternative method for conductive polymer solution. For a solution that contains magnetic material, the auxiliary magnetic field can be applied in the electrospinning process. However, the area and the length of the fiber resulted from electrical or magnetic alignment are limited compared to rotating collector–produced fiber [94]. Compared to disorderly fibers, highly aligned fibers are reported to have better mechanical properties and are more biocompatible [96].

1.5.2 Specialized morphologies

1.5.2.1 Ribbons and bleeding fibers

Ribbon-like fibers are formed due to the spinning of a high viscosity solution [97]. Higher voltage application on the polymer solution is also reported to produce thinner fibers due to the rapid electrospinning process [98]. Various electrospun polymers such as gelatin and polyethylene showed these flat-shaped fibers with the application of these particular process parameters. Gelatin solutions and Nylon-11 in formic acid solvent demonstrated these findings after 20 kV voltage was applied to the solution where flat ribbon-like fibers were formed [98]. The same report also found a high concentration of gelatin increases the viscosity of the solution and resulted in flat-shaped fibers. Increasing the applied voltage and solution polymer concentration allowed rapid evaporation of the solvent that led to flat or ribbon-like fibers formation. Besides, ribbon fibers showed a highly ordered orientation when compared to beaded fibers.

1.5.3 Wavy fibers

Wavy fibers are caused by bending instability during the electrospinning process. It is reported that when the collector speed is low, the fibers resulted from electrospun poly(ethylene oxide) can appear in the near-field electrospinning [99]. Furthermore, alternating current power (ACP) supply is also reported to affect the occurrence and amplitude of wavy fibers. The amplitude of the fibers itself has a linear correlation with collector speed and ACP voltage. The morphology of wavy fibers is affected by ACP frequency as well. Unlike ACP voltage, increasing ACP frequency causes a decreasing amplitude of the wavy fibers. Magnetic field–assisted electrospinning (MFAES) is another method that can be used to produce wavy fibers. Poly(D,L-lactic-co-glycolic acid) (PLGA) and poly(vinyl pyrrolidone)

(PVP) polymers were able to generate electrospun wavy fibers with MFAES method by increasing the flow rate [100]. The result from MFAES processing indicates that wavy fibers' fabrication is material independent and does not require magnetic content. The fibers also demonstrated biocompatibility with stem cells following the wavy fibers form. Due to the tunable properties and unique structures of wavy fibers, they have been used in various applications such as sensors, electromagnetic devices, and electronic products.

1.5.4 Porous fibers

Three-dimensional porous fibers can be beneficial for tissue engineering because they could facilitate cell seeding and nutrient diffusion. It was reported that porous electrospun fibers could be produced by the use of volatile solvents and rapid phase separation [101]. Electrospun PLLA fibers with dichloromethane volatile solvent were shown to have a regular pore structure. The pores were generated by rapid phase separation during the electrospinning where the solvent-rich area was transformed into pores. Changing the volatile solvent with a lower vapor pressure solvent such as chloroform decreased the pore formation on the fibers [102]. These pores can also be produced by adding porogen, using liquid collection methods, and applying controlled patterning by a conductive collector. Porogens that can be used during the electrospinning process are salts, polymers, or ice crystals. These porogens will be removed by dissolution or evaporation and resulting in 3D macroporous fibers. Liquid collection collects the electrospun fibers in a liquid bath and freezes the fiber stack to fabricate a 3D foamlike porous structure. However, porous fibers that were resulted from these methods are not evenly distributed. Controlled patterning can provide controllable geometry and size that will be beneficial for tissue engineering applications.

1.5.5 Beads

Beaded fiber formation has been reported as the result of axisymmetric instability by surface tension (Rayleigh instability) as well as an electrical force [97]. Solution viscosity is also reported as one of the main factors in the formation of the beads. Low polymer concentration solution leads to beaded fiber generation, while a higher concentration solution leads to smooth fiber formation [101]. Significantly, low polymer concentration could not be electrospun and resulted in droplets instead of fibers. This process is also known as electrospraying. The collecting distance contributes to beads formation on the fibers as well. Small collecting distance does not allow sufficient solvent evaporation and full stretching of the fiber that is resulting in beaded fiber formation [96]. Electrospinning experiments with polystyrene demonstrated that the morphology of bead formation on the fibers was affected by polymer concentration, applied voltage, and tip-to-collector distance [101]. The increase of the voltage gave rise to higher electrostatic repulsion force between a collector and capillary tip that caused higher jet drawing stress, which was resulting in smaller bead size. The same experiment also showed that increasing tip-to-collector distance would decrease the electrostatic force and drawing stress on the jet. As a result, the axis of the bead became larger.

1.6 Characterization of electrospun materials

1.6.1 Morphological characterization

The morphological characterization of electrospun fibers is mandatory during optimization and postfabrication, which begins with visualization of the individual fibers, fiber network, or electrospinning process by microscopy. Depending on the parameters needed to be observed, a certain type of microscope can be used for assessment. Initial assessment of fiber formation may be viewed using a standard compound microscope during the process of optimization without the need for laborious sample preparation requiring a scanning electron microscope (SEM). In a study by Reneker et al. [103], this technique was done to monitor the appearance of a "garland," a term coined for the columnar network of fibers which appear from the polymer propulsion jet, and how it is affected by modification of electrospinning parameters.

The high magnification and resolution of an SEM is essential in examining the fiber density and microstructure. As SEM gives a detailed three-dimensional view of the fibers, other morphological characteristics can also be evaluated such as the fiber surface, interconnectivity [104], orientation [105,106] (Fig. 1.8a1 and 2), and presence of pores [107,108] (Fig. 1.8b). Integral to these critical data is the careful preservation of the native state of the fibers. Samples with high moisture content, or when exposed to a biological fluid, must undergo critical point drying to prevent morphological alterations before gold or platinum coating and viewing. The high magnification of the SEM limits its area of vision; thus, the data derived from imaging must represent the whole sample.

Using a transmission electron microscope (TEM), the ultrathin sections of a sample can be viewed using atomic-level resolution and enable users to

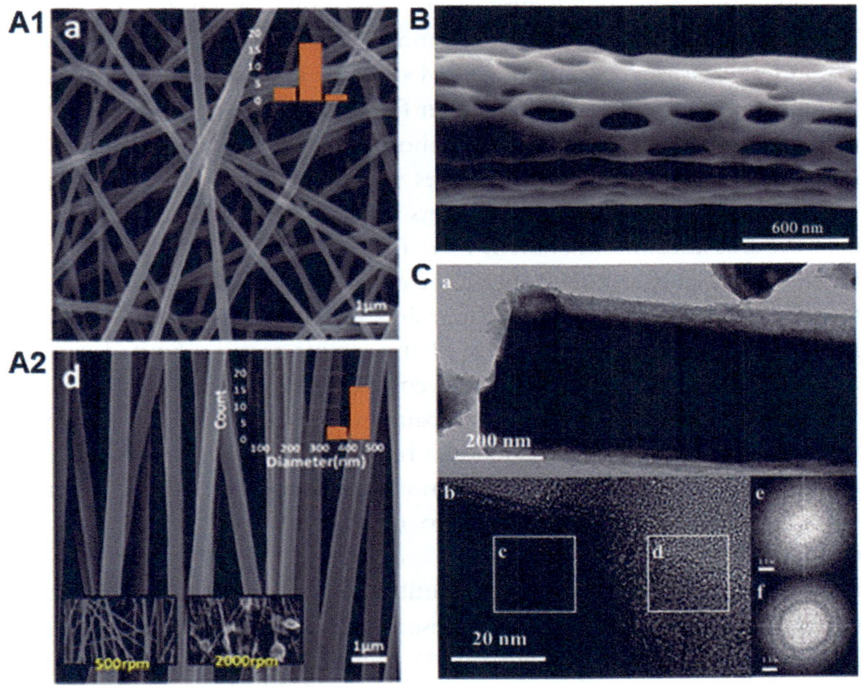

Figure 1.8 Morphological characterization of electrospun fibers using SEM and TEM: (a) SEM image of PU nanofibers: (1) randomly oriented and (2) aligned [106]; *Reproduced with permission from J.I. Kim, T.I. Hwang, L.E. Aguilar, C.H. Park, C.S. Kim, A controlled design of aligned and random nanofibers for 3D Bi-functionalized nerve conduits fabricated via a novel electrospinning set-up, Sci. Rep. 6 (1) (2016) 23761. https://doi.org/10.1038/srep23761; © 2016, The Author(s);* (b) Nanopore formation on an electrospun nanofiber surface [108a]; *Reproduced with permission from G.-M. Kim, G.H. Michler, P. Pötschke, Deformation processes of ultrahigh porous multiwalled carbon nanotubes/polycarbonate composite fibers prepared by electrospinning, Polymer 46 (18) (2005) 7346–7351. https://doi.org/10.1016/j.polymer.2005.06.008; Copyright © 2005 Elsevier Ltd.;* (c) TEM image of SiCN fibers (a and b), free carbon enrichment zone (c and e), and SiCN enrichment zone (d and f) [110]. *Reproduced with permission from F. Xiao, H. Sun, J. Li, X. Guo, H. Zhang, J. Lu, Z. Pan, J. Xu, Electrospinning preparation and electromagnetic wave absorption properties of SiCN fibers, Ceram. Int. 46 (8, Part B) (2020) 12773–12781. https://doi.org/10.1016/j.ceramint.2020.02.046; © 2020 Elsevier Ltd and Techna Group S.r.l.; PU,* polyurethane; *SEM,* scanning electron microscope; *TEM,* transmission electron microscope.

quantify picometer-scale measurements. The ultrahigh-resolution, cross-sectional view of the samples can determine different fiber attributes such as sample thickness, hollowness [109], and zoning of components [110]. Visual confirmation from micro- to nanosized loaded components into electrospun fibers can be done using TEM such as the detection of silver nanoparticles embedded in various polymer fibers [111–113]. The characteristic lattice network of biphasic calcium phosphate (BCP) nanoparticles loaded into electrospun nanofiber membranes was also verified using TEM [114]. The ultramicrostructure of SiCN fibers was visualized in TEM to differentiate the free carbon enrichment zone from SiCN enrichment zone [110] (Fig. 1.8c). Besides, optimization of the electrospinning solutions by characterization of a single SiO_2 nanowire using TEM imaging was also reported [115]. The two-dimensional view of the sample may be limited in some cases; thus, TEM images are usually complemented with surface imaging or analysis. The tedious sample preparation before TEM differentiates it with SEM where sample preparation is relatively minimal and less laborious. Additional sample processing and sectioning makes TEM samples prone to produce artifacts, which may lead to misinterpretation or misreading of results.

Atomic force microscopy (AFM) utilizes high-resolution surface sensing technology which can be effectively used to provide a topographical scan of a sample using a cantilever (Fig. 1.9a1) while providing quantitative information on the surface roughness, texture, general morphology, and approximation of the size of a particular area of focus where samples can be viewed in its native state and even in wet conditions [116]. Phase separation of polyurethane nanofibers was also visualized using AFM by comparing the distribution of hard segments between stretched and unstretched nanofibers [117] (Fig. 1.9a2). Xu et al. distinctly showed the structural evolution of chitosan–PEO electrospun fibers into columns, plates, micropores, bumps, and smooth surfaces (Fig. 1.9b) and bovine serum albumin loading by scanning the surface profile using AFM [118]. The surface charge of fiber can also be determined using AFM where the nonconducting phase appears less intense in color and not detected by traditional SEM observation [119].

1.6.2 Physical characterization

Hydrophilicity is a physical parameter of a material that allows it to interact positively with a liquid at a given temperature [120]. It is a desirable characteristic of electrospun fibers targeted for biomedical applications since the

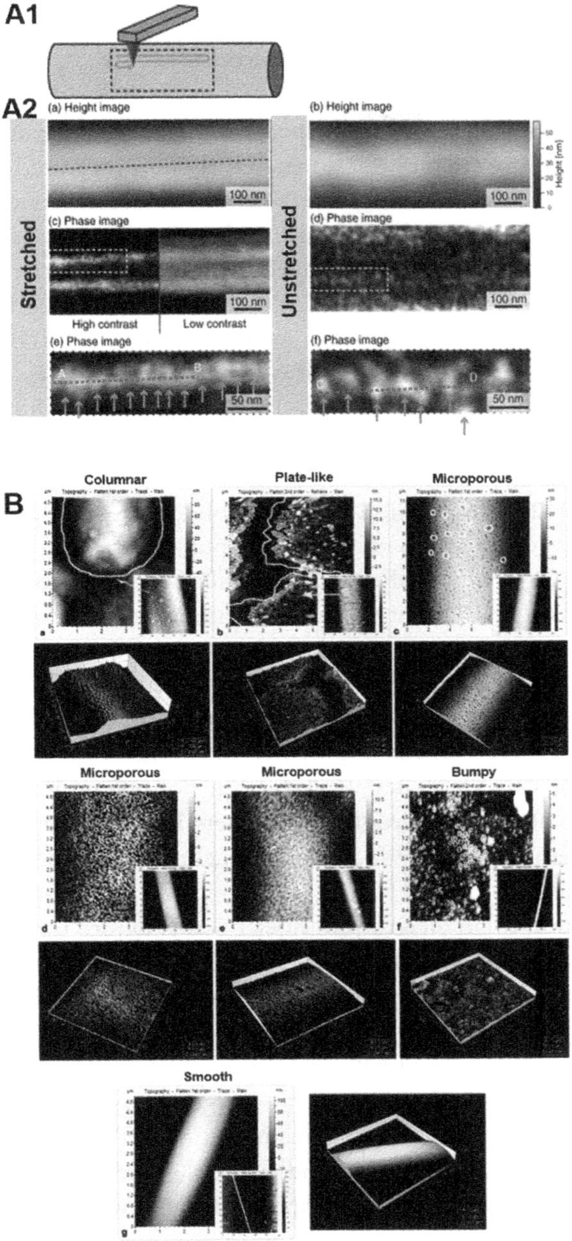

Figure 1.9 Morphological characterization of electrospun fibers using AFM: (a) Surface scanning of PU nanofibers: (1) Diagram of AFM cantilever scanning along the fiber axis and (2) AFM images of stretched and unstretched PU nanofibers. *Reproduced with permission from H. Sakamoto, H. Asakawa, T. Fukuma, S. Fujita, S.-i. Suye, Atomic force microscopy visualization of hard segment alignment in stretched polyurethane nanofibers prepared by electrospinning, Sci. Technol. Adv. Mater. 15 (1) (2014) 015008. https://doi.org/10.1088/1468-6996/15/1/015008; © 2014 National Institute for Materials Science*; (b) Structural evolution of chitosan–PEO jets through electrospinning using AFM topographies showing larger magnification morphologies of the surface (the full morphologies of jets are inserted in the lower right corner; the corresponding 3D images are shown

hydrophilicity of a scaffold affects the cell–material surface interactions and degradation. The wettability of a material is often measured by its contact angle, θ. This refers to the angle between the material surface and tangent to the dropped liquid on the material surface. Perfect wettability θ is equal to 0° when liquid is completely parallel to the material's surface; high wettability $0^\circ < \theta < 90$ degrees, and low wettability 90 degrees $< \theta < 180$ degrees when a 45 uL liquid is dropped and observed for 10 s [121]. In a study by Dorati et al. hydrophilicity was also evaluated by the ability of the electrospun scaffold to permeate Pullulan standards which is similar to the molecular weights of biologically important molecules (glucose, insulin, and high-molecular weight proteins) and measured by gel permeation chromatography [121]. In addition to a desirable contact angle, water permeability and water retention of an electrospun scaffold are also relevant as these predict the ability of the material to allow diffusion of essential nutrients to maintain cell viability. Water retention may be expressed as water absorption capacity or swelling ratio, although both will calculate the values from the dry weight and weight after immersion in the fluid after a certain time at a given temperature [122]. Improvement of the hydrophilic surface of electrospun fibers includes polymer blending [123–125], loading of biocompatible ceramic materials [126,127], postprocessing of electrospun fibers by a coating of hydrophilic polymers like polyvinyl alcohol [128] and polydopamine [129,130], and functionalization of phenylsulfonic acid by steam activation [131].

Modification of an electrospun fiber microstructure through the introduction of pores serves different specialized functions such as increased surface area, increased resorption, and aids in a compound release, improved contaminant adsorption, and heightened degradability. Direct measurement of the pores can be done visually using images obtained from high magnification microscopes and quantified by image analysis. Zhu et al. reported using at least five images taken at a magnification of 2,000*X* at random spots of a single sample [132]. This method is reliable when the evaluated images are representative of the whole sample and the sampling size is increased. Indirect methods include the evaluation of pore sizes by material intrusion

below the topographic images). The characteristic structures are highlighted by yellow curves or circles: columnar, plate-like, microporous, bumpy, and smooth; *Reproduced with permission from P. Xu, W. Li, H. Zhou, F. Pan, H. Xing, H. Liu, Investigations of the structural evolution of electrospun nanofibers using atomic force microscopy, RSC Adv. 2 (29) (2012) 11104–11110. https://doi.org/10.1039/C2RA20146A; © The Royal Society of Chemistry 2012. AFM*, atomic force microscopy; *PU*, polyurethane.

or calculation of the change in density. Mercury intrusion porosimetry quantifies the pore size, pore size distribution, and porosity of samples by permeabilization of the scaffold [133]. Due to safety issues with mercury use and handling, substitute material was proposed by Cortez Tornello et al. wherein they reported the use of liquid Vaseline as a wetting agent in liquid extrusion porosimetry [134]. Another method of quantification includes a method reported by Liu et al. where the pore sizes were calculated from the desorption branch of the adsorption isotherm [135]. In cases where specialized equipment is unavailable, porosity can be estimated by density calculations [122,132] or calculation of the ratio of the pore area to the whole area of the examined surface [136].

1.6.3 Chemical characterization

Chemical characterization of the polymers used for electrospinning and the final product after postprocessing delivers an in-depth understanding of the formed fibers, which affects other properties such as degradation and mechanical strength. The conventional methods of chemical characterization of electrospun fibers include Fourier transform infrared spectroscopy (FT-IR), X-ray diffraction spectroscopy (XRD), and energy-dispersive X-ray spectroscopy (EDS).

The long wavelengths of infrared (IR) light trigger vibration of molecular bonds when it passes through the electrospun fiber network, and since molecules absorb different frequencies of the IR, the absorbed part of the original IR beam will be detected and converted into a spectrum which aids in identifying compounds, notes differences in the composition, and confirms the presence of a certain molecule [137—139] or modifications after postprocessing [140]. FT-IR readings of electrospun fibers usually use the 4000-400 cm^{-1} absorption spectra where most organic and inorganic compounds are absorbed. FT-IR is highly advantageous in material characterization due to its sensitivity, selectivity, and accuracy. From an economical perspective, FT-IR is advantageous since it requires a small amount of sample, short time, and nonspecialized skills to operate, and low cost per analysis.

In XRD, the bombardment of incident X-rays to a sample provides integral information as the measured intensities and scattering angles of X-rays identify the signature atomic and molecular structure of a given sample. XRD is useful in identifying the crystal structure, quantifying the crystallite size, and comparing characteristics of crystallization of different ceramics embedded in the composite fibers with ceramic and polymer blends [139,141]. It is also used in evaluating texture orientation, identifying polymorphs, and detecting defects. While conventional use of XRD is done on ceramics, this mode of characterization can also be used in amorphous materials to determine successful integration in the electrospun fibers [142–144]. XRD was also used in differentiating two methods of fabrication in the incorporation of a compound [145] and postprocessing of samples [141,146].

EDS is a nondestructive approach in identifying and detecting the presence of certain elements of a compound loaded in electrospun nanofibers such as 45S5 Bioglass particle in polylactide–poly(ethylene glycol) blends [147], Zirconia elements in the Zirconia-based ceramic nanofibers [141], and BCP in polycaprolactone (PCL)/PLGA [114]. The EDS detector which is occasionally installed in an SEM can analyze the same surface during SEM imaging, thus reducing sample usage. The sampled area can be focused or enlarged by adjusting the magnification of the microscope. However, a high voltage in the range of 15–30 kV is recommended to stimulate enough X-rays for detection. Several elements have overlapping peaks; thus, prior knowledge of the elemental composition of a sample is needed to discern coinciding peaks for each element. Besides, some elements are not detectable in EDS, which will necessitate an alternative means for element identification.

1.6.4 Mechanical characterization

Measurement of the mechanical properties of a nanofiber membrane is typically done after the evaluation of morphological characteristics and confirmation of chemical components. The desired value of which is usually dictated by the final application of the electrospun product. The tensile test of an electrospun membrane is done using a universal testing machine to observe how it behaves under tension. To prepare for the evaluation, the dimensions of a sample are measured before attachment to grips where a known pull force using a load cell is applied. Throughout the test, the amount of force and elongation of the sample is measured and expressed as stress (the force applied per cross-sectional area) and strain (the change in length during force application) as seen in (Fig. 1.10a). The tensile strength of a material is the maximum force applied at a given area before it breaks or deforms. Fig. 1.10b shows the morphological changes in the fibers as it undergoes deformation during tensile testing. Other mechanical properties, which can be derived from the stress–strain curve, are elasticity, elastic modulus (Young's modulus), yield strength, and resilience.

A reasonable mechanical strength is desirable to ensure the stability of the material to withstand breakage and general stress during handling and target utilization. Conventional methods of improving the mechanical strength of electrospun fibers include cross-linking [148,149], heating [150,151], and combination with polymers or carbon nanotubes [127,152,153]. Conventionally, strips of the electrospun membrane are evaluated for tensile testing.

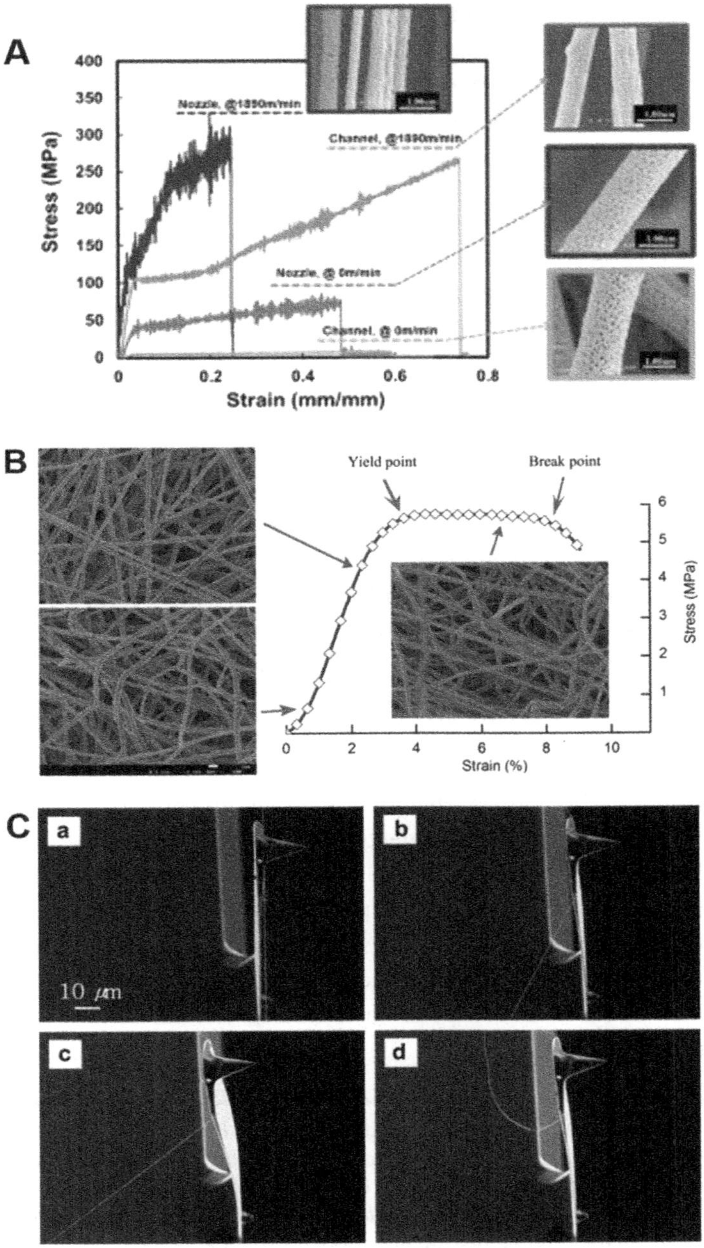

Figure 1.10 Mechanical characterization of electrospun nanofibers. (a) An example of stress–strain curves of different porous PLA nanofibers [136]. *Reproduced with permission from Y. Li, C.T. Lim, M. Kotaki, Study on structural and mechanical properties of porous PLA nanofibers electrospun by channel-based electrospinning system, Polymer 56 (2015) 572–580. https://doi.org/10.1016/j.polymer.2014.10.073; Copyright © 2014 Elsevier Ltd;* (b) SEM images during stretching of electrospun chitosan/poly(ethylene oxide) composite nanofibers reinforced with cellulose nanocrystals; *Reproduced with permission*

However, quantifying the mechanical strength of a single nanofiber is gaining interest as this will provide information on the behavior of a singular entity compared to the collective behavior of the fiber network [154]. In a study by Hwang et al. polyacrylonitrile nanofiber was "hooked" by a nanomanipulator and elongated by an AFM cantilever pulling in a transverse direction until it fractured and then measured [155] (Fig. 1.10c). Baker et al. also used the AFM to measure the tensile strength of a single PCL fiber and developed a strategy to anchor a single nanofiber on the substrate. PCL nanofiber was glued to the substrate and was similarly pulled by the AFM cantilever. The measured total elastic modulus of a single PCL nanofiber was 62 ± 26 MPa [156].

1.6.4.1 Other properties

Depending on the desired application of the fabricated electrospun fibers, additional properties are also characterized such as thermal stability (by differential scanning calorimetry (DSC) and thermogravimetric analysis (TGA)), chemical characterization (by Raman spectroscopy and nuclear magnetic resonance (NMR)), and evaluation of biocompatibility using in vitro assays or in vivo implantation using animal models.

The thermal stability of an electrospun fiber (made of polymer) as it undergoes chemical changes (and physical changes) can be measured by DSC. It is used to study a polymer's thermal transitions which include glass transition and crystallization and determining the temperature at which it melts. Combined polymers, changing polymer concentrations, and embedding nonpolymeric materials to electrospun fibers [139] can be differentiated with neat fibers since variation in the composition will alter the heat capacity and phase transitions of a certain sample [146]. TGA is another thermal characterization technique that measures the mass of a sample as a function of temperature at a given rate. The inert purge gas is used in this method to ensure that material decomposition is due to its reaction to the applied increasing temperature.

from D. Wang, W. Cheng, Q. Wang, J. Zang, Y. Zhang, G. Han, Preparation of electrospun chitosan/poly (ethylene oxide) composite nanofibers reinforced with cellulose nanocrystals: Structure, morphology, and mechanical behavior, Compos. Sci. Technol. 182 (2019), 107774. https://doi.org/10.1016/j.compscitech.2019.107774; © 2019 Elsevier Ltd; (c) Procedure of the nanotensile test: (a) fiber hookup, (b) fiber elongation, (c) further fiber elongation, and (d) fiber fracture and entanglement; *Reproduced with permission from D. Wang, W. Cheng, Q. Wang, J. Zang, Y. Zhang, G. Han, Preparation of electrospun chitosan/poly (ethylene oxide) composite nanofibers reinforced with cellulose nanocrystals: Structure, morphology, and mechanical behavior, Compos. Sci. Technol. 182 (2019), 107774. https://doi.org/10.1016/j.compscitech.2019.107774; © 2019 Elsevier Ltd;. PLA,* polylactic acid; *SEM*, scanning electron microscope.

Raman spectroscopy, like FTIR, detects for molecules present in electrospun fibers for chemical characterization. While FTIR measures the light absorbed, Raman spectroscopy quantifies the energy scattered by the vibrational bonds of molecules present in a sample which can give distinct peaks to identify increases in chemical concentration or changes in the chemical composition of a sample. On the other hand, NMR is highly useful for the detection of organic compounds present in electrospun fibers whether it is used as part of the spin solution or functionalization of biologically relevant molecules for biomaterial applications.

Assessment of the biocompatibility (or cytotoxicity) of an electrospun scaffold is necessary when its use is targeted for medical applications such as tissue engineering scaffold, drug delivery system, or for wound healing applications. *In vitro* cellular assays aim to determine a scaffold's ability to host cell viability and adhesion as a prerequisite to its implantation in an animal model. Cell viability in an electrospun scaffold can be quantified using metabolic assays such as reduction of MTT (3-(4,5-dimethylthiazol-2-yl)-2,5-diphenyltetrazolium bromide) substrate to purple formazan crystals by metabolically active cells or differential fluorescence staining of live and dead cells seeded on the electrospun scaffold using calcein AM and ethidium bromide. Electrospun scaffolds aimed for hemostatic application or as blood vessel stents are additionally evaluated for blood coagulation and compatibility properties.

The ability of a scaffold to host cell migration and tissue repair within a living organism is a definitive indication of its biocompatibility. The host—material interaction is complex and a favorable response will depend on the material, degradation by-products, and the host's inflammatory response. The choice of animal models and critical defects vary and are also dependent on the target application of the fabricated electrospun fiber.

1.7 Summary

This section outlined and discussed the critical factors involved in conducting electrospinning, a process for fibrous material fabrication via electrostatic forces. This process has been proven to reliably produce micro- and nanosized fibers suitable for industrial and medical applications. Electrospinning requires a fabrication setup with specific components: spinneret, electrical power supply, and a collector. Arrangement of these components facilitates the formation of fibers through electrical charge buildup and induction of an electrical field that exerts shearing forces that drive the formation of fibers between the spinneret and the collector. Different configurations of spinnerets, collectors, and auxiliary electrodes can be designed to modify the resulting nonwoven electrospun fibers and their corresponding material microarchitecture.

The formation of the fibers during electrospinning is influenced by several factors. Electrospinning variables such as the spinneret to collector distance/movement, applied voltage, flow rate, and collector geometry/configuration affect the resulting fiber formation and bulk material structure. Ambient factors such as humidity and temperature primarily influence the formation of fiber strands midair travel toward the designated collector. On the other hand, solution composition and property determine the potential for fiber formation and govern minimum electrospinning variables for electrospinning. Electrospinning has been utilized to mainly fabricate polymeric fibrous materials through either melt or solution-based systems. Fiber modification can be done by increasing polymer concentration for ribbon morphology or beading, ACP supply for wavy fibers, and the introduction of pores by solvent leaching, salt leaching, or formation of ice crystals as porogen. Other studies have also proven the usefulness of the electrospinning process using ceramic and/or composite-based materials.

The morphological, physical, chemical, and biocompatibility properties of an electrospun fiber scaffold determine its suitability for a given application. Visualization of the fibers through microscopy provides an in-depth analysis of its ultrastructure which can be used to explore certain attributes such as fiber thickness, hollowness, interconnectivity, or zoning of components. Porosity can also be visualized using microscopy but quantified by porosimetry or image analysis, while the hydrophilicity (or hydrophobicity) is measured by determination of the water contact angle or swelling studies. The native chemical composition and/or corresponding changes in fibers after fabrication or postfabrication treatment are evaluated by elemental analysis (EDS), detection of changes in vibration of functional groups (FTIR and Raman spectroscopy), crystalline peaks (XRD), or the molecular structure itself (NMR). Raw materials, polymer concentration, fiber morphology, and electrospinning conditions are among the factors which affect the mechanical properties of electrospun fibers. The tensile strength test determines the durability of an electrospun scaffold and can predict its stability during handling. In cases where thermal stability is a requirement, thermal transitions are evaluated using DSC or TGA. Electrospun scaffolds meant for biomedical applications are additionally evaluated for its biocompatibility to determine the cell—material dynamics in culture and host—material interactions when implanted in actual living organisms.

Acknowledgments

The authors would also like to acknowledge the funding of National Research Foundation of Korea (Program for UCL Eastman-Korea Dental Medicine Innovation Centre; 2018K1A4A3A0106425) and (NRF; 2018R1D1A1B07048020).

References

[1] W.E. Teo, S. Ramakrishna, A review on electrospinning design and nanofibre assemblies, Nanotechnology 17 (14) (2006) R89–R106.
[2] J. Doshi, D.H. Reneker, Electrospinning process and applications of electrospun fibers, J. Electrost. 35 (2) (1995) 151–160.
[3] Z.-M. Huang, Y.Z. Zhang, M. Kotaki, S. Ramakrishna, A review on polymer nanofibers by electrospinning and their applications in nanocomposites, Compos. Sci. Technol. 63 (15) (2003) 2223–2253.
[4] S.-H. Shin, O. Purevdorj, O. Castano, J.A. Planell, H.-W. Kim, A short review: recent advances in electrospinning for bone tissue regeneration, J. Tissue Eng. 3 (1) (2012), 2041731412443530.
[5] J. Xue, T. Wu, Y. Dai, Y. Xia, Electrospinning and electrospun nanofibers: methods, materials, and applications, Chem. Rev. 119 (8) (2019) 5298–5415.
[6] R.S. Barhate, S. Ramakrishna, Nanofibrous filtering media: filtration problems and solutions from tiny materials, J. Membr. Sci. 296 (1) (2007) 1–8.
[7] W.H. Carothers, Alkylene ester of polybasic acids, U.S. Pat. 2 (012) (1935) 267.
[8] W.H. Carothers, Linear condensation polymers, U.S. Pat. 2 (071) (1937) 250.
[9] C.J. Luo, S.D. Stoyanov, E. Stride, E. Pelan, M. Edirisinghe, Electrospinning versus fibre production methods: from specifics to technological convergence, Chem. Soc. Rev. 41 (13) (2012) 4708–4735.
[10] D.H. Reneker, I. Chun, Nanometre diameter fibres of polymer, produced by electrospinning, Nanotechnology 7 (3) (1996) 216–223.
[11] C.J.F. (US), Apparatus for Electrically Dispersing Fluids, Charles S. Farquhar,Ambrose eastman, United States, 1902.
[12] F. Anton, Process and Apparatus for Preparing Artificial Threads, Richard, Schreiber Gastell, Anton, Formhals, United States, 1934.
[13] H. Fong, I. Chun, D.H. Reneker, Beaded nanofibers formed during electrospinning, Polymer 40 (16) (1999) 4585–4592.
[14] M.G. Hajra, K. Mehta, G.G. Chase, Effects of humidity, temperature, and nanofibers on drop coalescence in glass fiber media, Separ. Purif. Technol. 30 (1) (2003) 79–88.
[15] H. Rodríguez-Tobías, G. Morales, D. Grande, Comprehensive review on electrospinning techniques as versatile approaches toward antimicrobial biopolymeric composite fibers, Mater. Sci. Eng. C 101 (2019) 306–322.
[16] L. Persano, A. Camposeo, C. Tekmen, D. Pisignano, Industrial upscaling of electrospinning and applications of polymer nanofibers: a review, Macromol. Mater. Eng. 298 (5) (2013) 504–520.
[17] T.D. Brown, P.D. Dalton, D.W. Hutmacher, Melt electrospinning today: an opportune time for an emerging polymer process, Prog. Polym. Sci. 56 (2016) 116–166.
[18] J. Lyons, C. Li, F. Ko, Melt-electrospinning part I: processing parameters and geometric properties, Polymer 45 (22) (2004) 7597–7603.
[19] N. Bhardwaj, S.C. Kundu, Electrospinning: a fascinating fiber fabrication technique, Biotechnol. Adv. 28 (3) (2010) 325–347.
[20] R. Sahay, V. Thavasi, S. Ramakrishna, Design modifications in electrospinning setup for advanced applications, J. Nanomater. 2011 (2011) 17, https://doi.org/10.1155/2011/317673.

[21] A. Balogh, R. Cselkó, B. Démuth, G. Verreck, J. Mensch, G. Marosi, Z.K. Nagy, Alternating current electrospinning for preparation of fibrous drug delivery systems, Int. J. Pharm. 495 (1) (2015) 75–80.
[22] A. Mirek, P. Korycka, M. Grzeczkowicz, D. Lewińska, Polymer fibers electrospun using pulsed voltage, Mater. Des. 183 (2019) 108106.
[23] S. Sarkar, S. Deevi, G. Tepper, Biased AC electrospinning of aligned polymer nanofibers, Macromol. Rapid Commun. 28 (2007) 1034–1039.
[24] R. Kessick, J. Fenn, G. Tepper, The use of AC potentials in electrospraying and electrospinning processes, Polymer 45 (2004) 2981–2984.
[25] S. Krzysztof, F.-N. Anna, L. Marcin, Three-dimensional computer models of electrospinning systems, Open Phys. 15 (1) (2017) 777–789.
[26] Z. Liu, K. Ju, Z. Wang, W. Li, H. Ke, J. He, Electrospun jets number and nanofiber morphology effected by voltage value: numerical simulation and experimental verification, Nano. Res. Lett. 14 (1) (2019) 310.
[27] Y. Xiangyu, C. Ye, P. Guo, Electric field manipulation for deposition control in near-field electrospinning, J. Manuf. Process. 30 (2017) 431–438.
[28] A. Rogina, Electrospinning process: versatile preparation method for biodegradable and natural polymers and biocomposite systems applied in tissue engineering and drug delivery, Appl. Surf. Sci. 296 (2014) 221–230.
[29] D. Li, Y. Wang, Y. Xia, Electrospinning of polymeric and ceramic nanofibers as uniaxially aligned arrays, Nano Lett. 3 (8) (2003) 1167–1171.
[30] J. Matthews, G. Wnek, G. Bowlin, Electrospin. Collag. Nanofib., Biomacromol. 3 (2002) 232–238.
[31] Y. Yokoyama, S. Hattori, C. Yoshikawa, Y. Yasuda, H. Koyama, T. Takato, H. Kobayashi, Novel wet electrospinning system for fabrication of spongiform nanofiber 3-dimensional fabric, Mater. Lett. 63 (9) (2009) 754–756.
[32] S.M. Park, S. Eom, W. Kim, D.S. Kim, Role of grounded liquid collectors in precise patterning of electrospun nanofiber mats, Langmuir 34 (1) (2018) 284–290.
[33] B. Tarus, N. Fadel, A. Al-Oufy, M. El-Messiry, Effect of polymer concentration on the morphology and mechanical characteristics of electrospun cellulose acetate and poly (vinyl chloride) nanofiber mats, Alexandria Eng. J. 55 (3) (2016) 2975–2984.
[34] V. Beachley, X. Wen, Effect of electrospinning parameters on the nanofiber diameter and length, Mater. Sci. Eng. C 29 (3) (2009) 663–668.
[35] P.D. Dalton, D. Grafahrend, K. Klinkhammer, D. Klee, M. Möller, Electrospinning of polymer melts: phenomenological observations, Polymer 48 (23) (2007) 6823–6833.
[36] S. Ramakrishna, K. Fujihara, W.-E. Teo, T. Yong, Z. Ma, R. Ramaseshan, Electrospun nanofibers: solving global issues, Mater. Today 9 (3) (2006) 40–50.
[37] S.L. Shenoy, W.D. Bates, H.L. Frisch, G.E. Wnek, Role of chain entanglements on fiber formation during electrospinning of polymer solutions: good solvent, non-specific polymer–polymer interaction limit, Polymer 46 (10) (2005) 3372–3384.
[38] T. Lin, X.G. Wang, 5 - controlling the morphologies of electrospun nanofibres, in: P.J. Brown, K. Stevens (Eds.), Nanofibers and Nanotechnology in Textiles, Woodhead Publishing, 2007, pp. 90–110.
[39] P. Kebarle, M. Peschke, On the mechanisms by which the charged droplets produced by electrospray lead to gas phase ions, Anal. Chim. Acta 406 (2000) 11–35.
[40] Y.M. Shin, M.M. Hohman, M.P. Brenner, G.C. Rutledge, Electrospinning: a whipping fluid jet generates submicron polymer fibers, Appl. Phys. Lett. 78 (8) (2001) 1149–1151.
[41] J.M. Deitzel, J. Kleinmeyer, D. Harris, N.C. Beck Tan, The effect of processing variables on the morphology of electrospun nanofibers and textiles, Polymer 42 (1) (2001) 261–272.

[42] S. Tungprapa, T. Puangparn, M. Weerasombut, I. Jangchud, P. Fakum, S. Semongkhol, C. Meechaisue, P. Supaphol, Electrospun cellulose acetate fibers: effect of solvent system on morphology and fiber diameter, Cellulose 14 (6) (2007) 563–575.
[43] A.L. Yarin, S. Koombhongse, D.H. Reneker, Taylor cone and jetting from liquid droplets in electrospinning of nanofibers, J. Appl. Phys. 90 (9) (2001) 4836–4846.
[44] G.C. Rutledge, S.V. Fridrikh, Formation of fibers by electrospinning, Adv. Drug Deliv. Rev. 59 (14) (2007) 1384–1391.
[45] D.H. Peregrine, Free liquid jets and films: hydrodynamics and rheology, By A. L. YARIN. Longman (in USA, Wiley), 1993. 446 pp. ISBN 0 582 10295 2. £68, J. Fluid Mech. 312 (1996) 408–409.
[46] V.A.G. Bailey, Electrostatic spraying of liquids, Von A. G. Bailey, Research Studies Press LTD Taunton, Somerset/John Wiley & Sons Inc, New York 1988, 197 Seiten, 24,75 $, Phys. Unserer Zeit 20 (5) (1989), 160-160.
[47] J.-Y. Zheng, M.-F. Zhuang, Z.-J. Yu, G.-F. Zheng, Y. Zhao, H. Wang, D.-H. Sun, The effect of surfactants on the diameter and morphology of electrospun ultrafine nanofiber, J. Nanomater. 2014 (2014) 689298.
[48] A. Abutaleb, D. Lolla, A. Aljuhani, H. Shin, J. Rajala, G. Chase, Effects of surfactants on the morphology and properties of electrospun polyetherimide fibers, Fibers 5 (2017) 33.
[49] L. Hristian, M. Chirita, L.R. Manea, I. Sandu, Influence of torsion degree and the elastomer content on yarn characteristics, Mater. Plast. 53 (4) (2016) 739–+.
[50] L.R. Manea, B. Cramariuc, V. Caunii, I. Sandu, Equipment for Obtaining Polimeric Nanofibers by Electrospinning Technology, 2015.
[51] V. Jacobs, R.D. Anandjiwala, M. Maaza, The influence of electrospinning parameters on the structural morphology and diameter of electrospun nanofibers, J. Appl. Polym. Sci. 115 (5) (2010) 3130–3136.
[52] G. Collins, J. Federici, Y. Imura, L. Catalani, Charge generation, charge transport, and residual charge in the electrospinning of polymers: a review of issues and complications, J. Appl. Phys. 111 (2012).
[53] N. Amariei, L.R. Manea, A.P. Bertea, A. Bertea, A. Popa, The influence of polymer solution on the properties of electrospun 3D nanostructures, IOP Conf. Ser. Mater. Sci. Eng. 209 (2017) 012092.
[54] L. Hristian, M. Ostafe, L. Manea, A. Leon, The Study about the Use of the Natural Fibres in Composite Materials, IOP Conference Series: Materials Science and Engineering, IOP Publishing, 2016, p. 032004.
[55] X. Zong, K. Kim, D. Fang, S. Ran, B.S. Hsiao, B. Chu, Structure and process relationship of electrospun bioabsorbable nanofiber membranes, Polymer 43 (16) (2002) 4403–4412.
[56] W.K. Son, J.H. Youk, T.S. Lee, W.H. Park, The effects of solution properties and polyelectrolyte on electrospinning of ultrafine poly(ethylene oxide) fibers, Polymer 45 (9) (2004) 2959–2966.
[57] J.S. Lee, K.H. Choi, H.D. Ghim, S.S. Kim, D.H. Chun, H.Y. Kim, W.S. Lyoo, Role of molecular weight of atactic poly(vinyl alcohol) (PVA) in the structure and properties of PVA nanofabric prepared by electrospinning, J. Appl. Polym. Sci. 93 (4) (2004) 1638–1646.
[58] W. Zuo, M. Zhu, W. Yang, H. Yu, Y. Chen, Y. Zhang, Experimental study on relationship between jet instability and formation of beaded fibers during electrospinning, Polym. Eng. Sci. 45 (5) (2005) 704–709.
[59] C. Mit-uppatham, M. Nithitanakul, P. Supaphol, Ultrafine electrospun polyamide-6 fibers: effect of solution conditions on morphology and average fiber diameter, Macromol. Chem. Phys. 205 (17) (2004) 2327–2338.

[60] Z. Ahmad, Polymeric Dielectric Materials, 2012.
[61] S. Machmudah, Wahyudiono, H. Kanda, M. Goto, Chapter 3 - hydrolysis of biopolymers in near-critical and subcritical water, in: H. Dominguez González, M.J. González Muñoz (Eds.), Water Extraction of Bioactive Compounds, Elsevier, 2017, pp. 69–107.
[62] J.F.d.l. Mora, The fluid dynamics of taylor cones, Annu. Rev. Fluid Mech. 39 (1) (2007) 217–243.
[63] G.I. Taylor, A.D. McEwan, L.N.J.d. Jong, Studies in electrohydrodynamics. I. The circulation produced in a drop by an electric field, Proc. Roy. Soc. Lond. Math. Phys. Sci. 291 (1425) (1966) 159–166.
[64] Y. Son, H. Kim, W. Mao, J. Park, D. Lee, H. Lee, H. Yoo, Hydro-nanofibrous mesh deep cell penetration: a strategy based on peeling of electrospun coaxial nanofibers, Nanoscale 10 (13) (2018) 6051–6059.
[65] J. Ju, Z. Shi, L. Fan, Y. Liang, W. Kang, B. Cheng, Preparation of elastomeric tree-like nanofiber membranes using thermoplastic polyurethane by one-step electrospinning, Mater. Lett. 205 (2017) 190–193.
[66] M. Hasanzadeh, B. Hadavi Moghadam, M. Moghadam Abatari, A. Haghi, On the production optimization of polyacrylonitrile electrospun nanofiber, Bulg. Chem. Commun. 45 (2013) 178–190.
[67] M. Hohman, M. Shin, G. Rutledge, M. Brenner, Electrospinning and electrically forced jets. I. Stability theory, Phy. Fluid. 13 (2001).
[68] S. Hao, N. Pingjuan, N. Pingfan, The auxiliary electrode can improve the electric field distribution of the roller electrostatic spinning, IOP Conf. Ser. Earth Environ. Sci. 358 (2019) 052077.
[69] D. Li, Y. Wang, Y. Xia, Electrospinning nanofibers as uniaxially aligned arrays and layer-by-layer stacked films, Adv. Mater. 16 (4) (2004) 361–366.
[70] A. Baji, Y.-W. Mai, S.-C. Wong, M. Abtahi, P. Chen, Electrospinning of polymer nanofibers: effects on oriented morphology, structures and tensile properties, Compos. Sci. Technol. 70 (5) (2010) 703–718.
[71] G.H. Kim, Electrospun PCL nanofibers with anisotropic mechanical properties as a biomedical scaffold, Biomed. Mater. 3 (2) (2008) 025010.
[72] M.M.L. Arras, C. Grasl, H. Bergmeister, H. Schima, Electrospinning of aligned fibers with adjustable orientation using auxiliary electrodes, Sci. Technol. Adv. Mater. 13 (3) (2012) 035008.
[73] J. Lee, S.Y. Lee, J. Jang, Y.H. Jeong, D.-W. Cho, Fabrication of patterned nanofibrous mats using direct-write electrospinning, Langmuir 28 (18) (2012) 7267–7275.
[74] D.H. Reneker, A.L. Yarin, H. Fong, S. Koombhongse, Bending instability of electrically charged liquid jets of polymer solutions in electrospinning, J. Appl. Phys. 87 (9) (2000) 4531–4547.
[75] J.J. Feng, Stretching of a straight electrically charged viscoelastic jet, J. Non-Newtonian Fluid Mech. 116 (1) (2003) 55–70.
[76] L.L. Barannyk, D.T. Papageorgiou, P.G. Petropoulos, Suppression of Rayleigh–Taylor instability using electric fields, Math. Comput. Simulat. 82 (6) (2012) 1008–1016.
[77] S.P. Shariatpanahi, D. Bonn, M.R. Ejtehadi, A.I. Zad, Electrical bending instability in electrospinning visco-elastic solutions, J. Polym. Sci. B Polym. Phys. 54 (11) (2016) 1036–1042.
[78] D.H. Reneker, A.L. Yarin, Electrospinning jets and polymer nanofibers, Polymer 49 (10) (2008) 2387–2425.
[79] T. Han, D.H. Reneker, A.L. Yarin, Buckling of jets in electrospinning, Polymer 48 (20) (2007) 6064–6076.

[80] C. Mingjun, Z. Youchen, L. Haoyi, L. Xiangnan, D. Yumei, M.M. Bubakir, Y. Weimin, An example of industrialization of melt electrospinning: polymer melt differential electrospinning, Advan. Indus. Eng. Polymer Res. 2 (3) (2019) 110–115.
[81] S. Liao, B. Langfield, N. Ristovski, C. Theodoropoulos, J. Hardt, K.A. Blackwood, S.D. Yambem, S.D. Gregory, M.A. Woodruff, S. Powell, Effect of Humid. Melt Electro. Polycaprolact. Scaffold. 17 (3–4) (2016) 173.
[82] K. Desai, K. Kit, Effect of spinning temperature and blend ratios on electrospun chitosan/poly(acrylamide) blends fibers, Polymer 49 (19) (2008) 4046–4050.
[83] F. Huang, Q. Wei, J. Wang, Y. Cai, Y. Huang, Effect of temperature on structure, morphology and crystallinity of PVDF nanofibers via, Electrospinning 8 (1) (2008) 152.
[84] O. Hardick, B. Stevens, D. Bracewell, Nanofiber fabrication in a temperature and humidity controlled environment for improved fibre consistency, Nat. Prec. (2010) 1.
[85] R.M. Nezarati, M.B. Eifert, E. Cosgriff-Hernandez, Effects of humidity and solution viscosity on electrospun fiber morphology, Tissue Eng. C Methods 19 (10) (2013) 810–819.
[86] S.B. Jo, U. Erdenebileg, K. Dashnyam, G.-Z. Jin, J.-R. Cha, A. El-Fiqi, J.C. Knowles, K.D. Patel, H.-H. Lee, J.-H. Lee, H.-W. Kim, Nano-graphene oxide/polyurethane nanofibers: mechanically flexible and myogenic stimulating matrix for skeletal tissue engineering, J. Tissue Eng. 11 (2020), 2041731419900424.
[87] R.K. Singh, K.D. Patel, J.H. Lee, E.-J. Lee, J.-H. Kim, T.-H. Kim, H.-W. Kim, Potential of magnetic nanofiber scaffolds with mechanical and biological properties applicable for bone regeneration, PloS One 9 (4) (2014) e91584-e91584.
[88] K.D. Patel, H.-W. Kim, J.C. Knowles, A. Poma, Molecularly Imprinted Polymers and Electrospinning: Manufacturing Convergence for Next-Level Applications, Advanced Functional Materials N/a(n/a) 2001955.
[89] M.S. Kang, J.-H. Kim, R.K. Singh, J.-H. Jang, H.-W. Kim, Therapeutic-designed electrospun bone scaffolds: mesoporous bioactive nanocarriers in hollow fiber composites to sequentially deliver dual growth factors, Acta Biomater. 16 (2015) 103–116.
[90] A. El-Fiqi, J.-H. Kim, H.-W. Kim, Osteoinductive fibrous scaffolds of biopolymer/mesoporous bioactive glass nanocarriers with excellent bioactivity and long-term delivery of osteogenic drug, ACS Appl. Mater. Interface. 7 (2) (2015) 1140–1152.
[91] K.D. Patel, T.-H. Kim, N. Mandakhbayar, R.K. Singh, J.-H. Jang, J.-H. Lee, H.-W. Kim, Coating biopolymer nanofibers with carbon nanotubes accelerates tissue healing and bone regeneration through orchestrated cell- and tissue-regulatory responses, Acta Biomater. 108 (2020) 97–110, https://doi.org/10.1016/j.actbio.2020.03.012.
[92] R.K. Singh, G.-Z. Jin, C. Mahapatra, K.D. Patel, W. Chrzanowski, H.-W. Kim, Mesoporous silica-layered biopolymer hybrid nanofibrous scaffold: a novel nanobiomatrix platform for therapeutics delivery and bone regeneration, ACS Appl. Mater. Interface. 7 (15) (2015) 8088–8098.
[93] R. Colquhoun, K.E. Tanner, Mechanical behaviour of degradable phosphate glass fibres and composites—a review, Biomed. Mater. 11 (1) (2015) 014105.
[94] B. Sun, X.-J. Jiang, S. Zhang, J.-C. Zhang, Y.-F. Li, Q.-Z. You, Y.-Z. Long, Electrospun anisotropic architectures and porous structures for tissue engineering, J. Mater. Chem. B 3 (27) (2015) 5389–5410.
[95] J.H. Wendorff, S. Agarwal, A. Greiner, Electrospinning: Materials, Processing, and Applications, Wiley, 2012.
[96] L. Yu, Z. Shao, L. Xu, High throughput preparation of aligned nanofibers using an improved, Bubble-Electrospin. 9 (12) (2017).

[97] T. Yoshioka, R. Dersch, M. Tsuji, A.K. Schaper, Orientation analysis of individual electrospun PE nanofibers by transmission electron microscopy, Polymer 51 (11) (2010) 2383–2389.

[98] F. Topuz, T. Uyar, Electrospinning of gelatin with tunable fiber morphology from round to flat/ribbon, Mater. Sci. Eng. C 80 (2017) 371–378.

[99] S. Miao, W. Zhu, N.J. Castro, M. Nowicki, X. Zhou, H. Cui, J.P. Fisher, L.G. Zhang, 4D printing smart biomedical scaffolds with novel soybean oil epoxidized acrylate, Sci. Rep. 6 (1) (2016) 27226.

[100] Y. Liu, X. Zhang, Y. Xia, H. Yang, Magnetic-field-assisted electrospinning of aligned straight and wavy polymeric nanofibers, Adv. Mater. 22 (22) (2010) 2454–2457.

[101] K.H. Lee, H.Y. Kim, H.J. Bang, Y.H. Jung, S.G. Lee, The change of bead morphology formed on electrospun polystyrene fibers, Polymer 44 (14) (2003) 4029–4034.

[102] M. Bognitzki, W. Czado, T. Frese, A. Schaper, M. Hellwig, M. Steinhart, A. Greiner, J.H. Wendorff, Nanostructured fibers via electrospinning, Adv. Mater. 13 (1) (2001) 70–72.

[103] D.H. Reneker, W. Kataphinan, A. Theron, E. Zussman, A.L. Yarin, Nanofiber garlands of polycaprolactone by electrospinning, Polymer 43 (25) (2002) 6785–6794.

[104] Y.-H. Hsu, C.-C. Lai, Y.-T. Peng, C.-T. Lo, Preparation and characterization of interconnected carbon nanofibers, Textil. Res. J. 85 (1) (2014) 3–12.

[105] C.-C. Yu, Y.-W. Chen, P.-Y. Yeh, Y.-S. Hsiao, W.-T. Lin, C.-W. Kuo, D.-Y. Chueh, Y.-W. You, J.-J. Shyue, Y.-C. Chang, P. Chen, Random and aligned electrospun PLGA nanofibers embedded in microfluidic chips for cancer cell isolation and integration with air foam technology for cell release, J. Nanobiotechnol. 17 (1) (2019) 31.

[106] J.I. Kim, T.I. Hwang, L.E. Aguilar, C.H. Park, C.S. Kim, A controlled design of aligned and random nanofibers for 3D Bi-functionalized nerve conduits fabricated via a novel electrospinning set-up, Sci. Rep. 6 (1) (2016) 23761.

[107] L.Y. Yeo, J.R. Friend, Electrospinning carbon nanotube polymer composite nanofibers, J. Exp. Nanosci. 1 (2) (2006) 177–209.

[108] W. Liu, L. Zhu, C. Huang, X. Jin, Direct electrospinning of ultrafine fibers with interconnected macropores enabled by in situ mixing microfluidics, ACS Appl. Mater. Interface. 8 (50) (2016) 34870–34878.

[108a] G.-M. Kim, G.H. Michler, P. Pötschke, Deformation processes of ultrahigh porous multiwalled carbon nanotubes/polycarbonate composite fibers prepared by electrospinning, Polymer 46 (18) (2005) 7346–7351.

[109] G. Poologasundarampillai, D. Wang, S. Li, J. Nakamura, R. Bradley, P.D. Lee, M.M. Stevens, D.S. McPhail, T. Kasuga, J.R. Jones, Cotton-wool-like bioactive glasses for bone regeneration, Acta Biomater. 10 (8) (2014) 3733–3746.

[110] F. Xiao, H. Sun, J. Li, X. Guo, H. Zhang, J. Lu, Z. Pan, J. Xu, Electrospinning preparation and electromagnetic wave absorption properties of SiCN fibers, Ceram. Int. 46 (8, Part B) (2020) 12773–12781.

[111] B. Yu, Y. Liu, G. Jiang, D. Liu, W. Yu, H. Chen, L. Li, Q. Huang, Preparation of electrospun Ag/g-C3N4 loaded composite carbon nanofibers for catalytic applications, Mater. Res. Express 4 (1) (2017) 015603.

[112] Z. Zhang, Y. Wu, Z. Wang, X. Zou, Y. Zhao, L. Sun, Fabrication of silver nanoparticles embedded into polyvinyl alcohol (Ag/PVA) composite nanofibrous films through electrospinning for antibacterial and surface-enhanced Raman scattering (SERS) activities, Mater. Sci. Eng. C 69 (2016) 462–469.

[113] C. Spagnol, E.H. Fragal, A.G.B. Pereira, C.V. Nakamura, E.C. Muniz, H.D.M. Follmann, R. Silva, A.F. Rubira, Cellulose nanowhiskers decorated with silver nanoparticles as an additive to antibacterial polymers membranes fabricated by electrospinning, J. Colloid Interface Sci. 531 (2018) 705–715.

[114] R.a. Franco, A. Sadiasa, H.S. Seo, B.-T. Lee, Biphasic calcium phosphate loading on polycaprolactone/poly(lacto-co-glycolic acid) membranes for improved tensile strength, in vitro biocompatibility, and in vivo tissue regeneration, J. Biomater. Appl. 28 (2013) 1164–1179.
[115] W. Matysiak, T. Tański, Analysis of the morphology, structure and optical properties of 1D SiO2 nanostructures obtained with sol-gel and electrospinning methods, Appl. Surf. Sci. 489 (2019) 34–43.
[116] Y.F. Dufrêne, T. Ando, R. Garcia, D. Alsteens, D. Martinez-Martin, A. Engel, C. Gerber, D.J. Müller, Imaging modes of atomic force microscopy for application in molecular and cell biology, Nat. Nanotechnol. 12 (4) (2017) 295–307.
[117] H. Sakamoto, H. Asakawa, T. Fukuma, S. Fujita, S.-i. Suye, Atomic force microscopy visualization of hard segment alignment in stretched polyurethane nanofibers prepared by electrospinning, Sci. Technol. Adv. Mater. 15 (1) (2014) 015008.
[118] P. Xu, W. Li, H. Zhou, F. Pan, H. Xing, H. Liu, Investigations of the structural evolution of electrospun nanofibers using atomic force microscopy, RSC Adv. 2 (29) (2012) 11104–11110.
[119] K. Desai, J.S. Lee, C. Sung, Nanocharacterization of electrospun nanofibers of polyaniline/poly methyl methacrylate blends using SEM, TEM and AFM, Microsc. Microanal. 10 (S02) (2004) 556–557.
[120] M. Kanduč, A. Schlaich, E. Schneck, R.R. Netz, Water-mediated interactions between hydrophilic and hydrophobic surfaces, Langmuir 32 (35) (2016) 8767–8782.
[121] R. Dorati, S. Pisani, G. Maffeis, B. Conti, T. Modena, E. Chiesa, G. Bruni, U.M. Musazzi, I. Genta, Study on hydrophilicity and degradability of chitosan/polylactide-co-polycaprolactone nanofibre blend electrospun membrane, Carbohydr. Polym. 199 (2018) 150–160.
[122] A.M. Deliormanlı, R. Konyalı, Bioactive glass/hydroxyapatite- containing electrospun poly (ε-Caprolactone) composite nanofibers for bone tissue engineering, J. Austral. Ceramic Soc. 55 (1) (2019) 247–256.
[123] Y. Ji, K. Liang, X. Shen, G.L. Bowlin, Electrospinning and characterization of chitin nanofibril/polycaprolactone nanocomposite fiber mats, Carbohydr. Polym. 101 (2014) 68–74.
[124] W. Cui, L. Cheng, H. Li, Y. Zhou, Y. Zhang, J. Chang, Preparation of hydrophilic poly(l-lactide) electrospun fibrous scaffolds modified with chitosan for enhanced cell biocompatibility, Polymer 53 (11) (2012) 2298–2305.
[125] A.D. Li, Z.Z. Sun, M. Zhou, X.X. Xu, J.Y. Ma, W. Zheng, H.M. Zhou, L. Li, Y.F. Zheng, Electrospun Chitosan-graft-PLGA nanofibres with significantly enhanced hydrophilicity and improved mechanical property, Colloids Surf. B Biointerface. 102 (2013) 674–681.
[126] A. Abdal-hay, H.R. Pant, J.K. Lim, Super-hydrophilic electrospun nylon-6/hydroxyapatite membrane for bone tissue engineering, Eur. Polym. J. 49 (6) (2013) 1314–1321.
[127] N.T. Ba Linh, Y.K. Min, B.-T. Lee, Hybrid hydroxyapatite nanoparticles-loaded PCL/GE blend fibers for bone tissue engineering, J. Biomater. Sci. Polym. Ed. 24 (5) (2013) 520–538.
[128] M.J. Park, R.R. Gonzales, A. Abdel-Wahab, S. Phuntsho, H.K. Shon, Hydrophilic polyvinyl alcohol coating on hydrophobic electrospun nanofiber membrane for high performance thin film composite forward osmosis membrane, Desalination 426 (2018) 50–59.
[129] L. Huang, J.T. Arena, S.S. Manickam, X. Jiang, B.G. Willis, J.R. McCutcheon, Improved mechanical properties and hydrophilicity of electrospun nanofiber membranes for filtration applications by dopamine modification, J. Membr. Sci. 460 (2014) 241–249.

[130] Y. Dong, J. Kong, S.L. Phua, C. Zhao, N.L. Thomas, X. Lu, Tailoring surface hydrophilicity of porous electrospun nanofibers to enhance capillary and push−pull effects for moisture wicking, ACS Appl. Mater. Interface. 6 (16) (2014) 14087−14095.
[131] Y. Bai, Z.-H. Huang, Z.-X. Zhang, F. Kang, Improvement of the hydrophilicity of electrospun porous carbon nanofibers by grafting phenylsulfonic acid groups, J. Colloid Interface Sci. 394 (2013) 177−182.
[132] X. Zhu, W. Cui, X. Li, Y. Jin, Electrospun fibrous mats with high porosity as potential scaffolds for skin tissue engineering, Biomacromolecules 9 (7) (2008) 1795−1801.
[133] S. Vitas, J.S. Segmehl, I. Burgert, E. Cabane, Porosity and pore size distribution of native and delignified beech wood determined by mercury intrusion porosimetry, Materials 12 (3) (2019).
[134] P.R. Cortez Tornello, P.C. Caracciolo, J.I. Igartúa Roselló, G.A. Abraham, Electrospun scaffolds with enlarged pore size: porosimetry analysis, Mater. Lett. 227 (2018) 191−193.
[135] Y. Liu, J. Luo, C. Helleu, M. Behr, H. Ba, T. Romero, A. Hébraud, G. Schlatter, O. Ersen, D.S. Su, C. Pham-Huu, Hierarchical porous carbon fibers/carbon nanofibers monolith from electrospinning/CVD processes as a high effective surface area support platform, J. Mater. Chem. 5 (5) (2017) 2151−2162.
[136] Y. Li, C.T. Lim, M. Kotaki, Study on structural and mechanical properties of porous PLA nanofibers electrospun by channel-based electrospinning system, Polymer 56 (2015) 572−580.
[137] D. Wang, Y. Yue, Q. Wang, W. Cheng, G. Han, Preparation of cellulose acetate-polyacrylonitrile composite nanofibers by multi-fluid mixing electrospinning method: morphology, wettability, and mechanical properties, Appl. Surf. Sci. 510 (2020) 145462.
[138] Y.E. Aguirre-Chagala, V. Altuzar, E. León-Sarabia, J.C. Tinoco-Magaña, J.M. Yañez-Limón, C. Mendoza-Barrera, Physicochemical properties of polycaprolactone/collagen/elastin nanofibers fabricated by electrospinning, Mater. Sci. Eng. C 76 (2017) 897−907.
[139] L. Siqueira, F.R. Passador, M.M. Costa, A.O. Lobo, E. Sousa, Influence of the addition of β-TCP on the morphology, thermal properties and cell viability of poly (lactic acid) fibers obtained by electrospinning, Mater. Sci. Eng. C 52 (2015) 135−143.
[140] E. Ranjbari, S. Bazgir, M.M.A. Shirazi, Needleless electrospinning of poly(acrylic acid) superabsorbent: fabrication, characterization and swelling behavior, Polym. Test. 84 (2020) 106403.
[141] S. Khalili, H.M. Chenari, Successful electrospinning fabrication of ZrO2 nanofibers: a detailed physical − chemical characterization study, J. Alloys Compd. 828 (2020) 154414.
[142] T. Ahmadi, A. Monshi, V. Mortazavi, M.H. Fathi, S. Sharifi, M. Kharaziha, L. Khazdooz, A. Zarei, M. Taghian Dehaghani, Fabrication and characterization of polycaprolactone fumarate/gelatin-based nanocomposite incorporated with silicon and magnesium co-doped fluorapatite nanoparticles using electrospinning method, Mater. Sci. Eng. C 106 (2020) 110172.
[143] S. Gautam, A.K. Dinda, N.C. Mishra, Fabrication and characterization of PCL/gelatin composite nanofibrous scaffold for tissue engineering applications by electrospinning method, Mater. Sci. Eng. C 33 (3) (2013) 1228−1235.
[144] L. Ma, X. Shi, X. Zhang, L. Li, Electrospinning of polycaprolacton/chitosan core-shell nanofibers by a stable emulsion system, Colloid. Surface. Physicochem. Eng. Aspect. 583 (2019) 123956.
[145] H. Lian, Z. Meng, Melt electrospinning vs. solution electrospinning: a comparative study of drug-loaded poly (ε-caprolactone) fibres, Mater. Sci. Eng. C 74 (2017) 117−123.

[146] E. Storti, C. Himcinschi, J. Kortus, C.G. Aneziris, Synthesis and characterization of calcium zirconate nanofibers produced by electrospinning, J. Eur. Ceram. Soc. 39 (16) (2019) 5338–5344.
[147] G. Hochleitner, M. Kessler, M. Schmitz, A.R. Boccaccini, J. Teßmar, J. Groll, Melt electrospinning writing of defined scaffolds using polylactide-poly(ethylene glycol) blends with 45S5 bioactive glass particles, Mater. Lett. 205 (2017) 257–260.
[148] S. Mohammadzadehmoghadam, Y. Dong, Fabrication and characterization of electrospun silk fibroin/gelatin scaffolds, Crosslink. With Glutaraldehyde Vapor 6 (91) (2019).
[149] D. Wang, W. Cheng, Q. Wang, J. Zang, Y. Zhang, G. Han, Preparation of electrospun chitosan/poly (ethylene oxide) composite nanofibers reinforced with cellulose nanocrystals: Structure, morphology, and mechanical behavior, Compos. Sci. Technol. 182 (2019), 107774.
[150] R.A. Franco, Y.K. Min, H.M. Yang, B.T. Lee, On stabilization of PVPA/PVA electrospun nanofiber membrane and its effect on material properties and biocompatibility, J. Nanomater. (2012) 2012.
[151] T.-N. Lam, C.-C. Wang, W.-C. Ko, J.-M. Wu, S.-N. Lai, W.-T. Chuang, C.-J. Su, C.-Y. Ma, M.-Y. Luo, Y.-J. Wang, E.W. Huang, Tuning mechanical properties of electrospun piezoelectric nanofibers by heat treatment, Materialia 8 (2019) 100461.
[152] M.S. Islam, A.N. Naz, M.N. Alam, A.K. Das, J.H. Yeum, Electrospun poly(vinyl alcohol)/silver nanoparticle/carbon nanotube multi-composite nanofiber mat: fabrication, characterization and evaluation of thermal, mechanical and antibacterial properties, Colloid Interface Sci. Commun. 35 (2020) 100247.
[153] X. Song, K. Zhang, Y. Song, Z. Duan, Q. Liu, Y. Liu, Morphology, microstructure and mechanical properties of electrospun alumina nanofibers prepared using different polymer templates: a comparative study, J. Alloys Compd. 829 (2020) 154502.
[154] S.Y. Chew, T.C. Hufnagel, C.T. Lim, K.W. Leong, Mechanical properties of single electrospun drug-encapsulated nanofibres, Nanotechnology 17 (15) (2006) 3880–3891.
[155] K.Y. Hwang, S.-D. Kim, Y.-W. Kim, W.-R. Yu, Mechanical characterization of nanofibers using a nanomanipulator and atomic force microscope cantilever in a scanning electron microscope, Polym. Test. 29 (3) (2010) 375–380.
[156] S.R. Baker, S. Banerjee, K. Bonin, M. Guthold, Determining the mechanical properties of electrospun poly-ε-caprolactone (PCL) nanofibers using AFM and a novel fiber anchoring technique, Mater. Sci. Eng. C 59 (2016) 203–212.

CHAPTER TWO

Advances and innovations in electrospinning technology

Pooya Davoodi[1,2,a] Elisabeth L. Gill[1,2] Wenyu Wang[1,2], Yan Yan Shery Huang[1,2]
[1]Department of Engineering, University of Cambridge, Cambridge, United Kingdom
[2]The Nanoscience Centre, University of Cambridge, Cambridge, United Kingdom

Abbreviations

2D Two-dimensional
3D Three-dimensional
AgNPs Silver nanoparticles
AM Additive manufacturing
CTS Critical translation speed
DC Direct current
FDM Fused deposition modeling
LEP Low-voltage electrospinning
MES Magnetic electrospinning
NFES Near-field electrospinning
PCL Polycaprolactone
PDLLA Poly-d,L-lactic acid
PDMS Polydimethylsiloxane
PEO Polyethylene glycol

2.1 Introduction

Fiber is a one-dimensional and high aspect ratio structure that widely exists in nature (i.e., spider silks and silkworm filaments) and has been extensively used in our daily life and industries, ranging from clothing fashion industry [1], wastewater treatment [2], to biomedical applications [3] and wearable electronics [4]. At a single thread level, individual fibers possess unique mechanical properties, including ultraflexibility, low bending resistance, and large surface-to-volume ratio; when processed into fiber mats or textiles, such large-scale fibrous structures could demonstrate bendability,

[a] Present address: School of Pharmacy and Bioengineering, Keele University, Keele, United Kingdom.

Biomedical Applications of Electrospinning and Electrospraying
ISBN: 978-0-12-822476-2
https://doi.org/10.1016/B978-0-12-822476-2.00004-2

stretchability, breathability, and high porosity, intriguing wide range applications in many areas. Numerous approaches have been developed to produce synthetic fibers with various materials, and among them, electrospinning is a broadly used and efficient method to produce micro-/nanoscaled fibers (fiber diameter ranges from 2 nm to several micrometers) [5]. Apart from electrospinning, most of other conventional fiber production approaches, such as wet and dry spinning, drag spinning, gel spinning, and three-dimensional (3D) printing, rely on the mechanical drawing or shear stresses alone to stretch and thin the fiber jet; thus, they usually struggle to produce ultrathin fibers with fiber diameter smaller than ~10 μm without causing fiber breakage [6]. Electrospinning utilizes strong static electrical forces to pull and stretch the polymer solutions or melts into thin jets, leading to final micro-/nanofiber deposition. Such phenomenon was first being discovered and described over a century ago [7], but not until the early 1900s that the term "electrospinning" had been officially proposed [8]. Since then, the research and studies about this versatile and simple fiber production technique have been growing significantly [9].

With recent developments in materials science and nanotechnology, new materials have been incorporated with the electrospinning technique, such as conducting materials, energy generating materials, and biocompatible and bioactive materials. Electrospun micro-/nanoscaled fibers that are functionalized with these new materials have not only retained the physical merits of ultrathin fibers, such as high aspect ratio, flexibility, directionality, and high porosity, but also opened up novel fibrous and textile device configurations and applications. For example, the use of piezoelectric polymers has enabled a range of inherently flexible and transparent energy harvesters and self-powered sensors [10,11]. Composite material fibers made with polymers and metals or ceramics have shown promising application potentials in novel sensing and optoelectronic devices [12,13]. At the same time, these emerging applications demand more precise, convenient, and customized control of the morphologies and patterns of the electrospun fibers. Therefore, efforts have been invested to modify and adapt the electrospinning setups and working conditions, and to combine fiber spinning with other advanced processing techniques (i.e., 3D printing and microfluidics).

In this chapter, we aim to provide a comprehensive description of the recent innovations and technical advances of electrospinning. In order to readers who are not familiar with electrospinning to effectively read this chapter, a brief introduction of the physical principles and basic setup designs of electrospinning is provided at the beginning, followed by discussions of major and universal experimental factors that could affect the fiber spinnability in the technique, including polymer solution properties, ambient, and operation parameters. Next, we focus on the recent application-driven advances and innovations in electrospinning technique. Various approaches to modify the conventional electrospinning setups to acquire controlled and designed fiber patterns will be discussed first, including modifying nozzle and collecting substrate, controlling and directing fiber deposition, and stabilizing fiber jet, followed by introducing novel electrospinning techniques that are combined with other polymer processing technologies, such as additive manufacturing (AM) and microfluidic devices.

2.2 Electrospinning: the underpinning physical principles

Electrospinning is similar to other spinning techniques in that a tensile force draws a fiber from a spinnable source; however, it differs in the manner of fiber initiation [14]. The majority of other spinning techniques utilize mechanical initiation in the form of spindles or mechanical dragging, whereas in electrospinning, this effect is substituted with Coulomb's force from the application of a strong electric field. Briefly, a viscous polymer solution or melt is fed through to a syringe needle at low flow rate until a droplet of solution collects at the tip. As shown in Fig. 2.1, a high electrical charge is

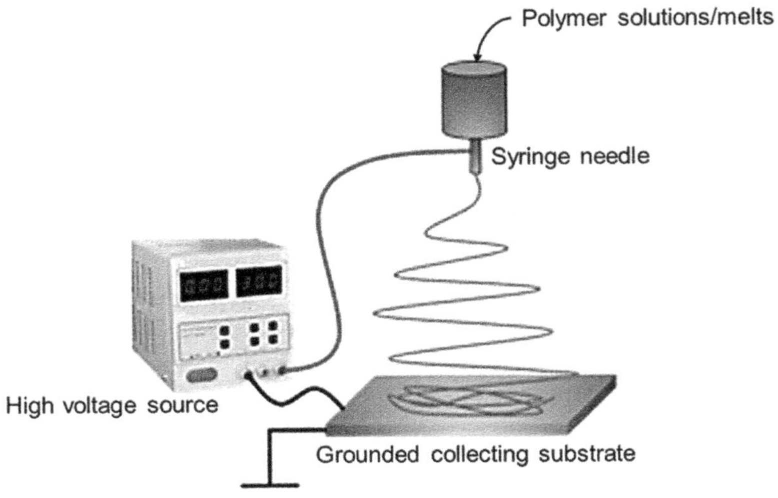

Figure 2.1 Schematic showing the basic setup configuration of electrospinning.

applied to the solution or melt either within the syringe or at the syringe needle, which is directed toward an oppositely charged collecting substrate. This exposes the droplet on the tip of the syringe to an electric field, exerting a tensile force in the same direction as the solution's internal electrostatic self-repulsion. A "Taylor cone" or deformation appears in the droplet just beyond the point where the resistive forces of droplet surface tension and solution/melt viscosity counterbalance the tensile force [6]. This formation initiates the ejection of a fine polymer jet from the apex of the cone toward the collecting substrate [15]. During the movement of the jet between the nozzle and the collecting substrate, the solvent vaporizes and a solid polymer fiber is collected. When the collecting substrate is greater than a few millimeters away, the self-repulsion of the polymer jet, due to Coulomb's force, gravity, and aerodynamic effects, causes chaotic bending instability [16,17]. This results in the polymer jet adopting a spinning motion that elongates the jet and consequently the collected fibers thin to a micro- to nanoscale, which concentrates the charge density within the fiber. Due to that bending instability [18,19], the deposition of fibers produced by conventional electrospinning creates random fiber packing.

Through careful optimization of the process instrumentation and working parameters of far-field electrospinning techniques, polymer fibers have been fabricated with diameters ranging between ~ 3 nm and a few micrometers [20]. Given the complexity of the process and high number of processing parameters, there is great scope for innovation with subtle variations extending product versatility. As one example, some have exploited the effect of the polymer jet splitting during transit to create such ultrafine fibers [21]. The section below thematically describes the influence of the key parameters and how these can be manipulated to create various fiber morphologies and fibrous designs.

2.3 Properties influencing spinnability of polymer solutions

Electrospinning setups typically include several basic parts: a high-voltage power supplier (usually a direct current power source), a conductive nozzle, a syringe pump used to control solution flow rate, and a grounded substrate for collecting fiber products [22]. During electrospinning, many factors can influence a jet movement and consequently the properties of final products. These factors include the following[22,23]: (a) solution properties (molecular weight, polymer molecule architecture, polymer concentration, solvent, conductivity, surface tension, and viscosity), (b) ambient parameters (temperature, relative humidity, airflow and pressure around the setup, and ambient gas), and (c) operating parameters (applied voltage, solution flow rate, nozzle material and geometry, substrate material and geometry, and the distance between a nozzle and substrate). Properties of the polymer solution should be the first consideration when determining the applied voltage and other experimental conditions for a desired fiber continuity and morphology.

2.3.1 Solution properties

Surface tension acts to minimize the energy at the air—solution interface through lowering the surface area and forming droplets [16], whereas viscosity acts as a resistive force to sudden changes in solution jet shape and maintains a smooth surface [24,25]. In the case of spun fibers, they oppose one another. At low polymer concentration, surface tension can overpower viscosity, causing a beaded fiber, bead-on-string, or nanoparticle morphology [26,27]. The reverse happens as polymer concentration, and therefore molecular entanglement increases. Viscous effects dominate and this favors the fabrication of smooth and defect-free fibers [28]. Hence, adequate polymer concentration is a prerequisite to attain fibers at all [29,30], as at a molecular level, there is a threshold concentration for entanglement [31,32]. Examples of the transition from bead-on-string morphology to smooth uniform fibers with increasing polymer concentration have been demonstrated, as exemplified in Fig. 2.2a—c [25,36,37]. This is also dependent on the molecular weight of the polymer as longer chain molecules favor entanglement more than short-chain alternatives. Fiber diameter also generally increases with increasing viscosity as this increases the resistance of the polymer jet to deformation by elongation [27]. Another critical balance of forces takes place on the ejected polymer jet as evaporation of the solvent takes place and it forms a fiber. Surface tension acts on the polymer jet to maintain a circular cross section, while the tensile force provided by the electric field stretches it. Sufficient polymer concentration is also required to prevent capillary breakage and Rayleigh instability [28], otherwise this also leads to beaded fibers.

The volatility of the chosen solvent affects the rate at which the fibers will solidify in the spinning process. Solvents with high volatility ensure that the fibers are dry upon reaching their collecting substrate and attain a circular cross section. Alternatively, in some situations, it can be desirable

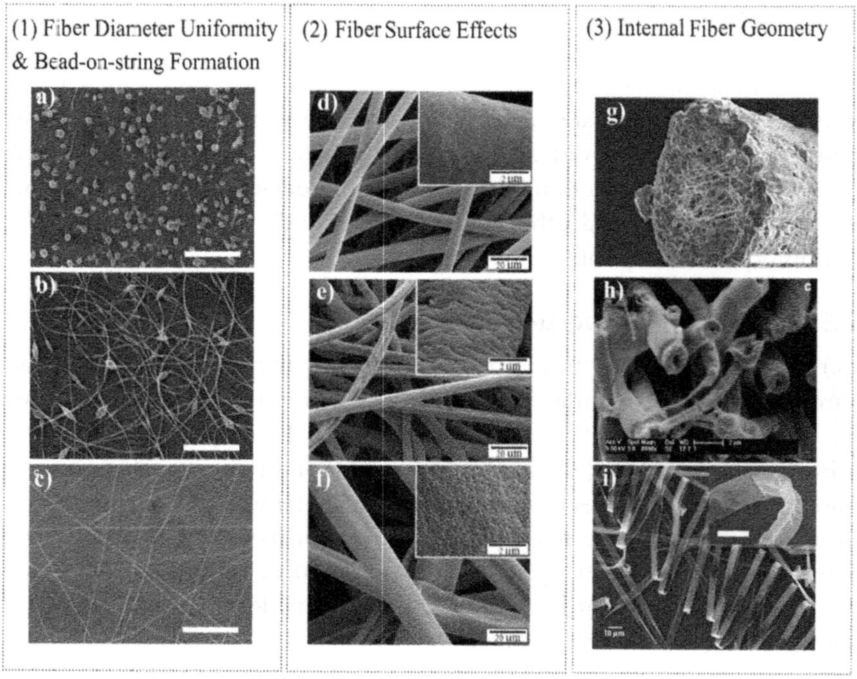

Figure 2.2 Control of electrospun fiber morphology. Polymer concentration and solution viscosity can lead to (a) electrosprayed beads, (b) bead-on-string, or (c) smooth fiber production [25]. Scales represent 5 μm. Solvent and atmospheric conditions can yield (d) smooth, (e) rough, and (f) nanoporous fiber surface morphologies [33]. Solvent conditions, nozzle configuration, and solution properties can be used to design internal fiber geometry, alternative to solid fibers, including (g) internal nanoporosity [34] (link: https://pubs.acs.org/doi/10.1021/acsami.8b17955), (h) hollow fibers [35], and (i) polymer ribbons [21]. Scales in (g) represent 1 μm, (h) 2 μm, and (i) 10 μm.

to have fibers spun wet, dry out gradually, and even merge with their neighbors to form mechanically strong interconnected fiber junctions [38]. At the other extreme, utilizing highly volatile solvents can design surface porosity and other surface textures on individual spun fibers through inducing phase separation during the process of fiber solidification. These nanoscale surface effects increase the fiber surface-to-volume ratio, a quality that is of interest for filtration and drug delivery applications for its efficacy in trapping small particles within nanopores (Fig. 2.2d–f) [33,39,40]. Manipulation of solvent properties can also extend to inducing porosity in fibers internally as was recently studied in, e.g., Fig. 2.2g [34].

Overall solution conductivity affects the surface free charge at the fiber surface, determining the charge density along the polymer jet [41]. It is essential to facilitate the electrostatic tensile force on the solution droplet and ensuing polymer jet to be characteristic of electrospinning. Increasing the solution conductivity is a direct way to increase the electrostatic tensile drawing force exerted on the polymer jet. This makes a solution more readily electrospun and increases the elongation effect on the polymer jet, which can be another strategy to decrease fiber diameter [42,43] and create a smooth fiber surface through maximizing the surface area [25]. Consequently, this also inherently increases the bending instability and disorder in the deposited fibers. This strategy has been explored by several groups through the addition of salt [44], such as NaCl [45], to enhance solution conductivity of PDLLA (poly-d,L-lactic acid) and other polymers. This demonstrated improved solution electrospinning behavior and yielded thinner fibers; furthermore, the addition of salt created surface roughness on the spun fibers.

2.3.2 Ambient parameters

The environmental factors that influence electrospinning processes can be logistically more challenging to control but undoubtedly have a considerable impact on spun fiber morphology [46–49]. These include surrounding temperature, humidity, and air velocity. Principally, this affects the rate of solvent evaporation. An increase in surrounding temperature has a complex overall effect: it increases the rate of evaporation, which can produce a rougher fiber surface. Localized heating of the polymer solution can also increase solution concentration and viscosity [47], and in some cases, this can be exploited to create thinner fibers [49]. Local airflow within a chemical safety hood is another indirect means to accelerate the rate of solvent evaporation, which like surrounding temperature may affect the fiber surface for some polymer solutions and be utilized to induce phase separation. Humidity can have varying effects on fiber topography through vapor-induced phase separation as shown by Moroni and et al. [46]. In the case of certain inorganic solutions that are immiscible in water, it can cause phase separation to the point at which the solution can no longer be spun [29]. Humidity can drastically change the solidification processes of polystyrene, for instance, and this can be exploited by smooth, porous, or wrinkled fibers [29,33,50]. Unlike ambient temperature and flow rate, which affect electrospinning processes more universally, the influence of humidity is more specific to the solution conditions.

2.3.3 Operating parameters

The operating conditions that affect electrospinning processes include the following: solution flow rate, nozzle tip size and geometry, the applied voltage, the electric field that creates with a distanced substrate, and the substrate conditions. Without an adequate polymer flow rate, electrospinning processes cannot be maintained. At excess, high flow rate will produce much thicker or even beaded fibers [51], partially due to the rate of solvent evaporation being reduced and a greater influence of surface tension. One study constructively used the effect of fiber beading through optimizing polycaprolactone (PCL) concentration, the applied voltage, and working distance to produce "self-assembled" honeycomb patterns [36]. In addition to voltage and working distance, nozzle conditions can also affect solution flow rate. The size of the electrospinning nozzle directly influences the size of the initial polymer jet and the nozzle conductivity also has some influence over the overall solution conductivity. If the solution receives electric charge from inside the syringe, a conductive nozzle might encourage charge dissipation before spinning takes place, whereas if charge is imparted at the nozzle, the nozzle conductivity is the sole component which determines efficient charge transfer. Various works have innovated nozzle design to create core—shell and hollow fiber morphologies with the use of sacrificial materials [35] (Fig. 2.2h).

The application of voltage to polymer solution is the key distinguishing feature of electrospinning from any other fiber spinning techniques. By definition, potential difference between the source and the collecting substrate provides the threshold tensile force required to initiate fiber formation. The electrostatic forces that a droplet of polymer solution experiences during the intrinsic Taylor cone formation of electrospinning are twofold: the tensile Coulomb force in the direction of the collection substrate and the repulsive force due to surface charge accumulation. Once a polymer jet is initiated, the electrostatic forces stretch the jet up until the point of complete solvent evaporation or when the fiber is collected. Aside from the aforementioned solution properties, the magnitude of the electrostatic force is a function of the electric field strength. Both the applied voltage and the working distance between the suspended droplet and collecting substrate determine that magnitude. Increasing the applied voltage has a clear effect on the spun fiber diameter [52]; however, this relationship is complex and subject to the other parameters. One can argue that increasing the applied voltage directly increases the tensile force on the polymer jet, so the stretching effect would be greater. Alternatively, a high voltage might accelerate the jet toward the collector so that the fiber is in transit for less time and accordingly is less stretched [53]. Another explanation could be that high voltages enhance the flow rate of a solution leading to thicker fibers, as the strength is simply pulling more material through the syringe. To support that, there is a clear correlation that at excess applied voltage, beaded fibers begin forming and there is an increase in "whipping" behavior of the polymer jet [43,51].

Altering the working distance is another direct means to manipulate the electric field and influence fiber diameter. As the working distance between the Taylor cone apex and collecting substrate increases, the electric field intensity decays in a rapid and nonlinear way [54]. It also largely determines the time that the polymer jet remains in transit, which effects the extent of the bending instability and evaporation rate of the solvent. Traditionally, electrospinning processes utilize a working distance between 10 and 20 cm to permit thorough solvent evaporation and collection of dry fibers. To create a sufficient electric field for fiber initiation, the applied voltage often is in a range of 10–40 kV, and the consequent bending instability generates fibers in a random network. When the applied voltage is high and the working distance is comparatively short, this generates a very intense electric field and can induce electric arcing, highlighting the importance of selecting experimental parameters within an optimal threshold.

2.4 Advances and innovations in electrospinning for application-driven research

The factors mentioned in the previous sections may play different roles in different electrospinning systems. Thus, depending on ultimate applications anticipated for a product, the process parameters can be precisely adjusted by an operator to control the properties of the final products. Further, to impose a more precise control on final products morphology, geometries, and arrangement, the electrospinning processes have been modified through the following:

(a) Redesigning and improving the traditional setups based on a particular application (e.g., modifying nozzle and collecting substrate, controlling and directing fiber deposition, and stabilizing jet).

(b) Transition from far-field electrospinning to high-resolution near-field electrospinning (NFES) of controlled fiber deposition.
(c) Transition from the use of high voltage to low voltage for continuous electrospinning fiber patterning.
(d) Transition from electrospinning to high-resolution electrowriting.
(e) Combining electrospinning with other polymer processing technologies such as AM and microfluidic devices.

2.4.1 Redesigning the traditional electrospinning

As shown in Fig. 2.3, the improvement of traditional electrospinning has been mainly focused on dispensing nozzles and collecting substrates. Therefore, in addition to a traditional single nozzle [55–57], coaxial [58,59] and triaxial nozzles [60,61], multinozzle [62,63], and side-by-side/multichannel nozzles [64] have been successfully introduced for the fabrication of core/shell, triaxial, multichannel, Janus, beaded [25], bead-on-string [65], necklacelike [66], colloidal [67], bamboolike [68], and ribbon fibers [21]. Along with these modifications, needleless electrospinning via rotating disk [69] and bubble formation [70] techniques have been also introduced to achieve nanofibrous structures. The proposed modifications on collecting substrates include various rotating collectors (e.g., rotating drums and disks, wire drums) [71], water bath [72], and a dynamic liquid substrate for collecting nanofiber yarns [73]. (These modifications were thoroughly reviewed elsewhere [6]).

Alternatively, the sensitivity of the electrospinning jet to local substrate electric field profile can be advantageously used to guide fiber deposition in 2D and even 3D. These methods focus on the final stages of the fiber-drawing process, pulling the traveling jet away from the region of bending instability, and directing it to a specific target electrostatically [74]. For instance, collection electrodes and collection substrates with ridges and micropillars, parallel electrodes [75], dual collecting rings [76], adding nanomaterials triggered and guided by auxiliary fields (e.g., magnetic field) to the polymer solution, and patterned conductive substrates [77] or sharp edges or pins electrodes to ground an incoming jet [74,78–80] have been successfully utilized to create aligned fibers [81,82].

As the formation of free-standing fibrous structures has found many applications in biomedical fields, the two simple fabrication methods of such structures are presented in details. The simplest approach for the deposition of aligned fibers on a substrate or over a narrow gap was proposed by

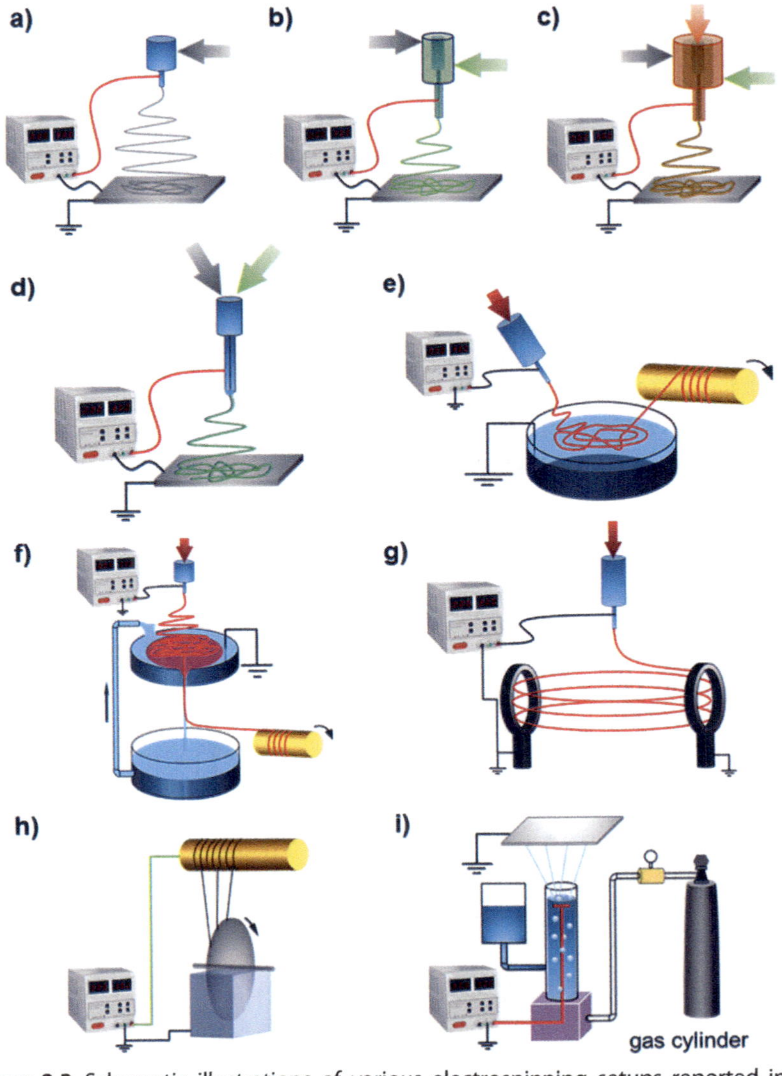

Figure 2.3 Schematic illustrations of various electrospinning setups reported in the literature: (a) traditional electrospinning setup, (b) coaxial electrospinning, (c) triaxial electrospinning, (d) multichannel electrospinning, (e) electrospinning via fiber collecting water bath, (f) a dynamic liquid substrate for collecting nanofiber yarns, (g) collecting aligned nanofiber using dual collections rings, (h) needleless disk electrospinning, and (i) needleless bubble electrospinning. *All schemes were redrawn with modifications.*

Xia et al. [83]. They changed the geometry of a grounded substrate from a flat surface into two conductors separated by a void gap (Fig. 2.4). Such a collector could be simply manufactured by placing two strips of electrical conductors such as highly doped silicon and metal bars together or by using two pieces of aluminum foil, where the gap could change up to several centimeters depending on the desired applications. In contrast to conventional electrospinning, in this configuration, the electric field lines are split into two fractions pointing toward the conductors at each side of the gap. This electrical field deviation imposes two sets of electric forces onto nanofibers and consequently aligns them uniaxially across the gap, where their longitudinal axes oriented perpendicular to collector edges. The stacking density of fibers deposited over a gap is proportional to the collection time and inversely depends on the gap width. The longer collection time and the narrower gap yield denser arrays. However, their results demonstrated

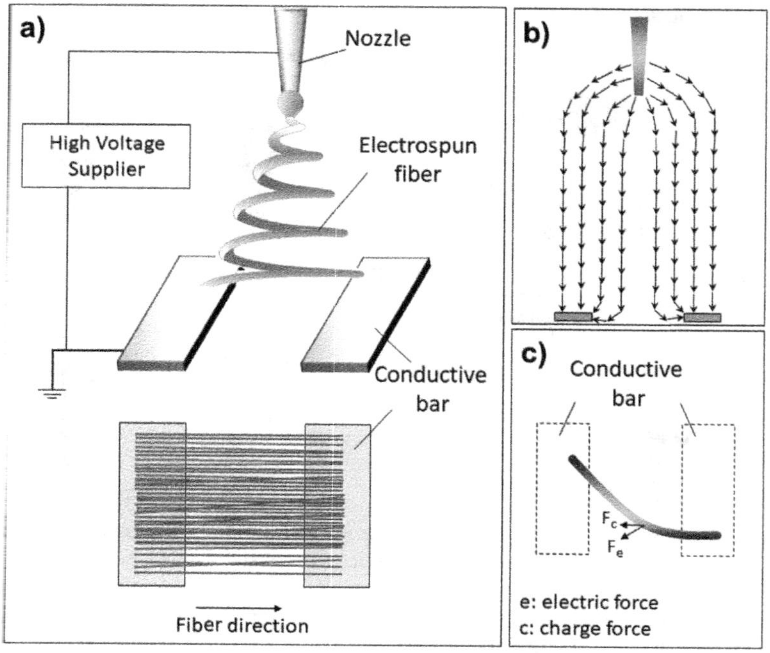

Figure 2.4 Schematic illustrations of the setup for electrospinning for generating uniaxially aligned nanofibers. (a) Modified setup configuration with the parallel conductive bars as collecting substrates. (b) Schematic illustration showing the distribution of static fields. (c) Schematic illustration showing the electric and charged forces exerting on the fiber jet.

that thinner fibers (diameter <150 nm) are quite unstable across a gap >1 cm, as the fibers cannot tolerate their own weight and electrostatic repulsion forces applied by other fibers. To deposit fibers across a wide gap beyond several micrometers, it was suggested to use a temporary and nongrounded substrate for supporting fibers. In addition to uniaxially aligning fibers, it would be also easy to fabricate a multilayer nanofiber structure by controlling the configuration of electrodes [9].

Another approach proposed for patterning aligned fibers is to directly manipulate the electrospinning process through incorporating stimuli-responsive materials such as magnetic nanoparticles to the solution and directing fiber orientation via applying an external stimulus (e.g., magnetic field) [84]. Therefore, magnetic electrospinning was reported as a facile and effective technique that could simply fabricate highly aligned fibers and multilayer lattices over a large area. The fiber meshes could also be easily transferred to other substrates or over microfluidic channels for more sophisticated applications. In this method, a small amount (>0.5 wt%) of magnetic nanoparticles was mixed with a polymer solution to magnetize it, and the solution is electrospun in the presence of a permanent magnetic field imposed by a pair of parallel-positioned permanent magnets. While both magnetic and electric fields can attract fibers to a collecting substrate, the magnetic field plays an essential role in aligning them over the gap between the two magnets (Fig. 2.5) [85,86].

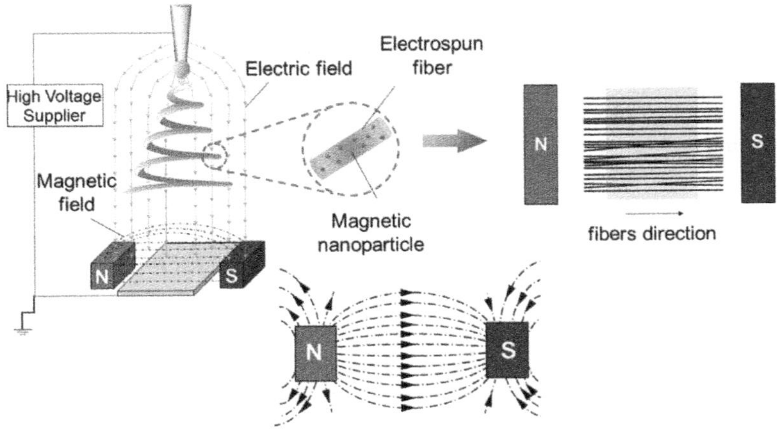

Figure 2.5 Schematic illustration of the setup used in the magnetic field–assisted electrospinning technique for fabricating aligned nanofibers.

Furthermore, to fabricate an electrospun fiber structure over a void gap with a curved geometry, researchers substituted solid collecting substrates with sacrificial conductive materials or an electrolyte [87]. The fluidic nature of the electrolyte provides flexibility in shaping the grounded collector and patterning according to the shape of a narrow channel. The ease of removing electrolytes after depositing fibers allows formation of a free-standing structure without conducting further mechanical or chemical peel-off processes for transferring fibers over the channel.

2.4.2 Transition from far-field to near-field electrospinning

High-resolution images of an electrospinning show that a polymer jet is made of three characteristic regions: a Taylor cone, proceeded by a stable straight region of around 10–30 mm, known as near-field region, before a bending instability takes effect [88] (Fig. 2.6).

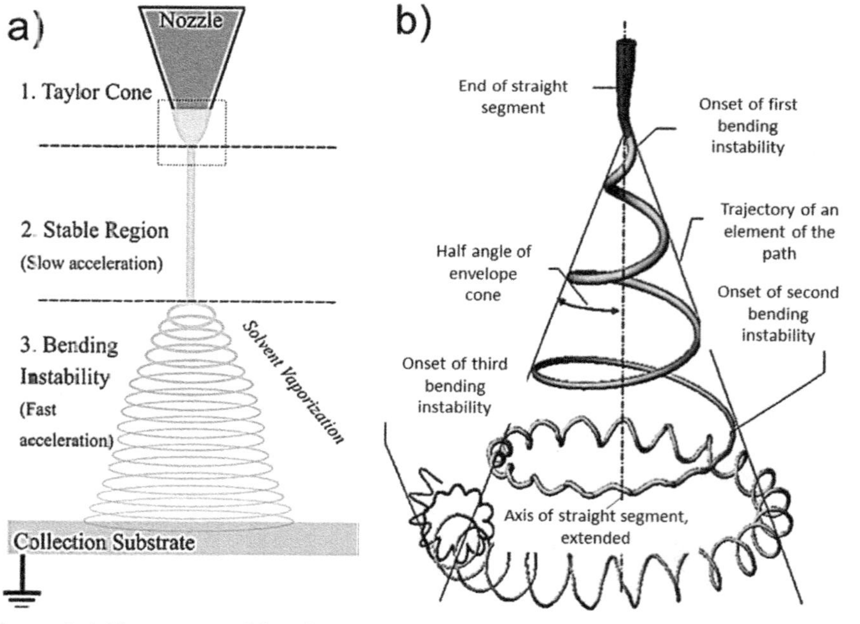

Figure 2.6 The region of bending instability characteristic of electrospinning techniques. (a) The point at which the bending instability establishes and its relation to jet stabilization strategies, (b) Solution jet path of traditional electrospinning. *Adapted from Reference Reneker, D.H., Yarin, A.L. (2008). Electrospinning jets and polymer nanofibers. Polymer 49(10), 2387–2425 under CC BY-NC-ND 3.0 license.*

In fact, the viscoelastic properties of the polymer jet should be able to overcome the Rayleigh instability which may break the jet into droplets [89,90], that is observed in electrospraying process [91–93]. As the polymer stream moves through the stable region, it creates a conductive path for the electric current to pass through. The velocity of the jet within this region was estimated to be ~1–15 m/s [94,95]. Therefore, the estimated critical length of the stable and straight jet can be calculated via Eq. (2.1):

$$L = \frac{4kQ^3}{\pi\rho^2 I^2}\left(\frac{1}{R_0^2} - \frac{1}{r_0^2}\right) \tag{2.1}$$

where $R_0 = (2\sigma Q/\pi k\rho E)^{1/3}$, σ is the surface tension, Q is the polymer solution flow rate, k is the electrical conductivity of the solution, ρ is the solution density, E is the electrical field strength, I is the current passing through the jet, and r_0 is the jet initial radius [96,97].

Based on the above information, the key to patterning electrospun fibers with greater precision is to dampen the influence of the chaotic jet bending instability on fibers. This can be achieved through redesigning the process around the stable region on the jet and preventing the bending instability from establishing in the first place. This is the central premise behind NFES [98], which reduces the distance between the Taylor cone and a collecting substrate to a millimeter scale as well as reducing the applied potential difference at the source by an order of magnitude. Thus, the overall electric field strength required for electrostatically driven fiber initiation is maintained. Adjusting these parameters enables direct writing of straight, coiled, or helical polymer fibers through matching the feed rate of solution with the translation speed of either the deposition substrate or the electrospinning spinneret itself. The ability to design the path of the translating component of NFES configurations allows drawing of complex 2D patterns in a versatile manner akin to 3D printing [99–101].

Omitting the region of bending instability does reduce the elongation effect on the polymer jet; thus, the fibers produced tend to be larger. Additionally, as the jet has a shorter travel distance, the solvent has less opportunity to evaporate and the fibers may still be wet immediately after patterning unless the solvent is volatile. In some cases, the wet fibers may adopt a semicircular cross section [102], as opposed to a rounded fiber or merge with neighboring fibers [38,103]. Another factor to consider is that the deposited fibers may retain some residual charge, which can act against achieving dense fiber alignment through repelling the incoming jet [104]. Use of coagulation baths as a collecting substrate is one strategy to avoid this issue while ensuring thorough removal of solvents [105].

2.4.3 Transition from high-voltage to low-voltage electrospinning

Another research direction developed using NFES to pattern fibers in 3D is to reduce the applied voltage further through initiating jet formation with high voltage to begin with before significantly lowering it [101] or the use of physical objects or "initiators" to draw out the polymer jet [99,106]. Here, both stabilized jet and substrate modification control and direct a patterning process. Bisht et al. developed a highly elastic polymer ink that can draw dry fibers spanning between micropatterned posts at voltages as low as 200V [99]. Recently, Huang et al. proposed a new technique in which a motorized XYZ-stage was integrated with NFES to fabricate and precisely position fibers over a gap of several millimeters [107–109]. To achieve this goal, they employed an initiator that facilitated the formation of the polymer jet under an applied voltage. Subsequently, fibers were drawn between the two initiators due to moving the nozzle between these initiators. A drawback of the proposed technique is the solvent evaporation from a predeposited solution that confines its application for patterning only across narrow gaps to lessen the adverse effect of solution drying [107–110].

Recent development in near-field techniques has further lowered the operating voltage to the range of 100V [108]. Low-voltage electrospinning patterning introduced by Huang's group utilizes both mechanical and electrical forces for fiber initiation process, in addition to the mechanical stretching of the fiber against a collection substrate (Fig. 2.7). The presence of the initiator can promote the onset of fiber jetting and enhance the fiber stretching and thinning process. When the initiator is close to the nozzle position, even at a voltage of around 100 V, the focusing of the electric field can locally reach ~2500 V/cm. As the substrate moves toward the center of the substrate, the electric field distribution becomes more symmetrical which allows fibers to be accurately deposited at a predetermined position. Lowering the applied voltage in electrostatic processing can minimize potential damages on bioactive components, provide greater flexibility and higher safety when combined with 3D printing mechanisms.

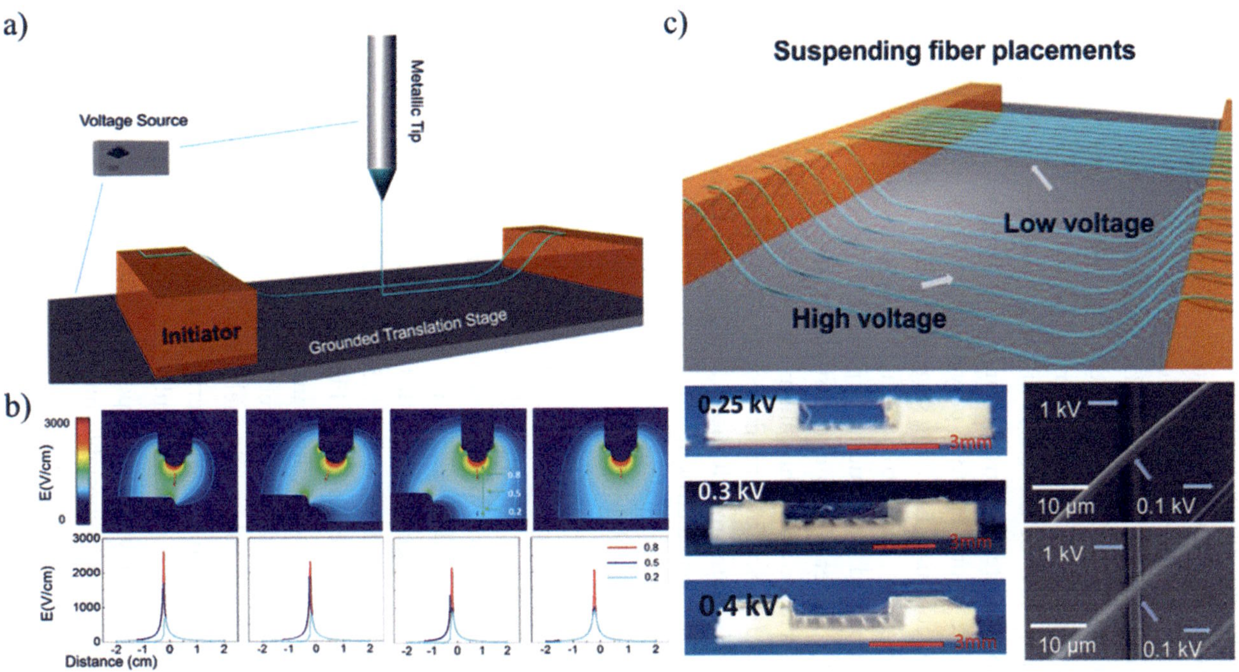

Figure 2.7 (a) Schematic illustration of figure low-voltage electrospinning setup; (b) Simulation of the electric field distribution with the moving of the initiator relative to the nozzle; (c) Schematic illustration of fiber deposition by adjusting the voltage application over a gap; (d) Fibrils bridging over a gap of 2 mm deep with a separation distance of 2.4–3.2 mm. Fibers were created using voltages of 0.25, 0.3, and 0.4 kV, respectively. SEM images show the effect of voltage on fiber deposition on the substrate (at 1 kV) and suspension (at 0.1 kV) over the gap. *Adapted from Reference Li, X., Li, Z., Wang, L., Ma, G., Meng, F., Pritchard, R.H., Gill, E.L., Liu, Y., Huang, Y.Y.S. (2016). Low-voltage continuous electrospinning patterning. ACS Appl. Mater. Interfaces 8(47), 32120–32131 under Creative Commons Attribution 4.0 International license-Open access.*

2.4.4 Transition from electrospinning to electrowriting

Scanning tip electrospinning, high-precision deposition electrospinning, and NFES are different direct writing solution electrospinning, in which an automated XYZ-stage is used as a collecting substrate [111]. The short collection distances between nozzles and substrates, together with moving stages presented in these techniques, yield a high relevance of fiber deposition in a predetermined fashion. However, the production rate in such techniques is extremely low of the order of 0.7 μg polymer per hour [112]. Researchers also reported electrospinning a PCL/dimethyl formamide/ methylene chloride solution into a polyethylene glycol (5 wt%) aqueous bath placed on an automated moving stage [113]. This technique produced fibrous structures with 205 ± 61 μm fiber diameter and rough surface morphology, compared to structures produced with fused deposition modeling (FDM). Lee et al. also demonstrated a new approach in which a cylindrical side electrode and a thin, sharp, and moving collector controlled fiber deposition [114]. Scaffolds produced via their method benefited from uniform fibers with submicron diameter and constant morphology.

Compared to solution electrospinning, melt electrospinning can produce fibers of several micrometers in diameter. Moreover, electrified jet in molten electrospinning does not exhibit dynamic motions observed in conventional electrospinning and reduces charge accumulation on deposited fibers, enabling more accurate stacking fibers. These advantages can be attributed to the lack of charge solvent and the higher viscosity of the fluid. In addition, the lack of chaotic motions in melt electrospinning significantly reduces complexities required for designing XYZ-stages, where straight fibers can be drawn for speeds ranging from ~8 to 20 mm/s compared to speeds (~50–150 mm/s) required in NFES [115]. Although melt electrospinning writing is the most similar technique to FDM, there are some important distinctions between these two methods including much smaller fiber diameter, lower pressure at the spinneret tip, and much larger distance between the nozzle and collector in melt electrospinning (Fig. 2.8).

The formation of a stable jet is a prerequisite for a controlled deposition of electrospun fibers on a stationary substrate. However, in the case of a moving platform, the formation and deposition of continuous and unbeaded fibers in a predictable and repeatable manner requires further adjustments and controls over key processing parameters including polymer flow rate in the nozzle, collector speed, electric field, while the viscosity and charge of the fluid define the properties of the molten polymer [117]. Polymer

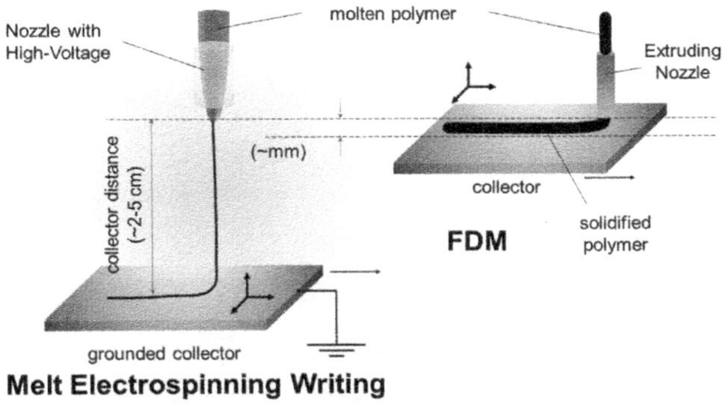

Figure 2.8 The distinctions between fused deposition modeling (FDM) and melt electrospinning writing. *Redrawn from Reference Dalton, P.D., Vaquette, C., Farrugia, B.L., Dargaville, T.R., Brown, T.D., Hutmacher, D.W. (2013). Electrospinning and additive manufacturing: converging technologies. Biomaterials Science 1(2), 171–185.*

melts with high viscosity and low conductivity are suitable for melt electrospinning writing applications to create 3D structures through controlled fiber patterning. Thus, all the parameters should be precisely and simultaneously tuned in order to fabricate highly ordered structures in laboratory scales and even in large scales.

For melt electrospinning writing (Fig. 2.9a), when polymer mass flows from the spinneret to the jet and then onto the collector are not adjusted, it may cause inconsistency and undesired sectional oscillation (known as "pulsing") of the fiber diameter or bead formation. Pulsing can affect the fiber deposition particularly when the moving stage changes the direction. In addition to the flow rate [120], accelerating voltage can cause pulsing effects and introduce artifacts into the printed construct due to the oscillation of jet flow rate. When the applied voltage is slightly lower than the optimized voltage at a fixed collector distance, the pulsing occurs as the forces which lead to jet stretching are not constant. This condition is even worse when the voltage is considerably lower and leads to the formation of long beads on fibers (Fig. 2.9b). Overall, to avoid these undesired process instabilities, the operator should limit the mass flow injected through the spinneret or stabilize the mass flow of the polymer jet via increasing the applied voltage which increases the electrical field strength [118].

To successfully deposit fibers on a moving substrate, the moving speed (S_c) should be higher than the ultimate jet speed (S_j), known as the critical translation speed, CTS. For a melt electrospinning writing setup operating well beyond CTS, the fiber can be stretched to obtain a submicron diameter size. On the other hand, for a transition speed below CTS, a jet buckling

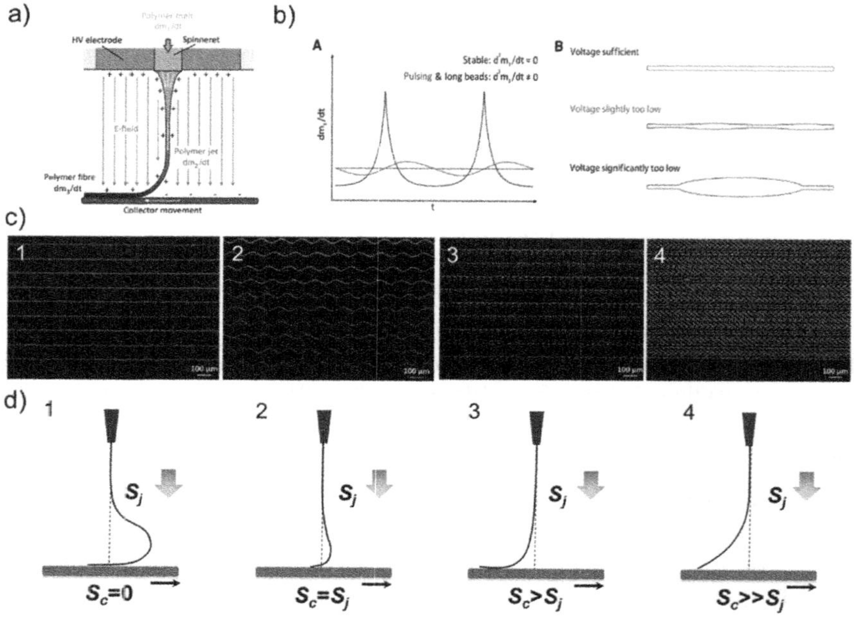

Figure 2.9 (a) The schematic illustration of melt electrospinning writing; (b) the effects of flow rate and voltage on the fiber geometry: (A) Mass flow rate deposited on the moving substrate (dm_3/dt) versus time. The dm_3/dt is proportional to the polymer flow rate of the jet. (B) The morphology of fibers collected on the moving substrate; (c) jet buckling and nonlinear patterns on the substrate. (d) Different scenarios for the relationship between jet speed (S_J) and collector speed (S_C). *Reproduced from Reference Gernot, H., Almoatazbellah, Y., Andrei, H., Jodie, N.H., Tomasz, J., Jürgen, G., Paul, D.D. (2016). Fibre pulsing during melt electrospinning writing. BioNanoMaterials 17(3–4), 159–171 under the Creative Commons CC BY-NC-ND 3.0 license; Redrawn from Reference Brown, T.D., Dalton, P.D., Hutmacher, D.W. (2011). Direct writing by way of melt electrospinning. Adv. Mater. 23(47), 5651–5657.*

occurs which yields a nonlinear pattern on the substrate. This may produce some of the typical shapes such as linear, sinusoidal, side loops, "figure of eight," and circular coiling [118,121], shown in Fig. 2.9c. Therefore, based on the relationship between collector speed and jet speed and the forces imposed on the jet stream, the jet profiles can be categorized into four different shapes, schematically illustrated in Fig. 2.9d. These shapes include the following:

- Case 1: When the collector speed is zero, $S_C = 0$, the jet vertically goes down and starts bending and forming a compressive heel near the collector due to buckling. This deforms the straight jet to a coil shape.

- Case 2: When the collector speed is equal to the jet speed ($S_C = S_J$), the compressive force decreases as the collector speed increases, which reduces the heel region and brings the point of deposition directly under the nozzle.
- Case 3: As the collector speed further increases ($S_C > S_J$), the contact point of the jet and the substrate moves behind that is the point vertically below the nozzle and causes a "lag" region due to a delay in responding to axial tensile force stretching the jet. The delay originates from the viscoelastic properties of the jet.
- Case 4. Upon increasing the collector speed, ($S_C >> S_J$), the lag region is extended, causing further stretching of the jet. However, this phenomenon causes undesirable effects on fibers geometry and location, and consequently affects the quality of final products.

Overall, as suggested by Hutmacher et al. [119], complex patterns and geometries can be produced via matching the translating speed of the collector to the jet speed.

2.4.5 Combining electrospinning with other polymer processing technologies

The combination of polymer processing techniques has also gained a great deal of attention in recent years, as these unique combinations can integrate the advantages of each method and overcome shortcomings observed for using an individual one. For instance, a combination of electrospinning and microfluidic devices could provide a unique opportunity for fabricating fiber meshes of different gradients where the concentrations of various functional agents (e.g., nanoparticles, biomolecules, therapeutic drugs) could be precisely controlled through a microfluidic chip [122]. The combination of AM and electrospinning can also be beneficial for precisely controlling fiber deposition and orientation, as well as pore sizes of scaffolds. Further discussion of such combined approaches have been provided in the following subsections.

2.4.5.1 Electrospinning and microfluidics

One of the major drawbacks of conventional electrospinning is the lack of ability to produce fibers matrices with desired gradients of different materials and physical and chemical signals. Common electrospinning techniques can only produce nanofibers with the same concentration, while matrices with various physicochemical properties are usually required for successfully mimicking tissue engineering constructs or drug delivery applications. To address this problem and to produce electrospun nanofibers containing gradients of compositions, biomolecules, active chemicals, and nanoparticles, researchers integrated a microfluidic technology with electrospinning [122]. This novel and flexible technique benefits from a Y-shaped microchannel with two inlets and one outlet, where the injection rates of the two different solutions were precisely controlled by a computer (Fig. 2.10). The outlet of the device was connected to a metal tube and subsequently to a thin conductive nozzle. Also, an XYZ-moving platform is used as a substrate to collect nanofibers with different concentrations within the spinning area. This approach enables the creation of matrices with spatially controlled gradients and enhanced functionalities suitable for studying spatial differentiation in mesenchymal stem cells or releasing therapeutic agents in a controlled and preprogrammed fashion.

The use of paper-based microfluidics devices has gained more attention in healthcare, food safety, environmental monitoring, and veterinary medicine [123,124] due to their low cost, simple and rapid fabrication process, compatibility with small volumes of sample, and ease of disposing by incineration with minor environmental consequences [125]. While most of paper-based devices are designed and fabricated in 2D, recently, 3D devices have been fabricated with more functions using paper materials through stacking 2D paper layers or paper origami [126–128]. However, these

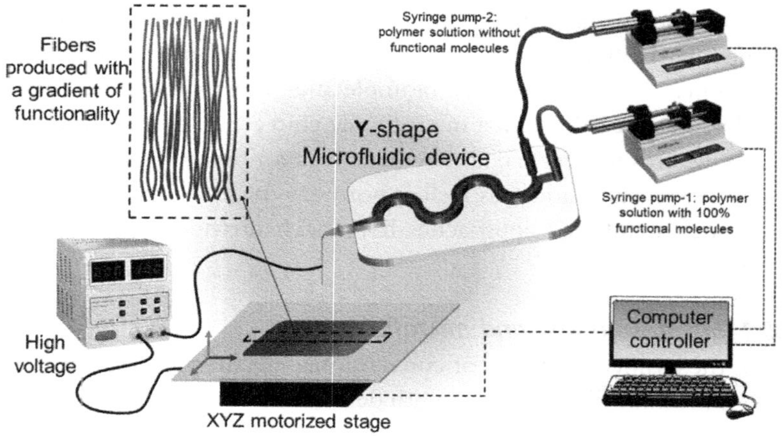

Figure 2.10 Schematic diagram of the platform used to produce nanofibers with different gradient. *Redrawn from Reference Zhang, X., Gao, X., Jiang, L., Qin, J. (2012). Flexible generation of gradient electrospinning nanofibers using a microfluidic assisted approach. Langmuir 28(26), 10026–10032.*

techniques are time consuming and labor-intensive, and the potential misalignment and discontinuity among paper layers and tape layers may affect device performance and confine the reproducibility of the process. Ref. [129] proposed a new technique in which a 3D nanofiber microfluidic device was fabricated using electrospinning and waxing processes controlled by a computer-guided trajectory (Fig. 2.11). The proposed technique could overcome the problems envisaged using old-fashioned methods.

Embedding micro-/nanofibrous structures into microfluidic chips can generate a complex microenvironment for cells for regulating phenotype expression in diagnosis [130], drug screening and discovery research, and tissue engineering applications [131,132]. While an electrospun polymer matrix simulates extracellular matrix for cells, an integrated microfluidic network provides a spatiotemporal liquid microenvironment through velocity and shear force imposed. The potential advantage of such devices was verified by investigating the alignment of neural stem cells in response to the orientation of 2D electrospun matrices versus microfluidic channels. This technique generated a controlled gradient of stromal cell—derived factor 1-alpha [133]. Liu et al. also fabricated a new device via embedding a patterned electrospun fibers into a polydimethylsiloxane (PDMS) microfluidic chip for hepatocyte culture [134]. Under optimized flow conditions, hepatocyte spheroids showed hepatocyte biliary and polarity excretion and

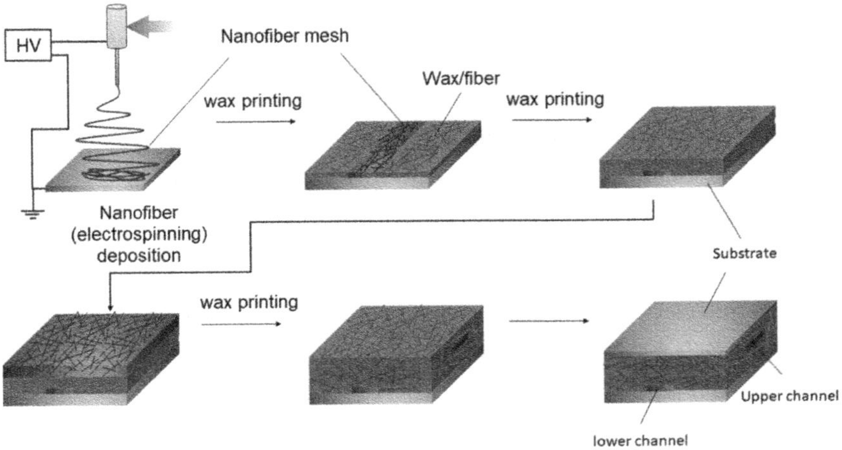

Figure 2.11 Multilayer construct with upper and lower flow channels: fabrication process includes electrospinning nanofibers and printing wax. *Redrawn from Ref. Chen, X., Mo, D., Gong, M. (2020). A flexible method for nanofiber-based 3d microfluidic device fabrication for water quality monitoring. Micromachines 11(3), 276.*

could preserve high levels of urea and albumin secretion for >15 days. The toxic effects of silver nanoparticles (AgNPs) were assessed using this organ-on-a-chip model, where the results indicated consistent and sensitive hepatotoxicity of AgNPs during the experiment.

Although culturing cells on electrospun fibers placed on a solid substrate, as described above, can provide valuable information about the cell attachment, proliferation, expansion, and differentiation, it is often desirable, particularly in biomedical and sensing domains, to utilize a free-standing fibrous micro-/nanostructures. Research findings have proved that a 3D cell culture coupled with online detection and analysis techniques can significantly improve our ability to mimic and understand in vivo systems [135]. Assembled over a channel gap, this novel architecture can provide a more realistic condition for investigating tissue—tissue interface, and for organ tissue engineering, such as liver and lung, where a biomimetic membrane will enable the transport of nutrients as well as wastes while mechanically supporting cells as porous and fibrous structure. However, due to the inherent nature of traditional electrospinning, fabrication of such microdevices still remains a challenge.

Compared to the techniques where fibers are directly generated over a void gap, the postmodifications of electrospun fibers through electromechanical processes [136,137] can be used for creating free-standing fibrous structures. In 2017, Hu et al. [138] introduced a universal, green, and straightforward strategy to produce micropatterned electrospun nanofibers. Their proposed approach utilized a solvent-loaded agarose hydrogel stamp for direct patterning of electrospun nanofibers on a substrate (Fig. 2.12). In general, this method involved the fabrication of an agarose hydrogel stamp by cast molding from a PDMS master. Then, agarose hydrogel stamp was submerged into a solvent—water mixture and subsequently placed over nanofiber meshes (randomly patterned or aligned nanofibers). As the organic solvent in the hydrogel stamp diffused to the nanofiber/stamp interface, it induced a localized coalescence of nanofibers and formed a thin membrane on the contacted zone. Finally, the patterned nanofibers were transferred onto a substrate for further processing. The substrate with patterned electrospun nanofibers was further utilized to spatially coordinate cell orientation in microfluidic devices. Using this technique, complex microstructures can be further fabricated via multistep alteration of microcontact patterning and electrospinning and used for several applications, particularly in biosensing, biomedical engineering, and lab-on-a-chip systems.

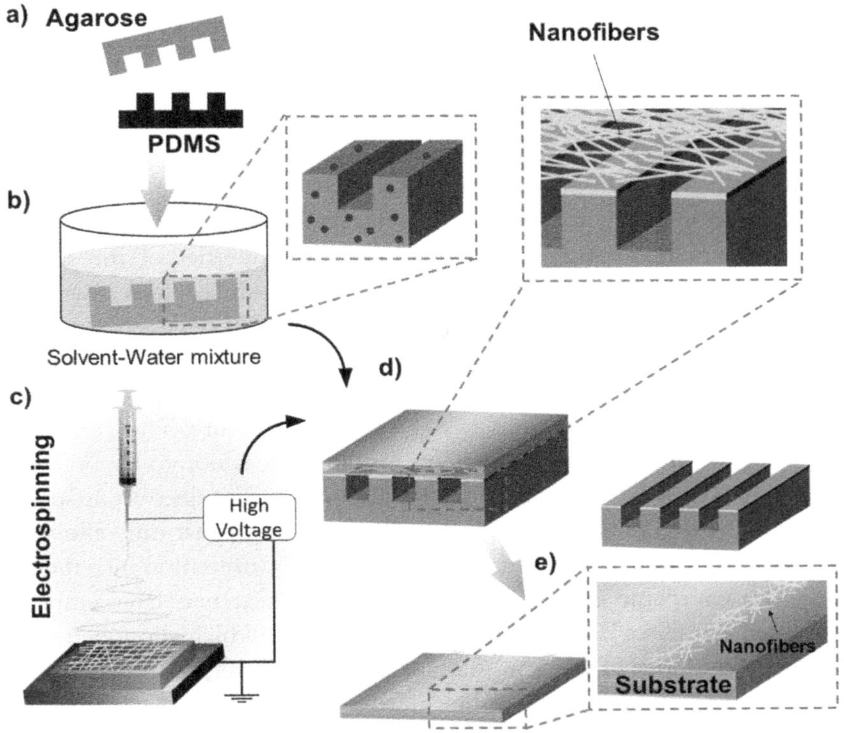

Figure 2.12 Patterning of electrospun nanofibers via solvent-loaded agarose hydrogel stamps. This process involves (a–b) fabrication of solvent-loaded agarose hydrogel, (c) electrospinning nanofibers, (d) contacting electrospun nanofibers with the hydrogel stamp, and (e) transferring nanofibers to a substrate. *Redrawn from Reference Hu, T., Li, Q., Dong, H., Xiao, W., Li, L., Cao, X. (2017). Patterning electrospun nanofibers via agarose hydrogel stamps to spatially coordinate cell orientation in microfluidic device. Small 13(3), 1602610.*

2.4.5.2 Electrospinning and additive manufacturing

A reliable and well-engineered scaffold plays a central role in tissue engineering and regenerative medicine. AM and electrospinning are two separate technologies extensively employed for manufacturing scaffolds in biomedical applications. However, a need to accurately control the pore size and spatial distribution of pores within scaffolds has motivated researchers to combine these two technologies to overcome deficiencies in each method. AM is abroad name for techniques in which an artificial construct is fabricated through layer-by-layer deposition of materials according to a computer-aided design. Although these techniques can precisely control pores and structure of scaffolds, they usually suffer from low filament resolution not suitable for tissue engineering. In contrast, solution electrospinning can generally produce fibers of different diameters.

As previously mentioned, electrospinning relies on a strong electric field imposed on a viscous fluid, including both polymer solutions and melts, to produce electrified jet passes through the air toward an oppositely charged collector. While electrospinning a polymer solution suffers from different levels of instability originating from inherent properties of the solution and surface charge density, melt electrospinning, which offers lower conductivity and higher viscosity, can produce fibers without such instabilities [139,140]. Further, the charge accumulated with the deposited fibers, especially in solution electrospinning, confines the number of layers which can be deposited and remain bound as one coherent structure. Thus, due to the size of fibers, the thickness of scaffolds produced does not go beyond a few millimeters [116,141]. In addition, typically, solution electrospun meshes have low porosity and form tightly packed structures that only allow cells to proliferate on the mesh surface and restrict cells infiltration into the scaffolds. To overcome some of these challenges, researchers have employed patterned substrates [142,143] or rotating mandrels which allow better prediction and control of the deposition of fibers. However, these processes still lack precisely controlled fiber depositions.

In 2008, researchers reported new fabrication methods via combining AM and electrospinning [144,145]. They fabricated bimodal scaffolds in which the main layers of the structure were formed via FDM, while electrospun fibers were deposited between each of those layers. These scaffolds exhibited large micropores for cells to infiltrate into as well as nanofibrous structures suitable for cell adhesion. Another study showed the advantages of combined electrospinning and FDM to produce tubular architectures for vascular tissue engineering. A more advanced technique has recently been introduced by Huang's group, where they reported the fabrication of intricate suspended fiber architectures. The individual fibers deposited by this technique approach the micrometer/submicrometer scale, while the ultimate height of suspended 3D fiber constructs can span over a centimeter (Fig. 2.13). They also showed an application of the fiber construct in 3D cell culture, where patterned fiber topography was utilized to guide the organization of suspended high-cellular density structures [107]. To further extend the application of 3D fiber constructs for standard biological

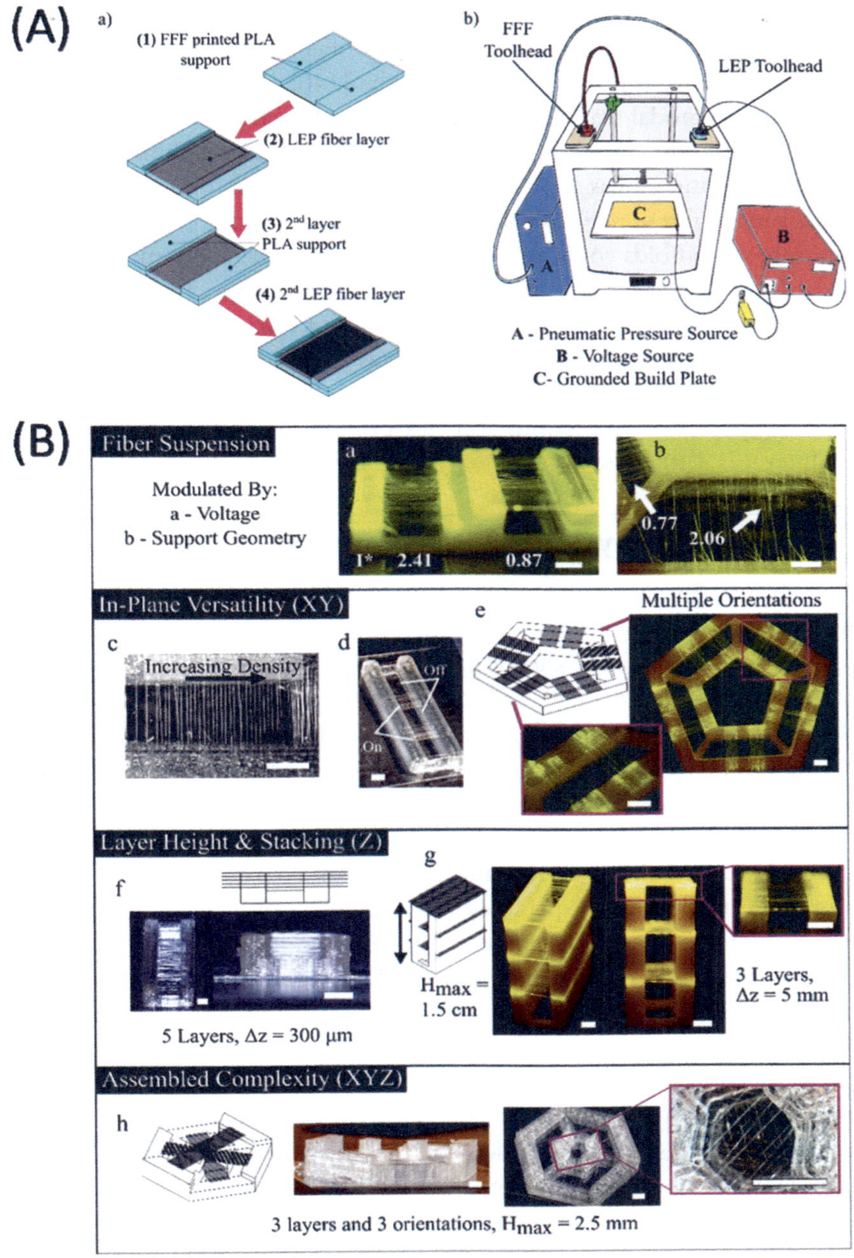

Figure 2.13 (a) Fabrication of bimodal 3D scaffolds via combining near-field electrospinning and additive manufacturing; (b) producing scaffolds of different geometries using the technique introduced in part (a). *Adapted from Reference Gill, E.L., Willis, S., Gerigk, M., Cohen, P., Zhang, D., Li, X., Huang, Y.Y.S. (2019). Fabrication of designable and suspended microfibers via low-voltage 3d micropatterning. ACS Appl. Mater. Interfaces 11(22), 19679–19690 under Creative Commons Attribution 4.0 International license-Open access.*

applications, 3D additive batch electrospinning has been developed to efficiently produce 3D hydrogel gelatin microfiber devices in a batch fashion with minimized sample-to-sample variance [146].

Besides bimodal scaffolds containing microfibrous and nanofibrous features distributed throughout the entire structure, the combination of AM and electrospinning has also been utilized to produce multiphasic constructs containing different regions with different pore size and porosity. Therefore, multiphasic scaffolds could produce adequate artificial tissue microenvironment for different cells to form a functional tissue unit. Hutmacher et al. [147] used this integrated technique to manufacture a multiphasic scaffold and to encapsulate biological agents such as proteins for promoting ectopic periodontal regeneration in rat models. Further details on the combinatorial approaches in electrospinning and 3D printing are covered separately in Chapter 12 of this book by Ameer et al. 2020.

2.5 Summary and future prospects

Electrospinning offers a myriad of design options for functional micro- and nanofiber production for a diverse range of applications. They can be adapted to process a large selection of polymers both of natural and synthetic origin. Other key advantages include that it processes materials in a highly efficient and throughput way. Fibers can be designed in a broad range of sizes [148], mesh porosities [149], and various fiber surface textures. Innovation in the experimental configurations can produce randomly organized fiber networks, highly ordered 2D patterns, and free-standing and stacked fibers. All these can be easily achieved through appropriate material selection, adjusting operating parameters, controlling ambient conditions, and redesigning collectors with particular geometries.

The integration of electrospinning with other manufacturing techniques such as microfluidics has led to enormous progress in tissue engineering and analytical devices for point-of-care diagnosis. It offers versatile advantages for the fabrication of multimaterial constructs with spatial gradients. These innovative and complex architectures could present applications as in vitro models for drug screening, toxicological studies, and cancer research. The combination of electrospinning and AM techniques could also bring a breakthrough for making well-designed constructs via accurately controlling fiber deposition in micro-/nanoscales. This novel combination can fill the need for bimodal and multiphasic scaffolds with systemic variations in morphology. While small-scale architectures are usually produced with solution electrospinning, these can also be produced via melt electrospinning combined with AM, which together provides higher resolution compared to FDM 3D printers.

Despite the existing achievements with electrospinning, the evolving end-use applications still demand new breakthroughs and improvements of this technique for improving material functionality and device integration. In particular, scaled-up productions for industry purposes and bench-to-bed customization for personalized equipment are of great interest, but yet to be fully addressed. Future developments of electrospinning and fiber production researches could be directed toward integrating with new materials and other advanced material processing and printing approaches.

References

[1] A.K. Yetisen, H. Qu, A. Manbachi, H. Butt, M.R. Dokmeci, J.P. Hinestroza, M. Skorobogatiy, A. Khademhosseini, S.H. Yun, Nanotechnology in textiles, ACS Nano. 10 (3) (2016) 3042–3068.
[2] C.R. Holkar, A.J. Jadhav, D.V. Pinjari, N.M. Mahamuni, A.B. Pandit, A critical review on textile wastewater treatments: possible approaches, J. Environ. Manag. 182 (2016) 351–366.
[3] S. Agarwal, J.H. Wendorff, A. Greiner, Use of electrospinning technique for biomedical applications, Polymer 49 (26) (2008) 5603–5621.
[4] J. Shi, S. Liu, L. Zhang, B. Yang, L. Shu, Y. Yang, M. Ren, Y. Wang, J. Chen, W. Chen, Y. Chai, X. Tao, Smart textile-integrated microelectronic systems for wearable applications, Adv. Mater. 32 (5) (2020) 1901958.
[5] N. Bhardwaj, S.C. Kundu, Electrospinning: a fascinating fiber fabrication technique, Biotechnol. Adv. 28 (3) (2010) 325–347.
[6] J. Xue, T. Wu, Y. Dai, Y. Xia, Electrospinning and electrospun nanofibers: methods, materials, and applications, Chem. Rev. 119 (8) (2019) 5298–5415.
[7] C.V. Boys, On the production, properties, and some suggested uses of the finest threads, Proc. Phys. Soc. Lond. 9 (1) (1887) 8–19.
[8] J. Doshi, D.H. Reneker, Electrospinning process and applications of electrospun fibers, J. Electrost. 35 (2) (1995) 151–160.
[9] D. Li, Y. Xia, Electrospinning of nanofibers: reinventing the wheel? Adv. Mater. 16 (14) (2004) 1151–1170.
[10] C. Chang, V.H. Tran, J. Wang, Y.-K. Fuh, L. Lin, Direct-write piezoelectric polymeric nanogenerator with high energy conversion efficiency, Nano. Lett. 10 (2) (2010) 726–731.
[11] W. Wang, P.N. Stipp, K. Ouaras, S. Fathi, Y.Y.S. Huang, Broad bandwidth, self-powered acoustic sensor created by dynamic near-field electrospinning of suspended, transparent piezoelectric nanofiber mesh, Small 16 (28) (2020) 2000581.
[12] Y. Huang, X. Bai, M. Zhou, S. Liao, Z. Yu, Y. Wang, H. Wu, Large-scale spinning of silver nanofibers as flexible and reliable conductors, Nano. Lett. 16 (9) (2016) 5846–5851.

[13] W. Wenyu, O. Karim, L.,R. Alexandra, L. Xia, G. Magda, N. Tobias, M. George, H. Yan Yan Shery, Inflight fluidic fibre printing towards array and 3d optoelectronic and sensing architectures, Sci. Adv. 6 (40) (2020) eaba0931.
[14] T.D. Brown, P.D. Dalton, D.W. Hutmacher, Melt electrospinning today: an opportune time for an emerging polymer process, Prog. Polym. Sci. 56 (2016) 116–166.
[15] R.T. Collins, J.J. Jones, M.T. Harris, O.A. Basaran, Electrohydrodynamic tip streaming and emission of charged drops from liquid cones, Nat. Phys. 4 (2) (2008) 149–154.
[16] D.H. Reneker, A.L. Yarin, Electrospinning jets and polymer nanofibers, Polymer 49 (10) (2008) 2387–2425.
[17] T. Subbiah, G.S. Bhat, R.W. Tock, S. Parameswaran, S.S. Ramkumar, Electrospinning of nanofibers, J. Appl. Polym. Sci. 96 (2) (2005) 557–569.
[18] C.J. Luo, S.D. Stoyanov, E. Stride, E. Pelan, M. Edirisinghe, Electrospinning versus fibre production methods: from specifics to technological convergence, Chem. Soc. Rev. 41 (13) (2012) 4708–4735.
[19] D.H. Reneker, A.L. Yarin, H. Fong, S. Koombhongse, Bending instability of electrically charged liquid jets of polymer solutions in electrospinning, J. Appl. Phys. 87 (9) (2000) 4531–4547.
[20] Z.-M. Huang, Y.Z. Zhang, M. Kotaki, S. Ramakrishna, A review on polymer nanofibers by electrospinning and their applications in nanocomposites, Compos. Sci. Technol. 63 (15) (2003) 2223–2253.
[21] S. Koombhongse, W. Liu, D.H. Reneker, Flat polymer ribbons and other shapes by electrospinning, J. Polym. Sci. B Polym. Phys. 39 (21) (2001) 2598–2606.
[22] G. Yang, X. Li, Y. He, J. Ma, G. Ni, S. Zhou, From nano to micro to macro: electrospun hierarchically structured polymeric fibers for biomedical applications, Prog. Polym. Sci. 81 (2018) 80–113.
[23] S. Chen, R. Li, X. Li, J. Xie, Electrospinning: an enabling nanotechnology platform for drug delivery and regenerative medicine, Adv. Drug Deliv. Rev. 132 (2018b) 188–213.
[24] C. Drew, X. Wang, L.A. Samuelson, J. Kumar, The effect of viscosity and filler on electrospun fiber morphology, J. Macromol. Sci., Part A 40 (12) (2003) 1415–1422.
[25] H. Fong, I. Chun, D.H. Reneker, Beaded nanofibers formed during electrospinning, Polymer 40 (16) (1999) 4585–4592.
[26] T. Jarusuwannapoom, W. Hongrojjanawiwat, S. Jitjaicham, L. Wannatong, M. Nithitanakul, C. Pattamaprom, P. Koombhongse, R. Rangkupan, P. Supaphol, Effect of solvents on electro-spinnability of polystyrene solutions and morphological appearance of resulting electrospun polystyrene fibers, Eur. Polym. J. 41 (3) (2005) 409–421.
[27] C.S. Ki, D.H. Baek, K.D. Gang, K.H. Lee, I.C. Um, Y.H. Park, Characterization of gelatin nanofiber prepared from gelatin–formic acid solution, Polymer 46 (14) (2005) 5094–5102.
[28] P. Gupta, C. Elkins, T.E. Long, G.L. Wilkes, Electrospinning of linear homopolymers of poly(methyl methacrylate): exploring relationships between fiber formation, viscosity, molecular weight and concentration in a good solvent, Polymer 46 (13) (2005) 4799–4810.
[29] C.L. Casper, J.S. Stephens, N.G. Tassi, D.B. Chase, J.F. Rabolt, Controlling surface morphology of electrospun polystyrene fibers: Effect of humidity and molecular weight in the electrospinning process, Macromolecules 37 (2) (2004) 573–578.
[30] G.C. Rutledge, S.V. Fridrikh, Formation of fibers by electrospinning, Adv. Drug Deliv. Rev. 59 (14) (2007) 1384–1391.

[31] H. Nie, A. He, J. Zheng, S. Xu, J. Li, C.C. Han, Effects of chain conformation and entanglement on the electrospinning of pure alginate, Biomacromolecules 9 (5) (2008) 1362–1365.
[32] S.L. Shenoy, W.D. Bates, H.L. Frisch, G.E. Wnek, Role of chain entanglements on fiber formation during electrospinning of polymer solutions: good solvent, non-specific polymer–polymer interaction limit, Polymer 46 (10) (2005) 3372–3384.
[33] J. Lin, B. Ding, J. Yu, Y. Hsieh, Direct fabrication of highly nanoporous polystyrene fibers via electrospinning, ACS Appl. Mater. Interface. 2 (2) (2010) 521–528.
[34] A. Omidinia-Anarkoli, R. Rimal, Y. Chandorkar, D.B. Gehlen, J.C. Rose, K. Rahimi, T. Haraszti, L. De Laporte, Solvent-induced nanotopographies of single microfibers regulate cell mechanotransduction, ACS Appl. Mater. Interface. 11 (8) (2019) 7671–7685.
[35] F.-L. Zhou, P.L. Hubbard, S.J. Eichhorn, G.J.M. Parker, Jet deposition in near-field electrospinning of patterned polycaprolactone and sugar-polycaprolactone core–shell fibres, Polymer 52 (16) (2011) 3603–3610.
[36] T. Yao, H. Chen, P. Samal, S. Giselbrecht, M.B. Baker, L. Moroni, Self-assembly of electrospun nanofibers into gradient honeycomb structures, Mater. Des. 168 (2019) 107614.
[37] X. Zong, K. Kim, D. Fang, S. Ran, B.S. Hsiao, B. Chu, Structure and process relationship of electrospun bioabsorbable nanofiber membranes, Polymer 43 (16) (2002) 4403–4412.
[38] R. Middleton, X. Li, J. Shepherd, Z. Li, W. Wang, S.M. Best, R.E. Cameron, Y.Y.S. Huang, Near-field electrospinning patterning polycaprolactone and polycaprolactone/collagen interconnected fiber membrane, Macromol. Mater. Eng. 303 (2) (2018) 1700463.
[39] M. Bognitzki, W. Czado, T. Frese, A. Schaper, M. Hellwig, M. Steinhart, A. Greiner, J.H. Wendorff, Nanostructured fibers via electrospinning, Adv. Mater. 13 (1) (2001) 70–72.
[40] Y. Hong, X. Chen, X. Jing, H. Fan, B. Guo, Z. Gu, X. Zhang, Preparation, bioactivity, and drug release of hierarchical nanoporous bioactive glass ultrathin fibers, Adv. Mater. 22 (6) (2010) 754–758.
[41] N. Amariei, L.R. Manea, A.P. Bertea, A. Bertea, A. Popa, The influence of polymer solution on the properties of electrospun 3d nanostructures, IOP Conf. Ser. Mater. Sci. Eng. 209 (2017) 012092.
[42] I.S. Chronakis, S. Grapenson, A. Jakob, Conductive polypyrrole nanofibers via electrospinning: electrical and morphological properties, Polymer 47 (5) (2006) 1597–1603.
[43] C. Mit-uppatham, M. Nithitanakul, P. Supaphol, Ultrafine electrospun polyamide-6 fibers: effect of solution conditions on morphology and average fiber diameter, Macromol. Chem. Phys. 205 (17) (2004) 2327–2338.
[44] M.M. Demir, I. Yilgor, E. Yilgor, B. Erman, Electrospinning of polyurethane fibers, Polymer 43 (11) (2002) 3303–3309.
[45] C. Huang, S. Chen, C. Lai, D.H. Reneker, H. Qiu, Y. Ye, H. Hou, Electrospun polymer nanofibres with small diameters, Nanotechnology 17 (6) (2006) 1558–1563.
[46] H. Chen, X. Huang, M. Zhang, F. Damanik, M.B. Baker, A. Leferink, H. Yuan, R. Truckenmüller, C. van Blitterswijk, L. Moroni, Tailoring surface nanoroughness of electrospun scaffolds for skeletal tissue engineering, Acta Biomater. 59 (2017a) 82–93.
[47] S. De Vrieze, T. Van Camp, A. Nelvig, B. Hagström, P. Westbroek, K. De Clerck, The effect of temperature and humidity on electrospinning, J. Mater. Sci. 44 (5) (2009) 1357–1362.

[48] J. Pelipenko, J. Kristl, B. Janković, S. Baumgartner, P. Kocbek, The impact of relative humidity during electrospinning on the morphology and mechanical properties of nanofibers, Int. J. Pharm. 456 (1) (2013) 125–134.
[49] C. Wang, H.-S. Chien, C.-H. Hsu, Y.-C. Wang, C.-T. Wang, H.-A. Lu, Electrospinning of polyacrylonitrile solutions at elevated temperatures, Macromolecules 40 (22) (2007) 7973–7983.
[50] P. Lu, Y. Xia, Maneuvering the internal porosity and surface morphology of electrospun polystyrene yarns by controlling the solvent and relative humidity, Langmuir 29 (23) (2013) 7070–7078.
[51] W. Zuo, M. Zhu, W. Yang, H. Yu, Y. Chen, Y. Zhang, Experimental study on relationship between jet instability and formation of beaded fibers during electrospinning, Polym. Eng. Sci. 45 (5) (2005) 704–709.
[52] C.J. Thompson, G.G. Chase, A.L. Yarin, D.H. Reneker, Effects of parameters on nanofiber diameter determined from electrospinning model, Polymer 48 (23) (2007) 6913–6922.
[53] C. Zhang, X. Yuan, L. Wu, Y. Han, J. Sheng, Study on morphology of electrospun poly(vinyl alcohol) mats, Eur. Polym. J. 41 (3) (2005) 423–432.
[54] J. Doshi, D.H. Reneker, Electrospinning Process and Applications of Electrospun Fibers, Conference Record of the 1993 IEEE Industry Applications Conference Twenty-Eighth IAS Annual Meeting, vol. 1693, 1993, pp. 1698–1703.
[55] S. Chen, S.K. Boda, S.K. Batra, X. Li, J. Xie, Emerging roles of electrospun nanofibers in cancer research, Advanced Healthcare Materials 7 (6) (2018a) 1701024.
[56] K. Ghaseminezhad, M. Zare, S. Lashkarara, M. Yousefzadeh, J. Aghazadeh Mohandesi, Fabrication of althea officinalis loaded electrospun nanofibrous scaffold for potential application of skin tissue engineering, J. Appl. Polym. Sci. 137 (16) (2020) 48587.
[57] Z. Tashi, M. Zare, N. Parvin, Application of phytic-acid as an in-situ crosslinking agent in electrospun gelatin-based scaffolds for skin tissue engineering, Mater. Lett. 264 (2020) 127275.
[58] I.G. Loscertales, A. Barrero, I. Guerrero, R. Cortijo, M. Marquez, A.M. Gañán-Calvo, Micro/nano encapsulation via electrified coaxial liquid jets, Science 295 (5560) (2002) 1695–1698.
[59] L. Xiaoyan, H. Tao, W. Yitao, C. Xiao, H. Yiyong, Y. Dengguang, Innovation Training-From Analogy to Deepen Comprehension and to Innovation with Modified Coaxial Electrospinning as an Example, 2018 2nd International Conference on Management, Education and Social Science (ICMESS 2018), Atlantis Press, 2018.
[60] D. Han, A.J. Steckl, Triaxial electrospun nanofiber membranes for controlled dual release of functional molecules, ACS Appl. Mater. Interfaces 5 (16) (2013) 8241–8245.
[61] A. Khalf, K. Singarapu, S.V. Madihally, Influence of solvent characteristics in triaxial electrospun fiber formation, React. Funct. Polym. 90 (2015) 36–46.
[62] J. Jiang, G. Zheng, X. Wang, W. Li, G. Kang, H. Chen, S. Guo, J. Liu, Arced multinozzle electrospinning spinneret for high-throughput production of nanofibers, Micromachines 11 (1) (2020) 27.
[63] G. Zheng, J. Jiang, D. Chen, J. Liu, Y. Liu, J. Zheng, X. Wang, W. Li, Multinozzle high efficiency electrospinning with the constraint of sheath gas, J. Appl. Polym. Sci. 136 (22) (2019) 47574.
[64] N. Wang, H. Chen, L. Lin, Y. Zhao, X. Cao, Y. Song, L. Jiang, Multicomponent phase change microfibers prepared by temperature control multifluidic electrospinning, Macromol. Rapid Commun. 31 (18) (2010) 1622–1627.

[65] X. Tian, H. Bai, Y. Zheng, L. Jiang, Bio-inspired heterostructured bead-on-string fibers that respond to environmental wetting, Adv. Funct. Mater. 21 (8) (2011) 1398–1402.
[66] Y. Jin, D. Yang, D. Kang, X. Jiang, Fabrication of necklace-like structures via electrospinning, Langmuir 26 (2) (2010) 1186–1190.
[67] W. Yuan, K.-Q. Zhang, Structural evolution of electrospun composite fibers from the blend of polyvinyl alcohol and polymer nanoparticles, Langmuir 28 (43) (2012) 15418–15424.
[68] Y. Sun, R.B. Sills, X. Hu, Z.W. Seh, X. Xiao, H. Xu, W. Luo, H. Jin, Y. Xin, T. Li, Z. Zhang, J. Zhou, W. Cai, Y. Huang, Y. Cui, A bamboo-inspired nanostructure design for flexible, foldable, and twistable energy storage devices, Nano. Lett. 15 (6) (2015) 3899–3906.
[69] H. Niu, T. Lin, X. Wang, Needleless electrospinning. I. A comparison of cylinder and disk nozzles, J. Appl. Polym. Sci. 114 (6) (2009) 3524–3530.
[70] R. Yang, J. He, L. Xu, J. Yu, Bubble-electrospinning for fabricating nanofibers, Polymer 50 (24) (2009) 5846–5850.
[71] A. Becker, H. Zernetsch, M. Mueller, B. Glasmacher, A novel coaxial nozzle for in-process adjustment of electrospun scaffolds' fiber diameter, Curr. Direct. Biomed. Eng. 1 (1) (2015) 104–107.
[72] E. Smit, U. Bűttner, R.D. Sanderson, Continuous yarns from electrospun fibers, Polymer 46 (8) (2005) 2419–2423.
[73] W.-E. Teo, R. Gopal, R. Ramaseshan, K. Fujihara, S. Ramakrishna, A dynamic liquid support system for continuous electrospun yarn fabrication, Polymer 48 (12) (2007) 3400–3405.
[74] R. Solberg, Position-controlled Deposition for Electrospinning, Department Mechanical Engineering, 2007.
[75] D. Li, Y. Wang, Y. Xia, Electrospinning nanofibers as uniaxially aligned arrays and layer-by-layer stacked films, Adv. Mater. 16 (4) (2004) 361–366.
[76] P.D. Dalton, D. Klee, M. Möller, Electrospinning with dual collection rings, Polymer 46 (3) (2005) 611–614.
[77] T.D. Brown, F. Edin, N. Detta, A.D. Skelton, D.W. Hutmacher, P.D. Dalton, Melt electrospinning of poly(ε-caprolactone) scaffolds: phenomenological observations associated with collection and direct writing, Mater. Sci. Eng. C 45 (2014) 698–708.
[78] B. Sundaray, V. Subramanian, T.S. Natarajan, R.-Z. Xiang, C.-C. Chang, W.-S. Fann, Electrospinning of continuous aligned polymer fibers, Appl. Phys. Lett. 84 (7) (2004) 1222–1224.
[79] W.E. Teo, M. Kotaki, X.M. Mo, S. Ramakrishna, Porous tubular structures with controlled fibre orientation using a modified electrospinning method, Nanotechnology 16 (6) (2005) 918–924.
[80] A. Theron, E. Zussman, A.L. Yarin, Electrostatic field-assisted alignment of electrospun nanofibres, Nanotechnology 12 (3) (2001) 384–390.
[81] S.A. Harfenist, S.D. Cambron, E.W. Nelson, S.M. Berry, A.W. Isham, M.M. Crain, K.M. Walsh, R.S. Keynton, R.W. Cohn, Direct drawing of suspended filamentary micro- and nanostructures from liquid polymers, Nano. Lett. 4 (10) (2004) 1931–1937.
[82] Y. Liu, G. Ma, D. Fang, J. Xu, H. Zhang, J. Nie, Effects of solution properties and electric field on the electrospinning of hyaluronic acid, Carbohydr. Polym. 83 (2) (2011) 1011–1015.
[83] D. Li, Y. Wang, Y. Xia, Electrospinning of polymeric and ceramic nanofibers as uniaxially aligned arrays, Nano. Lett. 3 (8) (2003) 1167–1171.

[84] X. Chen, L. Cheng, H. Li, A. Barhoum, Y. Zhang, X. He, W. Yang, M.M. Bubakir, H. Chen, Magnetic nanofibers: unique properties, fabrication techniques, and emerging applications, Chemistry 3 (31) (2018c) 9127–9143.
[85] Y. Liu, X. Zhang, Y. Xia, H. Yang, Magnetic-field-assisted electrospinning of aligned straight and wavy polymeric nanofibers, Adv. Mater. 22 (22) (2010) 2454–2457.
[86] D. Yang, B. Lu, Y. Zhao, X. Jiang, Fabrication of aligned fibrous arrays by magnetic electrospinning, Adv. Mater. 19 (21) (2007) 3702–3706.
[87] S.M. Park, S. Eom, W. Kim, D.S. Kim, Role of grounded liquid collectors in precise patterning of electrospun nanofiber mats, Langmuir 34 (1) (2018) 284–290.
[88] Y. Xin, D.H. Reneker, Hierarchical polystyrene patterns produced by electrospinning, Polymer 53 (19) (2012) 4254–4261.
[89] D. Duft, T. Achtzehn, R. Müller, B.A. Huber, T. Leisner, Rayleigh jets from levitated microdroplets, Nature 421 (6919) (2003), 128-128.
[90] D.H. Reneker, H. Fong, Polymeric Nanofibers, ACS Publications, 2006.
[91] L.K. Lim, J. Hua, C.-H. Wang, K.A. Smith, Numerical simulation of cone-jet formation in electrohydrodynamic atomization, AIChE J. 57 (1) (2011) 57–78.
[92] J. Xie, J. Jiang, P. Davoodi, M.P. Srinivasan, C.-H. Wang, Electrohydrodynamic atomization: a two-decade effort to produce and process micro-/nanoparticulate materials, Chem. Eng. Sci. 125 (2015) 32–57.
[93] W.-C. Yan, P. Davoodi, Y.W. Tong, C.-H. Wang, Computational study of core-shell droplet formation in coaxial electrohydrodynamic atomization process, AICHE J. 62 (12) (2016) 4259–4276.
[94] M.E. Helgeson, K.N. Grammatikos, J.M. Deitzel, N.J. Wagner, Theory and kinematic measurements of the mechanics of stable electrospun polymer jets, Polymer 49 (12) (2008) 2924–2936.
[95] D.H. Reneker, W. Kataphinan, A. Theron, E. Zussman, A.L. Yarin, Nanofiber garlands of polycaprolactone by electrospinning, Polymer 43 (25) (2002) 6785–6794.
[96] A.M. Gañán-Calvo, Cone-jet analytical extension of taylor's electrostatic solution and the asymptotic universal scaling laws in electrospraying, Phys. Rev. Lett. 79 (2) (1997) 217–220.
[97] J.-H. He, Y. Wu, W.-W. Zuo, Critical length of straight jet in electrospinning, Polymer 46 (26) (2005) 12637–12640.
[98] D. Sun, C. Chang, S. Li, L. Lin, Near-field electrospinning, Nano. Lett. 6 (4) (2006) 839–842.
[99] G.S. Bisht, G. Canton, A. Mirsepassi, L. Kulinsky, S. Oh, D. Dunn-Rankin, M.J. Madou, Controlled continuous patterning of polymeric nanofibers on three-dimensional substrates using low-voltage near-field electrospinning, Nano. Lett. 11 (4) (2011) 1831–1837.
[100] H. Chen, A.d.B.F.B. Malheiro, C. van Blitterswijk, C. Mota, P.A. Wieringa, L. Moroni, Direct writing electrospinning of scaffolds with multidimensional fiber architecture for hierarchical tissue engineering, ACS Appl. Mater. Interfaces 9 (44) (2017b) 38187–38200.
[101] Y. Huang, Y. Duan, Y. Ding, N. Bu, Y. Pan, N. Lu, Z. Yin, Versatile, kinetically controlled, high precision electrohydrodynamic writing of micro/nanofibers, Sci. Rep. 4 (1) (2014) 5949.
[102] N. Xue, X. Li, C. Bertulli, Z. Li, A. Patharagulpong, A. Sadok, Y.Y.S. Huang, Rapid patterning of 1-d collagenous topography as an ecm protein fibril platform for image cytometry, PloS One 9 (4) (2014) e93590.
[103] Y.M. Shin, M.M. Hohman, M.P. Brenner, G.C. Rutledge, Experimental characterization of electrospinning: the electrically forced jet and instabilities, Polymer 42 (25) (2001) 09955–09967.

[104] G. Zheng, W. Li, X. Wang, D. Wu, D. Sun, L. Lin, Precision deposition of a nanofibre by near-field electrospinning, J. Phys. Appl. Phys. 43 (41) (2010) 415501.
[105] L. Kong, G.R. Ziegler, Rheological aspects in fabricating pullulan fibers by electro-wet-spinning, Food Hydrocolloids 38 (2014) 220—226.
[106] R. Chang, J. Nam, W. Sun, Effects of dispensing pressure and nozzle diameter on cell survival from solid freeform fabrication—based direct cell writing, Tissue Eng. 14 (1) (2008) 41—48.
[107] E.L. Gill, S. Willis, M. Gerigk, P. Cohen, D. Zhang, X. Li, Y.Y.S. Huang, Fabrication of designable and suspended microfibers via low-voltage 3d micropatterning, ACS Appl. Mater. Interface. 11 (22) (2019) 19679—19690.
[108] X. Li, Z. Li, L. Wang, G. Ma, F. Meng, R.H. Pritchard, E.L. Gill, Y. Liu, Y.Y.S. Huang, Low-voltage continuous electrospinning patterning, ACS Appl. Mater. Interface. 8 (47) (2016) 32120—32131.
[109] Z. Li, I.M. Lei, P. Davoodi, L. Huleihel, Y.Y.S. Huang, Solution formulation and rheology for fabricating extracellular matrix-derived fibers using low-voltage electrospinning patterning, ACS Biomater. Sci. Eng. 5 (7) (2019) 3676—3684.
[110] Z. Li, J. Tuffin, I.M. Lei, F.S. Ruggeri, N.S. Lewis, E.L. Gill, T. Savin, L. Huleihel, S.F. Badylak, T. Knowles, S.C. Satchell, G.I. Welsh, M.A. Saleem, Y.Y.S. Huang, Solution fibre spinning technique for the fabrication of tuneable decellularised matrix-laden fibres and fibrous micromembranes, Acta Biomater. 78 (2018) 111—122.
[111] J.A. Lewis, Direct ink writing of 3d functional materials, Adv. Funct. Mater. 16 (17) (2006) 2193—2204.
[112] C. Hellmann, J. Belardi, R. Dersch, A. Greiner, J.H. Wendorff, S. Bahnmueller, High precision deposition electrospinning of nanofibers and nanofiber nonwovens, Polymer 50 (5) (2009) 1197—1205.
[113] S.H. Ahn, H.J. Lee, G.H. Kim, Polycaprolactone scaffolds fabricated with an advanced electrohydrodynamic direct-printing method for bone tissue regeneration, Biomacromolecules 12 (12) (2011) 4256—4263.
[114] J. Lee, S.Y. Lee, J. Jang, Y.H. Jeong, D.-W. Cho, Fabrication of patterned nanofibrous mats using direct-write electrospinning, Langmuir 28 (18) (2012) 7267—7275.
[115] E. Zhmayev, D. Cho, Y. Lak Joo, Electrohydrodynamic quenching in polymer melt electrospinning, Phys. Fluid. 23 (7) (2011) 073102.
[116] P.D. Dalton, C. Vaquette, B.L. Farrugia, T.R. Dargaville, T.D. Brown, D.W. Hutmacher, Electrospinning and additive manufacturing: converging technologies, Biomaterial. Sci. 1 (2) (2013) 171—185.
[117] C.B. Dayan, F. Afghah, B.S. Okan, M. Yıldız, Y. Menceloglu, M. Culha, B. Koc, Modeling 3d melt electrospinning writing by response surface methodology, Mater. Des. 148 (2018) 87—95.
[118] H. Gernot, Y. Almoatazbellah, H. Andrei, N.H. Jodie, J. Tomasz, G. Jürgen, D.D. Paul, Fibre pulsing during melt electrospinning writing, BioNanoMaterials 17 (3—4) (2016) 159—171.
[119] T.D. Brown, P.D. Dalton, D.W. Hutmacher, Direct writing by way of melt electrospinning, Adv. Mater. 23 (47) (2011) 5651—5657.
[120] F.M. Au - Wunner, O. Au - Bas, N.T. Au - Saidy, P.D. Au - Dalton, E.M.D.-J. Au - Pardo, D.W. Au - Hutmacher, Melt electrospinning writing of three-dimensional poly(ε-caprolactone) scaffolds with controllable morphologies for tissue engineering applications, JoVE 130 (2017) e56289.
[121] T. Jungst, M.L. Muerza-Cascante, T.D. Brown, M. Standfest, D.W. Hutmacher, J. Groll, P.D. Dalton, Melt electrospinning onto cylinders: effects of rotational velocity and collector diameter on morphology of tubular structures, Polym. Int. 64 (9) (2015) 1086—1095.

[122] X. Zhang, X. Gao, L. Jiang, J. Qin, Flexible generation of gradient electrospinning nanofibers using a microfluidic assisted approach, Langmuir 28 (26) (2012) 10026–10032.
[123] H.N. Chan, Y. Shu, B. Xiong, Y. Chen, Y. Chen, Q. Tian, S.A. Michael, B. Shen, H. Wu, Simple, cost-effective 3d printed microfluidic components for disposable, point-of-care colorimetric analysis, ACS Sens. 1 (3) (2016) 227–234.
[124] A.K. Yetisen, M.S. Akram, C.R. Lowe, Paper-based microfluidic point-of-care diagnostic devices, Lab Chip 13 (12) (2013) 2210–2251.
[125] Y. Zhang, L. Zhang, K. Cui, S. Ge, X. Cheng, M. Yan, J. Yu, H. Liu, Flexible electronics based on micro/nanostructured paper, Adv. Mater. 30 (51) (2018) 1801588.
[126] L. Ge, S. Wang, X. Song, S. Ge, J. Yu, 3d origami-based multifunction-integrated immunodevice: low-cost and multiplexed sandwich chemiluminescence immunoassay on microfluidic paper-based analytical device, Lab Chip 12 (17) (2012) 3150–3158.
[127] A.W. Martinez, S.T. Phillips, G.M. Whitesides, Three-dimensional microfluidic devices fabricated in layered paper and tape, Proc. Natl. Acad. Sci. U. S. A. 105 (50) (2008) 19606–19611.
[128] J. Reboud, G. Xu, A. Garrett, M. Adriko, Z. Yang, E.M. Tukahebwa, C. Rowell, J.M. Cooper, Paper-based microfluidics for DNA diagnostics of malaria in low resource underserved rural communities, Proc. Natl. Acad. Sci. U. S. A. 116 (11) (2019) 4834–4842.
[129] X. Chen, D. Mo, M. Gong, A flexible method for nanofiber-based 3d microfluidic device fabrication for water quality monitoring, Micromachines 11 (3) (2020) 276.
[130] Z. Rezaei, M. Mahmoudifard, Pivotal role of electrospun nanofibers in microfluidic diagnostic systems – a review, J. Mater. Chem. B 7 (30) (2019) 4602–4619.
[131] Z. He, N. Ranganathan, P. Li, Evaluating nanomedicine with microfluidics, Nanotechnology 29 (49) (2018) 492001.
[132] Y. Liu, K. Hu, Y. Wang, Primary hepatocytes cultured on a fiber-embedded pdms chip to study drug metabolism, Polymers 9 (6) (2017) 215.
[133] P. Wallin, C. Zandén, B. Carlberg, N. Hellström Erkenstam, J. Liu, J. Gold, A method to integrate patterned electrospun fibers with microfluidic systems to generate complex microenvironments for cell culture applications, Biomicrofluidics 6 (2) (2012) 024131.
[134] Y. Liu, S. Wang, Y. Wang, Patterned fibers embedded microfluidic chips based on pla and pdms for ag nanoparticle safety testing, Polymers 8 (11) (2016) 402.
[135] A.D. Castiaux, D.M. Spence, R.S. Martin, Review of 3d cell culture with analysis in microfluidic systems, Analyt. Method. 11 (33) (2019) 4220–4232.
[136] B. Carlberg, T. Wang, J. Liu, Direct photolithographic patterning of electrospun films for defined nanofibrillar microarchitectures, Langmuir 26 (4) (2010) 2235–2239.
[137] Y. Liu, L. Zhang, H. Li, S. Yan, J. Yu, J. Weng, X. Li, Electrospun fibrous mats on lithographically micropatterned collectors to control cellular behaviors, Langmuir 28 (49) (2012) 17134–17142.
[138] T. Hu, Q. Li, H. Dong, W. Xiao, L. Li, X. Cao, Patterning electrospun nanofibers via agarose hydrogel stamps to spatially coordinate cell orientation in microfluidic device, Small 13 (3) (2017) 1602610.
[139] P.D. Dalton, D. Grafahrend, K. Klinkhammer, D. Klee, M. Möller, Electrospinning of polymer melts: phenomenological observations, Polymer 48 (23) (2007) 6823–6833.
[140] H. Zhou, T.B. Green, Y.L. Joo, The thermal effects on electrospinning of polylactic acid melts, Polymer 47 (21) (2006) 7497–7505.
[141] C. Vaquette, J. Cooper-White, The use of an electrostatic lens to enhance the efficiency of the electrospinning process, Cell Tissue Res. 347 (3) (2012) 815–826.

[142] C. Vaquette, J.J. Cooper-White, Increasing electrospun scaffold pore size with tailored collectors for improved cell penetration, Acta Biomater. 7 (6) (2011) 2544–2557.

[143] D. Zhang, J. Chang, Patterning of electrospun fibers using electroconductive templates, Adv. Mater. 19 (21) (2007) 3664–3667.

[144] G. Kim, J. Son, S. Park, W. Kim, Hybrid process for fabricating 3d hierarchical scaffolds combining rapid prototyping and electrospinning, Macromol. Rapid Commun. 29 (19) (2008) 1577–1581.

[145] S.H. Park, T.G. Kim, H.C. Kim, D.-Y. Yang, T.G. Park, Development of dual scale scaffolds via direct polymer melt deposition and electrospinning for applications in tissue regeneration, Acta Biomater. 4 (5) (2008) 1198–1207.

[146] E.L. Gill, W. Wang, R. Liu, Y.Y.S. Huang, Additive batch electrospinning patterning of tethered gelatin hydrogel fibres with swelling-induced fibre curling, Addit. Manufact. 36 (2020) 101456.

[147] C. Vaquette, W. Fan, Y. Xiao, S. Hamlet, D.W. Hutmacher, S. Ivanovski, A biphasic scaffold design combined with cell sheet technology for simultaneous regeneration of alveolar bone/periodontal ligament complex, Biomaterial. 33 (22) (2012) 5560–5573.

[148] Z. Wang, Y. Cui, J. Wang, X. Yang, Y. Wu, K. Wang, X. Gao, D. Li, Y. Li, X.-L. Zheng, Y. Zhu, D. Kong, Q. Zhao, The effect of thick fibers and large pores of electrospun poly(ε-caprolactone) vascular grafts on macrophage polarization and arterial regeneration, Biomaterials 35 (22) (2014) 5700–5710.

[149] A. Hrynevich, B.Ş. Elçi, J.N. Haigh, R. McMaster, A. Youssef, C. Blum, T. Blunk, G. Hochleitner, J. Groll, P.D. Dalton, Dimension-based design of melt electrowritten scaffolds, Small 14 (22) (2018) 1800232.

CHAPTER THREE

Electrospun materials as scaffolds in tissue engineering and regenerative medicine

Aakriti Aggarwal, Mahesh Kumar Sah
Department of Biotechnology, Dr. B. R. Ambedkar National Institute of Technology, Jalandhar, Punjab, India

Abbreviations

ECM Extracellular matrix
ES Electrospinning
FAP Fluorohydroxyapatite
HAP Hydroxyapatite
MSCs Mesenchymal stem cells
PHB Polyhydroxybutarate
PLA Poly(lactic acid)

3.1 Introduction

Tissue and organ failure can occur from trauma, injury, systemic disorders, infection, or other conditions. According to a recent report by the World Health Organization, organ failure leads to about a million deaths in the United States alone, while the statistics are much larger on the global front. Global Observatory of Donation and Transplantation statistics estimates 126,670 organ transplants annually [1]. Lack of organ availability and the need to meet increased organ demand have led to the employment of other treatment options like surgical repair and chemotherapy, besides transplantation. However, none of these can fully recover the structure and functionality of major organ/damaged tissue. Tissue engineering has emerged as an alternative and promising technique to overcome the drawbacks of transplantation in medical practice. Therefore, using tissue-engineered transplants would deal with most of the limitations of direct transplantation and avoid conditions of rejection and disease transmission in addition to the need of donors. The field of tissue engineering aims to develop complex 3D tissue composite systems that mimic the morphology,

Biomedical Applications of Electrospinning and Electrospraying
ISBN: 978-0-12-822476-2
https://doi.org/10.1016/B978-0-12-822476-2.00005-4

architecture, and microenvironments of the target tissue. These constructs are designed to restore, replace, or improve function of body organs [2]. The basis of tissue engineering lies in populating the scaffold with the cells and the regulatory factors. The scaffolds provide structural integrity to the growing cells; which in turn populate the scaffold and secrete the components of the extracellular matrix (ECM)—the natural environment of the cells. The regulatory or signaling molecules help to induce several mechanisms, such as cell adhesion, proliferation, antigen presentation, and activation of explicit pathways, necessary for appropriate tissue development [3,4].

The utility of scaffolds that have been developed from a wide range of natural and synthetic polymers is a key challenge for successful implementation in tissue engineering [5,6]. Natural polymers are advantageous in terms of hydrophilicity, bioactivity, and structural similarity with ECM [6]. Variations arising in their isolation from biological sources and inefficient mechanical properties [7] are the bottlenecks for their wide-scale use. The synthetic polymers overcome the above-mentioned drawbacks by showing high levels of fiber reproducibility and mechanical strength [4]. They are, however, limited due to the acidic nature of their by-products and a difficult attachment with different biological moieties [7]. Apart from the composition of the scaffold, its architecture also plays a key role in its functionality. Hierarchical micro- and nanoscale morphologies provide significant mechanical strength, and porous 3D structures enhance cell adhesion, infiltration (penetration of cells deep within the scaffolds), cell migration, and vascularization (formation of blood vessels to meet nutritional needs of the growing cells) [2,8]. A proper balance between its mechanical function and transport of regulatory molecules is essential for creating an appropriate anatomical tissue [8]. Most of the conventional strategies [2] for scaffold fabrication like *porogen extraction* [9], *freeze-drying* [10], *phase separation* [11], *foaming* [12], *sintering* [13], *etc.*, can form highly interconnected and porous scaffolds. However, the techniques suffer from inherent limitations and also face difficulties in tailoring and reproducing different scaffold properties [14]. An attractive method, electrospinning, was reintroduced after Reneker et al. demonstrated the synthesis of nanoscale polymeric fibers using this technique Since its first biomedical application (elastomeric vascular prosthesis, from polyurethane elastomer) in 1978 by Annis et al. [3], this technique has gained considerable interest, for it serves as a potential candidate for synthesizing nonwoven fibers with dimensions similar to that of fibers of the ECM [15]. It uses electrostatic forces to produce a versatile range of polymeric fibers, which can then be processed to form scaffolds for tissue engineering. The polymeric fibers can be customized, depending on the type of tissue to be regenerated in its scaffold. The fibers' geometry can be changed by altering the electrospinning process parameters viz. electric field applied, the flow rate of solution, the needle and collector interspace, metallic needle diameter, and speed of the collector drum; and solution characteristics (concentration, viscosity, and conductivity) [16,17,18,19]. Usually, the electrospun fibrous scaffolds consist of randomly arranged fibers. Such scaffolds fare well for bone and skin tissue repair as they are consistent with their natural microstructure [20]. However, for the regeneration of tissues of heart, nerves, etc., the electrospun fibers need to replicate certain particular alignments for guiding effective cell growth and function. The work by Gnavi et al. affirmed that fibers' orientation played a key role for proper cell development [21]. Another important aspect of tissues, such as bones, is the presence of hierarchical structures. The structures vary in their size, ranging from micro-to nanoscale [22]. Hence, it is imperative to design scaffolds with hierarchical structures, for providing an optimal environment to the growing cells. Simple and inexpensive experimental setup, applicability to a wide variety of both natural and synthetic materials, ease in formation of nanoscale and highly porous nonwoven fibers, well-shaped structures (mats, meshes, tubes, etc.) in addition to its effective surface modification strategies make the technique of electrospinning more favorable among others [3,4].

This chapter discusses different electrospinning techniques for fabricating tissue-specific scaffolds (Fig. 3.1), providing an overview of the different electrospun forms and their applications in tissue reengineering. The computer-aided designing of 3D scaffolds, and their realization, is a process-dependent phenomenon which is briefly explained. A comprehensive study on regenerating various types of hard and soft tissues, using processing and postprocessing methods of electrospinning technology, gives a detailed insight on the structure—function relationship of the biomimicking scaffold. Importance of scaffold architecture and its surface modification to house different types of cells and enhance cell—cell interaction is well elaborated. The gradient designing of the scaffolds have been given a special mention. This chapter also reviews a variety of polymeric materials, electrospun into desired morphologies for efficient tissue engineering. Finally, the market of a few remarkable tissue-engineered products developed with electrospinning method is enlightened in terms of enhancing the healthcare sector.

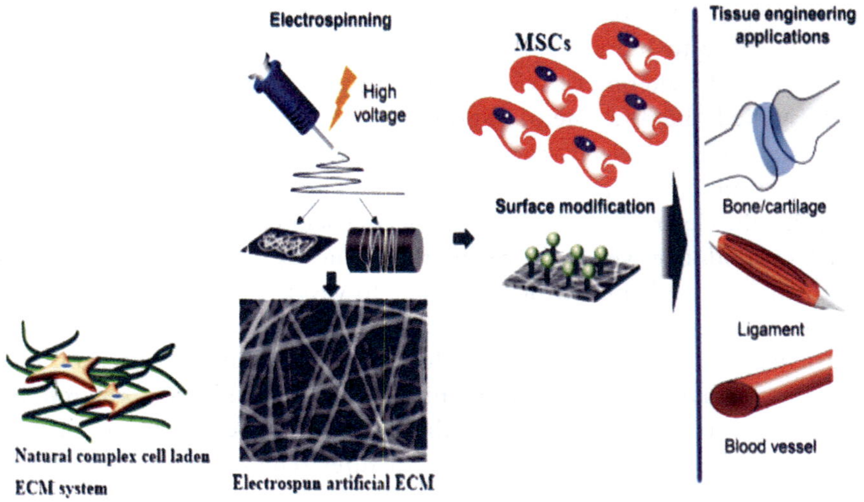

Figure 3.1 Cell-laden electrospun matrices developed for hard and soft tissue engineering applications closely mimicking the structure and function of natural complex system. *Figure is reproduced with modification. Modified from S. Nemati, S. Kim, Y. Shin, H. Shin, Current progress in application of polymeric nanofibers to tissue engineering, Nano Convergence 6 (1) (2019). https://doi.org/10.1186/s40580-019-0209-y.*

3.2 Electrospun scaffold as artificial ECM for tissue regeneration

The resemblance of the 3D scaffold structures to the native environment of various tissue types is well studied and exploited extensively in the field of tissue engineering. We now discuss the different types of electrospun scaffolds, their fabrication, and use in reengineering various types of hard and soft tissues.

3.2.1 Hard tissue engineering

3.2.1.1 Bone tissue engineering

Bone defects and injuries are the major causal agents for high morbidity, thereby impairing the health and quality of life. The main property of the bone that is the load-bearing in the human skeletal system arises from its hierarchical organization of nano-, micro-, and macrosized structures. This organized structure is also responsible for providing the bone tissue with reversible and irreversible mechanical energy dissipation, thus preventing fractures [23]. *Dual extrusion electrospinning* is used to produce highly aligned and alternating micro- and nanofibrous structures. The multiple layers of fibers get deposited onto a rotating collector drum, after passing through the spinnerets of a two-syringe system. The solution concentration and viscosity can be modified to achieve the desire fiber dimensions [15]. This method was used to fabricate a nanofibrous mat comprising eggshell-based hydroxyapatite (HAP) nanoparticles and poly(lactic acid) (PLA). The scaffold was studied for its ability to support the human osteoblasts and good cell attachment and differentiation was visible with the scaffold [24].

A recent study showed enhanced cell proliferation and diffusion of MG-63 osteoblast-like cells cultured in the scaffold comprising 3D helical assembly of polycaprolactone (PCL) nanofibers, as compared to its 2D forms. This architecture was obtained by using a helical-shaped collector in *micropatterned collector—based electrospinning*, and the process showed successful fabrication of similarly shaped scaffolds (Fig. 3.2) [25,26]. The mineral content of the bone also promotes various physiochemical characteristics, required for its proper functioning. Thus, it becomes imperative to design scaffolds with optimum mechanical strength for bone tissue engineering.

A new method for bone tissue repair by the group of Roya Sedghi involved the grafting of PCL over the chitosan backbone, using the copper (I)-catalyzed azide-alkyne cycloaddition reaction [27]. The copolymer after

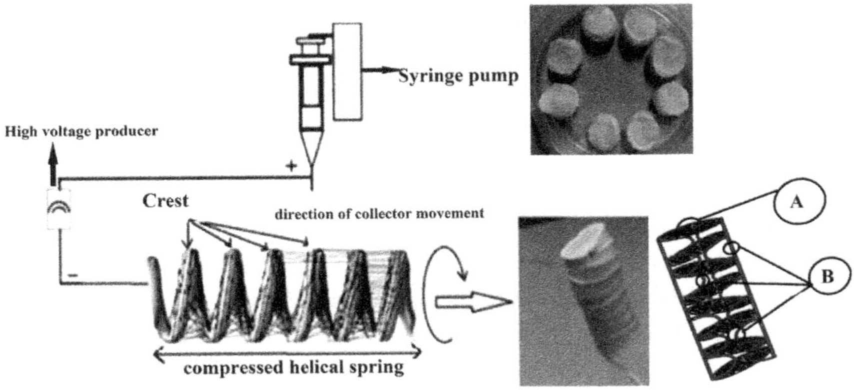

Figure 3.2 Nanofiber deposition across the spring crests and covering the spring all around. The method used for fabricating similarly shaped scaffolds for load-bearing tissue engineering [25,26]. A and B signify the filled and void regions in scaffold ultimately give rising to helical compressible spring design for better load-bearing capacity. *Data from F. Hejazi, H. Mirzadeh, N. Contessi, M. Tanzi, S. Faré, Novel class of collector in electrospinning device for the fabrication of 3D nanofibrous structure of large defect load-bearing tissue engineering application, J. Biomed. Mater. Res. 105 (5) (2017) 1535—1548. https://doi.org/10.1002/jbm.a.35822.*

enrichment with Mg-doped HAP nanoparticles was processed into nanofibers via electrospinning, and the process optimized to obtain uniform, bead-free fibrous scaffold. Improved adherence of MG-63 osteoblast-like cells to the fabricated scaffold and its higher mechanical strength was attributed to the presence of a triazole ring in the polymer. The ring's polarity caused presumable hydrogen bonding between the cells and the fibers, thus making the scaffold surface highly bioactive [27]. Alizarin red staining confirmed the production of calcium by the osteoblast cells, proving the suitability of the developed electrospun construct for osteogenic differentiation. The mechanical properties of the scaffolds containing 5 wt% Mg-doped HAP nanofibers showed similarity with that of the cancellous bone, thus establishing its utility for cancellous bone repair and regeneration [27].

A recent development in the field of electrospinning, near-field electrospinning, is highly researched for its ability to produce nanofibers [28,15]. The technique uses a programmed movable spinneret, and its distance from the collector is very small (a few millimeters ~5), unlike conventional electrospinning that utilizes a working distance in the range of centimeters [29]. This was utilized for the formation of a nanofibrous 3D scaffold as reported by Kolan et al. by using PCL/borate bioactive glass composite. 20wt% borate bioactive glass provided the scaffold with enhanced angiogenic characteristics. The mesenchymal stem cells (from human adipose) showed a high degree of cell proliferation when seeded in these scaffolds, which displayed structural similarities to the cancellous bone in terms of porosity and wide pore distribution [30]. Surface modification of the electrospun fibers in addition to their nanodimensionality is highly desired for improving cell—scaffold interaction [31].

In a recent report, electrospun polyurethane nanofibers were modified by *ultrasonication* for consequent adsorption with cellulose nanofibrils (CNFs) [32]. This technique utilizes the mechanical separation of polymeric nanofibers to further incorporate the desired moieties in the tissue engineering construct. These composite nanofibers were further coated with polydopamine, leading to core—shell morphology [32]. The CNFs were able to align the polydopamine along the fiber direction, and promoted inter- and intramolecular hydrogen bonding in it. The polyurethane/CNFs/polydopamine scaffold thus exhibited improved strength and biocompatibility toward the growing mouse embryonic osteoblast cells, in comparison to polyurethane/CNFs scaffolds. This versatile ultrasonication technique used in combination with electrospinning can prove advantageous in tuning the scaffolds for tissue-specific applications [32].

3.2.1.2 Dental tissue engineering

Dental caries and untreated periodontal diseases may lead to a decrease in the pulp—dentin complex, tissue destruction, and eventual loss of the tooth [33]. The hardest mineralized tissue of the human body is the dental enamel and is prone to a lot of wear and tear. Damage to the tooth may also arise from certain biological disorders, making it imperative to custom-design scaffolds for efficient repair [33]. The high mechanical strength of the enamel stems from the arrangement of the apatite crystals into prisms, and the further ordered alignment of these prisms [34]. The reengineering of dental tissues is limited owing to difficulties in mimicking the alignment and movement of the enamel forming cells (ameloblasts), during the assembly of HAP crystals into enamel prisms [34]. Periodontal reconstruction is based on the effective regeneration of cementum, which in turn guides the morphology of the HAP crystals [35]. The electrospun fibers are being extensively studied to provide effective and well adaptable scaffolds for regenerating the tooth [33].

In one of the studies, cementum protein 1 was entrapped in a hybrid scaffold, constructed by electrospinning PCL/collagen type 1/poly(ethylene glycol) modified with amorphous calcium phosphate. This multiphase construct, with nanofibrous mesh morphology, was cocultured with human periodontal ligament cells [35]. The cells displayed good adherence and a spindle-shaped morphology after 7 days of culture. The scaffold could induce cementogenic differentiation of the seeded cells, which was assessed by the presence of certain gene markers. When tested in calvarial defects of rats, mineralization, uniform bone density, and presence of cementum like tissue was observed after 8 weeks of implantation. The results proved the potential of this hybrid scaffold in regenerating the cementum [35]. The guided tissue regeneration membranes are known to prevent the penetration of the connective tissue into the surrounding bony defects. This creates an optimum niche for the regeneration of alveolar bone and periodontal ligaments, which grow slower in comparison to the connective tissues [36]. *Ultrasonication in combination with electrospinning* was used to obtain poly-5D/95L-lactide (PLA95) fibers loaded with β-TCP powders. These microsized electrospun membranes were placed in the bony defects of a pig model and were also studied in the clinical trials comparing with the commercially available PLA dental membrane (PLA; *Epi-Guide*, Kensey Nash Corp., Exton, PA, USA, [36]). The studies on the animal model showed notable differences in before and after surgery cementum and bone height, and almost similar results were obtained, when compared with the Epi-Guide in the clinical trials [36].

Incorporating gradient designs in the fabricated scaffolds are well known to enhance their biomimicking ability. Poly(3-hydroxybutyrate-co-4-hydroxybutyrate) (PHB) matrix was incorporated with fluorohydroxyapatite (FAP) filler to fabricate composition-gradient films [37]. Thin, uniform layers of PHB/FAP with different weight ratios were electrospun over each other, keeping the interval of 30 min. The morphology studies showed nonuniform diameters of PHB fibers (microdimensional), which resulted from the entwinement of the fibers around the hexagonal prisms of FAP [37] (Fig. 3.3). Higher FAP content lead to reinforced fibers, on account of increased entwinement; thus, preventing slipping of individual fiber strands on top of each other. The mouse fibroblasts showed good adhesion and proliferation in these scaffolds, suggesting its potential in tooth tissue engineering [37].

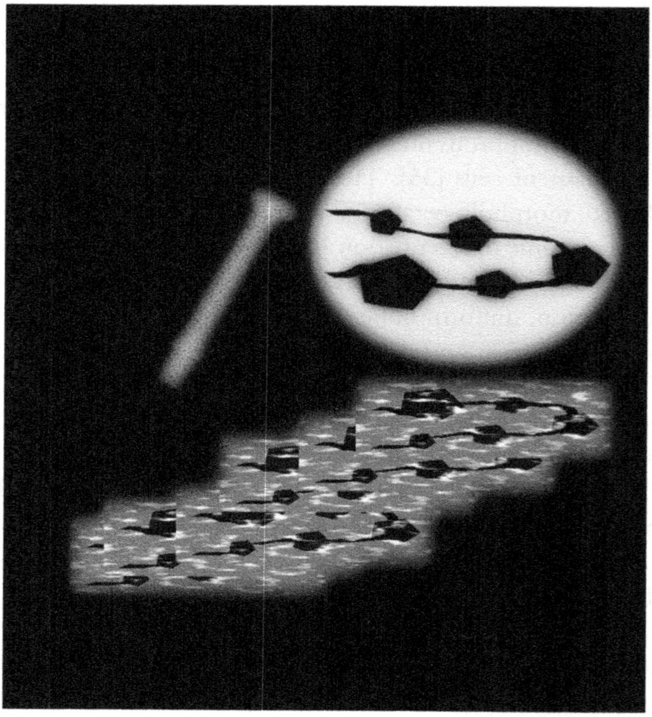

Figure 3.3 Incorporating stacked arrangement of electrospun PHB layers with hexagonal FAP prisms reinforcing the scaffold architecture for tooth tissue engineering. *Modified from D. Zhao, Y. Wang, R. Xu, G. Wu, L. Zhang, D. Yu, F. Cui, D. Chen, W. Tian, Composition-graded films of fluoroapatite/PHB fabricated via electrospinning for tissue engineering, J. Bioact. Compat. Polym. 22 (4) (2007) 379–393. https://doi.org/10.1177/0883911507079802.*

3.2.2 Soft tissue engineering

3.2.2.1 Skin tissue engineering

Skin is the largest organ in the humans, responsible for a lot of functions including regulation of body temperature, immunity, body fluids etc. It is the most affected surface from environmental damage, involving wounds, burns, and ulcers. Tissue-engineered skin, a substitute to the natural skin, should be able to promote wound healing and establish proper vascular networks, in addition to other characteristic functions. It should also be able to prevent "scarring," i.e., should be able to integrate with the natural skin efficiently without leaving the after-marks. Coherent integration ensures the property of "touch perception" to be retained at the wound site [38]. The scaffolds used for regenerating skin appendages should meet appropriate physical and chemical features, leading to desired tissue reconstruction. The nanofibrous scaffold structure helps to improve cell adhesion and proliferation [38], while porosity and 3D architecture generate higher cell infiltration [39]. Cell infiltration aids the development of layered constructs, which is an essential requirement in the formation of skin tissues. The scaffold surface must present different functional moieties to the seeded cells. This ensures required chemical interactions with various cytokines and growth factors, which are known for their potential in wound healing and tissue regeneration [39,40].

Sandri et al. employed glycosaminoglycans (chondroitin sulfate and hyaluronic acid, constituents of the ECM) and chitosan blends for developing nanofibrous scaffolds to be used in wound-healing applications. Pullulan was linked to chitosan, making it easier to electrospin with both the glycosaminoglycans [38]. The morphological studies showed smooth and well-shaped nanofibers, making them suitable for designing well-aligned scaffolds. The electrospun scaffolds were seeded with normal human dermal fibroblasts and endothelial cells, with in vitro investigations revealing enhanced cell proliferation and wound-healing properties. The strong interaction of glycosaminoglycans with the growth factors enhanced cell proliferation and chitosan provided the desired antimicrobial and wound-healing properties [38]. Citric acid, used along with the polymer blends during the process of electrospinning, served as the cross-linker between two oppositely charged polymers, thus rendering aqueous insolubility to the fabricated scaffold. The chitosan/chondroitin sulfate scaffold showed better results in wound healing of murine lesions. This in vivo study highlighted the restoration of epidermal layers and collagen fibers at dermal—epidermal boundary, keratinization, and absence of wound exudate and abnormal dilation of blood vessels. The histological studies on these scaffolds showed their complete elimination, owing to biodegradability of chitosan by lysozyme [38].

A highly characteristic feature of the native skin, i.e., the presence of depressions over its surface, was incorporated by the group of Powell et al. which studied the fabrication of collagen scaffolds by employing the patterning technique of *laser irradiation with electrospinning* [41]. This technique is used to obtain uniformly shaped porous structures in the polymeric scaffolds. The laser beam is focused on the desired spot, thus melting the fibers at the local region without disturbing the overall fiber morphology [42]. The human fibroblasts—seeded scaffolds were exposed to laser beams, thus creating well-spaced groove structures with architecture similar to that of rete ridges (Fig. 3.4). Rete ridges are the interdigitations in the skin which contribute toward homeostasis and cell adhesion. These scaffolds were studied for their skin regeneration ability in athymic mice, and the tissue-engineered skin showed the presence of stable ridges along with improved barrier function and epidermal growth [41].

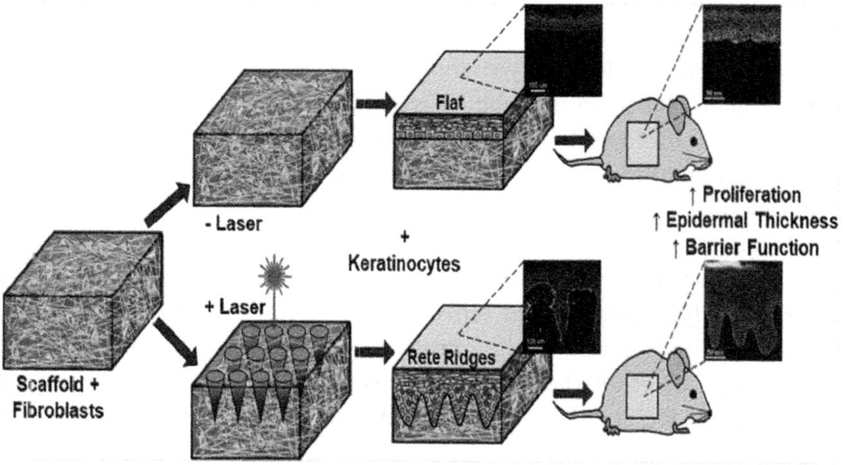

Figure 3.4 Concentration of keratinocytes and formation of rete ridge-like projections into the dermis with a continuous basement membrane by day 11, Scale bar = 100 μm [41]. *From B. Blackstone, M. Malara, M. Baumann, K. McFarland, D. Supp, H. Powell, Fractional CO_2 laser micropatterning of cell-seeded electrospun collagen scaffolds enables rete ridge formation in 3D engineered skin, Acta Biomnterialia 102 (2007) 287–297. https://doi.Org/10.1016/j.actbio.2019.11.051.*

In another study, *porogen leaching* was used in combination with melt electrospinning to form porous 3D scaffolds. It involves the addition of porogens like salt and ice crystals to the electrospinning polymer solution. The porogens can then be leached out of the collector surface by solvent dissolution [42]. This cost-effective method can be employed with different polymer melts and the resultant fibers can be easily customized and processed to match its end usage. The team of Luciana Sartore developed porous PLA scaffolds using this cell-friendly technique. They used sodium polyacrylate particles as porogen during the melt electrospinning procedure and then leached out these particles under aqueous environment. The cell line of mouse embryonic fibroblasts showed good cell adhesion and proliferation in these scaffolds [43]. The scaffold's ability to promote vascularization is another essential feature that is looked into during designing the scaffold.

Investigations on electrospinning polycarbonate-based polyurethane blended with gelatin revealed the formation of mechanically fit scaffolds to be used for creating skin constructs [44]. The cospinning of the polymers produced microsized fibers, with their density being in the range of a few micrometers. The optimum mechanical strength and controlled degradation rate were achieved by using 20% polyurethane with 80% gelatin. The swelling capacity of this scaffold, which can serve as a measure of the amount of wound exudate absorbed by the scaffold, was also quantified. The *in vivo* studies on mouse wounds showed enhanced cell growth at the wound site, increased cell infiltration, and lesser number of macrophages, as compared to *INTEGRA*, the well-established matrix for skin regeneration [44]. This initial study will pave a new way for the production of improved skin regenerating matrices.

3.2.2.2 Kidney tissue engineering

According to the International Society of Nephrology, kidney disease is estimated to affect around 850 million people worldwide. It is one of the leading causes of death in the United States, as reported by the Centers for Disease Control and Prevention. Renal tissue regeneration aims to incorporate optimum scaffold porosity and all the complex pathways required for recapitulating a fully functional kidney [45]. Decellularized tissues are commonly used vehicles for culturing kidney cells. Despite huge advancement in this area, the formidable process of decellularization accompanied by the poor mechanical strength of the resultants led to the studies on using different polymeric fibers for renal tissue engineering [46]. Callanan et al.

studied the multipopulation of rat kidney cells on the electrospun PLA fibrous scaffolds [46]. By utilizing the technique of *cryogenic electrospinning* and varying the concentration of PLA, the research group fabricated different sized fibers and studied the corresponding cell behavior [46]. Cryogenic electrospinning involves the use of a freezing collector in place of the conventional metal collector. The collector is connected to a cooling pump to achieve freezing temperatures. The method serves in fabricating a hierarchy of pores over the fibers' surface [47]. All the scaffolds designed thereof supported cell growth, with variations arising only in terms of cell infiltration and mechanical strength. The larger sized fibers promoted deeper cell penetration, owing to greater porosity, on the cost of decreased mechanical properties [48].

Electrospun nanofiber meshes prove to be significant for developing scaffolds for regenerating kidney tissues. The porosity imparts the required diffusion to the engineered construct, while functionalization of fibers contributes toward its resemblance to the ECM. In one of the recent studies, PCL was electrospun into tubular nanofibrous scaffolds and functionalized with L-3,4-dihydroxyphenylalanine (L-DOPA) and collagen IV to achieve aqueous insolubility [49]. The inner diameter of the tubular structure was in correspondence to the needle diameter of the electrospinning setup (Fig. 3.5). Proximal tubule cell lines, with two different sizes, were injected in the scaffolds and investigated for cell proliferation, functionality, and viability. The microscopic images showed that the adherence and growth of smaller-sized cells were dependent on the density of nanofibers, which in turn is a function of polymeric concentration used for electrospinning [49]. Tightly packed nanofibers promoted close placement of the cells, thus preventing leakage during selective transport of metabolites. The functionality of the constructs was measured by conducting transport studies on the added cationic and anionic fluorescein solutes. Swift diffusion of these solutes from the tubular wall toward the inner layers confirmed their efficiency (Fig. 3.5). The scaffolds remained fully functional until 3 weeks, suggesting their potential to continuously eliminate metabolic waste from the body [49].

Various studies on bioartificial kidneys (BAKs) suggest its efficacy in the treatment of acute renal failures in animal models. They involve the development of proximal tubule mimicking constructs as they can circumvent the presently used dialysis treatment by performing the important renal functions of transportation, reabsorption, and toxin secretion. These BAKs utilize a membranous scaffold, for assembling the proximal tubule cells in a

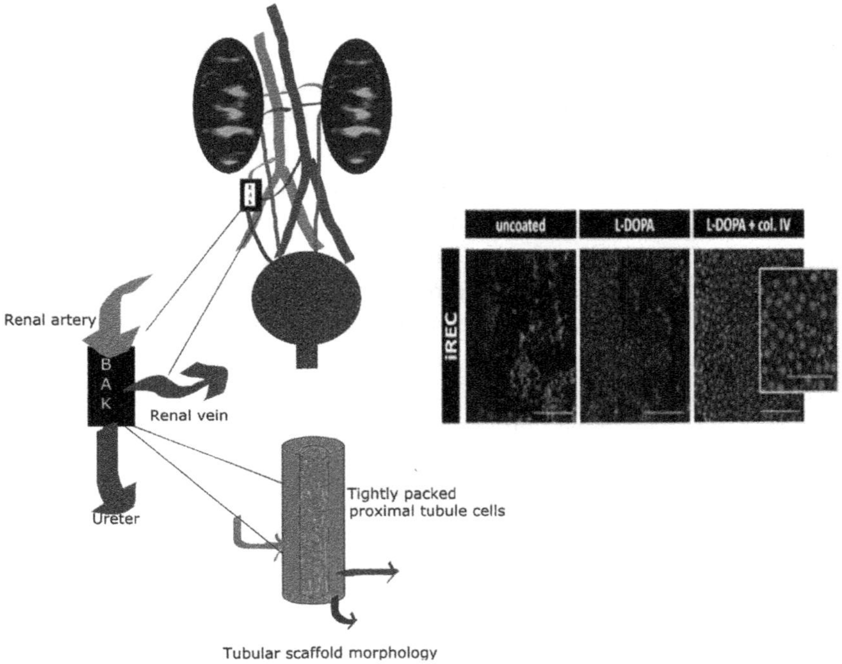

Figure 3.5 BAK Electrospun PCL scaffolds for use in BAKs Polycaprolactone were electrospun into tubular nanofibrous scaffolds and functionalized with L-3,4-dihydroxyphenylalanine (L-DOPA) and collagen IV to achieve aqueous insolubility [49]. *From K. Jansen, M. Castilho, S. Aarts, M. Kaminski, S. Lienkamp, R. Pichler, J. Malda, T. Vermonden, J. Jansen, R. Masereeuw, Fabrication of kidney proximal tubule grafts using biofunctionalized electrospun polymer scaffolds, Macromol. Biosci. 19 (2) (2019). https://doi.org/10.1002/mabi.201800412.*

monolayer. It is also essential that the cells differentiate in a proper manner that leads to the formation of tight junctions. They facilitate the renal functions by lowering the leakiness of the epithelium. Another important factor to be looked into is the optimal ECM, which can sustain the monolayers for a long period of time, thus proving its role in the treatment of chronic renal failure [50]. Nuno M. Neves studied the behavior of Human Kidney cell lines (HK-2) upon their seeding in electrospun PCL scaffolds. Decellularized kidney ECM was coelectrospun with PCL, and these membrane structures allowed for enhanced cell growth and proliferation as compared with pure PCL scaffolds. They also demonstrated the presence and increase in the content of zona-occludens 1, with increasing concentrations of the decellularized kidney ECM. Zona-occludens 1 is an epithelial marker, which regulates the formation of tightly packed arrangement of the renal cells [51], an essential requirement for producing successful BAKs [50].

3.2.2.3 Neural tissue engineering

Injury to the spinal cord results in loss of motor, sensory, and autonomic functions; associated with the site of injury and deteriorates patient's physical and psychological health [52]. Though the regenerative therapies have shown promising results in *in vivo* models, the efficiency in clinical trials is quite less, owing to the limited regenerative capacity of the spinal cord and complex innate structure. The scaffolds for neural tissue engineering must possess a high degree of permeability and 3D orientation of fibers for promoting cell migration and directing axonal elongation [53]. A recent study by Rao et al. showed the fabrication of 3D PLA/silk fibroin scaffolds using the technique of *gas foaming along with electrospinning* [54]. This strategy is effectively used to develop fluffy and porous 3D scaffolds from 2D structures (Fig. 3.6). The technique works on the principle of difference in gas solubility in different solvents. The gas molecules move toward the solvent having more affinity for it, thus leaving behind spaces in the native region. The percentage porosity achieved can be controlled by altering the time of

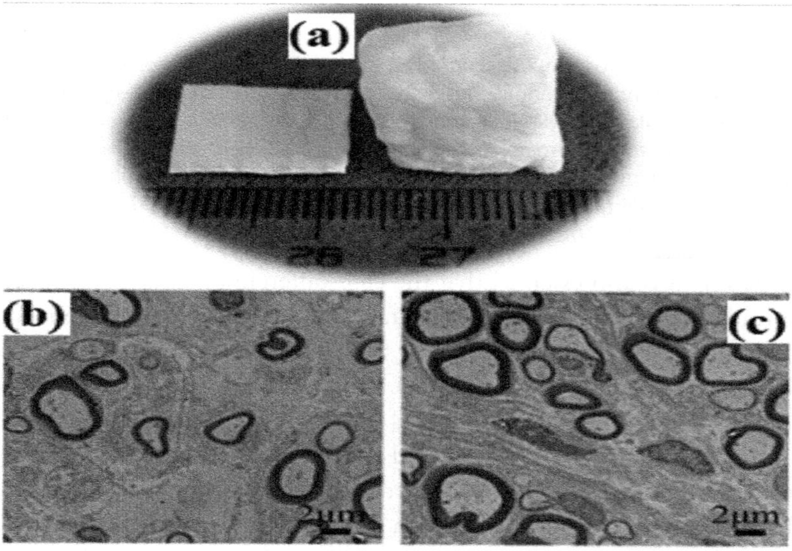

Figure 3.6 Morphology of SF/PLA 3D nanofiber scaffold (a). Density of myelinated axons in (b) hollow chitosan nerve guiding conduits, and (c) 3D PLA/Silk Fibroin scaffolds as filler in chitosan nerve guiding conduits. *From F. Rao, Z. Yuan, M. Li, F. Yu, X. Fang, B. Jiang, Y. Wen, P. Zhang, Expanded 3D nanofibre sponge scaffolds by gas-foaming technique enhance peripheral nerve regeneration, Artificial Cells, Nanomed. Biotechnol. 47 (1) (2019) 491–500. https://doi.org/10.1080/21691401.2018.1557669.*

exposure of the scaffold with the solvent. A 10-mm long sciatic nerve defect in rats was bridged by using the 3D PLA/silk fibroin scaffolds as filler in chitosan nerve guiding conduits, and these proved to be more efficient for the proliferation of Schwann cells than the hollow conduits. Assessment of the regenerated nerve fibers after 12 weeks of implantation showed a higher density of the nerve fibers in the filled conduits (Fig. 3.6). The expansion proved helpful in designing an oriented and layered structure, which was successful in providing guiding cues to the seeded cells [54]. In another instance, a group of researchers collected protein-encapsulated silk electrospun fibers; and repeated this process of forming core—shell structures with varying protein concentrations. They obtained a double gradient of fiber density and bioactive molecules. The process was tedious and unsuitable for obtaining a continuous graded pattern [53]. Various studies are attempting the fabrication of biomimicking scaffolds, along with gradient design to fully recapitulate the native cellular microenvironment.

Incorporating the architectural similarities of the natural proteins with the nanofibers and an aligned topography for directional cell growth, the group of Nune et al. coelectrospun [55] poly(lactic-co-glycolic acid), PLGA, with self-assembling peptide sequences (SAPs). These SAPs favor easy functionalization due to the presence of designer motifs and elicit a negligible immune response. RADA-16-I hydrogels with self-assembled bone marrow homing peptide-1 [56] blend with PLGA scaffolds were studied for their efficiency in peripheral nerve regeneration. Rat Schwann cells showed enhanced cell infiltration in these electrospun constructs as compared to the surface-modified PLGA scaffolds. The higher gene expression of neural-specific markers like neural cell adhesion molecule, peripheral myelin protein 22 (PMP22), and glial fibrillary acidic protein also confirmed the potential on the use of the electrospun constructs for axonal regeneration and functional nerve recovery [55]. A close look at the physiological and anatomical characteristics of the spinal cord led the investigators to consider hydrogel-based scaffolds with high water retention capacity and variable mechanical properties. Chen et al. developed gelatin-methacryloyl (GelMA) hydrogel fibers by first photo-cross-linking the methacryloyl groups with gelatin, and then electrospinning the resultant solution [57]. The fibers were collected in an aligned manner, hence making the scaffold optimum for seeding the bone mesenchymal stem cells. The results from the *in vitro* experiments confirmed a significant cell growth, proliferation, differentiation, and directional axonal extension. The *in vivo* studies on T9 spinal cord injured rats confirmed the promotion of vascularization, suppression of glial scar, and the scaffold's good antideforming capacity. The bioinspired viscoelastic scaffold can serve to reengineer injured spinal cord tissues; even in the absence of bony spinal canal [57]. Another combinatorial approach of neuroprotection and neuroregeneration was closely examined by the team of Silvia Rossi, for the treatment of spinal cord injury. A scaffold based on alginate and poly(ethylene oxide) was formed by electrospinning [58]. The fibers were first cross-linked with the Sigma1 receptor agonist, RC-33, a neuroprotective drug; and then embedded in chitosan layers, which imparted controlled degradation rate to the scaffold. Initial studies on human neuroblastoma cell line confirmed cell viability and scaffold biocompatibility. The ongoing research in tuned drug release in the "nerve-injured" simulated environment will bring forth the efficacy of this novel approach [58].

3.2.2.4 Cardiac tissue engineering

The global population is witnessing an alarming increase in cardiovascular diseases, with myocardial infarction (MI) being one of the leading causes of injury to the heart. The human heart possesses a fractional ability to regenerate due to its complex anatomy and cell cycle arrest [59,60]. Various studies have shown the positive impact of c-kit + stem cells on the cardiac repair. Stem cells derived from the bone marrow express cluster of differentiation 117 (c kit) as their surface marker. MI in mice leads to an increase in the number of these cells and can be magnetically sorted from the bone marrow. The major hindrance to this stem cell therapy approach is the poor rate of survival among these bone marrow–derived cells [61]. The blend of silk fibroin and poly(L-lactic acid-co-caprolactone) was electrospun to form nanofibrous sheets and were studied for enhancing the survival rate of c-kit + cells in mice, after confirming the scaffold's success in *in vitro* experiments. Transplantation of the c-kit + seeded scaffolds showed a reduction of infarct size and prevention of myocardial damage, suggesting their efficiency in MI treatment [61].

Biomaterials for cardiac tissue engineering should be able to acquire optimum mechanical strength and degradability in its scaffold form. These essential prerequisites in a scaffold in addition to its ability to provide an environment favorable for the cells' continuous beating determine their fate in *in vitro* and *in vivo* applications [62]. Schlatter's research group investigated the poly(glycerol sebacate), PGS, and PLA blend after electrospinning to achieve the desired fiber dimensions and strength [63]. The fibers were heat treated, before their incubation with commercial Matrigel solution to obtain the required fiber densities and enhance surface functionalization in the PGS-PLA mats. This promoted cell adhesion and proliferation among the seeded neonatal cardiomyocytes (from rat). The *in vivo* assessment comprised of suturing these mats on the ventricular surface of mice. The mat structure maintained a good integrity for 4 weeks, and also triggered low inflammatory response at the implanted site; all hinting toward its suitability in cardiac tissue engineering [63].

The recent progress in cardiac tissue engineering has involved the use of cardiomyocytes derived from human pluripotent stem cells, which has brought an upsurge in mimicking the heart's microenvironment [64]. An important characteristic that needs special mention is the ability of the tissue construct to recapitulate the natural heartbeat. Enhanced cell—cell communication was demonstrated by Liu et al. by employing *micropatterned collector—based electrospinning* [65]. This technique focuses on the use of a prepatterned collector for the deposition of polymeric fibers. The collector surface is modified with desirable geometric cues of varying sizes, using lithographic techniques. The pattern is thus replicated over the fiber surface, for obtaining hierarchical fibrous scaffolds. Poly(ethylene glycol)-poly(DL-lactide) electrospun fibers were deposited over a square, rectangle, and honeycomb-patterned collector, to obtain similar shaped fibrous sheets to be assembled in a stratified manner for fabricating the desired scaffold [65]. Presence of multiwalled carbon nanotubes was able to provide the scaffold with conductive properties. Cardiomyoblasts, cardiac fibroblasts, and endothelial cells were cocultured over these scaffolds and the cardiomyoblasts cultured in honeycomb-shaped scaffolds achieved spontaneous beating at the rate of 101 ± 12 times/min after coculturing for 5 days. The beating rates closely resembled that of adults and neonatal rats. Continuous and synchronous beating at 94 ± 8 times/min after 15 days of culture highlights the use of this strategy for developing efficient cardiac patches [65]. Thus, integrating a sensor to evaluate the tissue's contractile performance also becomes essential during scaffold fabrication. Working on these parameters, Dvir et al. hypothesized mechanical deformations in the scaffold induced by cardiomyocytes' contractile action [66] (Fig. 3.7). They utilized the inherent mechanoresponsive property of poly(vinylidene fluoride) (PVDF) by electrospinning a comonomer, trifluoroethylene (TrFE), to obtain tunable piezoelectric PVDF scaffolds. The highly aligned fibers promoted cell growth and elongation of the seeded human pluripotent stem cells. These cells matured into cardiomyocytes in 40 days and the corresponding contractile action could be well measured by the scaffold during this phase. Additional studies on the enhanced maturation of cardiomyocytes in a "voltage-generating scaffold" can lead to progress in optimizing cell differentiation [66].

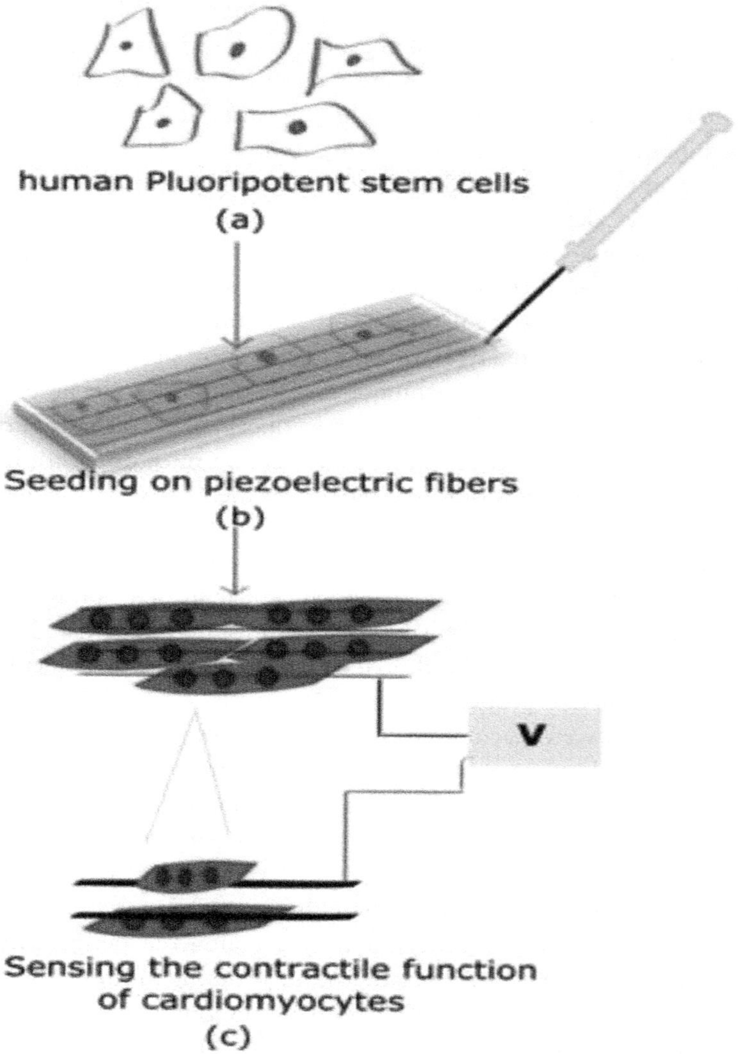

Figure 3.7 Electrospun piezoelectric PVDF scaffolds for reengineering of cardiac tissues. Integrating a sensor to evaluate the tissue's contractile performance also becomes essential during scaffold fabrication. Mechanical deformations in the scaffold induced by cardiomyocytes' contractile action [66]. *Modified from N. Adadi, M. Yadid, I. Gal, M. Asulin, R. Feiner, R. Edri, T. Dvir, Electrospun fibrous PVDF-TrFe scaffolds for cardiac tissue engineering, differentiation, and maturation, Adv. Mater. Technol. 5 (3) (2020). https://doi.org/10.1002/admt.201900820.*

3.2.2.5 Tendon, ligament, and skeletal muscle tissue engineering

Dysfunctional tendons and ligaments are one of the most commonly observed aging effects and have a high incidence of occurrence in sports injuries. They account for about 30% of all the musculoskeletal problems globally [67] with muscle diseases, trauma, and tumor ablations making up the rest. The location and function of the tendons and ligaments contribute toward their varied shapes and sizes. Apart from incorporating these morphological features, providing high elasticity and high mechanical strength is imperative in the design of successful scaffolds [68]. A method for imparting high mechanical strength to the fibers is *Temperature-Assisted Electrospinning*. Melt electrospinning technology focuses on the use of polymer melts, instead of polymeric solvents for the production of fibrous scaffolds. This is beneficial in preventing environmental pollution in comparison to solution electrospinning, due to the absence of solvent evaporation. The fibers produced are free from residual toxic solvents and higher in mechanical strength [69].

Gwiazda et al. utilized the technique of *melt electrospinning writing* to produce highly aligned PCL scaffolds for ligament tissue engineering [70]. They constructed scaffolds with aligned, crimped, and random fiber topologies to study the growth of seeded human mesenchymal stem cells (hMSC). The aligned scaffolds could steer the cell growth in the fiber direction for up to 4 weeks, which was not seen in the case of crimped scaffolds (Fig. 3.8). The mechanical tests showed high values of resilience under conditions of cyclic stretching, which is extremely favorable for engineering anterior cruciate ligament that helps to provide rotational stability to the knee joints [70].

Control on the orientation of electrospun nanofibers into well-defined shapes and directional alignment have favored the successful regeneration of many tissues. In another study on tendon and ligament injuries, Cai et al. investigated and compared the random and dual-layer of aligned-random silk fibroin/poly(L-lactic acid-co-e-caprolactone) (P(LLA-CL)) nanofibrous scaffolds for reintegrating the ruptured Achilles tendon to the bone in the rabbit model (Fig. 3.9). The studies showed increased maturation and improved organization of the collagen between the tendon and the bone, and new bone formation after 12 weeks in the aligned-random scaffolds; when compared with the random scaffold [71]. The dual-layer scaffolds also fared well on the mechanical front such as load-bearing and stiffness. The results proved the use of multilayer scaffolds in interfacial tissue engineering, as they effectively mimic the gradient microstructure of tendon, fibrocartilage, calcified fibrocartilage, and bone, for the tendon-to-bone healing [71].

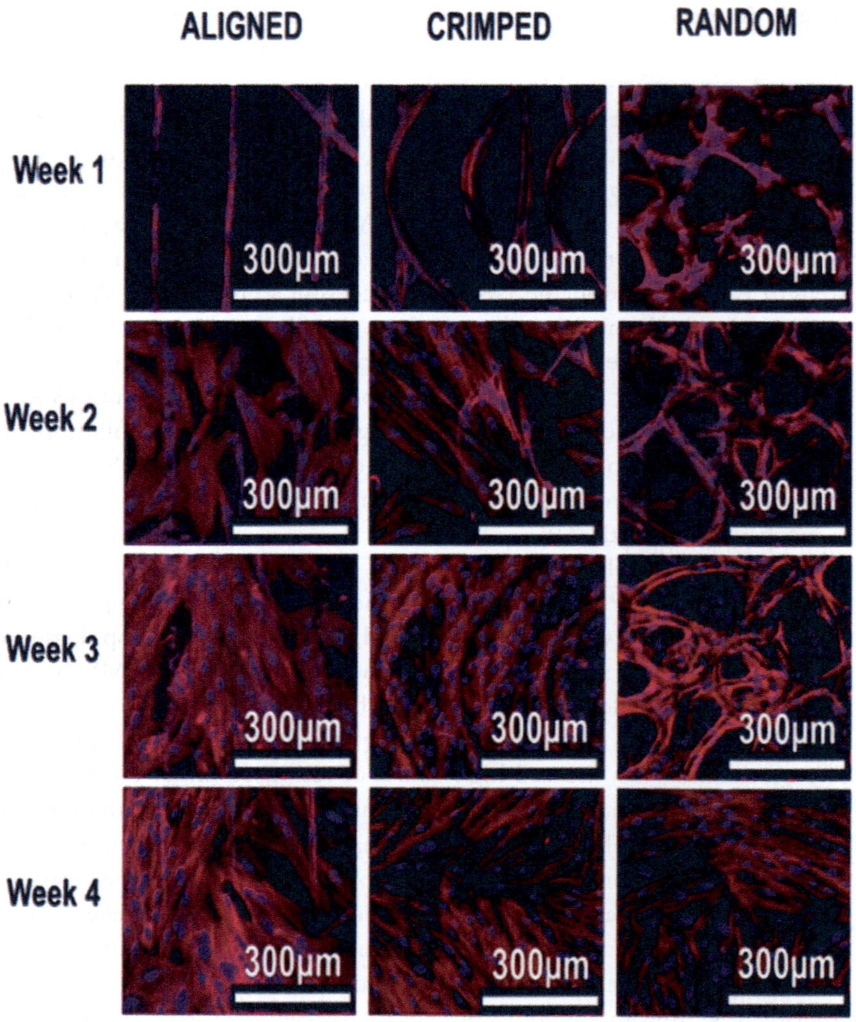

Figure 3.8 Confocal imaging of in vitro cell culture after 4 weeks depicting cell proliferation. DAPI stained the nuclei blue, while Phalloidin stained the actin filaments red. *Reproduced from M. Gwiazda, S. Kumar, W. Swieszkowski, S. Ivanovski, C. Vaquette, The effect of melt electrospun writing fiber orientation onto cellular organization and mechanical properties for application in Anterior Cruciate Ligament tissue engineering. J. Mech. Beha. Biomed. Mater. (2020), 104. https://doi.Org/10.1016/j.jmbbm.2020.1036317.*

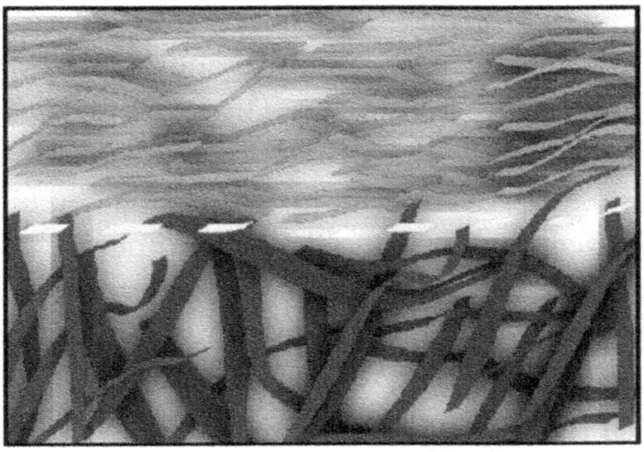

Figure 3.9 Dual layered randomly aligned nanofibrous scaffold.

The presence of natural micro-/nanostructures in the ECM of skeletal muscles was closely mimicked by the group of Chen et al. They developed a 3D scaffold by *melt electrowriting* microgroove structure on top of electrospun PCL nanofibers. The grooves were placed in parallel and perpendicular directions to the well-aligned PCL nanomeshes, and these scaffolds were studied and compared for their effects on the alignment, elongation, and differentiation of the H9c2 myoblast cells into myotubes. The PCL nanofibers were also coated with gold (Au) nanoparticles, which acted as an electroactive cue for enhancing myogenic differentiation. The results indicated the parallel arrangement of the microgrooves, with the unidirectional PCL nanofibers to fare well in comparison to their perpendicular counterparts. The increase in thickness of the Au coating leads to enhanced scaffold conductivity, which results in better transfer of electrical signal between the cells. The spacing between the microgrooves was also analyzed, and the results demonstrated their significance in elongation and orientation of myotubes [72].

Various studies on musculoskeletal tissue engineering highlight the importance of incorporating the complex phenomenon of muscle contraction within the designed scaffolds, for advancing in this field.

3.2.3 Specialized tissue engineering

3.2.3.1 Reproductive tissue Engineering

A highly emerging field, REPROTEN (Reproductive Tissue Engineering) [73], is helping to restore the functionality of diseased and injured reproductive tissues, which may ultimately lead to infertility and end-stage organ failure. This causes a high emotional and physical discomfort among people, resulting in a highly stressful life. The scaffolds used in REPROTEN technology are in most of the cases patient customized. They involve the use of invasive methods to derive patients' cells to be seeded in the highly interconnected and macroporous scaffolds; later implanting the entire tissue construct in the abnormal organ. In many of the cases, application of the stem cells for designing the construct has shown much better results, and it also circumvents the possibility of extracting diseased cells [74].

Studying the treatment options for pelvic organ prolapse (POP)—a disorder mainly arising from vaginal birth injury—a research group developed electrospun poly L-lactic acid-co-poly ε-caprolactone nanofibrous mesh (P nanomesh) (Fig. 3.10) and seeded them with endometrial mesenchymal stem cells [75]. These biodegradable scaffolds, in comparison to the recently FDA banned nonbiodegradable polypropylene transvaginal meshes, have been reported as an efficient alternative for POP repair, which includes improvement in urine and bowel motion, sexual functions, etc. The fabricated scaffolds were able to eliminate inflammatory and undesirable foreign body response, highly prominent in the case of polypropylene meshes. They were also able to replicate the gradient micro–nano architecture of the native vaginal tissue, as opposed to the banned meshes. The *in vivo* studies on the tissue construct showed increased ECM expression, angiogenesis, cell adhesion, and repair after 6 weeks of implantation in mice [75].

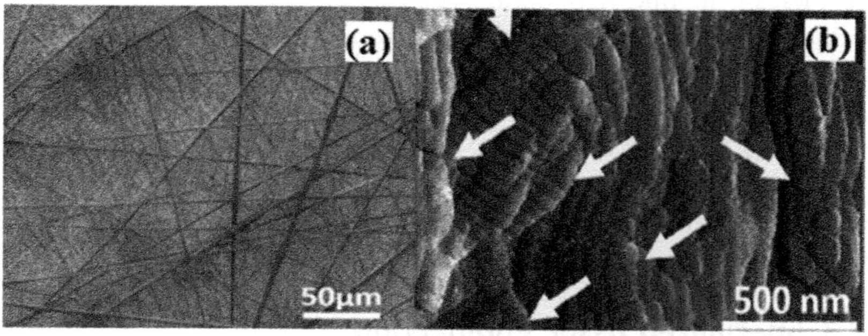

Figure 3.10 Scanning electron micrograph of PLCL nanofiber mesh structure at 1000 × magnification (a), showing close resemblance with the human vaginal microstructure (b) comprised of collagen fibril structures denoted by yellow arrows. *Figure reproduced from S. Mukherjee, S. Darzi, K. Paul, F. Cousins, J. Werkmeister, C. Gargett, Electrospun nanofiber meshes with endometrial MSCs modulate foreign body response by increased angiogenesis, matrix synthesis, and mnti-inflammatory gene expression in mice: implication in pelvic floor. Fron. Pharmacol. 11 (2020). https://doi.org/10.3389/fphar.2020.00353.*

In another study attempting to solve infertility problems in males, which affects almost 7% of the global male population, spermatogonial stem cells (SSCs) were used for fabricating a bioengineered tissue construct [76]. The neonatal SSCs are well known for their pluripotency and were hence chosen for seeding in the electrospun PVA/agar scaffolds. A layered topology of well-interconnected, uniform, and randomly oriented nanofibers supplemented with growth factors proved to be effective in maintaining undifferentiated mouse SSCs [76]. The scaffold was able to promote cell proliferation and renewability, in addition to directing the cells into well-differentiated cell lineages; all pointing toward its potential in treating infertility, especially in males with an azoospermic condition (spermless semen) [76].

3.2.3.2 Salivary glands

Damage to the salivary glands results from radiation therapies, tumors, and some autoimmune disorders. It leads to loss of saliva production, which is highly detrimental to the swallowing, speaking, digestion, and oral health of the patients. Restoration of the salivary function depends on the efficiency of polarization and formation of tight junctions in the salivary epithelial cells. The ability of the scaffold to effectively mimic the basement membrane and the ECM is an essential prerequisite for activating various cell—signaling pathways for successful glandular regeneration [77].

Castracane et al. studied the electrospun elastin-poly-lactic-co-glycolic acid (PLGA) nanofiber scaffolds for regenerating the salivary glands. They prepared two different sets of scaffolds; first by *blend electrospinning* of elastin and PLGA, and second by chemical conjugation of elastin onto the electrospun PLGA nanofibers. The scaffolds were seeded with SIMS, mouse ductal submandibular epithelial cell line, and were compared for their efficiency. The results demonstrated better elasticity, wettability, and epithelial cell self-organization into clusters in case of the blend—electrospun scaffolds. The formation of tight junctions visualized through the biomarker protein Zona Occludin-1, and the polarization of salivary epithelial cells could only be seen in the case of these scaffolds. This was believed to be affected by the uniform distribution of elastin in the PLGA nanofibers (by blend electrospinning), which renders the scaffold with improved elastic and mechanical characteristics, essential for proper cell function [77].

Another attempt in developing bioartificial salivary glands was carried out by the group of Koh et al. They fabricated electrospun PCL nanofibrous sheets and integrated them into a hydrogel solution (comprised of 2-hydroxy-2- methylpropiophenone and poly(ethylene glycol)-diacrylate), by directly pouring the solution over the PCL sheets. An array of microwells, with nanofibrous base and hydrogel walls, was obtained by performing the technique of photolithography. This 3D scaffold was seeded with human single clonal salivary gland stem cells (hSGSCs), and was studied for its efficacy in directing the stem cells toward the formation of salivary organoids. For comparative studies, the hSGSCs were also grown simultaneously in plastic petridishes, floating culture, and Matrigel. At first, these stem cells aggregated to form 3D spheroids in all the types of culture conditions, barring the plastic ones. Their numbers were relatively higher in the 3D microwells (Fig. 3.11). The spheroid morphology activates the stem cells for further differentiation into organoid structures. The resulting organoids were studied for the expression of ductal and acinar markers; some of the most important proteins required for the proper functioning of the salivary glands. The results proved the success of 3D microwells when compared

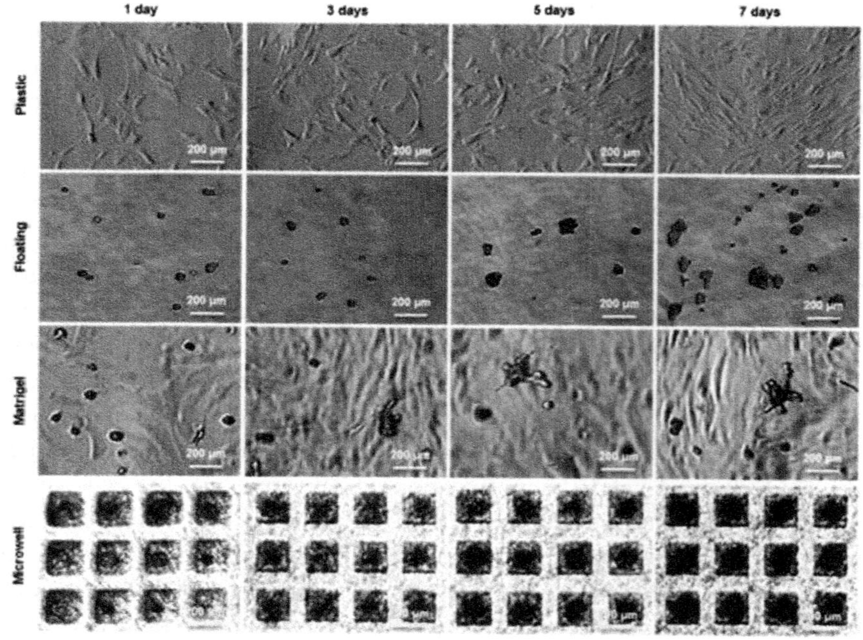

Figure 3.11 In vitro time dependency of hSGSCs to aggregate and assemble into 3D spheroids induced by floating, matrigel, and microwell scaffolds. (Scale bars = 200 μm) [78]. *From H. Shin, H. Hong, W. Koh, J. Lim, Organotypic 3D culture in nanoscaffold microwells supports salivary gland stem-cell-based organization, ACS Biomater. Sci. Eng. 4(12) (2018) 4311–4320. https://doi.org/10.1021/acsbiomaterials.8b00894.*

with its traditional culturing counterparts. The organoids obtained from the 3D microwells were transplanted into Non-obese Diabetic/Severe Combined Immunodeficient (NOD/SCID) mice salivary glands and studied for its effects in the transplanted area. After 14 days of transplantation, the organoids showed successful engrafting and neovascularization (Fig. 3.12). These electrospun 3D microwells can prove to be useful for efficient reengineering of the salivary glands [78].

3.2.3.3 Pancreatic islets

The autoimmune destruction of pancreatic beta cells is the causal agent of diabetes type I. It is one of the most common endocrine diseases and leads to insulin deficiency. Amputation of the lower limbs, kidney failure, and blindness are some of the chronic complications arising in people suffering from diabetes [79]. Successful regeneration of the islet cells is highly dependent on the pore sizes, their interconnectivity, composition of the scaffolds, and extent and efficiency of vascularization in the implanted constructs upon engraftment [80,81].

In one of the studies, conjunctiva mesenchymal stem cells were seeded in both natural and synthetic electrospun scaffolds, and investigated for their differentiation into insulin-producing cells (IPCs). Silk fibroin and poly(L-lactic) acid were electrospun into nanofibrous scaffolds with uniform, aligned, and bead-free nanofibers. The morphological studies showed the

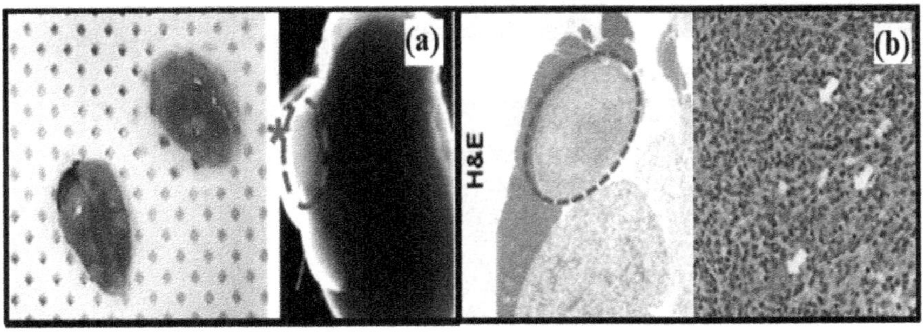

Figure 3.12 In vivo transplant of assembled and aggregated 3D spheroids from hSGSCs in the microwell culture. Hydrogel-encapsulated 3D spheroids transplanted under submandibular capsule (a). H&E stained histological micrographs of after transplanted spheroid after 14 days (b). Capillaries in the neovasculature are clearly visible and marked with the arrow [78]. *From H. Shin, H. Hong, W. Koh, J. Lim, Organotypic 3D culture in nanoscaffold microwells supports salivary gland stem-cell-based organization. ACS Biomat. Sci. Eng. 4 (12) (2018) 4311–4320. https://doi.org/10.1021/acsbiomaterials.8b00894.*

gradual condensation of stem cell clusters into cells similar to pancreatic islets. The results indicated the presence of specific pancreatic tissue genes such as insulin, glucagon, etc., in both the type of scaffolds, with a significant higher expression seen in PLLA scaffolds. Exposing the scaffolds with different glucose concentrations resulted in higher insulin secretion by the cells of the PLLA scaffold, which proved its higher efficiency in differentiating the stem cells into functional IPCs [82]. The group of Nair et al. demonstrated the structure—function relationship of the poly(ε-caprolactone) blended with poly (ε-caprolactone)-b-poly (tetrahydrofuran)-b-poly (ε-caprolactone) electrospun scaffold. They utilized *micropatterned collector-based electrospinning* technique to fabricate 2D membranes with a varying range of pore sizes (24—250 μm and 24—190 μm). The membranes were further layered to form 3D scaffolds. Rat adipose mesenchymal stem cells were cultured on these small and large lattice scaffolds (Fig. 3.13) and were studied for their ability to differentiate into functional Islet-like cells (ILCs). After 20 days of culturing, clusters of ILCs with a diameter of 51.95 ± 10.90 μm were visible in the large lattice scaffolds, as opposed to

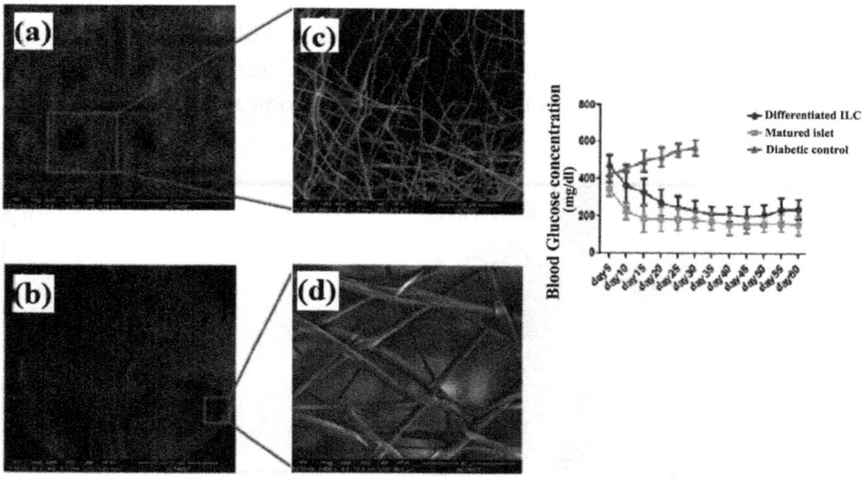

Figure 3.13 ESEM of small lattice and large lattice scaffold (a), (b); Fibers formed in the interspacing of small lattice and large lattice scaffold (c), (d). Time-dependent control of blood glucose levels in a diabetic rat model after implantation. *Modified figure from R. Anitha, D. Vaikkath, S. Shenoy, P. Nair, Tissue-engineered islet-like cell clusters generated from adipose tissue-derived stem cells on three-dimensional electrospun scaffolds can reverse diabetes in an experimental rat model and the role of porosity of scaffolds on cluster differentiation. J. Biomed. Mater. Res. 108 (3) (2020) 749—759. https://doi.org/10.1002/jbm.a.36854.*

ILC clusters with a diameter of 16.35 ± 3.86 μm in small lattice scaffolds. The in vivo studies were carried out in a rat model by transplanting ILC clusters of large lattice scaffolds. Mature islet seeded scaffolds were also implanted for comparative studies. Lowering of blood glucose levels was observed after 15 days by the mature islets, whereas it was regulated after 30 days in case of engineered ILC clusters. The studies also showed continuous release of insulin by the ILC clusters, which is necessary for controlling hyperglycemia (Fig. 3.13). Explantation after 60 days showed the presence of blood vessels in the ILCs, thus proving the potential of "large lattice ILCs" in tissue-engineered pancreatic islets [80].

The discussion in this section reveals the high potential of electrospinning technique in regenerating anatomically complex tissues by incorporating various gradient designs in the scaffolds and embedding them with appropriate functional moieties. Table 3.1 gives a brief account of the various types of electrospinning materials used for reengineering different types of tissues. Next, we discuss the market of electrospun materials; highlighting their role in the field of tissue engineering.

3.3 Commercial electrospun grafts

The detailed studies on the tissue engineering scaffolds via electrospinning and its high success rate opened this field for its industry scale-up. The industry custom designs the scaffolds to match the required commercial applications. *Nanofiber solutions* produces aligned or random PCL nanofibers to be integrated into different types of cell culture vessels. *NanoAligned*^{TM} is designed to mimic the white matter within the brain, the central nervous system, the cardiac tissue, the skeletal muscle, etc., while *NanoECM* is designed for working with stem cells. The company also develops veterinary products for wound healing, *NanoCare* and injectable fibers, *NanoWhiskers* [100]. *Neotherix* [101] innovates bioresorbable scaffolds for soft tissue repair and therapy. The company has evolved greatly with its scaffolds for periodontal diseases and skin cancer. Versatility in the forms of electrospun polymeric fibers is achieved by *AVflo* by Nicast company [102] specialized for creating single or multilayered meshes, films, gels, and coatings. Its unique nanofibrous graft, *AVflo* is made of medical-grade biocompatible poly(carbonate—urea) urethane, PCU, and proves to be a superior alternative to hemodialysis. A highly cost-effective methodology for developing multilayered and blended nanofibers is adopted by the Stellenbosch Nanofiber Company. Their patented Ball ElectroSpinning Technology, *SNC*

Table 3.1 The fibrous scaffold morphology achieved via different ES techniques.

S. No.	Electrospinning type	Fiber morphology	Materials used	Tissues engineering applications	Reference
1.	Dual extrusion ES	Aligned and alternating micro- and nanofibers	PLA/HAP	Human osteoblasts	[24]
		Aligned nanofibers	Chitosan/PLA/human-like collagen	Vascular tissue engineering	[83]
		Porous nanofibers	PCL/tricalcium phosphate nanoparticles	Mouse preosteoblast cells	[84]
		Microfibrous mats	Chitosan-*g*-oligo/polylactide copolymer, containing collagen/gelatin proteins	Potential for hollow organ tissues of trachea, urethra, etc.	[85]
		Microfibers	Poly(ethylene oxide terephthalate)/poly(butylene terephthalate) (PEOT/PBT) copolymer	Human mesenchymal stem cells hMSCs and human immortalized dermal keratinocyte HaCaT cell line	[86]
2.	Melt ES	Porous microtubes	PCL	Primary human osteoblasts, mesothelial cells, mouse osteoblasts	[87]
		Micro- and nanofibers	Poly(L-lactide-co-E–caprolactone)	Vascular tissue engineering	[88]
		Aligned, crimped, and random topologies	PCL	Ligament tissue engineering	[70]

		Microfibers	PCL	Osteoblasts (MG63), keratinocytes (HaCaT), and fibroblasts	[89]
		Microfibers	PCL	Endometrial mesenchymal stem/stromal cells (eMSCs)	[90]
3.	Cryogenic ES	Hierarchy of pores, ranging from micrometer to nanometer in size	PCL	Rat kidney cells	[46]
		Microfibers	PCL	Human kidney epithelial cells	[48]
		Porous microfibers	Silk	Human foreskin fibroblasts, human oral keratinocyte, human foreskin keratinocytes	[91]
		Porous microfibers	Poly(D,L-lactide)	Fibroblasts	[92]
		Porous microfibers	Poly(lactide-co-glycolide)	Human mesenchymal stem cells	[93]
4.	Micropatterned collector–based ES	Hierarchical fibers with varying geometric cues	PCL	MG-63 osteoblast-like cells	[25]
		Hierarchical fibrous scaffolds	Poly(ethylene glycol)-poly(D,L-lactide)	Cardiomyoblasts, cardiac fibroblasts, and endothelial cells	[65]
		Smooth-random and aligned nanofibers	Polyamide-66	Chondrocytes	[94]
		Patterned microfibers			[95]

(Continued)

Table 3.1 The fibrous scaffold morphology achieved via different ES techniques.—cont'd

S. No.	Electrospinning type	Fiber morphology	Materials used	Tissues engineering applications	Reference
			Poly(ethylene glycol)-poly(D,L-lactide)	Coculture of hepatocytes with fibroblasts and endothelial cell	
		Aligned microfibers	Copper sulfide nanoparticles—PLA/PCL	Human dermal fibroblasts, human umbilical vein endothelial cells, skin tumor cells	[96]
5.	Near-field ES	Porous nanofibers	PCL/borate bioactive glass composite	Mesenchymal stem cells	[30]
		Aligned microfibers	Alginate/poly(ethylene oxide)	Human embryonic kidney cells	[97]
		Random and aligned microfibers	PCL/collagen	Human periodontal ligament stem cells	[35]
		3D microfibers	Polydioxanone (PDO)	Human gingival fibroblasts	[98]
		Nano- and microfibers	M13 bacteriophage	Highly potential candidates for tissue regeneration	[29]
		Orthogonally aligned and interconnected microfibers	PCL/collagen	Highly potential candidates for tissue regeneration	[99]

BEST utilizes self-optimization and self-arrangement of the jets by employing its free surface spinning property. Depending on the type of polymer and solvent, it is able to achieve the production rate up to kilograms per hour. The company extends its services for tissue engineering scaffolds and wound dressings [103].

PolyRemedy also addresses the issues related to wound repair and management by combining healthcare information technology with personalized therapeutics. They offer *HealSmart Dressings* made from their patented fiber technology [104]. A versatile range of nanofibrous products, manufactured at BioSurfaces Inc., are being successfully used in the 3D tissue biofabrication. Many of its implantable products like *NuSpun*—Vascular Graft for kidney disease, Small-Diameter Artificial Artery, Artificial Heart Assist Device Conduit, etc., have completed the preclinical trials [105]. *3D Insert*, commercialized by *3DBiotek*, is a highly porous scaffold ideal for early drug screening of oncology. PCL, polystyrene, and poly(lactic-co-glycolic) acid are the polymers mainly used for its fabrication. The insert utilizes the gradient micro- and nanoscale architecture to reproduce the conditions suitable for cancer epithelium and stroma tissue growth. It is well suited for epithelial—stromal invasion studies [106].

The recent and ongoing research in the field of 3D electrospinning is being continuously implemented in the industry to bring out more effective tissue-engineered products. New researches in this field are focused on imparting "smart" characteristics to the electrospun fibers.

3.4 Conclusion and future perspectives

A number of hard and soft tissues are being successfully regenerated in the electrospun scaffolds, owing to varied and well-optimized process conditions in this technique. The use of electrospun scaffolds in the new field of REPROTEN and cancer therapy is showing promising results. Studies have also shown the incorporation of native cellular features; such as the rete ridges in the reengineered skin tissue. Another study into skin tissue engineering involved the use of ionic liquids for dissolution of the biopolymer straight from its source, thus ensuring reduced carbon footprint with minimal wastes. This green method has paved way for the development of nanofibrous patches, which efficiently release various drugs like gentamycin sulfate for treatment of different skin conditions like wounds, eczema, burns, etc. Developments in this sustainable technology of utilizing ionic liquids are presently being employed by Mari-Signum, Mid-Atlantic; which can lead to high quality, low-cost scaffolds; that could be exploited in a number of tissue engineering applications. Self-standing 3D scaffold structures are obtained by the recent development in 3D Electrospinning machine which reads the computer-generated code, containing instructions on the flow rate of the polymer, the movement of the nozzle, its path and speed; the working distance between the nozzle and the collector, the movement of the collector, voltage, and time. Control on the orientation of electrospun nanofibers into well-defined shapes and directional alignment have favored the successful regeneration of many tissues.

Adding a fourth dimension to the 3D scaffolds can bring about a huge change in the field of tissue engineering. These smart materials, the 4D scaffolds, can perform a certain function on encountering an external stimulus. They can, for example, release insulin on sudden increase or decrease in blood glucose levels, thus enhancing the rate of patient's survival. Their ability to bring a revolution in the field of healthcare cannot be looked upon. The progressing field of developing tissue-engineered engrafts with the aid of electrospinning technology has greatly influenced its successful implementation for tissue and organ functionality restoration. Efforts are still on among research groups for the development of more closely biomimicking and advanced hierarchical artificial tissue support system for complex tissues and tissue sites with the integration of electrospinning technology.

Conflict of interest

The authors declare no conflict of interest.

Acknowledgment

We acknowledge the support from MHRD (Govt. of India) to Ms. Aakriti Aggarwal, one of the coauthors for the completion of this chapter.

References

[1] S.K. Chandrasekhar, F.G. Thankam, D.K. Agrawal, J.C. Ouseph, Interface biology of stem cell—driven tissue engineering, in: Biointegration of Medical Implant Materials, Elsevier, 2020, pp. 19—44, https://doi.org/10.1016/B978-0-08-102680-9.00002-0.

[2] A. Eltom, G. Zhong, A. Muhammad, Scaffold techniques and designs in tissue engineering functions and purposes: a review [WWW document], Ann. Mater. Sci. Eng. 2019 (2019), https://doi.org/10.1155/2019/3429527. Article ID 3429527.

[3] J. Lannutti, D. Reneker, T. Ma, D. Tomasko, D. Farson, Electrospinning for tissue engineering scaffolds, Mater. Sci. Eng. C, Next Gen. Biomater. 27 (2007) 504—509, https://doi.org/10.1016/j.msec.2006.05.019.

[4] Y. Li, T. Bou-Akl, Electrospinning in tissue engineering, Electrospinning - Mater. Tech. Biomed. Appl. (2016) 117—139, https://doi.org/10.5772/65836.

[5] U.K. Roopavath, M.K. Sah, B.B. Panigrahi, S.N. Rath, Mechanochemically synthesized phase stable and biocompatible β-tricalcium phosphate from avian eggshell for the development of tissue ingrowth system, Ceram. Int. 45 (10) (2019) 12910–12919.
[6] M.K. Sah, S.N. Rath, Soluble eggshell membrane: a natural protein to improve the properties of biomaterials used for tissue engineering applications, Mater. Sci. Eng. C 67 (2016) 807–821.
[7] S. Yang, K.-F. Leong, Z. Du, C.-K. Chua, The design of scaffolds for use in tissue engineering. Part I. Traditional factors, Tissue Eng. 7 (2001) 679–689, https://doi.org/10.1089/107632701753337645.
[8] S.J. Hollister, Porous scaffold design for tissue engineering, Nat. Mater. 4 (2005) 518–524, https://doi.org/10.1038/nmat1421.
[9] C. Agrawal, J. McKinney, D. Huang, K. Athanasiou, The use of the vibrating particle technique to fabricate highly porous and permeable biodegradable scaffolds, in: C. Agrawal, J. Parr, S. Lin (Eds.), Synthetic Bioabsorbable Polymers for Implants. ASTM International, 100 Barr Harbor Drive, PO Box C700, West Conshohocken, PA, 2000, https://doi.org/10.1520/STP15303S, 19428-2959, pp. 99–99–16.
[10] L. Roseti, V. Parisi, M. Petretta, C. Cavallo, G. Desando, I. Bartolotti, B. Grigolo, Scaffolds for bone tissue engineering: state of the art and new perspectives, Mater. Sci. Eng. C Mater. Biol. Appl. 78 (2017) 1246–1262, https://doi.org/10.1016/j.msec.2017.05.017.
[11] Y.S. Nam, T.G. Park, Porous biodegradable polymeric scaffolds prepared by thermally induced phase separation, J. Biomed. Mater. Res. 47 (1999) 8–17, https://doi.org/10.1002/(SICI)1097-4636(199910)47:1<8::AID-JBM2>3.0.CO;2-L.
[12] O.A. Abdelaal, S.M. Darwish, Review of rapid prototyping techniques for tissue engineering scaffolds fabrication, in: Characterization and Development of Biosystems and Biomaterials, Springer, 2013, pp. 33–54.
[13] J.T. Rimell, P.M. Marquis, Selective laser sintering of ultra high molecular weight polyethylene for clinical applications, J. Biomed. Mater. Res. 53 (2000) 414–420.
[14] P. Zhao, H. Gu, H.-Y. Mi, C. Rao, J. Fu, L.-S. Turng, Fabrication of scaffolds in tissue engineering: a review, Front. Mech. Eng. 1–13 (2017), https://doi.org/10.1007/s11465-018-0496-8.
[15] I. Jun, H.-S. Han, J.R. Edwards, H. Jeon, Electrospun fibrous scaffolds for tissue engineering: viewpoints on architecture and fabrication, Int. J. Mol. Sci. 19 (2018) 745, https://doi.org/10.3390/ijms19030745.
[16] D.M. Correia, C. Ribeiro, J.C. Ferreira, G. Botelho, J.L.G. Ribelles, S. Lanceros-Méndez, V. Sencadas, Influence of electrospinning parameters on poly (hydroxybutyrate) electrospun membranes fiber size and distribution, Polym. Eng. Sci. 54 (2014) 1608–1617.
[17] M. Mirjalili, S. Zohoori, Review for application of electrospinning and electrospun nanofibers technology in textile industry, J. Nanostructure Chem. 6 (2016) 207–213.
[18] A.S. Motamedi, H. Mirzadeh, F. Hajiesmaeilbaigi, S. Bagheri-Khoulenjani, M. Shokrgozar, Effect of electrospinning parameters on morphological properties of PVDF nanofibrous scaffolds, Prog. Biomater. 6 (2017) 113–123.
[19] M. Zafar, S. Najeeb, Z. Khurshid, M. Vazirzadeh, S. Zohaib, B. Najeeb, F. Sefat, Potential of electrospun nanofibers for biomedical and dental applications, Materials 9 (2016) 73.
[20] S. Chen, B. Liu, M.A. Carlson, A.F. Gombart, D.A. Reilly, J. Xie, Recent advances in electrospun nanofibers for wound healing, Nanomedicine 12 (2017) 1335–1352.

[21] S. Gnavi, B.E. Fornasari, C. Tonda-Turo, R. Laurano, M. Zanetti, G. Ciardelli, S. Geuna, The effect of electrospun gelatin fibers alignment on schwann cell and axon behavior and organization in the perspective of artificial nerve design, Int. J. Mol. Sci. 16 (2015) 12925−12942.
[22] N. Reznikov, R. Shahar, S. Weiner, Bone hierarchical structure in three dimensions, Acta Biomater. 10 (2014) 3815−3826.
[23] H. Qu, H. Fu, Z. Han, Y. Sun, Biomaterials for bone tissue engineering scaffolds: a review, RSC Adv. 9 (2019) 26252−26262, https://doi.org/10.1039/C9RA05214C.
[24] V.A. Apalangya, V.K. Rangari, B.J. Tiimob, S. Jeelani, T. Samuel, Eggshell based nano-engineered hydroxyapatite and poly(lactic) acid electrospun fibers as potential tissue scaffold [WWW document], Int. J. Biomater. 2019 (2019), https://doi.org/10.1155/2019/6762575. Article ID 6762575.
[25] F. Hejazi, H. Mirzadeh, N. Contessi, M.C. Tanzi, S. Faré, Novel class of collector in electrospinning device for the fabrication of 3D nanofibrous structure for large defect load-bearing tissue engineering application: helical spring collector for highly porous 3D electrospun scaffolds, J. Biomed. Mater. Res. 105 (2017) 1535−1548, https://doi.org/10.1002/jbm.a.35822.
[26] Y. Zhou, Z. Hu, D. Du, G.Z. Tan, The effects of collector geometry on the internal structure of the 3D nanofiber scaffold fabricated by divergent electrospinning, Int. J. Adv. Manuf. Technol. 100 (2019) 3045−3054, https://doi.org/10.1007/s00170-018-2899-4.
[27] R. Sedghi, A. Shaabani, N. Sayyari, Electrospun triazole-based chitosan nanofibers as a novel scaffolds for bone tissue repair and regeneration, Carbohydr. Polym. 230 (2020) 115707, https://doi.org/10.1016/j.carbpol.2019.115707.
[28] Alexander R. Nagle, Cormac D. Fay, Zhigang Xie, Gordan G. Wallance, Xungai Wang, Micheal J. Higgins., A direct 3D suspension near-field electrospinning technique for the fabrication of polymer nanoarrays, Nanotechnology 30 (2019), https://doi.org/10.1088/1361-6528/ab011b, 195301−195301.
[29] R. Sugimoto, J. Hun Lee, J.-H. Lee, H.-E. Jin, S. Young Yoo, S.-W. Lee, Bacteriophage nanofiber fabrication using near field electrospinning, RSC Adv. 9 (2019) 39111−39118, https://doi.org/10.1039/C9RA07510K.
[30] K. Kolan, J. Li, S. Roberts, J. Semon, J. Park, D. Day, M.-C. Leu, Near-field electrospinning of a polymer/bioactive glass composite to fabricate 3D biomimetic structures, Int. J. Bioprinting 5 (2019), https://doi.org/10.18063/ijb.v5i1.163.
[31] B. Zhang, N. Kasoju, Q. Li, J. Ma, A. Yang, Z. Cui, H. Wang, H. Ye, Effect of substrate topography and chemistry on human mesenchymal stem cell markers: a transcriptome study, Inter. J. Stem Cells 12 (1) (2019) 84.
[32] Z. Cui, J. Lin, C. Zhan, J. Wu, S. Shen, J. Si, Q. Wang, Biomimetic composite scaffolds based on surface modification of polydopamine on ultrasonication induced cellulose nanofibrils (CNF) adsorbing onto electrospun thermoplastic polyurethane (TPU) nanofibers, J. Biomater. Sci. Polym. Ed. (2020) 561−577.
[33] S.-J. Seo, H.-W. Kim, J.-H. Lee, Electrospun nanofibers applications in dentistry, J. Nanomater. 2016 (2016) 1−7, https://doi.org/10.1155/2016/5931946.
[34] G.M. Ahmed, E.A. Abouauf, N. AbuBakr, C.E. Dörfer, K.F. El-Sayed, Tissue engineering approaches for enamel, dentin, and pulp regeneration: an update [WWW document], Stem Cell. Int. 2020 (2020), https://doi.org/10.1155/2020/5734539. Article ID 5734539.
[35] X. Chen, Y. Liu, L. Miao, Y. Wang, S. Ren, X. Yang, Y. Hu, W. Sun, Controlled release of recombinant human cementum protein 1 from electrospun multiphasic scaffold for cementum regeneration, Int. J. Nanomed. 11 (2016) 3145−3158, https://doi.org/10.2147/IJN.S104324.

[36] C.-C. Chen, S.-Y. Lee, N.-C. Teng, H.-T. Hu, P.-C. Huang, J.-C. Yang, In vitro and in vivo studies of hydrophilic electrospun PLA95/β-TCP membranes for guided tissue regeneration (GTR) applications, Nanomaterials 9 (2019) 599, https://doi.org/10.3390/nano9040599.
[37] D.M. Zhao, Y.X. Wang, R.W. Xu, G. Wu, L.Q. Zhang, D.S. Yu, F.Z. Cui, D.F. Chen, W. Tian, Composition-graded films of fluoroapatite/PHB fabricated via electrospinning for tissue engineering, J. Bioact. Compat Polym. 22 (2007) 379–393, https://doi.org/10.1177/0883911507079802.
[38] G. Sandri, S. Rossi, M.C. Bonferoni, D. Miele, A. Faccendini, E. Del Favero, E. Di Cola, A. Icaro Cornaglia, C. Boselli, T. Luxbacher, L. Malavasi, L. Cantu', F. Ferrari, Chitosan/glycosaminoglycan scaffolds for skin reparation, Carbohydr. Polym. 220 (2019) 219–227, https://doi.org/10.1016/j.carbpol.2019.05.069.
[39] J.M. Ameer, A.K. PR, N. Kasoju, Strategies to tune electrospun scaffold porosity for effective cell response in tissue engineering, J. Funct. Biomater. 10 (2019) 30.
[40] T. Weng, P. Wu, W. Zhang, Y. Zheng, Q. Li, R. Jin, H. Chen, C. You, S. Guo, C. Han, X. Wang, Regeneration of skin appendages and nerves: current status and further challenges, J. Transl. Med. 18 (2020) 53, https://doi.org/10.1186/s12967-020-02248-5.
[41] B.N. Blackstone, M.M. Malara, M.E. Baumann, K.L. McFarland, D.M. Supp, H.M. Powell, Fractional CO_2 laser micropatterning of cell-seeded electrospun collagen scaffolds enables rete ridge formation in 3D engineered skin, Acta Biomater. 102 (2020) 287–297, https://doi.org/10.1016/j.actbio.2019.11.051.
[42] S. Bongiovanni Abel, F. Montini Ballarin, G.A. Abraham, Combination of electrospinning with other techniques for the fabrication of 3D polymeric and composite nanofibrous scaffolds with improved cellular interactions, Nanotechnology 31 (2020) 172002, https://doi.org/10.1088/1361-6528/ab6ab4.
[43] L. Sartore, S. Pandini, K. Dey, F. Bignotti, F. Chiellini, A versatile cell-friendly approach to produce PLA-based 3D micro-macro-porous blends for tissue engineering scaffolds, Materialia 9 (2020) 100615, https://doi.org/10.1016/j.mtla.2020.100615.
[44] M. Sheikholeslam, M.E.E. Wright, N. Cheng, H.H. Oh, Y. Wang, A.K. Datu, J.P. Santerre, S. Amini-Nik, M.G. Jeschke, Electrospun polyurethane–gelatin composite: a new tissue-engineered scaffold for application in skin regeneration and repair of complex wounds, ACS Biomater. Sci. Eng. 6 (2020) 505–516, https://doi.org/10.1021/acsbiomaterials.9b00861.
[45] A.F. Tarantal, C.A. Batchelder, Scaffolds for kidney tissue engineering, in: Handbook of Tissue Engineering Scaffolds, Volume Two, Elsevier, 2019, pp. 477–492, https://doi.org/10.1016/B978-0-08-102561-1.00020-8.
[46] T.P. Burton, A. Callanan, A non-woven path: electrospun poly(lactic acid) scaffolds for kidney tissue engineering, Tissue Eng. Regen. Med. 15 (2018) 301–310, https://doi.org/10.1007/s13770-017-0107-5.
[47] W. Li, L. Shi, K. Zhou, X. Zhang, I. Ullah, H. Ou, W. Zhang, T. Wu, Facile fabrication of porous polymer fibers via cryogenic electrospinning system, J. Mater. Process. Technol. 266 (2019) 551–557, https://doi.org/10.1016/j.jmatprotec.2018.11.035.
[48] T.P. Burton, A. Corcoran, A. Callanan, The effect of electrospun polycaprolactone scaffold morphology on human kidney epithelial cells, Biomed. Mater. 13 (2017) 015006, https://doi.org/10.1088/1748-605X/aa8dde.
[49] K. Jansen, M. Castilho, S. Aarts, M.M. Kaminski, S.S. Lienkamp, R. Pichler, J. Malda, T. Vermonden, J. Jansen, R. Masereeuw, Fabrication of kidney proximal tubule grafts using biofunctionalized electrospun polymer scaffolds, Macromol. Biosci. 19 (2019) 1800412, https://doi.org/10.1002/mabi.201800412.

[50] H. Zhang, F. Tasnim, J.Y. Ying, D. Zink, The impact of extracellular matrix coatings on the performance of human renal cells applied in bioartificial kidneys, Biomaterials 30 (2009) 2899–2911.

[51] R. Sobreiro-Almeida, D. Fonseca, N. Neves, Extracellular matrix electrospun membranes for mimicking natural renal filtration barriers, Mater. Sci. Eng. C 103 (2019) 109866. 6. https://doi.org/10.1016/j.msec.2019.109866.

[52] N. Ashammakhi, H.-J. Kim, A. Ehsanipour, R.D. Bierman, O. Kaarela, C. Xue, A. Khademhosseini, S.K. Seidlits, Regenerative therapies for spinal cord injury, Tissue Eng. B Rev. 25 (2019) 471–491, https://doi.org/10.1089/ten.teb.2019.0182.

[53] X. Li, Z. Chen, H. Zhang, Y. Zhuang, H. Shen, Y. Chen, Y. Zhao, B. Chen, Z. Xiao, J. Dai, Aligned scaffolds with biomolecular gradients for regenerative medicine, Polymers 11 (2019) 341, https://doi.org/10.3390/polym11020341.

[54] F. Rao, Z. Yuan, M. Li, F. Yu, X. Fang, B. Jiang, Y. Wen, P. Zhang, Expanded 3D nanofibre sponge scaffolds by gas-foaming technique enhance peripheral nerve regeneration, Artif. Cells Nanomedicine Biotechnol 47 (2019) 491–500, https://doi.org/10.1080/21691401.2018.1557669.

[55] M. Nune, A. Subramanian, U.M. Krishnan, S. Sethuraman, Peptide nanostructures on nanofibers for peripheral nerve regeneration, J. Tissue Eng. Regen. Med. term 2860 (2019), https://doi.org/10.1002/term.2860.

[56] T.C. Holmes, S. de Lacalle, X. Su, G. Liu, A. Rich, S. Zhang, Extensive neurite outgrowth and active synapse formation on self-assembling peptide scaffolds, Proc. Natl. Acad. Sci. Unit. States Am. 97 (2000) 6728–6733.

[57] C. Chen, J. Tang, Y. Gu, L. Liu, X. Liu, L. Deng, C. Martins, B. Sarmento, W. Cui, L. Chen, Bioinspired hydrogel electrospun fibers for spinal cord regeneration, Adv. Funct. Mater. 29 (2019) 1806899, https://doi.org/10.1002/adfm.201806899.

[58] B. Vigani, S. Rossi, G. Sandri, M.C. Bonferoni, M. Rui, S. Collina, F. Fagiani, C. Lanni, F. Ferrari, Dual-functioning scaffolds for the treatment of spinal cord injury: alginate nanofibers loaded with the Sigma 1 receptor (S1R) agonist RC-33 in chitosan films, Mar. Drugs 18 (2019) 21, https://doi.org/10.3390/md18010021.

[59] H. Juul Belling, W. Hofmeister, D.C. Andersen, A systematic exposition of methods used for quantification of heart regeneration after apex resection in zebrafish, Cells 9 (2020) 548, https://doi.org/10.3390/cells9030548.

[60] H. Sadek, E.N. Olson, Toward the goal of human heart regeneration, Cell Stem Cell 26 (2020) 7–16, https://doi.org/10.1016/j.stem.2019.12.004.

[61] M. Du, J. Gu, J. Wang, Y. Xue, Y. Ma, X. Mo, S. Xue, Silk fibroin/poly(L-lactic acid-co-ε-caprolactone) electrospun nanofibrous scaffolds exert a protective effect following myocardial infarction, Exp. Ther. Med. 17 (5) (2019) 3989–3998, https://doi.org/10.3892/etm.2019.7405.

[62] A. Bar, S. Cohen, Inducing endogenous cardiac regeneration: can biomaterials connect the dots? Front. Bioeng. Biotechnol. 8 (2020) https://doi.org/10.3389/fbioe.2020.00126.

[63] F. Flaig, H. Ragot, A. Simon, G. Revet, M. Kitsara, L. Kitasato, A. Hébraud, O. Agbulut, G. Schlatter, Design of functional electrospun scaffolds based on poly(-glycerol sebacate) elastomer and poly(lactic acid) for cardiac tissue engineering, ACS Biomater. Sci. Eng. Acsbiomaterials 6 (4) (2020) 2388–2400, https://doi.org/10.1021/acsbiomaterials.0c00243, 0c00243.

[64] M. Coffee, S. Biswanath, E. Bolesani, R. Zweigerdt, Heart muscle tissue engineering, in: B. Brand-Saberi (Ed.), Essential Current Concepts in Stem Cell Biology, Learning Materials in Biosciences, Springer International Publishing, Cham, 2020, pp. 99–121, https://doi.org/10.1007/978-3-030-33923-4_6.

[65] Y. Liu, G. Xu, J. Wei, Q. Wu, X. Li, Cardiomyocyte coculture on layered fibrous scaffolds assembled from micropatterned electrospun mats, Mater. Sci. Eng. C 81 (2017) 500–510, https://doi.org/10.1016/j.msec.2017.08.042.
[66] N. Adadi, M. Yadid, I. Gal, M. Asulin, R. Feiner, R. Edri, T. Dvir, Electrospun fibrous PVDF-TrFe scaffolds for cardiac tissue engineering, differentiation, and maturation, Adv. Mater. Technol. 5 (2020) 1900820, https://doi.org/10.1002/admt.201900820.
[67] W.L. Lim, L.L. Liau, M.H. Ng, S.R. Chowdhury, J.X. Law, Current progress in tendon and ligament tissue engineering, Tissue Eng. Regen. Med. 16 (2019) 549–571, https://doi.org/10.1007/s13770-019-00196-w.
[68] D. Ramos, M.S. Peach, A.D. Mazzocca, X. Yu, S.G. Kumbar, Tendon tissue engineering, in: Regenerative Engineering of Musculoskeletal Tissues and Interfaces, Elsevier, 2015, pp. 195–217, https://doi.org/10.1016/B978-1-78242-301-0.00008-2.
[69] W. Yang, H. Li, X. Chen, Melt electrospinning, in: Electrospinning: Nanofabrication and Applications, Elsevier, 2019, pp. 339–361, https://doi.org/10.1016/B978-0-323-51270-1.00011-X.
[70] M. Gwiazda, S. Kumar, W. Świeszkowski, S. Ivanovski, C. Vaquette, The effect of melt electrospun writing fiber orientation onto cellular organization and mechanical properties for application in Anterior Cruciate Ligament tissue engineering, J. Mech. Behav. Biomed. Mater. 104 (2020) 103631, https://doi.org/10.1016/j.jmbbm.2020.103631.
[71] J. Cai, J. Wang, K. Ye, D. Li, C. Ai, D. Sheng, W. Jin, X. Liu, Y. Zhi, J. Jiang, J. Chen, X. Mo, S. Chen, Dual-layer aligned-random nanofibrous scaffolds for improving gradient microstructure of tendon-to-bone healing in a rabbit extra-articular model, Int. J. Nanomed. 13 (2018) 3481–3492, https://doi.org/10.2147/IJN.S165633.
[72] Y. Zhang, Z. Zhang, Y. Wang, Y. Su, M. Chen, 3D myotube guidance on hierarchically organized anisotropic and conductive fibers for skeletal muscle tissue engineering, Mater. Sci. Eng. C 116 (2020) 111070. https://doi.org/10.1016/j.msec.2020.111070.
[73] H. Campo, X. Santamaria, I. Cervelló, C. Simón, Scaffolds for bioengineered uterus, in: Handbook of Tissue Engineering Scaffolds, Volume Two, Elsevier, 2019, pp. 283–316, https://doi.org/10.1016/B978-0-08-102561-1.00011-7.
[74] Y. Jahanbani, S. Davaran, M. Ghahremani-Nasab, L. Aghebati-Maleki, M. Yousefi, Scaffold-based tissue engineering approaches in treating infertility, Life Sci. 240 (2020) 117066, https://doi.org/10.1016/j.lfs.2019.117066.
[75] S. Mukherjee, S. Darzi, K. Paul, F.L. Cousins, J.A. Werkmeister, C.E. Gargett, Electrospun nanofiber meshes with endometrial MSCs modulate foreign body response by increased angiogenesis, matrix synthesis, and anti-inflammatory gene expression in mice: implication in pelvic floor, Front. Pharmacol. 11 (2020), https://doi.org/10.3389/fphar.2020.00353.
[76] M.Z. Kashani, Z. Bagher, H.R. Asgari, M. Najafi, M. Koruji, F. Mehraein, Differentiation of neonate mouse spermatogonial stem cells on three-dimensional agar/polyvinyl alcohol nanofiber scaffold, Syst. Biol. Reprod. Med. 0 (2020) 1–14, https://doi.org/10.1080/19396368.2020.1725927.
[77] Z.I. Foraida, T. Kamaldinov, D.A. Nelson, M. Larsen, J. Castracane, Elastin-PLGA hybrid electrospun nanofiber scaffolds for salivary epithelial cell self-organization and polarization, Acta Biomater. 62 (2017) 116–127, https://doi.org/10.1016/j.actbio.2017.08.009.

[78] H.-S. Shin, H.J. Hong, W.-G. Koh, J.-Y. Lim, Organotypic 3D culture in Nanoscaffold microwells supports salivary gland stem-cell-based organization, ACS Biomater. Sci. Eng. 4 (2018) 4311–4320, https://doi.org/10.1021/acsbiomaterials.8b00894.
[79] M. Ojaghi, F. Soleimanifar, A. Kazemi, M. Ghollasi, M. Soleimani, N. Nasoohi, S.E. Enderami, Electrospun poly-l-lactic acid/polyvinyl alcohol nanofibers improved insulin-producing cell differentiation potential of human adipose-derived mesenchymal stem cells, J. Cell. Biochem. 120 (2019) 9917–9926, https://doi.org/10.1002/jcb.28274.
[80] R. Anitha, D. Vaikkath, S.J. Shenoy, P.D. Nair, Tissue-engineered islet-like cell clusters generated from adipose tissue-derived stem cells on three-dimensional electrospun scaffolds can reverse diabetes in an experimental rat model and the role of porosity of scaffolds on cluster differentiation, J. Biomed. Mater. Res. 108 (2020) 749–759, https://doi.org/10.1002/jbm.a.36854.
[81] N. Kasoju, J. George, H. Ye, Z. Cui, Sacrificial core-based electrospinning: a facile and versatile approach to fabricate devices for potential cell and tissue encapsulation applications, Nanomaterials 8 (2018) 863.
[82] G. Barati, A. rahmani, S. Nadri, In vitro differentiation of conjunctiva mesenchymal stem cells into insulin producing cells on natural and synthetic electrospun scaffolds, Biologicals 62 (2019) 33–38, https://doi.org/10.1016/j.biologicals.2019.10.004.
[83] C. Zhu, X. Ma, L. Xian, Y. Zhou, D. Fan, Characterization of a co-electrospun scaffold of HLC/CS/PLA for vascular tissue engineering, Bio Med. Mater. Eng. 24 (2014) 1999–2005, https://doi.org/10.3233/BME-141009.
[84] C. Erisken, D.M. Kalyon, H. Wang, Functionally graded electrospun polycaprolactone and β-tricalcium phosphate nanocomposites for tissue engineering applications, Biomaterials 29 (2008) 4065–4073, https://doi.org/10.1016/j.biomaterials.2008.06.022.
[85] S. Demina, T.,S. Kuryanova, A.,A. Aksenova, N.,G. Shubnyy, A.,N. Popyrina, T.,V. Sokovikov, Y.,V. Istranova, E.,L. Ivanov, P.,S. Timashev, P.,T.A. Akopova, Chitosan- g -oligo/polylactide copolymer non-woven fibrous mats containing protein: from solid-state synthesis to electrospinning, RSC Adv. 9 (2019) 37652–37659, https://doi.org/10.1039/C9RA07667K.
[86] C. Günday, S. Anand, H.B. Gencer, S. Munafò, L. Moroni, A. Fusco, G. Donnarumma, C. Ricci, P.C. Hatir, N.G. Türeli, A.E. Türeli, C. Mota, S. Danti, Ciprofloxacin-loaded polymeric nanoparticles incorporated electrospun fibers for drug delivery in tissue engineering applications, Drug Deliv. Transl. Res (2020) 706–720, https://doi.org/10.1007/s13346-020-00736-1.
[87] T.D. Brown, A. Slotosch, L. Thibaudeau, A. Taubenberger, D. Loessner, C. Vaquette, P.D. Dalton, D.W. Hutmacher, Design and fabrication of tubular scaffolds via direct writing in a melt electrospinning mode, Biointerphases 7 (2012) 13, https://doi.org/10.1007/s13758-011-0013-7.
[88] S. Chung, N.P. Ingle, G.A. Montero, S.H. Kim, M.W. King, Bioresorbable elastomeric vascular tissue engineering scaffolds via melt spinning and electrospinning, Acta Biomater. 6 (2010) 1958–1967, https://doi.org/10.1016/j.actbio.2009.12.007.
[89] A. Fuchs, A. Youssef, A. Seher, S. Hartmann, R.C. Brands, U.D.A. Müller-Richter, A.C. Kübler, C. Linz, A new multilayered membrane for tissue engineering of oral hard- and soft tissue by means of melt electrospinning writing and film casting – an in vitro study, J. Cranio-Maxillo-Fac. Surg. 47 (2019) 695–703, https://doi.org/10.1016/j.jcms.2019.01.043.
[90] K. Paul, S. Darzi, G. Mcphee, M.D. Borgo, J.A. Werkmeister, C.E. Gargett, S. Mukherjee, 3D Bioprinted Endometrial Stem Cells on Melt Electrospun PCL Meshes for Pelvic Floor Application Promote Anti-inflammatory Responses in Mice (SSRN Scholarly Paper No. ID 3387674), Social Science Research Network, Rochester, NY, 2019.

[91] A.A. Bulysheva, G.L. Bowlin, A.J. Klingelhutz, W.A. Yeudall, Low-temperature electrospun silk scaffold for in vitro mucosal modeling, J. Biomed. Mater. Res. A (2012) 757–767, https://doi.org/10.1002/jbm.a.33288.
[92] M.F. Leong, M.Z. Rasheed, T.C. Lim, K.S. Chian, In vitro cell infiltration and in vivo cell infiltration and vascularization in a fibrous, highly porous poly(D,L-lactide) scaffold fabricated by cryogenic electrospinning technique, J. Biomed. Mater. Res. 91 (1) (2009) 231–240, https://doi.org/10.1002/jbm.a.32208.
[93] O.D. Schneider, D. Mohn, R. Fuhrer, K. Klein, K. Kämpf, K.M. Nuss, M. Sidler, K. Zlinszky, B. von Rechenberg, W.J. Stark, Biocompatibility and bone formation of flexible, cotton wool-like PLGA/calcium phosphate nanocomposites in sheep, Open Orthop. J. 5 (2011) 63.
[94] N.S. Hosseini, N. Bölgen, N. Khenoussi, Ş.N. Yılmaz, D. Yetkin, A.H. Hekmati, L. Schacher, D. Adolphe, Novel 3D electrospun polyamide scaffolds prepared by 3D printed collectors and their interaction with chondrocytes, Int. J. Polym. Mater. Polym. Biomater. 67 (2018) 143–150, https://doi.org/10.1080/00914037.2017.1309541.
[95] Y. Liu, J. Wei, J. Lu, D. Lei, S. Yan, X. Li, Micropatterned coculture of hepatocytes on electrospun fibers as a potential in vitro model for predictive drug metabolism, Mater. Sci. Eng. C 63 (2016) 475–484, https://doi.org/10.1016/j.msec.2016.03.025.
[96] X. Wang, F. Lv, T. Li, Y. Han, Z. Yi, M. Liu, J. Chang, C. Wu, Electrospun Micropatterned Nanocomposites Incorporated with Cu2S Nanoflowers for Skin Tumor Therapy and Wound Healing [WWW Document], 2017, https://doi.org/10.1021/acsnano.7b05858.
[97] Y.-K. Fuh, Y.-C. Wu, Z.-Y. He, Z.-M. Huang, W.-W. Hu, The control of cell orientation using biodegradable alginate fibers fabricated by near-field electrospinning, Mater. Sci. Eng. C 62 (2016) 879–887, https://doi.org/10.1016/j.msec.2016.02.028.
[98] W.E. King, Y. Gillespie, K.L. Gilbert, G. Bowlin, Characterization of polydioxanone in near-field electrospinning, Polymers 12 (2020) 1, https://doi.org/10.3390/polym12010001.
[99] R. Middleton, X. Li, J. Shepherd, Z. Li, W. Wang, S.M. Best, R.E. Cameron, Y.Y.S. Huang, Near-field electrospinning patterning polycaprolactone and polycaprolactone/collagen interconnected fiber membrane, Macromol. Mater. Eng. 303 (2018) 1700463, https://doi.org/10.1002/mame.201700463.
[100] K. Dockman, Nanofiber solutions::3-D cell culture for a 3-D world, Nanofiber Solut (2020). URL, https://nanofibersolutions.com/technology/. accessed 4.14.20.
[101] Neotherix, Regenerative Scaffolds for Tissue Repair | Technology [WWW Document], 2020. URL, http://www.neotherix.com/technology.php. accessed 4.14.20.
[102] M. Ferraresso, E.M. Bortolani, G. Amnon, A two-year experience with a rapid access, self-sealing, polycarbonate urethane nanofiber vascular access graft for hemodialysis, J. Vasc. Access 17 (2016) 210–214.
[103] Electrospun Nanofiber Materials for the Biomedical Industry, SNC Fibers [WWW Document], SNC, 2020. URL, https://sncfibers.com. accessed 4.15.20.
[104] PolyRemedy, Personalized Dressings, 2020. URL, http://www.polyremedy.com/personalized-dressings/. accessed 4.24.20.
[105] Advanced Technologies [WWW Document], Biosurfaces, 2020. URL, https://www.biosurfaces.us/advanced-applications. accessed 4.15.20.
[106] 3D Biotek, 3D Insert Nanomesh [WWW Document], 2020. URL, http://3dbiotek.com/prod_3dnanomesh.aspx. accessed 4.15.20.

CHAPTER FOUR

From nonwoven fibers to woven nanotextiles: electrospinning in drug delivery

C.R. Reshmi, Shantikumar V. Nair, Deepthy Menon
Amrita Centre for Nanosciences and Molecular Medicine, Amrita Vishwa Vidyapeetham, Kochi, Kerala, India

Abbreviations

5-FU 5-fluorouracil
ALN Alendronate
CA Cellulose acetate
CEF Cephalexin
CTA Cetyltrimethylammonium bromide
DDS Drug delivery systems
DEX Dexamethasone
DOX Doxorubicin
EDC/NHS N-(3-dimethylaminopropyl)-N′-ethylcarbodiimide hydrochloride/ N-hydroxysuccinimide
HCPT Hydrophobic drug hydroxycamptothecin
HNTs Hallosite nanotubes
IMC Indomethacin
KAB Keyacid blue
KAU Keyacid uranine
LCST Lower critical solution temperature
NaCMC Sodium carboxymethyl cellulose
nHAp Nanohydroxyapatite
O/W Oil-in-water
PCL Poly(ε-caprolactone)
PDS Polydioxanone
PEG Poly(ethylene glycol)
PgP Poly(lactide-co-glycolide)-graft-polyethyleneimine
PL-DS Lecithin containing diclofenac sodium
PLGA Poly(L-lactide-co-glycolide)
PLLA Poly(L-lactic acid)
PMMA Poly(methylmethacrylate)
PNIPAM Poly(N-isopropyl acrylamide)
PTX Paclitaxel
PU Polyurethane
PVA Poly(vinyl alcohol)

Biomedical Applications of Electrospinning and Electrospraying
ISBN: 978-0-12-822476-2
https://doi.org/10.1016/B978-0-12-822476-2.00003-0

PVP Poly(vinyl pyrrolidine)
SDBS Sodium dodecylbenzenesulfonate
Span 80 Sorbitan monooleate
THY Thymol
TP Hydrophilic drug tea polyphenol
Tβ4 Thymosin beta-4
W/O Water-in-oil

4.1 Introduction

Implantable drug delivery systems (DDSs) have attracted immense interest for the site-specific delivery of therapeutic agents in a spatiotemporal manner. Localized drug delivery facilitated by such DDSs helps to avoid any unnecessary exposure of drug to nontarget tissues and also prevents systemic toxicity. Functional materials in various forms are utilized as implantable DDSs which include micro-/nanofibrous membranes [1], hydrogels [2], microporous scaffolds [3], microspheres/beads [4], etc. Among these, nonwoven micro-/nanofibrous membranes developed by electrospinning have gained considerable attention owing to the controlled and sustained drug release offered by these matrices [5]. Additionally, electrospun membranes have the unique advantages of high surface area-to-volume ratio, nanoscale architecture, good flexibility, suitability to incorporate different types of drugs in a wide range of polymers, etc [6]. Also, this matrix provides tunable drug-loading efficiency by altering the electrospinning process, choice of polymer and solvent [7].

Electrospun matrices have been successfully utilized as the platform for delivering a wide variety of therapeutic agents such as the antiinflammatory [8], antimicrobial [9], anticancer [10], cardiovascular [11], antihistamine [12], and gastrointestinal drugs [13]. The process of electrospinning does not compromise the bioactivity of drugs, and it also provides controlled and sustained drug release at the therapeutic site [14]. Moreover, encapsulation of the drugs within polymeric nanofibers protect them from degradation in adverse environments (e.g., stomach acid and intestinal fluid), with reduced side effects [15]. Easy tunability in drug loading and release through control of polymer type, membrane morphology, and architecture is yet another attractive feature of electrospun matrices over other conventional DDS [16,17]. These flexible nonwoven membranes find utility for drug delivery to any part of the human body ranging from the skin [9] to bone [18], as well as various body cavities which include the buccal [19], ocular [20], and peritoneal cavities [21], brain [5], etc., wherein site-specific drug delivery at high concentrations is desired. A recent trend in electrospinning for drug delivery has shown a paradigm shift from nonwoven to the woven matrices, wherein bundled nanofibers are used to generate nanotextiles by the textile technology techniques of braiding, knitting, weaving, etc [22]. Such novel systems aid in two ways: (i) provide enhanced mechanical properties for site-specific applications and (ii) offer tunable drug release via modulations of the weaving architecture.

This chapter mainly reviews the diverse electrospinning processing strategies utilized for the delivery of drugs, factors that influence drug delivery rate, and kinetics and the applications that demand localized drug delivery using such implants. How the traditional textile techniques that transform nanofibers to nanotextiles influence the drug release kinetics and its applicability in mechanically demanding situations is also discussed.

4.2 Key factors influencing drug release in electrospun DDS

The drug-releasing characteristics can be tuned by varying the hydrophilicity/phobicity of polymer, choice of solvents, drug solubility, drug—polymer interaction, polymer degradation, degree of cross-linking, fiber alignment, fiber diameter, etc. A schematic representation of drug-releasing behavior from electrospun fibers with reference to the properties of base polymer, drug, solvent, and fiber morphology is depicted in Fig. 4.1.

4.2.1 Polymer characteristics

Properties of the polymer such as its hydrophilicity and hydrophobicity have a major role in influencing drug release. The key mechanisms that dictate drug release from polymeric matrices are drug diffusion and polymer degradation. Accordingly, hydrophobic polymers such as poly(ε-caprolactone) (PCL), poly(L-lactic acid) (PLLA), poly(L-lactide-co-glycolide) (PLGA), polydioxanone (PDS), poly(methylmethacrylate) (PMMA), polyurethane (PU), etc., which exhibit poor interaction with water result in a comparatively slow, controlled, and thereby long-term drug release profile. Hydrophilic polymers such as poly(vinyl alcohol) (PVA), poly(ethylene glycol) (PEG), poly(vinyl pyrrolidine) (PVP), chitosan, sodium carboxymethyl cellulose, gelatin, etc., on the contrary, show burst release at initial time periods, which can be attributed to the fiber swelling, drug diffusion, polymer erosion, or dissolution. This drug release pattern can

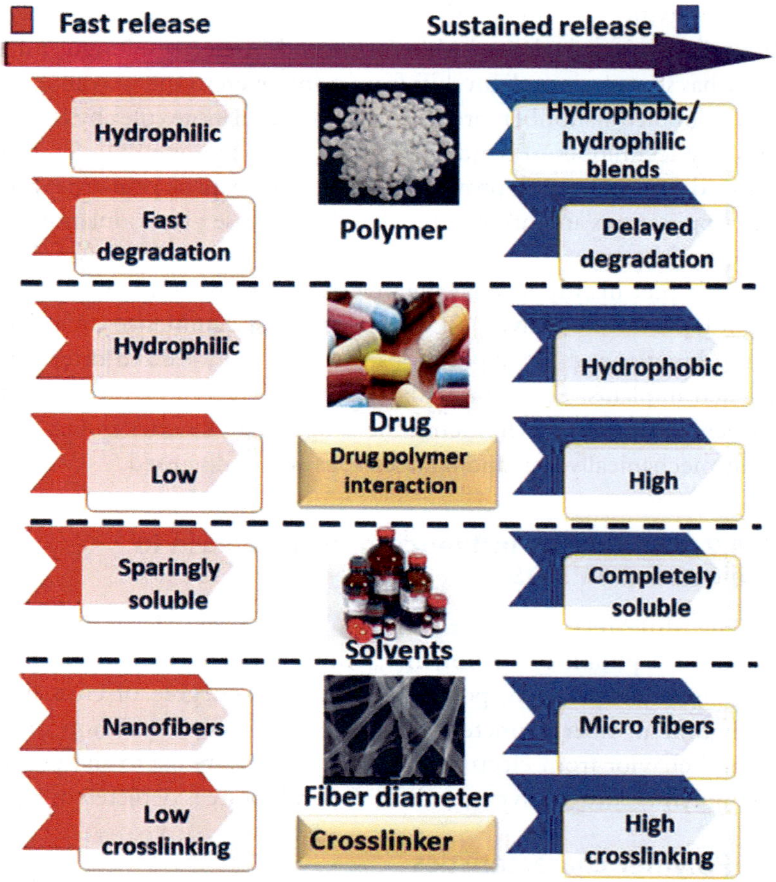

Figure 4.1 Schematic representation of drug-releasing behavior from electrospun fibers with reference to the properties of base polymer, drug, solvent, and fiber morphology.

be tuned by opting for a blend of hydrophobic and hydrophilic polymers. Yet another factor that critically influences drug release is the crystallinity of polymers. Highly crystalline polymers display poor access to water compared to its amorphous counterparts, thereby yielding a slower drug release profile.

Degradation of the polymeric electrospun matrix does not have a direct effect on the burst release of loaded drugs, although it affects the long-term drug release. Polymeric degradation mainly depends upon its molecular weight and hydrophilicity. It is in general accepted that polymers with high molecular weight and low hydrophilicity show delayed degradation. Hence, choice of the polymer is an essential criterion to formulate sustained drug delivery electrospun DDS. Polymeric membrane with lower degradation rate shows longer periods of sustained release, although complete release of the drug from this matrix is difficult. For example, electrospun membranes fabricated using PLGA revealed a zero-order drug release kinetics of Paclitaxel for more than 80 days from PLGA 85:15, whereas PLGA 50:50 showed a relatively burst release [23]. Here the higher glycolic component of the copolymer (50:50) with its rich ester groups offers a sudden release.

4.2.2 Solvent characteristics

Drug solubility in the solvent—polymer system has a direct effect on drug distribution and release characteristics from electrospun fibers. High solubility and interaction between drug and polymer impart uniform distribution throughout the fiber, which minimizes burst release. Several solvent combinations are also tried to improve drug solubility. Drugs with poor solubility tend to recrystallize or agglomerate as well as distribute nonuniformly in the polymeric matrix, leading to erratic patterns of release. Generally, hydrophilic drug molecules dissolve in aqueous medium/polar solvents and hydrophobic drugs dissolve in organic solvents/nonpolar medium. Electrospinning solvent volatility also has a vital role in influencing the drug release pattern. Solvents with high volatility have a tendency to immediately recrystallize the drug molecules on the surface of fibers, leading to a burst release [24]. Hence, an appropriate choice of solvent mixtures can be used to rectify this problem.

4.2.3 Drug characteristics

The solubility of drug is another criterion which directly impacts the release behavior. Generally, hydrophilic drugs display high aqueous solubility, and thereby a faster diffusion from polymeric matrices than that of hydrophobic drugs. In general, hydrophilic drug molecules that are surface bound to the polymeric fibers exhibit sudden release to the external medium, followed by diffusion. A comparison of the drug release behavior of water-insoluble drug doxorubicin and its water-soluble derivative doxorubicin hydrochloride from PLLA electrospun DDS revealed burst release up to 70% for the hydrophilic derivative, in contrast to a zero-order release kinetics with only 20% burst for doxorubicin [25]. The crystallinity of loaded drugs in nanofibers also dictate the release characteristics by its tendency to immobilize on the fiber surface, which trigger burst release. Meanwhile, amorphous drug molecules easily get encapsulated within the fibers and display sustained release.

4.2.4 Drug–polymer interaction

Generally, any kind of drug–polymer interactions (weak chemical bonding such as van der Waals interaction, hydrogen bonding, or ionic interactions) within electrospun DDS will lead to the formation of a stable drug/polymer complex. Such an interaction will minimize burst release and lead to a slow and sustained release profile [20]. For example, PLLA/paclitaxel electrospun DDS showed zero-order kinetics with minimum burst release due to the hydrogen bonding interaction between the polymer and drug [24]. Sufficient degree of cross-linking is essential only for hydrophilic electrospun polymeric DDS to minimize burst release. Hydrophilic polymers such as PVA, gelatin, collagen, chitosan, etc., require matrix stabilization using various types of cross-linkers such as glutaraldehyde, tripolyphosphate, sodium trimetaphosphate, ethylene diamine carbodiimide, and N-hydroxy succinimide, for fabricating stable DDS that exhibit sustained drug release. In a specific study, gelatin electrospun DDS cross-linked with an optimal concentration of glutaraldehyde (5%) showed sustained release of rhodamine [26]. Another study using a hydrophilic blend of chitosan and polyethylene oxide loaded with ranitidine and cross-linked with the anionic cross-linker tripolyphosphate revealed improved mechanical and drug release behaviors. This matrix showed only 40% burst release within 3 h than that of non–cross-linked matrix which showed nearly 100% burst at 3 h [27]. These studies confirm the effect of degree of cross-linking in modulating release kinetics.

4.2.5 Fiber characteristics

A reduction in fiber diameter from micron- to nanoscale enhances the surface area-to-volume ratio, which in turn increases the interaction of DDS with the biological milieu. This in turn results in high localized drug concentrations from the fibers within shorter durations [28]. Alignment of micro-/nanofibers in electrospun membranes is a major criterion which impacts the drug release pattern. It is proven that a nonwoven membrane with random fiber alignment is beneficial for water intake and drug release than that of aligned membranes [29]. Hence, diffusion of drugs from aligned membranes is in general less, which in turn provides a sustained rate of drug release.

4.3 Drug-loading strategies in the development of electrospun DDS

4.3.1 Electrospinning drug-loaded polymer solutions

Direct encapsulation of drug in electrospun polymeric matrix is a simple one-step process commonly used to fabricate DDS. The drug—polymer mixture blended in a common solvent is directly electrospun through a single nozzle. A schematic representation of the simple electrospinning process is shown in Fig. 4.2. Drug-loading efficiency and its uniformity within nanofibers are highly dependent on the drug—polymer compatibility and solubility in electrospun solvent. Generally, compatibility and solubility follow the principle "like dissolves like." For example, hydrophobic drugs are clearly compatible and miscible with hydrophobic polymers and solvents, while hydrophilic drugs mostly prefer hydrophilic polymers and solvents [30].

A few of such simple drug/polymer blend electrospun DDSs have demonstrated potential in vivo. Rapamycin-loaded PCL nanofibrous membranes when utilized as stent coatings to inhibit inflammation and tissue hyperplasia showed sustained drug release for 30 days, with minimum burst release [31]. In another study, vancomycin-loaded, biodegradable PLGA nanofibrous membranes used in the treatment of brain infection released high drug concentrations for greater than 8 weeks in the cerebral cavity of rats [32]. In a tissue regeneration study using melatonin-loaded aligned PCL electrospun fibrous membranes, it was observed that long-term melatonin release significantly promoted the chondrogenic differentiation of human bone marrow—derived mesenchymal stem cells [33]. A very common observation of drug release from simple electrospun membranes is the rapid drug release, which ranges from 30% to as high as 70%—80%,

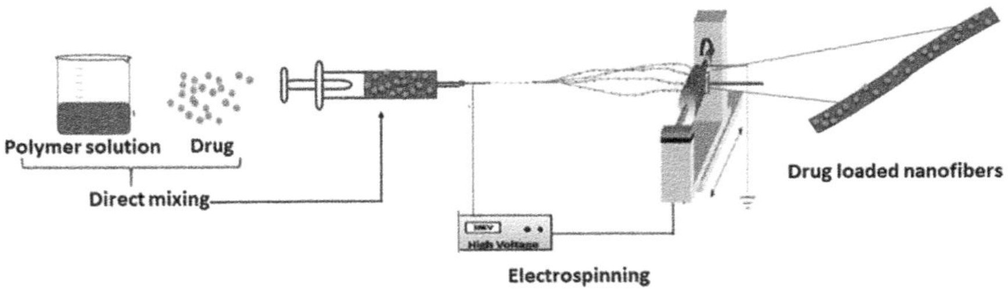

Figure 4.2 Schematic illustration of direct loading of drug molecule via simple electrospinning.

depending upon the choice of polymers. Several strategies have been adopted to minimize this initial burst such as the use of appropriate polymer blends, drug encapsulation within nanocarriers, layer-by-layer spinning, core—sheath geometry, etc. In general, low initial burst would help to avoid any undesired toxicity related to high drug concentrations and is hence widely advocated.

4.3.2 Electrospinning drug-loaded polymer blends

Blending of different polymers with variable degradation rates to fabricate electrospun DDS is a plausible strategy to tune both the drug-loading capacity and drug release pattern. A schematic representation of blend electrospinning is shown in Fig. 4.3. Generally, hydrophilic polymers blended with hydrophobic polymers can help to sustain drug release over long durations [34]. Normal hydrophilic and easily biodegradable polymers such as alginate, chitosan, gelatin, collagen, hyaluronic acid, and PEG when blended with hydrophobic nonbiodegradable (PU, PMMA) or delayed degradable polymers (PCL, PLLA, PDS) as electrospun matrices can prolong drug release over 2—3 months. To obtain uniform blends, the most important criterion is the selection of a common solvent wherein both the polymers are completely soluble. For example, PCL blended with gelatin in dichloromethane:dimethylformamide mixture aided the enhancement of the systemic availability of metronidazole for guided tissue regeneration [35]. The incorporation of gelatin in PCL improved the hydrophilicity, biocompatibility, and biodegradation rate, which influenced the drug release kinetics. The presence of gelatin accelerated drug diffusion from the matrix through swollen channels, which helped to achieve sustained metronidazole release till ~20 days, with a burst release (~40%) due to the incorporation of gelatin.

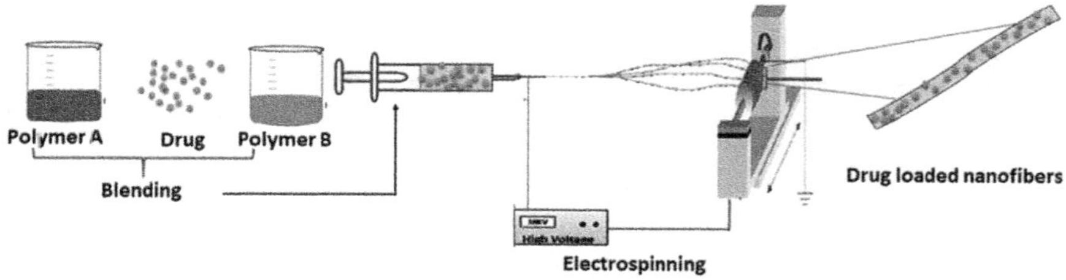

Figure 4.3 Schematic illustration of drug-loaded blend electrospinning process.

PLGA (75:25) blended with its own block copolymer of PLA-b-PEG (50:50) helped to enhance matrix hydrophilicity and stability [36]. A bilayer DDS-releasing carbazochrome sodium sulfonate (CA) and tinidazole (TI) in different layers was developed to prevent abdominal adhesion. This DDS showed high bioavailability of both drugs in a short period, without compromising structural stability and functionality of the antiadhesion membrane. In another study, PLGA/PDS electrospun membranes loaded with an antibacterial drug ciprofloxacin hydrochloride to prevent intraabdominal infection displayed accelerated drug diffusion. The comparatively high hydrophilic PDS component accelerated fiber swelling and displayed first-order release kinetics, with adequate antibacterial activity for 15 days [37]. Flexible electrospun membranes fabricated by simple blending of PLGA, PCL, and PLA loaded with chemotherapeutics have demonstrated their potential for localized chemotherapy. An antiglioma drug, Temozolamide, loaded within a blend of three bulk-eroding polymers, viz., PLGA, PCL, and PLA, could offer sustained drug release in rat brain from hours to months, by a mere tuning of the polymer blend ratio [38]. In situations that demanded burst release of drugs from DDS, as in chronic wound dressings, electrospun membranes were developed by blending two hydrophilic polymers. For example, PVA and chitosan were blended together for the release of the antibacterial drug tranexamic acid, and this DDS showed a high burst release of ~90% within 30 min [39].

However, electrospinning of polymer blends also could not completely address the problem of burst release in biological conditions due to the minimal chemical interactions between the drug and the polymer, or the absence of any protective layer above the drug-loaded fibers to prevent burst release of surface crystallized drug molecules. To circumvent these disadvantages a different kind of blend spinning, viz., emulsion electrospinning, is introduced to fabricate electrospun DDS.

4.3.3 Electrospinning drug-loaded polymer emulsions

Emulsion electrospinning is a type of blend electrospinning where the same or different polymers in different phases (water or oil) are blended together using a stabilizer. A schematic representation of emulsion electrospinning is depicted in Fig. 4.4. Here, two phases are stabilized by stirring, sonication, or via addition of surfactants. Emulsion electrospinning is done following the same principles of conventional emulsion preparation, wherein the drug molecules are encapsulated in the "dispersed phase," which is surrounded

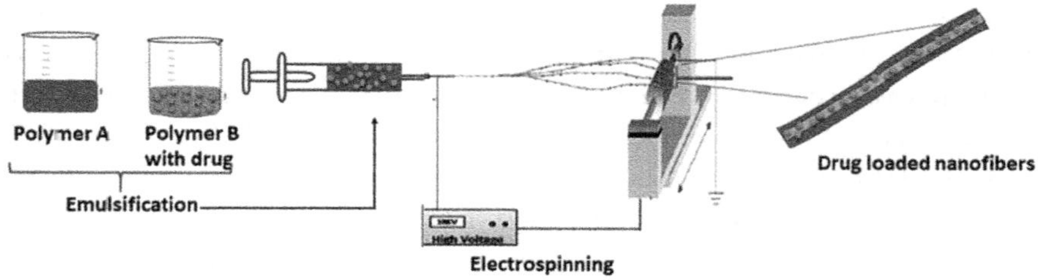

Figure 4.4 Schematic illustration of drug-loaded emulsion electrospinning process.

by a continuous dispersion medium [40]. During electrospinning of a water-in-oil (W/O) emulsion, the polymer oil phase and drug droplets in water elongate and transform into core–sheath structured nano-/microfibers. The oil phase evaporates quickly during the stretching and solidifies faster than that of aqueous phase, which results in the encapsulation of hydrophilic drug inside the fibers. This geometry with an inner drug-loaded core and an outer sheath minimizes burst release. Alternatively, using an oil-in-water (O/W) emulsion for electrospinning provides an inner core of a hydrophilic polymer and an outer sheath of drug-loaded hydrophobic polymer. These techniques can also be effectively utilized for the simultaneous encapsulation of hydrophilic drugs in hydrophobic polymer and vice-versa. High drug-loading efficiency and uniform distribution can be attained in emulsion electrospinning by the incorporation of an appropriate surfactant, which homogenizes the drug–polymer emulsion [40]. Drug release behavior from emulsion electrospun fibers can be easily altered by varying the surfactants or emulsifiers used as well as the oil and water phases. Such fibrous membranes have the potential to be utilized as controllable drug encapsulation/release depots with low burst release, by minimizing precipitation of the drug molecule on the fiber surface.

As an example, hydrophobic and hydrophilic drugs, viz., Cefradine and 5-fluorouracil (5-FU), respectively, were loaded in PLGA electrospun membranes by the technique of emulsion electrospinning. The hydrophobic drug Cefradine was dissolved in the organic phase with PLGA and 5-FU in gelatin in water. This emulsion was stabilized by stirring. The nanofibers formed displayed a minimum burst release due to the inherent core–sheath architecture of emulsion electrospun fibers [41]. In another study, dual drug–loaded emulsion electrospun DDS was fabricated by incorporation of metformin hydrochloride or metoprolol tartrate in PCL/poly (3-hydroxybutyric acid-co-3-hydroxyvaleric acid) blends [42].

This polymer—drug emulsion was stabilized by introducing a surfactant, viz., sorbitan monooleate (Span 80). This system exhibited minimum burst release of 40% in 2 h, compared to normal blended electrospun nanofibers with a burst of 80% in 2 h. This study confirms the benefit of emulsion electrospinning to control burst release over normal blend spinning. In another study, a green emulsion electrospinning method was introduced for loading ciprofloxacin sulfate in PVA/dextran blends, where the drug loaded in oil phase was dissolved in edible oil [43]. This DDS showed a nearly zero-order kinetics with 20% burst release, whereas simple blends showed nearly 80% burst release. Similarly, combinations of surfactants were used to produce a stable drug—polymer emulsion. This DDS based on poly(ethylene oxide) (PEO) stabilized with two surfactants, viz., cetyltrimethylammonium bromide (CTAB) and sodium dodecylbenzenesulfonate (SDBS), was designed for the dual delivery of a hydrophilic drug 5-FU and hydrophobic drug Paeonolum [44]. Drug release behaviors of the membrane fabricated with increased molar ratios of CTAB/SDBS surfactant combinations demonstrated an enhanced release of 5-FU, with a slow release of Paeonolum. Thus, the behavior of drug release from emulsion electrospun DDS can be effectively controlled by varying the type of emulsion used, surfactant concentration and its combination, and the type of drug.

4.3.4 Coaxial electrospinning of drug-loaded polymer solutions

Coaxial electrospinning is considered to be another promising strategy for designing core—sheath nanofibers. It involves the simultaneous flow of two different polymer solutions as a core and sheath from two different capillaries (inner and outer) to form a fiber structure (Fig. 4.5). Generally, the sheath is fabricated with high molecular weight polymer which can act as

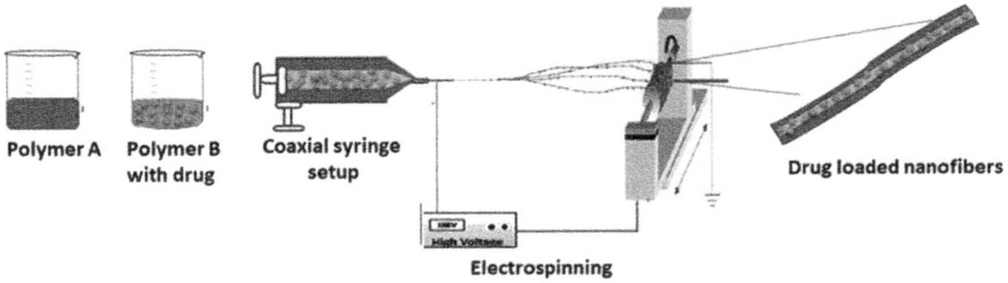

Figure 4.5 Schematic illustration of drug-loaded coaxial electrospinning process.

a physical barrier for the drug-loaded core to provide sustained release kinetics. Multiple drugs can be loaded using coaxial electrospinning by encapsulating different drugs in the sheath and core separately. In the case of single drug-loaded core–sheath electrospun membranes, the drug molecules are homogeneously distributed in the core of fibers, with the outer polymer sheath functioning as a protection to minimize burst release. In coaxial electrospinning, the electric charges mainly locate in the outer sheath than the core, thereby protecting the therapeutic molecules from structural instabilities and degradation [45].

In another coaxial system fabricated using PEO/thiolated chitosan loaded with low molecular weight drug tenofovir covered with PLA sheath, a steady release of the low molecular weight drug was attained for 10 days [46]. Coaxial electrospun DDS made using levetiracetam-loaded PLGA as core and PLGA sheath exhibited a linear drug release for over 20 days [47]. If the core–sheath membranes are loaded with dual drugs, the typical drug release pattern would be an initial burst release from the sheath, followed by a sustained release from the core. PVA and gelatin coaxial electrospun DDS were fabricated for dual drug delivery of lysozyme and phenytoin sodium [48]. The sheath was designed by phenytoin sodium–loaded gelatin and core with lysosome-loaded gelatin/PVA. This system showed independent dual and sustained release of the therapeutics with two types of release kinetics, including non-Fickian diffusion at the early stage, followed by Fickian diffusion of the drugs. Recently, another modified technique, viz., triaxial electrospinning, which utilizes similar principles of coaxial electrospinning, has been introduced. The morphology of triaxial nanofibers contains three layers: core, middle layer, and sheath, which provide different drug release patterns from each individual layer. Variations in the drug release pattern from coaxial and triaxial system were studied with PCL and PVP loaded with two dyes keyacid blue (KAB) and keyacid uranine (KAU) [49]. In both coaxial and triaxial assemblies, PVP/KAB blue was designed as the core and PVP/KAU as the sheath. In triaxial system, an additional PCL middle layer was provided. Both the coaxial and triaxial designs showed a similar release from the sheath. However, the release from the core of triaxial system showed a delayed release of 24 h, owing to the PCL layer acting as a barrier which delays drug diffusion from the core. In another study, ethyl cellulose–based triaxial electrospun DDS was fabricated by loading gradient concentrations of the drug ketoprofen to attain zero-order release kinetics [50]. The drug concentration gradually increased in each layer from the outer to the inner layer. This triaxial design of electrospun fibers was successful in attaining zero-order release kinetics for over 20 h despite drug loading in a highly hydrophilic polymer matrix. These studies proved that the release of therapeutic molecules is sustainable, with a statistically lower burst release for coaxial electrospinning than blend electrospinning.

4.3.5 Electrospinning drug-loaded nanocomposites

Electrospun nanocomposite membranes have attracted immense interest in the fabrication of DDS. Generally, two types of nanoparticles are loaded into electrospun nanocomposite DDS, viz., drug-loaded nanoparticles or non–drug-loaded nanoparticles. A schematic representation of composite electrospinning is shown in Fig. 4.6. Non–drug-loaded nanoparticles in electrospun DDS impart alterations in mechanical strength, hydrophilicity/phobicity, drug release rates, etc. This is due to the barrier effect offered by these particles, which minimizes the exposure of drug molecules to the surrounding biological milieu, resulting in minimized drug diffusion. Different kinds of nanoclays such as montmorillonite [51], hallosite [52], hydroxyapatite [53], and silica nanoparticles [54] have been explored in this category. For example, dexamethasone-loaded PLA/nanoclay electrospun DDS showed a slight change in drug delivery pattern due to the enhanced barrier effect of the dispersed nanosheet [55]. Similarly, amoxicillin-loaded PCL/nano-hydroxyapatite (nHAP) electrospun dental implants exhibited improved mechanical properties, osteoconductivity, and osteoinductivity, with only a slight variation in drug release with increasing nHAP concentration in the matrix [56].

Recently, embedding of drug-loaded micro- and nanoparticles into electrospun membranes emerged as an effective strategy to modulate drug release kinetics. Here, both polymeric and inorganic micro-/nanoparticles act as drug reservoirs, where the drug molecule is protected firstly within

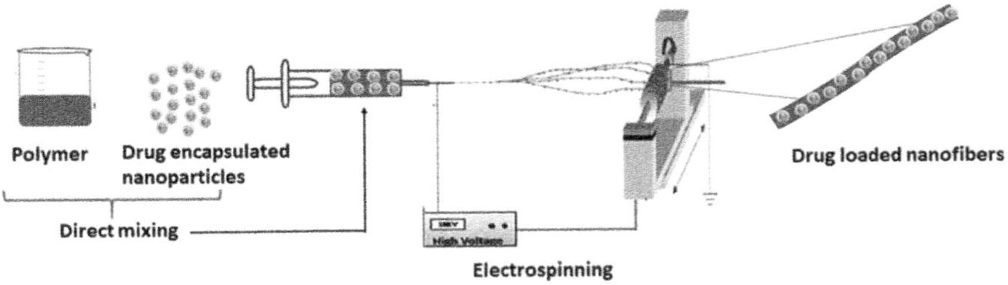

Figure 4.6 Schematic illustration of drug-loaded composite electrospinning process.

the shell of the nanocarrier, and secondly by the host fibrous matrix, thereby minimizing burst release. Stable emulsion of drug-encapsulated micro-/nanoparticles is prepared either by continuous stirring or sonication, and thereafter subjected to a single-step electrospinning process. Paclitaxel (PTX)-encapsulated mesoporous silica nanoparticles embedded in electrospun PLA was designed as a stent coating for controlled drug release [57]. This system showed sustained release of PTX for 63 days without burst release, thereby inhibiting stenosis caused by smooth muscle hyperplasia. In another study, halloysite nanotubes with diameter ~50 nm loaded with metronidazole were embedded in PCL/gelatin microfibers for bone tissue engineering [52]. The drug-encapsulated composite nanofibers showed a sustained drug release for over 20 days, in comparison to direct drug administration that lasted for only 4 days. Likewise, alendronate (ALN)-loaded mesoporous silicate nanoparticle (MSN) was embedded in PCL/gelatin nanofibers to achieve sustained delivery of ALN, imparting a synergistic effect with MSNs in bone remodeling [58]. ALN directly loaded within PCL/gelatin matrix showed a burst release, with nearly 60% release within 5 days, whereas the encapsulated ALN showed only 20% release at the same time point, with minimal burst. Gelatin nanospheres utilized as vancomycin reservoirs embedded within silk fibroin nanofibers exhibited sustained release of vancomycin than that of nanosphere-free membranes [59].

Programmed release of multiple drugs can also be attained using composite electrospinning. For example, core/shell silica nanoparticle embedded in PCL/gelatin electrospun DDS was designed for the dual drug delivery of indomethacin (IMC) and doxorubicin (DOX). Herein, the DDS was designed in such a way that IMC released fast, followed by a delayed release of DOX [60]. Another composite electrospun DDS fabricated with high concentration of osteogenic drug dexamethasone (DEX)-loaded mesoporous bioactive glass nanoparticles embedded in PCL/gelatin nanofibers showed a linear drug release kinetics up to 28 days [61]. This system exhibited a rapid DEX release up to ~30% within 24 h, whereas the simple electrospun PCL/gelatin membrane showed ~80% release at the same time point. Hallosite nanotubes (HNTs) are widely studied as nanoreservoirs for the fabrication of composite electrospun DDS. For example, tetracycline hydrochloride encapsulated in HNTs embedded within PLGA nanofibers loaded with the same drug acted as a double container DDS. Direct tetracycline loading into PLGA matrix exhibited ~90% burst release within 1 day, whereas drug-encapsulated

HNT-embedded PLGA had only about 15% release [62]. HNT/cephalexin (CEF)-encapsulated system incorporated in alginate electrospun membranes studied for antimicrobial protection showed sustained drug release up to 7 days [63]. In HNT/CEF-encapsulated system, the drug molecules penetrated into the lumen space of HNT and also got deposited on the outer walls with ~30 wt% loading capacity. Aminopropyltriethoxysilane or 3-glycidoxypropyltrimethoxysilane—modified HNT was studied as a nanocapsule for curcumin loading. The nanocapsule-embedded PCL/PEO-blended nanofibers revealed a slow release profile [64]. Despite the versatile release kinetics observed for composite electrospun DDS, it displays low drug-loading efficiency, which remains a major challenge.

4.3.6 Layer-by-layer electrospinning of drug-loaded polymer solutions

The cross-sectional morphology of layered electrospun membrane consists of typically three independent layers, with the drug-loaded layer sandwiched between two other non—drug-loaded electrospun layers (Fig. 4.7). This minimizes the direct exposure of drug-loaded fibers with the biological milieu, resulting in minimum burst release with a linear release pattern. Layered electrospinning is generally adapted for minimizing the burst release from hydrophilic electrospun membranes. For example, gelatin as layered electrospun DDS showed minimum burst and controlled drug-releasing pattern, where the non—drug-loaded gelatin fibers acted as barrier layers for the drug-loaded middle layer [65]. The burst release of curcumin from PCL/chitosan composite electrospun membrane was minimized (to ~ 15%) by designing a three-layered sandwich electrospun DDS which facilitated sustained release for about 15 days

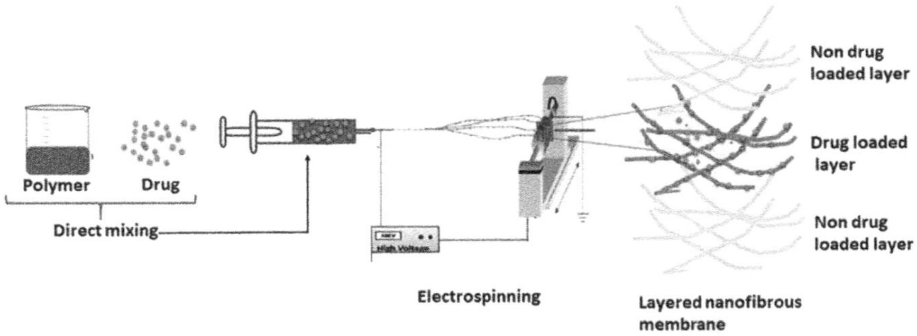

Figure 4.7 Schematic representation of layered electrospinning.

[66]. In another example, burst release of ~50% for tetracycline could be successfully reduced to 10% followed by a sustained release for more than 15 days by designing a PCL/PEVA/PCL-layered electrospun system [67]. One of the major criteria that dictates the release pattern in layered electrospinning is the thickness of the protective layer present above and below the drug-laden membrane. Minimum burst, with a delayed release, is attainable with increase in the protective layer thickness.

4.3.7 Postspinning drug loading onto electrospun matrices

The most commonly utilized postspinning drug-loading strategies in electrospun nanofibrous membranes include physical adsorption and chemical surface modification.

4.3.7.1 Physical adsorption of drugs

Physical adsorption of drug is a simple one-step post electrospinning process where the as-spun membrane is immersed in stable drug-loaded solution followed by drying (Fig. 4.8). Generally, there exists no chemical interactions between the polymer matrix and the drug molecules. The major drawback of this process is the recrystallization of drug particles on the membrane surface which leads to a burst release. Therefore, this technique is only useful for fabricating short-term drug release DDS with high burst release. As an example, antibiotic ornidazole dip coated on PCL membrane showed a high burst release within few hours [68]. Hence, this technique of absorptive drug loading is inadequate if high drug concentrations require to be sustained locally or the drug release need to be controlled for extended time periods. In this scenario, instead of adsorption, surface functionalization of drug molecules via chemical linkages is a preferred method for fabricating long-term DDS.

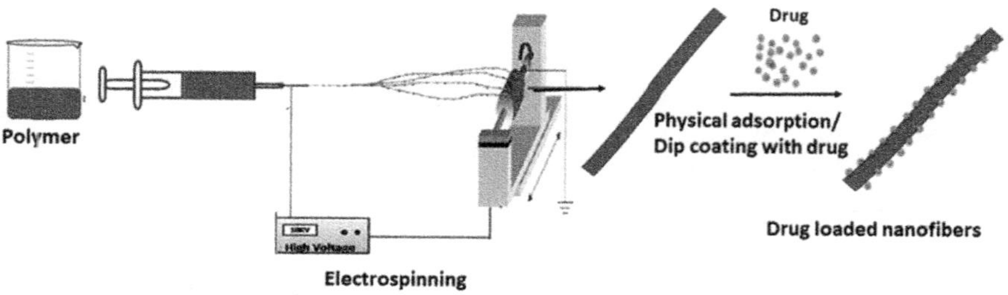

Figure 4.8 Depiction of the post electrospinning strategies utilized for drug loading by physical adsorption.

4.3.7.2 Surface functionalization

Surface functionalization/immobilization is the most effective post electrospinning technique to load drug/therapeutic agents on the surface of nanofibers to attain long-term sustained release [69]. Surface conjugation between polymer and drug can be achieved through various types of chemical linkages such as hydrogen, ionic, and/or covalent bonds. A schematic representation of surface functionalized electrospun membrane is depicted in Fig. 4.9. Numerous patterns of drug release can be achieved by varying the interactions/bonds between the fiber surface and the drug. Appropriate chemical modification should be undertaken on the nanofibrous surface by introducing reactive functional groups, prior to chemical bonding with drug molecules. The nanofibrous surface is generally functionalized with carboxyl and amine groups by hydrolysis using mild base and/or acid solution. For example, active −COOH groups were formed on polyester nanofibers after treating with aqueous alkaline solution [70]. Further, biomolecules such as heparin were immobilized onto the nanofiber surface, majorly by means of N-(3-dimethylaminopropyl)-N′-ethylcarbodiimide hydrochloride/N-hydroxysuccinimide (EDC/NHS) coupling chemistry [71]. However, surface functionalized electrospun membranes are not widely studied for the fabrication of DDS, because of the vigorous reaction conditions required for producing reactive groups on the fibrous surface. This can adversely affect the bioactivity of drug molecules and perhaps also impair the fiber morphology.

4.3.8 Combinatorial approaches in electrospun DDS

In addition to the methods of combining nanoparticles with electrospun fibers to obtain composite electrospun DDS, different electrospinning processes can also be coalesced to obtain tunability in drug release kinetics. For

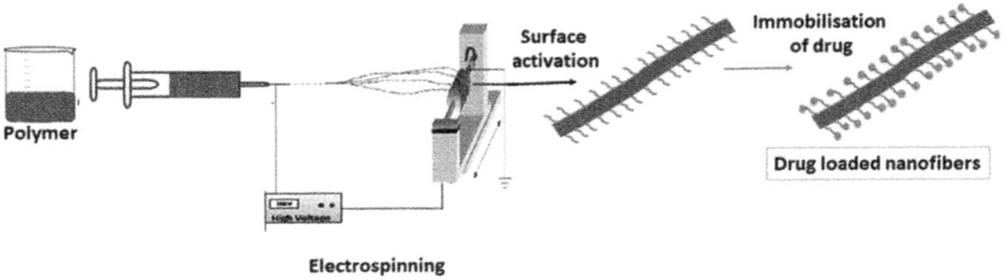

Figure 4.9 Depiction of the post electrospinning strategies utilized for drug loading by surface functionalization.

example, by adopting a combination of blending with surface modification strategies, stimuli-responsive DDSs were developed for the release of ketoprofen. PVA/PAA-blended electrospun membranes loaded with ketoprofen were surface functionalized by oxyfluorination and conjugated with MWCNTs to induce electric-stimuli–responsive DDS [72]. Likewise, blend and composite electrospinning processes can be coupled together for developing pH-sensitive DDS. In one such study, graphene oxide (GO) and TiO_2 nanoparticles were dispersed in doxorubicin-loaded chitosan/poly (lactic acid) (PLA) blends, yielding a pH-sensitive drug release [73]. Similarly, combining coaxial and emulsion electrospinning processes is an effective way to simultaneously load hydrophilic and hydrophobic drugs. A localized drug delivery patch developed using the hydrophobic drug hydroxycamptothecin (HCPT) and hydrophilic drug tea polyphenol (TP) was loaded as shell and core, respectively, in mPEG-b-PLGA nanofibers by utilizing emulsion and coaxial electrospinning [74]. The core–sheath architecture of the fibers facilitated an initial HCPT release, followed by the release of TP in a sustained manner for 15 days. Thus, based on the requirement of the drug release pattern and the duration of release, different polymer systems having varied degradation kinetics can be electrospun by adopting a combination of diverse techniques detailed earlier. Table 4.1 enlists the merits and demerits of the various electrospinning techniques in developing DDSs.

4.4 Mechanism of drug release from electrospun DDS

The mechanism of drug release from fiber-based DDSs is highly influenced by the choice of the polymer and drug. Generally, biodegradable polymers exhibit the following phenomena during various time points of drug release: (i) swelling of fibers, (ii) diffusion of drug molecules, (iii) erosion of fiber, and (iv) matrix degradation. Additionally, stimuli-responsive materials exhibit a specific kind of drug release based on the stimulus provided.

In the case of both biodegradable hydrophilic and hydrophobic polymeric electrospun membranes, dissolution of surface-bound drug molecules is the first step that occurs during drug release. Depending on the solubility of the drug in aqueous medium, this step can get completed within minutes to hours, and results in the burst release process. In the next step, diffusion of drug molecules occurs from within the fibers, which generally prolongs for days. Concurrently, the direct contact of the polymeric matrix with the

Table 4.1 Merits and demerits of various techniques of electrospinning for DDS fabrication: a comparison.

Electrospinning process	Merits in drug delivery	Demerits in drug delivery
Simple electrospinning (direct blending of drug)	• Simple technique • High drug-loading capacity	• Burst release
Blend electrospinning	• Simple technique • High drug-loading capacity • Easy to modulate drug release pattern	• Burst release
Emulsion electrospinning	• Simple technique • High drug-loading capacity • Controllable burst release • Tunability in release kinetics through variations in sheath thickness • Ability to coload hydrophilic/phobic drugs • Suitable for dual drug delivery	• Nonuniformity in core—sheath morphology
Coaxial electrospinning	• High drug-loading capacity • Controllable burst release • Tunability in release kinetics through variations in sheath thickness • Ability to coload hydrophilic/phobic drugs • Suitable for dual drug delivery	• Cumtrun -1bersome technique • Nonuniformity in core—sheath morphology
Composite electrospinning	• Simple process • Modulation of mechanical properties • Controlled drug release	• Preliminary burst release • Low drug-loading capacity for drug-loaded nanoparticles in fibers
Layer-by-layer electrospinning	• Minimum burst release • Tunability in drug release	• Multistep process
Nanoyarns and nanotextiles	• High mechanical strength • Amenable to postprocessing through textile techniques • Scaffolds of diverse geometries possible • Can easily alter the drug release kinetics • Dual drug delivery	• Difficulty in scalability

surrounding aqueous environment can lead to fiber swelling. This phenomenon, which varies depending upon the crystallinity and hydrophilicity of the polymer, facilitates convective transport of drug molecules through the gel into the medium [16]. Polymer erosion is the third stage, wherein surface degradation of fibers get initiated, followed by prolonged to bulk erosion. In this stage, almost 100% of the loaded drug permeates into the medium. A schematic representation of these drug-releasing steps is shown in Fig. 4.10a.

In the case of coaxial and emulsion electrospun membranes, the phenomenon of surface dissolution of drug molecule is not observed due to the core—sheath architecture. The first step of drug release here is the diffusion of drug from the core of the fiber toward the sheath, and thereafter from the sheath to the outside (Fig. 4.10b). In the second step, surface erosion followed by bulk erosion happen, which dictate the kinetics of drug release. Drug-loaded composite electrospun membranes also show a similar mechanism of drug release as given in Fig. 4.10c and d. Herein, the inorganic nanoparticles dispersed in the fibrous matrix can provide a shielding effect and thereby a tortuous pathway for drug release (Fig. 4.10c). For drug-encapsulated nanoparticles, release is delayed due to the diffusion of drug molecules across multiple barriers provided by the encapsulating nanoparticle and also the fibrous matrix. In the case of nondegradable polymers, drug delivery is mainly controlled by diffusion of drug molecules through the interstitial space within fibers.

Several mathematical models have been used to analyze the drug release profiles from nanofibrous membranes viz. zero-order, first-order, Higuchi, particle diffusion model, Hixson—Crowell model, and power law equation (Korsmeyer—Peppas equation) [75]. Till date, none of the existing models could fully describe the entire release kinetics from fibrous membranes. Hence, concerted efforts are underway to develop advanced mathematical models which can reliably and suitably predict the drug release kinetics from fibrous DDSs.

4.5 Trends in electrospun DDS

4.5.1 Porous electrospun DDS

Porous electrospun membrane DDS is another class of fibrous matrix that has attracted widespread interest due to its large surface area, which facilitates enhanced bioavailability of drugs in specific sites. Porous electrospun nano-/microfibers can be fabricated in three major ways: (i) use of a

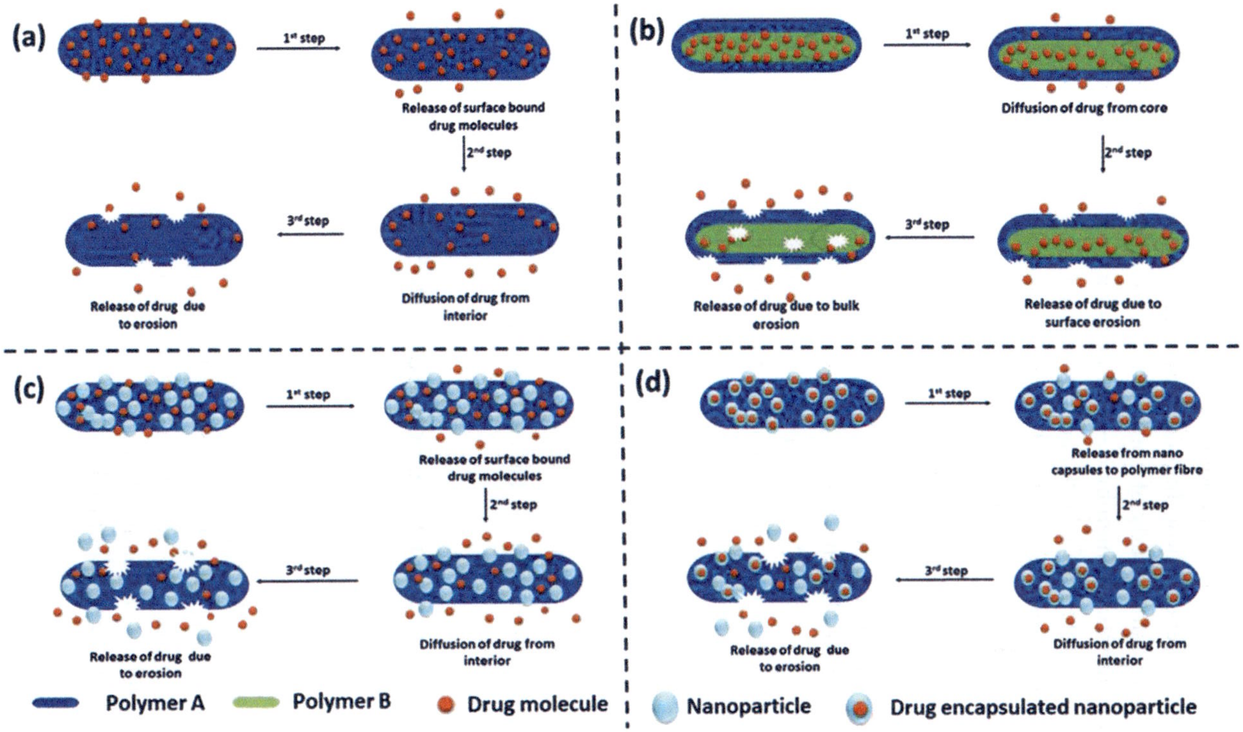

Figure 4.10 Schematic representation of drug release mechanisms from different types of electrospun membranes: (a) simple and blend, (b) emulsion and coaxial, (c) nanocomposite, and (d) nanocomposite electrospun fibers loaded with drug-encapsulated nanoparticles.

low boiling point solvent such as dichloromethane (BP: 39.6°C), (ii) increased atmospheric humidity during electrospinning process, and (iii) direct deposition of nanofibers into water [76]. Porous electrospun membranes generally show higher burst drug release compared to normal fibers. A comparative study of porous PLA/PEG coaxial electrospun membrane with nonporous membranes revealed that porous fibers released two times higher content of salicylic acid, facilitated by the easy penetration of water molecules into the matrix [77]. Such porous electrospun DDS thus find use in applications which demand high rate of drug elution in a short time. For example, PLLA-aligned porous fibers loaded with asiatic acid were designed for accelerated drug release in diabetic wounds [78]. In another study, PLLA porous electrospun membrane embedded with mesoporous silica nanoparticles containing dimethyloxalylglycine functioned as nanoreservoirs for diabetic wound healing [79]. Likewise, chemotherapeutic drug—loaded CuS/DOX nanocapsules dispersed in PCL/PLA electrospun membrane pores exhibited chemophotothermal synergistic melanoma therapy and wound healing [80]. Cellulose acetate (CA) porous nanofibers containing thymol (THY) for sustained drug release were prepared by coelectrospinning technique. Herein, the ellipsoidal-shaped nanopores on the surface of electrospun fibers trapped a part of air at the interface, resulting in enhanced hydrophobicity of the fibrous membranes. The higher specific surface area of porous THY-loaded CA fibrous membranes contributed to a higher drug utilization for enhanced antibacterial activity, with concurrent biocompatibility [81].

4.5.2 Stimuli-responsive electrospun DDS

Stimuli-responsive electrospun DDSs are highly beneficial for attaining programmed drug release in response to external stimuli such as temperature, pH, light, enzymes, etc. Among them, thermoresponsive electrospun DDS based on thermoresponsive polymers, specifically, poly(N-isopropyl acrylamide) (PNIPAM), is widely explored due to its lower critical solution temperature (LCST) of 32°C. LCST of PNIPAM can be tuned by varying the polymer molecular weight or copolymerization. In one such study, stimuli-responsive core/sheath electrospun fibers were fabricated using PNIPAM as the sheath and PCL as the core [82]. Due to the thermoresponsive nature of PNIPAM, these fibers displayed a hydrophilic surface at 20°C and hydrophobicity at 40°C. This in turn regulated the diffusion of water into the matrix, which then dictated the drug release kinetics. In another study, temperature-dependent swelling was observed for rhodamine-loaded poly(vinyl caprolactam co-hydroxymethyl acrylamide) nanofibers [83]. Fibers developed using this polymer showed swelling below LCST and shrinkage above, which regulated the temperature-dependent rhodamine release. Thus, temperature-dependent fiber shrinkage normally enhances the drug release, while swelling decreases it.

pH-responsive electrospun DDSs have been fabricated by polymers possessing excess amine or carboxylic surface functionalities. For example, PVA-PAA and dextran/PAA-based electrospun fibers reported a high swelling ratio at alkaline pH, thereby acting as pH-responsive DDS [84]. This system exhibited a pH-dependent swelling property due to the protonation of surface-exposed functional groups and ionization, which leads to intermolecular repulsion. Thereby the nanofibers become swollen and provides drug diffusion pathways. In another study, poly(N-isopropyl acrylamide-co-methacrylic acid-co-vinylpyrrolidone)-loaded DOX nanofibrous system showed pH-responsive release of DOX, with higher drug release at a pH of 5.4 versus 7.4 [85]. Here, apart from swelling, the stimuli-responsive drug release behavior is dictated by a pH-responsive polymer dissolution. For instance, drug release kinetics from a pH-sensitive polymer—lecithin nanocomposite core—sheath fibrous matrix developed using ES100 and lecithin containing diclofenac sodium (PL-DS) showed a stepwise release behavior. For this system, dissolution of the ES100 layer was followed by conversion of the core PL—DS into submicron-sized particles at a pH above 7. Further, a gradual release of the remaining DS from the PL-DS particles was observed by diffusion. At a pH below 7, the fibers displayed controlled drug release than that above 7 [86]. Labile group containing poly(D,L-lactide)-poly(ethylene glycol) electrospun membrane loaded with paracetamol also behaved as pH stimuli-responsive DDS. The acid labile moieties such as acetal groups present in the electrospun fibers underwent dissolution at pH 4 which facilitated paracetamol release [87].

Similarly, multi-responsive DDSs have been designed using PNIPAM electrospun membranes loaded with DOX/silica-coated gold nanorods. This system showed temperature-responsive wettability, typically hydrophilic at room temperature, and hydrophobic at 40°C. Further, illumination of NIR radiation resulted in a localized increase in temperature of the electrospun membrane, which resulted in a decrease in fiber diameter with accelerated DOX release [88].

4.5.3 Nanotextile-based drug delivery system

Nonwoven electrospun membranes fabricated using diverse methods display a wide range of drug release patterns. However, the main disadvantage of this nonwoven matrix is its compromised mechanical properties, which preclude its use as localized drug delivery depots in cavities such as the peritoneum, eye, etc., where the implants have to be sutured. In this scenario, implantable, suturable matrices based on nanofibrous textiles have an edge over simple nonwoven electrospun membranes [16]. To facilitate development of such woven matrices, different textile technology techniques such as yarning, weaving, knitting, and braiding have been utilized [89]. A schematic representation of the modified electrospinning setup for fabricating yarns and the products formed thereafter is depicted in Fig. 4.11a. For this, the nanofibers need to be bundled together to form continuous yarns (which are constituted of hundreds to thousands of fibers—Fig. 4.11b and c) through modifications in the electrospinning process [90,91]. Such yarns are flexible, elastic, and mechanically strong and can be loaded with drugs or

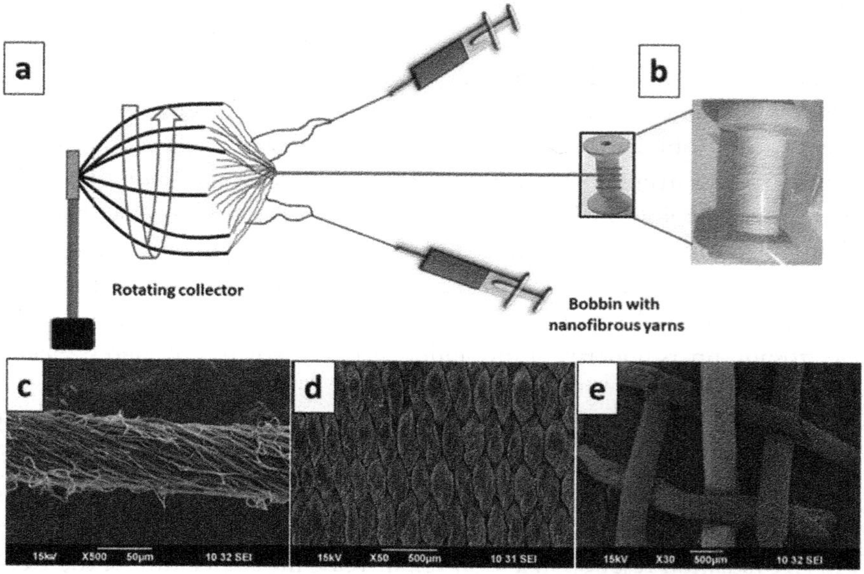

Figure 4.11 (a) Graphical representation of nanofibrous yarning process, (b) Photograph of nanofibrous yarn spool. Electron micrographs of (c) electrospun yarns and woven nanotextiles of (d) higher and (e) lower packing densities.

any other biomolecules [92] and are well suited for conventional weaving/knitting processes. By combining the textile technology processes of yarning, braiding, or plying with electrospinning, drug-eluting implantable matrices can be fabricated.

As an example, cefazolin-loaded PLLA and PLLA/PVA yarns were studied to analyze the variation in drug release pattern with respect to change in twist rates and crystallinity of the fibers in the yarns. The total amount of drug released from PLLA/PVA blended yarns was significantly higher than pure PLLA, with the blend composition and twist rate of PLLA/PVA yarns dictating the duration of drug release [93]. Likewise, curcumin-loaded PEG-PLA-PCL—based core—sheath yarns were studied for their application as drug-eluting sutures. It was concluded that electrospun yarns with finer fiber diameters in the core displayed higher drug release, with more initial release [94]. Vascular sutures were also developed by electrospinning of PLGA/PEO/poly(lactide-co-glycolide)-graft-polyethyleneimine (PgP) blends and immobilized with heparin to minimize thrombogenicity and excess cell proliferation. These yarns exhibited a sustained release over 20 days from PgP fibers, with a burst release of 60% within 4 h from PLGA/PEO. Therefore, this nanofiber yarn matrix offered a basis for the development of microvascular sutures having anticoagulant activity [95]. In another study, blend and coaxial electrospun tetracycline hydrochloride—loaded yarns were fabricated using the base polymer PLLA. The yarns formed by coaxial electrospinning showed minimal burst, with a sustained release profile than that of simple blended yarns [96]. Thymosin beta-4 (Tβ4)-loaded PLGA nanofibers were coated onto PLA microfibrous yarns to generate PLGA/PLA hybrid yarns for tendon tissue engineering. This hybrid yarn system exhibited sustained drug release for nearly 28 days [97].

Drug-loaded nanofiber sutures were also developed by braiding aligned PLLA nanofibers loaded with Cefotaxime sodium [98]. PLLA nanofibrous sutures displayed a sustained drug release exceeding 2 weeks, with efficient antibacterial activity. Core—sheath drug-eluting sutures were also fabricated using PLLA core yarns wrapped with PLGA nanofibers loaded with drugs of different chemical nature, viz., aceclofenac and insulin [92]. These yarns possessed sufficient mechanical strength and high drug-loading capacity and provided sustained release lasting 10 days. Majority of the studies reported thus far on drug delivery are based on electrospun yarns. Utilization of the weaving technique in combination with electrospun yarns is sparse, perhaps owing to its poor mechanical properties. This can be improved by different postyarning strategies such as hot-stretching, plying, etc [90]. In a recent study, by utilizing drug-eluting yarns, nanotextile fabrics were developed by the textile technique of weaving as shown in Fig. 4.11d [16]. In this study, PDS electrospun yarns loaded with PTX were developed as fabrics of different packing densities, which in turn modulated the drug release kinetics. These woven nanotextiles, owing to its specific architecture wherein drug molecules get entrapped within the tightly twisted nanofibrous bundles, could sustain drug release for typically 2–3 months in vitro. Loosely woven implants (Fig. 4.11e) outperformed tightly woven ones (Fig. 4.11d) and showed sustained release in the peritoneal cavity of mice for time durations exceeding 2 months [17]. Such an implantable drug-eluting matrix can find immense applications as controlled drug delivery depots—a field with immense potential, yet to be explored in depth.

4.5.4 Bioelectrospinning and beyond

In addition to the utility of electrospinning in fabricating nonwoven and woven electrospun matrices for drug delivery, this technique can also be extended to include encapsulation of biologics such as RNA, DNA, growth factors, etc. In one such work, siRNA-loaded PCL electrospun membranes could provide sustained long-term siRNA delivery for 28 days at the tumor site. This electrospun RNA delivery matrix exhibited 30.9% gene knockdown efficiency in vitro, pointing to its utility for long-term gene silencing applications [99]. In another study, PCL electrospun fibers were loaded with plasmid DNA/small/short hairpin RNA (shRNA) to inhibit the cell cycle–specific protein Cdk2. This matrix could deliver the bioactive plasmid DNA for over 21 days, leading to 40% decrease in the proliferation of MCF-7 breast cancer cells [100]. A bone regenerative growth factor (BMP-2) loaded in coaxial nanofibers of PLA/PVA blends was studied for bone regeneration application [101]. A biomimetic nanocomposite scaffold reinforced with electrospun yarns and loaded with a cocktail of growth factors (BMP-2 and ONO-1301) displayed fast release of ONO-1301 and a slow and controlled release of BMP-2, with augmented bone regeneration in vivo [102,103]. Controlled delivery of multiple growth factors can be considered an effective approach in nerve regeneration. In this context, PLLA core–shell nanofibers loaded with vascular endothelial growth factor (VEGF) and recombinant human nerve growth factor (NGF) in the shell and core, respectively, via emulsion electrospinning were studied for vascular regeneration. VEGF and NGF showed a sequential release profile, wherein VEFG was released in the initial phase, while NGF release prolonged for nearly a month, thereby offering synergistic effect on nerve tissue regeneration [104]. In another study, PCL emulsion electrospinning was employed for loading dual therapeutic agents (NGF and BSA) for vascular regeneration. Here BSA acted as a stabilizer and realized sustained release of NGF for almost 1 month [105]. Synergistic therapy is a new facet in the design of an electrospun DDS. In this aspect, a gene/drug dual delivery system was prepared by emulsion electrospinning using PLGA as the base matrix, which combines RNA interference and chemotherapy for brain tumor therapy. The emulsion was prepared using PTX/PEG mixture in PLGA as the oil phase and PEI/DNA nanoparticles as the aqueous phase, resulting in a core–shell matrix which provided controlled gene/drug release and thereby better tumor inhibition [106].

4.6 Summary and future prospects

Electrospun polymer micro-/nanofibers with variable fiber size, design, and alignment have advanced the field of drug delivery in a significant way. A wide variety of drug-loaded biodegradable polymers, blends, and composites have been successfully developed by the technique of electrospinning. These systems exhibit high drug-loading capacity and retain the bioactivity of the loaded drugs. Diverse drug-loading techniques adopted include blending, compositing, emulsion/coaxial electrospinning, physical adsorption, and surface functionalization. Fibrous polymeric matrices designed via physical adsorption or blend electrospinning typically follow a burst release pattern, while emulsion, coaxial, layered, and composite electrospinning display controlled release kinetics. Programmable drug release in response to external stimuli such as heat, pH, light, etc., is attainable using a special class of stimuli-responsive electrospun DDS. Drug release kinetics can also be modified by altering the architecture from nonwoven fiber to woven nanotextile geometry.

Despite the technological progress achieved thus far, what remains as a challenge is the large-scale industrial production of nanofibers with defined morphological and mechanical characteristics that can be tailored to suit the desired application. For this reason, no commercial therapeutic electrospun products are yet available in the clinics. Hence, to optimally utilize the potential of this technology and exploit the benefits of nanoscale architecture of electrospun matrices in drug delivery, it is indispensable to innovate novel and facile means of translating the technology for developing reproducible and scalable products, that conform to the standards of stability and safety, with long shelf-life.

References

[1] M.I. Shekh, J. Amirian, F.J. Stadler, B. Du, Y. Zhu, Oxidized chitosan modified electrospun scaffolds for controllable release of acyclovir, Int. J. Biol. Macromol. 151 (2020) 787–796.
[2] D. Ding, Z. Zhu, R. Li, X. Li, W. Wu, X. Jiang, B. Liu, Nanospheres-incorporated implantable hydrogel as a trans-tissue drug delivery system, ACS Nano 5 (4) (2011) 2520–2534.
[3] H.P. Dang, T. Shabab, A. Shafiee, Q.C. Peiffer, K. Fox, N. Tran, T.R. Dargaville, D.W. Hutmacher, P.A. Tran, 3D printed dual macro-, microscale porous network as a tissue engineering scaffold with drug delivering function, Biofabrication 11 (3) (2019) 035014.
[4] M. Scholz, T. Reske, F. Böhmer, A. Hornung, N. Grabow, H. Lang, In vitro chlorhexidine release from alginate based microbeads for periodontal therapy, PloS One 12 (10) (2017) e0185562.
[5] D. Han, R. Serra, N. Gorelick, U. Fatima, C.G. Eberhart, H. Brem, B. Tyler, A.J. Steckl, Multi-layered core-sheath fiber membranes for controlled drug release in the local treatment of brain tumor, Sci. Rep. 9 (1) (2019) 17936.
[6] S. Chen, J.V. John, A. McCarthy, J. Xie, New forms of electrospun nanofiber materials for biomedical applications, J. Mater. Chem. B 8 (2020) 3733–3746.
[7] H.S. Sofi, A. Abdal-hay, S. Ivanovski, Y.S. Zhang, F.A. Sheikh, Electrospun nanofibers for the delivery of active drugs through nasal, oral and vaginal mucosa: current status and future perspectives, Mater. Sci. Eng. C 111 (2020) 110756.
[8] C. Hu, S. Liu, Y. Zhang, B. Li, H. Yang, C. Fan, W. Cui, Long-term drug release from electrospun fibers for in vivo inflammation prevention in the prevention of peritendinous adhesions, Acta Biomater. 9 (7) (2013) 7381–7388.
[9] C.R. Reshmi, T. Menon, A. Binoy, N. Mishra, K.K. Elyas, A. Sujith, Poly(L-lactide-co-caprolactone)/collagen electrospun mat: potential for wound dressing and controlled drug delivery, Int. J. Polym. Mater. Polym. Biomater. 66 (13) (2017) 645–657.
[10] W. Li, X.N. Tan, T. Luo, X. Huang, Q. Wang, Y.J. Yang, M.J. Wang, L.F. Liu, Formation of pH-responsive drug-delivery systems by electrospinning of vesicle-templated nanocapsule solutions, RSC Adv. 6 (48) (2016) 42589–42595.
[11] B. Singh, T. Garg, A.K. Goyal, G. Rath, Development, optimization, and characterization of polymeric electrospun nanofiber: a new attempt in sublingual delivery of nicorandil for the management of angina pectoris, Artif. Cells, Nanomed. Biotechnol. 44 (6) (2016) 1498–1507.
[12] G.L. Pérez-González, L.J. Villarreal-Gómez, A. Serrano-Medina, E.J. Torres-Martínez, J.M. Cornejo-Bravo, Mucoadhesive electrospun nanofibers for drug delivery systems: applications of polymers and the parameters' roles, Int. J. Nanomed. 14 (2019) 5271–5285.
[13] E.M. Hoffmann, A. Breitenbach, J. Breitkreutz, Advances in orodispersible films for drug delivery, Expet Opin. Drug Deliv. 8 (3) (2011) 299–316.
[14] R. Qiu, J. Li, D. Sun, H. Li, F. Qian, L. Wang, 20(S)-ginsenoside Rg3-loaded electrospun membranes to prevent postoperative peritoneal adhesion, Biomed. Microdevices 21 (4) (2019) 78.

[15] X. Feng, J. Li, X. Zhang, T. Liu, J. Ding, X. Chen, Electrospun polymer micro/nanofibers as pharmaceutical repositories for healthcare, J. Contr. Release 302 (2019) 19–41.
[16] S. Padmakumar, B. Paul-Prasanth, K. Pavithran, D.K. Vijaykumar, A. Rajanbabu, T.B. Sivanarayanan, E. Kadakia, M.M. Amiji, S.V. Nair, D. Menon, Long-term drug delivery using implantable electrospun woven polymeric nanotextiles, Nanomed. Nanotechnol. Biol. Med. 15 (1) (2019) 274–284.
[17] S. Padmakumar, N.N. Parayath, S.V. Nair, D. Menon, M.M. Amiji, Enhanced antitumor efficacy and safety with metronomic intraperitoneal chemotherapy for metastatic ovarian cancer using biodegradable nanotextile implants, J. Contr. Release 305 (2019) 29–40.
[18] L. Yin, K. Wang, X. Lv, R. Sun, S. Yang, Y. Yang, Y. Liu, J. Liu, J. Zhou, Z. Yu, The fabrication of an ICA-SF/PLCL nanofibrous membrane by coaxial electrospinning and its effect on bone regeneration in vitro and in vivo, Sci. Rep. 7 (1) (2017) 8616.
[19] H.E. Colley, Z. Said, M.E. Santocildes-Romero, S.R. Baker, K. D'Apice, J. Hansen, L.S. Madsen, M.H. Thornhill, P.V. Hatton, C. Murdoch, Pre-clinical evaluation of novel mucoadhesive bilayer patches for local delivery of clobetasol-17-propionate to the oral mucosa, Biomaterials 178 (2018) 134–146.
[20] E.J. Torres-Martinez, J.M. Cornejo Bravo, A. Serrano Medina, G.L. Pérez González, L.J. Villarreal Gómez, A summary of electrospun nanofibers as drug delivery system: drugs loaded and biopolymers used as matrices, Curr. Drug Deliv. 15 (10) (2018) 1360–1374.
[21] S. Boroumand, S. Hosseini, M. Salehi, R. Faridi Majidi, Drug-loaded electrospun nanofibrous sheets as barriers against postsurgical adhesions in mice model, Nanomed. Res. J. 2 (1) (2017) 64–72.
[22] T. Walsh, L. Karperien, S.M.H. Dabiri, M. Akbari, Fiber-based microphysiological systems: a powerful tool for high throughput drug screening, Microphysiol. Syst. 3 (2019).
[23] D. Carson, Y. Jiang, K.A. Woodrow, Tunable release of multiclass anti-HIV drugs that are water-soluble and loaded at high drug content in polyester blended electrospun fibers, Pharm. Res. 33 (1) (2016) 125–136.
[24] J. Zeng, L. Yang, Q. Liang, X. Zhang, H. Guan, X. Xu, X. Chen, X. Jing, Influence of the drug compatibility with polymer solution on the release kinetics of electrospun fiber formulation, J. Contr. Release 105 (1–2) (2005) 43–51.
[25] Q. Zhao, B. Wang, R. Liu, M. Gong, M. Dong, M. Fang, T. Jiang, Drug release behavior of doxorubicin hydrochloride-loaded poly(L-lactic acid)/hydroxyapatite/gelatin by surface modification of hydroxyapatite, J. Nanosci. Nanotechnol. 18 (10) (2018) 7225–7230.
[26] S. Nagarajan, L. Soussan, M. Bechelany, C. Teyssier, V. Cavaillès, C. Pochat-Bohatier, P. Miele, N. Kalkura, J.-M. Janot, S. Balme, Novel biocompatible electrospun gelatin fiber mats with antibiotic drug delivery properties, J. Mater. Chem. B 4 (6) (2016) 1134–1141.
[27] B. Darbasizadeh, H. Motasadizadeh, B. Foroughi-Nia, H. Farhadnejad, Tripolyphosphate-crosslinked chitosan/poly (ethylene oxide) electrospun nanofibrous mats as a floating gastro-retentive delivery system for ranitidine hydrochloride, J. Pharmaceut. Biomed. Anal. 153 (2018) 63–75.
[28] J. Wu, Z. Zhang, J.g. Gu, W. Zhou, X. Liang, G. Zhou, C.C. Han, S. Xu, Y. Liu, Mechanism of a long-term controlled drug release system based on simple blended electrospun fibers, J. Contr. Release 320 (2020) 337–346.

[29] M. Eslamian, M. Khorrami, N. Yi, S. Majd, M.R. Abidian, Electrospinning of highly aligned fibers for drug delivery applications, J. Mater. Chem. B 7 (2) (2019) 224−232.
[30] S. Chen, S.K. Boda, S.K. Batra, X. Li, J. Xie, Emerging roles of electrospun nanofibers in cancer research, Adv. Healthc. Mater. 7 (6) (2018) 1701024.
[31] Y. Zhu, L. Edmonds, X. Zhao, X. Chen, C. Hu, Y. Cheng, W. Cui, In vitro and in vivo evaluation of rapamycin-eluting nanofibers coated on cardia stents, RSC Adv. 4 (65) (2014) 34405−34411.
[32] Y.-Y. Tseng, Y.-C. Kao, J.-Y. Liao, W.-A. Chen, S.-J. Liu, Biodegradable drug-eluting poly[lactic-co-glycol acid] nanofibers for the sustainable delivery of vancomycin to brain tissue: in vitro and in vivo studies, ACS Chem. Neurosci. 4 (9) (2013) 1314−1321.
[33] W. Song, Z. Ma, C. Wang, H. Li, Y. He, Pro-chondrogenic and immunomodulatory melatonin-loaded electrospun membranes for tendon-to-bone healing, J. Mater. Chem. B 7 (42) (2019) 6564−6575.
[34] S.P.,R.C.R.,S.P. Sundaran, A. Binoy, N. Mishra, S. A, In-vitro evaluation on drug release kinetics and antibacterial activity of dextran modified polyurethane fibrous membrane, Int. J. Biol. Macromol. 126 (2019) 717−730.
[35] J. Xue, M. He, Y. Liang, A. Crawford, P. Coates, D. Chen, R. Shi, L. Zhang, Fabrication and evaluation of electrospun PCL−gelatin micro-/nanofiber membranes for anti-infective GTR implants, J. Mater. Chem. B 2 (39) (2014) 6867−6877.
[36] H. Wang, M. Li, J. Hu, C. Wang, S. Xu, C.C. Han, Multiple targeted drugs carrying biodegradable membrane barrier: anti-adhesion, hemostasis, and anti-infection, Biomacromolecules 14 (4) (2013) 954−961.
[37] Z. Zhang, J. Tang, H. Wang, Q. Xia, S. Xu, C.C. Han, Controlled antibiotics release system through simple blended electrospun fibers for sustained antibacterial effects, ACS Appl. Mater. Interfaces 7 (48) (2015) 26400−26404.
[38] R. Ramachandran, V.R. Junnuthula, G.S. Gowd, A. Ashokan, J. Thomas, R. Peethambaran, A. Thomas, A.K.K. Unni, D. Panikar, S.V. Nair, M. Koyakutty, Theranostic 3-dimensional nano brain-implant for prolonged and localized treatment of recurrent glioma, Sci. Rep. 7 (1) (2017) 43271.
[39] P. Sasmal, P. Datta, Tranexamic acid-loaded chitosan electrospun nanofibers as drug delivery system for hemorrhage control applications, J. Drug Deliv. Sci. Technol. 52 (2019) 559−567.
[40] N. Nikmaram, S. Roohinejad, S. Hashemi, M. Koubaa, F.J. Barba, A. Abbaspourrad, R. Greiner, Emulsion-based systems for fabrication of electrospun nanofibers: food, pharmaceutical and biomedical applications, RSC Adv. 7 (46) (2017) 28951−28964.
[41] J. Hu, J. Wei, W. Liu, Y. Chen, Preparation and characterization of electrospun PLGA/gelatin nanofibers as a drug delivery system by emulsion electrospinning, J. Biomater. Sci. Polym. Ed. 24 (8) (2013) 972−985.
[42] J. Hu, M.P. Prabhakaran, L. Tian, X. Ding, S. Ramakrishna, Drug-loaded emulsion electrospun nanofibers: characterization, drug release and in vitro biocompatibility, RSC Adv. 5 (121) (2015) 100256−100267.
[43] A.M. Moydeen, M.S. Ali Padusha, E.F. Aboelfetoh, S.S. Al-Deyab, M.H. El-Newehy, Fabrication of electrospun poly(vinyl alcohol)/dextran nanofibers via emulsion process as drug delivery system: kinetics and in vitro release study, Int. J. Biol. Macromol. 116 (2018) 1250−1259.
[44] W. Li, T. Luo, Y. Yang, X. Tan, L. Liu, formation of controllable hydrophilic/hydrophobic drug delivery systems by electrospinning of vesicles, Langmuir 31 (18) (2015) 5141−5146.
[45] H. Qu, S. Wei, Z. Guo, Coaxial electrospun nanostructures and their applications, J. Mater. Chem. 1 (38) (2013) 11513−11528.

[46] J. Meng, V. Agrahari, M.J. Ezoulin, C. Zhang, S.S. Purohit, A. Molteni, D. Dim, N.A. Oyler, B.-B.C. Youan, Tenofovir containing thiolated chitosan core/shell nanofibers: in vitro and in vivo evaluations, Mol. Pharm. 13 (12) (2016) 4129–4140.
[47] L. Viry, S.E. Moulton, T. Romeo, C. Suhr, D. Mawad, M. Cook, G.G. Wallace, Emulsion-coaxial electrospinning: designing novel architectures for sustained release of highly soluble low molecular weight drugs, J. Mater. Chem. 22 (22) (2012) 11347–11353.
[48] N. Zandi, R. Lotfi, E. Tamjid, M.A. Shokrgozar, A. Simchi, Core-sheath gelatin based electrospun nanofibers for dual delivery release of biomolecules and therapeutics, Mater. Sci. Eng. C 108 (2020) 110432.
[49] D. Han, A.J. Steckl, Triaxial electrospun nanofiber membranes for controlled dual release of functional molecules, ACS Appl. Mater. Interfaces 5 (16) (2013) 8241–8245.
[50] D.-G. Yu, X.-Y. Li, X. Wang, J.-H. Yang, S.W.A. Bligh, G.R. Williams, Nanofibers fabricated using triaxial electrospinning as zero order drug delivery systems, ACS Appl. Mater. Interfaces 7 (33) (2015) 18891–18897.
[51] S.P. Sundaran, S. T, S. Athiyanathil, "Nano in micro" architecture composite membranes for controlled drug delivery, Appl. Clay Sci. 166 (2018) 262–275.
[52] J. Xue, Y. Niu, M. Gong, R. Shi, D. Chen, L. Zhang, Y. Lvov, Electrospun microfiber membranes embedded with drug-loaded clay nanotubes for sustained antimicrobial protection, ACS Nano 9 (2) (2015) 1600–1612.
[53] M.I. Hassan, N. Sultana, Characterization, drug loading and antibacterial activity of nanohydroxyapatite/polycaprolactone (nHA/PCL) electrospun membrane, 3 Biotech 7 (4) (2017) 249.
[54] C. Xu, Y. Cao, C. Lei, Z. Li, T. Kumeria, A.K. Meka, J. Xu, J. Liu, C. Yan, L. Luo, A. Khademhosseini, A. Popat, Y. He, Q. Ye, Polymer–mesoporous silica nanoparticle core–shell nanofibers as a dual-drug-delivery system for guided tissue regeneration, ACS Appl. Nano Mater. 3 (2) (2020) 1457–1467.
[55] S. Kumar, A.P. Singh, S. Senapati, P. Maiti, Controlling drug delivery using nanosheet-embedded electrospun fibers for efficient tumor treatment, Appl. Biomater. 2 (2) (2019) 884–894.
[56] G. Furtos, G. Rivero, S. Rapuntean, G.A. Abraham, Amoxicillin-loaded electrospun nanocomposite membranes for dental applications, J. Biomed. Mater. Res. B Appl. Biomater. 105 (5) (2017) 966–976.
[57] Y. Zhang, J. Wang, J. Xiao, T. Fang, N. Hu, M. Li, L. Deng, Y. Cheng, Y. Zhu, W. Cui, An electrospun fiber-covered stent with programmable dual drug release for endothelialization acceleration and lumen stenosis prevention, Acta Biomater. 94 (2019) 295–305.
[58] Y. Wang, W. Cui, X. Zhao, S. Wen, Y. Sun, J. Han, H. Zhang, Bone remodeling-inspired dual delivery electrospun nanofibers for promoting bone regeneration, Nanoscale 11 (1) (2019) 60–71.
[59] J. Song, A. Klymov, J. Shao, Y. Zhang, W. Ji, E. Kolwijck, J.A. Jansen, S.C.G. Leeuwenburgh, F. Yang, Electrospun nanofibrous silk fibroin membranes containing gelatin nanospheres for controlled delivery of biomolecules, Adv. Healthc. Mater. 6 (14) (2017) 1700014.
[60] Z. Hou, X. Li, C. Li, Y. Dai, P.a. Ma, X. Zhang, X. Kang, Z. Cheng, J. Lin, Electrospun upconversion composite fibers as dual drugs delivery system with individual release properties, Langmuir 29 (30) (2013) 9473–9482.
[61] A. El-Fiqi, J.-H. Kim, H.-W. Kim, Osteoinductive fibrous scaffolds of biopolymer/mesoporous bioactive glass nanocarriers with excellent bioactivity and long-term delivery of osteogenic drug, ACS Appl. Mater. Interfaces 7 (2) (2015) 1140–1152.

[62] R. Qi, R. Guo, M. Shen, X. Cao, L. Zhang, J. Xu, J. Yu, X. Shi, Electrospun poly(-lactic-co-glycolic acid)/halloysite nanotube composite nanofibers for drug encapsulation and sustained release, J. Mater. Chem. 20 (47) (2010) 10622–10629.
[63] R.T. De Silva, R.K. Dissanayake, M.M.M.G.P.G. Mantilaka, W.P.S.L. Wijesinghe, S.S. Kaleel, T.N. Premachandra, L. Weerasinghe, G.A.J. Amaratunga, K.M.N. de Silva, Drug-loaded halloysite nanotube-reinforced electrospun alginate-based nanofibrous scaffolds with sustained antimicrobial protection, ACS Appl. Mater. Interfaces 10 (40) (2018) 33913–33922.
[64] Y.E. Bulbul, M. Okur, F. Demirtas-Korkmaz, N. Dilsiz, Development of PCL/PEO electrospun fibrous membranes blended with silane-modified halloysite nanotube as a curcumin release system, Appl. Clay Sci. 186 (2020) 105430.
[65] A. Laha, C.S. Sharma, S. Majumdar, Sustained drug release from multi-layered sequentially crosslinked electrospun gelatin nanofiber mesh, Mater. Sci. Eng. C 76 (2017) 782–786.
[66] R. Cr, S. Ps, M. O, S. Pp, S. A, Nanochitosan enriched poly ε-caprolactone electrospun wound dressing membranes: a fine tuning of physicochemical properties, hemocompatibility and curcumin release profile, Int. J. Biol. Macromol. 108 (2018) 1261–1272.
[67] N. Alhusein, I.S. Blagbrough, P.A. De Bank, Electrospun matrices for localised controlled drug delivery: release of tetracycline hydrochloride from layers of polycaprolactone and poly(ethylene-co-vinyl acetate), Drug Deliv. Trans. Res. 2 (6) (2012) 477–488.
[68] N. Bölgen, İ. Vargel, P. Korkusuz, Y.Z. Menceloğlu, E. Pişkin, In vivo performance of antibiotic embedded electrospun PCL membranes for prevention of abdominal adhesions, J. Biomed. Mater. Res. B Appl. Biomater. 81B (2) (2007) 530–543.
[69] P. Sagitha, C.R. Reshmi, S.P. Sundaran, A. Sujith, Recent advances in post-modification strategies of polymeric electrospun membranes, Eur. Polym. J. 105 (2018) 227–249.
[70] C. He, W. Nie, W. Feng, Engineering of biomimetic nanofibrous matrices for drug delivery and tissue engineering, J. Mater. Chem. B 2 (45) (2014) 7828–7848.
[71] K.T. Kurpinski, J.T. Stephenson, R.R.R. Janairo, H. Lee, S. Li, The effect of fiber alignment and heparin coating on cell infiltration into nanofibrous PLLA scaffolds, Biomaterials 31 (13) (2010) 3536–3542.
[72] J. Yun, J.S. Im, Y.-S. Lee, H.-I. Kim, Electro-responsive transdermal drug delivery behavior of PVA/PAA/MWCNT nanofibers, Eur. Polym. J. 47 (10) (2011) 1893–1902.
[73] S. Samadi, M. Moradkhani, H. Beheshti, M. Irani, M. Aliabadi, Fabrication of chitosan/poly(lactic acid)/graphene oxide/TiO_2 composite nanofibrous scaffolds for sustained delivery of doxorubicin and treatment of lung cancer, Int. J. Biol. Macromol. 110 (2018) 416–424.
[74] J. Li, W. Xu, D. Li, T. Liu, Y.S. Zhang, J. Ding, X. Chen, Locally deployable nanofiber patch for sequential drug delivery in treatment of primary and advanced orthotopic hepatomas, ACS Nano 12 (7) (2018) 6685–6699.
[75] Y. Fu, W.J. Kao, Drug release kinetics and transport mechanisms of non-degradable and degradable polymeric delivery systems, Expet Opin. Drug Deliv. 7 (4) (2010) 429–444.
[76] F.E. Ahmed, B.S. Lalia, R. Hashaikeh, A review on electrospinning for membrane fabrication: challenges and applications, Desalination 356 (2015) 15–30.
[77] T.T.T. Nguyen, C. Ghosh, S.-G. Hwang, N. Chanunpanich, J.S. Park, Porous core/sheath composite nanofibers fabricated by coaxial electrospinning as a potential mat for drug release system, Int. J. Pharm. 439 (1) (2012) 296–306.

[78] Y. Han, Y. Jiang, Y. Li, M. Wang, T. Fan, M. Liu, Q. Ke, H. Xu, Z. Yi, An aligned porous electrospun fibrous scaffold with embedded asiatic acid for accelerating diabetic wound healing, J. Mater. Chem. B 7 (40) (2019) 6125–6138.
[79] X. Ren, Y. Han, J. Wang, Y. Jiang, Z. Yi, H. Xu, Q. Ke, An aligned porous electrospun fibrous membrane with controlled drug delivery – an efficient strategy to accelerate diabetic wound healing with improved angiogenesis, Acta Biomater. 70 (2018) 140–153.
[80] Z. Yuan, K. Zhang, X. Jiao, Y. Cheng, Y. Zhang, P. Zhang, X. Zhang, Y. Wen, A controllable local drug delivery system based on porous fibers for synergistic treatment of melanoma and promoting wound healing, Biomater. Sci. 7 (12) (2019) 5084–5096.
[81] Y. Chen, Y. Qiu, W. Chen, Q. Wei, Electrospun thymol-loaded porous cellulose acetate fibers with potential biomedical applications, Mater. Sci. Eng. C 109 (2020) 110536.
[82] M. Chen, M. Dong, R. Havelund, V.R. Regina, R.L. Meyer, F. Besenbacher, P. Kingshott, Thermo-responsive core–sheath electrospun nanofibers from poly (N-isopropylacrylamide)/polycaprolactone blends, Chem. Mater. 22 (14) (2010) 4214–4221.
[83] E. González, M.W. Frey, Synthesis, characterization and electrospinning of poly(vinyl caprolactam-co-hydroxymethyl acrylamide) to create stimuli-responsive nanofibers, Polymer 108 (2017) 154–162.
[84] K.I. Jahan, A. Goponenko, Y. Dzenis, Electrospun nanofibrous materials as stimuli-responsive polymerized hydrogels, Macromol. Symp. 365 (1) (2016) 118–127.
[85] R. Salehi, M. Irani, M. Eskandani, K. Nowruzi, S. Davaran, I. Haririan, Interaction, controlled release, and antitumor activity of doxorubicin hydrochloride from pH-sensitive P(NIPAAm-MAA-VP) nanofibrous scaffolds prepared by green electrospinning, Int. J. Polym. Mater. Polym. Biomater. 63 (12) (2014) 609–619.
[86] C. Yang, D.-G. Yu, D. Pan, X.-K. Liu, X. Wang, S.W.A. Bligh, G.R. Williams, Electrospun pH-sensitive core–shell polymer nanocomposites fabricated using a tri-axial process, Acta Biomater. 35 (2016) 77–86.
[87] W. Cui, X. Li, X. Zhu, G. Yu, S. Zhou, J. Weng, Investigation of drug release and matrix degradation of electrospun poly(DL-lactide) fibers with paracetanol inoculation, Biomacromolecules 7 (5) (2006) 1623–1629.
[88] Y.F. Li, P. Slemming-Adamsen, J. Wang, J. Song, X. Wang, Y. Yu, M. Dong, C. Chen, F. Besenbacher, M. Chen, Light responsive hybrid nanofibres for on-demand therapeutic drug and cell delivery, J. Tissue Eng. Regen. Med. 11 (8) (2017) 2411–2420.
[89] A. Baji, K. Agarwal, S.V. Oopath, Emerging developments in the use of electrospun fibers and membranes for protective clothing applications, Polymers 12 (2) (2020) 492.
[90] J. Joseph, S.V. Nair, D. Menon, Integrating substrateless electrospinning with textile technology for creating biodegradable three-dimensional structures, Nano Lett. 15 (8) (2015) 5420–5426.
[91] Y. Yang, Y. Zhao, Z. Quan, H. Zhang, X. Qin, R. Wang, J. Yu, An efficient hybrid strategy for composite yarns of micro-/nano-fibers, Mater. Des. 184 (2019) 108196.
[92] S. Padmakumar, J. Joseph, M.H. Neppalli, S.E. Mathew, S.V. Nair, S.A. Shankarappa, D. Menon, Electrospun polymeric core–sheath yarns as drug eluting surgical sutures, ACS Appl. Mater. Interfaces 8 (11) (2016) 6925–6934.
[93] H. Maleki, A.A. Gharehaghaji, T. Toliyat, P.J. Dijkstra, Drug release behavior of electrospun twisted yarns as implantable medical devices, Biofabrication 8 (3) (2016) 035019.

[94] E. Sharifisamani, F. Mousazadegan, R. Bagherzadeh, M. Latifi, PEG-PLA-PCL based electrospun yarns with curcumin control release property as suture, Polym. Eng. Sci. 60 (7) (2020) 1520–1529.
[95] S. Bae, M.J. DiBalsi, N. Meilinger, C. Zhang, E. Beal, G. Korneva, R.O. Brown, K.G. Kornev, J.S. Lee, Heparin-eluting electrospun nanofiber yarns for antithrombotic vascular sutures, ACS Appl. Mater. Interfaces 10 (10) (2018) 8426–8435.
[96] C.L. He, Z.M. Huang, X.J. Han, Fabrication of drug-loaded electrospun aligned fibrous threads for suture applications, J. Biomed. Mater. Res. 89 (1) (2009) 80–95.
[97] S. Wu, R. Zhou, F. Zhou, P.N. Streubel, S. Chen, B. Duan, Electrospun thymosin beta-4 loaded PLGA/PLA nanofiber/microfiber hybrid yarns for tendon tissue engineering application, Mater. Sci. Eng. C Mater. Biol. Appl. 106 (2020) 110268.
[98] W. Hu, Z.M. Huang, X.Y. Liu, Development of braided drug-loaded nanofiber sutures, Nanotechnology 21 (31) (2010) 315104.
[99] P.-o. Rujitanaroj, Y.-C. Wang, J. Wang, S.Y. Chew, Nanofiber-mediated controlled release of siRNA complexes for long term gene-silencing applications, Biomaterials 32 (25) (2011) 5915–5923.
[100] C. Achille, S. Sundaresh, B. Chu, M. Hadjiargyrou, Cdk2 silencing via a DNA/PCL electrospun scaffold suppresses proliferation and increases death of breast cancer cells, PloS One 7 (12) (2012) e52356.
[101] T.N. da Silva, R.P. Gonçalves, C.L. Rocha, B.S. Archanjo, C.A.G. Barboza, M.B.R. Pierre, F. Reynaud, P.H. de Souza Picciani, Controlling burst effect with PLA/PVA coaxial electrospun scaffolds loaded with BMP-2 for bone guided regeneration, Mater. Sci. Eng. C 97 (2019) 602–612.
[102] S. Kuttappan, J.-i. Jo, C.K. Sabu, D. Menon, Y. Tabata, M.B. Nair, Bioinspired nanocomposite fibrous scaffold mediated delivery of ONO-1301 and BMP2 enhance bone regeneration in critical sized defect, Mater. Sci. Eng. C 110 (2020) 110591.
[103] S. Kuttappan, J.-i. Jo, D. Menon, T. Ishimoto, T. Nakano, S.V. Nair, Y. Tabata, M.B. Nair, ONO-1301 loaded nanocomposite scaffolds modulate cAMP mediated signaling and induce new bone formation in critical sized bone defect, Biomater. Sci. 8 (3) (2020) 884–896.
[104] B. Xia, Y. Lv, Dual-delivery of VEGF and NGF by emulsion electrospun nanofibrous scaffold for peripheral nerve regeneration, Mater. Sci. Eng. C 82 (2018) 253–264.
[105] J. Hu, L. Tian, M.P. Prabhakaran, X. Ding, S. Ramakrishna, Fabrication of nerve growth factor encapsulated aligned poly(ε-caprolactone) nanofibers and their assessment as a potential neural tissue engineering scaffold, Polymers 8 (2) (2016) 54.
[106] C. Lei, Y. Cui, L. Zheng, P.K.-H. Chow, C.-H. Wang, Development of a gene/drug dual delivery system for brain tumor therapy: potent inhibition via RNA interference and synergistic effects, Biomaterials 34 (30) (2013) 7483–7494.

CHAPTER FIVE

Electrospun nanomaterials as biosensors in diagnostics and beyond

Gang Wei
College of Chemistry and Chemical Engineering, Qingdao University, Qingdao, Shandong Province, PR China

Abbreviations

BSA Bovine serum albumin
CFU Colony-forming unit
CNFs Carbon nanofibers
CNT Carbon nanotubes
GCE Glassy carbon electrode
GO Graphene oxide
MMP-9 Matrix metalloproteinases-9
PAA Poly(acrylic acid)
PAN Polyacrylonitrile
PDA Polydiacetylene
PEO Poly(ethylene oxide)
PMMA Poly(methyl methacrylate)
PVA Poly(vinyl alcohol)
PVDF Polyvinylidene difluoride
PVP Polyvinylpyrrolidone
QGDs Graphene quantum dots
RGO Reduced graphene oxide
SERS Surface-enhanced Raman scattering
SPR Surface plasmon resonance

5.1 Introduction

In 1996, Reneker et al. fabricated ultrafine polymer nanofibers (NFs) with diameters ranging from nm to μm by electrospinning and first proved that electrospinning could be a simple and effective technique to prepare nanofibrous materials [1]. Since then, electrospinning has been utilized as a new strategy to fabricate various materials in the fields of materials science, biomaterials, tissue engineering, biomedicine, sensors/biosensors, and

Biomedical Applications of Electrospinning and Electrospraying
ISBN: 978-0-12-822476-2
https://doi.org/10.1016/B978-0-12-822476-2.00002-9

environmental science [2—7]. In recent years, sensors and biosensors have been widely used in the fields of bioanalysis, biomedicine, food science, and environmental science due to their high sensitivity, good selectivity, and high detection ability [8—10]. With the development of materials science and nanotechnology, various functional nanoparticles such as nanoparticles, NFs, carbon nanotubes (CNTs), and two-dimensional materials (like graphene and MoS_2) have been used for the fabrication of biosensors [11,12], in which the one-dimensional nanomaterials including CNTs, polymer NFs, and carbon NFs (CNFs) exhibited very high potential to improve the sensing performance of the fabricated biosensors ascribed to the high aspect ratio and surface area of NFs [13—15].

However, previous studies indicated that the use of simple electrospun polymer NFs for biosensors has very limited efficiency as the polymer substrates could not provide satisfied optical, electronic, and chemical properties for creating sensitive signals [16]. To solve this problem, two typical potential methods have been used to improve the potential of electrospinning toward biosensors applications. One way is to make the posttreatment like carbonization on the electrospun polymer NFs to obtain CNFs, which show wider applications and better performances for the fabrication of biosensors. The other method is to modify the electrospun polymer NFs with functional nanomaterials or building blocks, including biomolecules, nanoparticles, quantum dots, carbon materials, and others to enhance the optical, electronic, and chemical properties of polymer NFs for biosensing application [6,17]. In this case, the conjugation of nanomaterials or building blocks with electrospun polymer NFs has synergistic effects toward the final biosensing performance. Through both methods, various polymer NF- and CNF-based hybrid nanomaterials have been created with electrospinning and used for the fabrication of electrochemical, fluorescent, electrochemiluminescence, colorimetric, electronic, surface plasma resonance (SPR), and other sensors, which exhibited high sensitivity and selectivity, good stability, as well as low detection limit for the determination of biological analytes [18,19].

In this chapter, we would like to present recent advancements in the preparation of electrospun functional fibrous nanomaterials for the fabrication of various biosensor platforms with high performance. The design and electrospinning synthesis of fibrous nanomaterials by conjugating zero-, one-, and two-dimensional building blocks to polymer NF are introduced. In addition, the fabrication of biosensor platforms with electrospun nanomaterials for detecting DNA, RNA, proteins, small molecules, drugs, organisms, and others is demonstrated and discussed in detail.

5.2 Functional nanomaterials by electrospinning

In this section, the formation of functional nanomaterials by introducing zero-, one-, and two-dimensional building blocks onto electrospun polymer NFs through pretreatment and posttreatment methods is demonstrated and discussed briefly.

5.2.1 Formation of zero-dimensional building blocks on polymer nanofibers

In order to improve the physical, chemical, and mechanical properties of electrospun polymer NF, previously, a lot of studies have been performed by incorporating metal nanoparticles [20—22], quantum dots [23], and bimetallic nanoparticles [24] onto polymer NFs to prepare one-dimensional hybrid nanomaterials.

For instance, Celebioglu et al. demonstrated the one-step green synthesis of silver nanoparticles (AgNPs) embedded in the electrospun cyclodextrin NFs [20]. Firstly, cyclodextrin NFs were produced by electrospinning cyclodextrin in DMF solution, and then $AgNO_3$ solution with different concentration was added to promote the in situ green synthesis of AgNPs due to the high reduction ability and stability of cyclodextrin molecules toward silver ions. With the similar method, Li and coworkers obtained platinum nanoparticles (PtNPs) along electrospun polyacrylonitrile (PAN) NFs through electrostatic assembling of negative-charged PtNPs on positive-modified PAN NFs [21]. In another study, Liu et al. reported the self-assembly of as-prepared gold nanoparticles (AuNPs) on electrospun three-dimensional poly(acrylic acid)/poly(vinyl alcohol) (PAA/PVA) nanofibrous membrane by electrostatic interactions between nanoparticles and NFs [22]. Besides the posttreatment of NFs for the conjugation of nanoparticles, the electrospinning mixed solution of polymers and nanoparticles to hybrid NFs has also been reported. In a typical study, Zhang and coworkers prepared PVA/graphene quantum dots (GQDs) nanofibrous membranes by electrospinning mixed GQDs and PVA together [23] and found that the formed PVA/GQD membranes exhibited fluorescent and catalytic properties.

Bimetallic nanoparticles have also been conjugated onto electrospun nanomaterials for advanced applications. For example, Huang et al. introduced a facile method for the formation of Ag—Pt bimetallic nanoparticles on electrospun CNFs [24], as shown in Fig. 5.1. In their work, PAN/polyvinylpyrrolidone (PVP) NFs were firstly produced by electrospinning blend PAN/PVP solution, and then nanoporous PAN NFs were obtained by

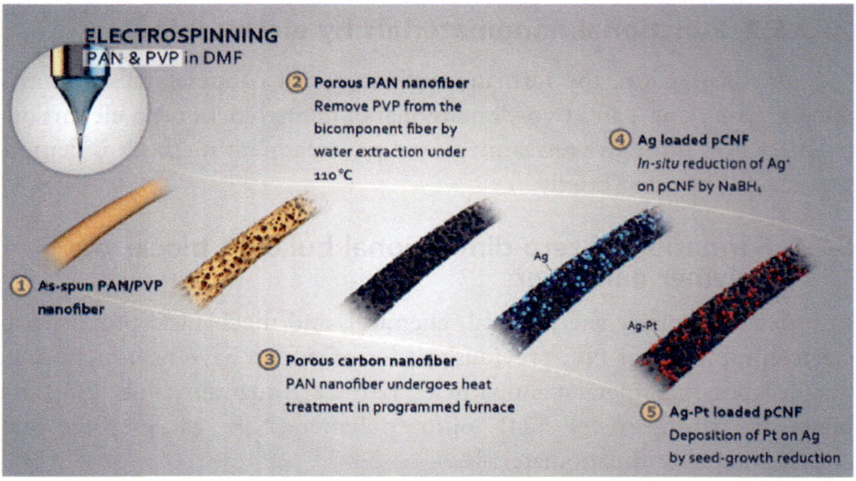

Figure 5.1 Electrospinning formation of bimetallic Ag−Pt nanoparticles on pCNFs. *Reprinted with permission from Y.P. Huang, Y.E. Miao, S.S. Ji, W.W. Tjiu, T.X. Liu, Electrospun carbon nanofibers decorated with Ag-Pt bimetallic nanoparticles for selective detection of dopamine, ACS Appl. Mater. Interfaces 6(15) (2014) 12449−12456. Copyright 2014, American Chemical Society.*

removing PVP component by subsequent water extraction and heat treatment under 110°C. After that, the formed nanoporous PAN NFs were transferred to porous CNFs (pCNFs) by heat treatment, which were then used for the ionic binding of Ag^+ and chemical reduction to create AgNPs. Finally, the formation of Ag−Pt-loaded pCNFs was achieved by Ag-based seed growth. This study presented an effective strategy for the production of electrospun CNFs and bimetallic nanoparticles by ionic reduction and seed growth, and the complex hybrid NFs with porous structure revealed high potentials in electrocatalytic and sensor fields ascribed to the syngenetic effects of CNFs and bimetals.

With the abovementioned strategies, metal oxide nanoparticles [25], metal/metal oxide nanoparticles [26], and others [27] have also been produced by electrospinning and postchemical treatments. For instance, Zheng et al. reported the preparation of Ag/CuO NFs by electrospinning $AgNO_3$ and $Cu(NO_3)_2$ with PVP onto the surface of indium tin oxide, following with oxidization to Ag/CuO and subsequent annealing in air to remove PVP component. It was found that the structure and catalytic properties of the produced Ag/CuO NFs were affected by some factors like the electrospinning time, NaOH concentration, Ag/Cu molar ratio, and the calcinations temperature.

5.2.2 Formation of one-dimensional building blocks on polymer nanofibers

It is possible to improve the electrical, optical, and mechanical properties of electrospun polymer NFs by introducing one-dimensional building blocks into the NF matrix. CNTs have been used as excellent candidates for this aim by electrospinning mixed polymer and CNT solution.

Previously, Mercante et al. reported a simple strategy to prepare CNT-functionalized polymer NFs by first electrospinning polymer NFs and then assembling CNTs onto the surface of NFs [28]. It was found that high-density CNTs were adsorbed onto the surface of NFs, and the synergistic effects of CNTs and NFs improved the material performance of bio/chemical sensors. However, the dispersity and orientation of CNTs in the fabricated polymer NFs along the long axis are two main challenges for the electrospinning synthesis. Previously, Su and coworkers developed an improved electrospinning technique to obtain poly(ethylene oxide) (PEO)−CNT hybrid NFs by controlling the orientations of CNTs in PEO NFs [29]. Their results indicated that both the uniaxially and biaxially oriented CNT-based hybrid NFs exhibited better tensile strength, modulus, and electrical conductivity than the CNT random-oriented NFs. In a further study, they demonstrated the successful preparation of polyvinylidene difluoride (PVDF) NFs that doped with CNTs and PtNPs by electrospinning PVDF, CNTs, and PtNPs together [30]. The created hybrid nanofibrous membrane revealed potential applications in high-performance biosensing and electrochemical catalysis.

With the similar technique, Paul and coworkers synthesized electrospun multiwalled CNTs (MWCNTs)-embedded ZnO nanowires by a simple and low-cost electrospinning method [31]. In their work, the used polymer, PAN, could mediate the formation of high-density ZnO nanoparticles in the mixed solution under a suitable reaction temperature, and therefore the hybrids PAN−ZnO and PAN−MWCNT−ZnO NFs were synthesized by directly electrospinning the mixed precursor solution of PAN, MWCNTs, and ZnAC, as shown in Fig. 5.2a. The synthesized PAN−MWCNT−ZnO NFs exhibited uniform distribution of MWCNTs and a diameter of 185−200 nm (Fig. 5.2b). After the calcination at a critical temperature, the MWCNTs-embedded ZnO nanowires were obtained finally (Fig. 5.2c). It is interesting that the one-step calcination created enough functional −COOH groups on the surface of MWCNT−ZnO nanowires, which could be further utilized as binding sites to conjugate covalently with

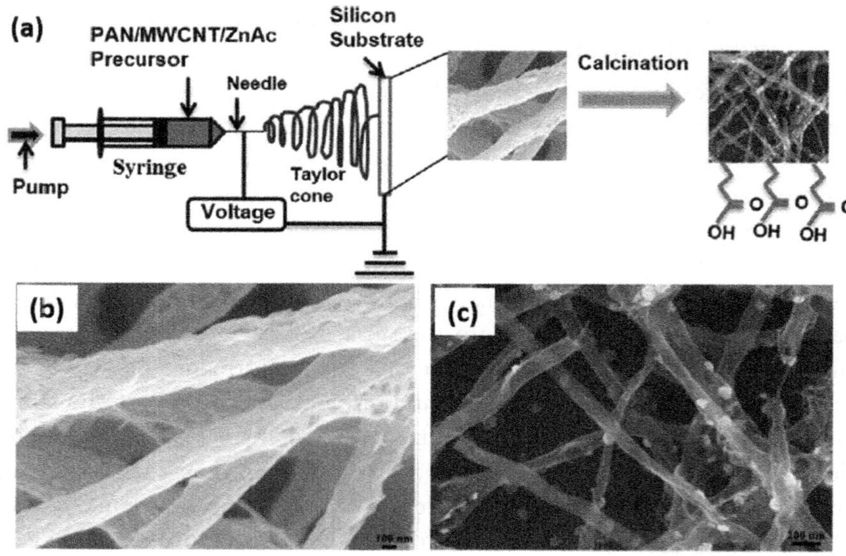

Figure 5.2 Electrospinning preparation of MWCNT–ZnO nanowires: (a) Electrospinning process of PAN–MWCNT–ZnO nanowires and the calcination to MWCNT–ZnO nanowires. (b,c) SEM images of electrospun PAN–MWCNT–ZnO nanowires before (b) and after (c) calcination. *Reproduced with permission from K.B. Paul, V. Singh, S.R.K. Vanjari, S.G. Singh, One step biofunctionalized electrospun multiwalled carbon nanotubes embedded zinc oxide nanowire interface for highly sensitive detection of carcinoma antigen-125, Biosens. Bioelectron. 88 (2017) 144–152. Copyright 2017, Elsevier B.V.*

antibody without any chemical modification, which shows high potentials for the fabrication of immunosensors for the detection of cancer biomarkers.

Besides CNTs, other metal oxide NFs have also been created by electrospinning and posttreatment methods [32,33]. For example, Kim et al. demonstrated the electrospun synthesis of TiO_2 NFs and the subsequent growth of RuO_2 nanowires on the surface of TiO_2 NFs [32]. In another case, Liu et al. reported the hydrothermal synthesis of binary $NiCo_2O_4$ nanoneedles on the electrospun CNFs [33]. Both electrospun-based hybrid nanomaterials have been used for the fabrication of nonenzymatic electrochemical biosensors for sensitive detection of ascorbic acid and glucose, respectively.

5.2.3 Formation of two-dimensional building blocks on polymer nanofibers

Two-dimensional materials have shown wide applications in the fields of materials science, nanotechnology, tissue engineering, biomedicine, analytical science, energy storage, and environmental science. Recently, with the development of two-dimensional materials, some two-dimensional building blocks, such as graphene oxide (GO), reduced GO (RGO), MoS_2, $Ti_3C_2T_X$, and $Ni(OH)_2$ nanosheets, have been utilized in electrospinning with polymers to form functional hybrid NFs.

Mishra et al. presented the deposition of GO/PVA composite NFs onto screen-printed carbon electrodes by an electrospinning process [34], in which the GO was dispersed in PVA-diluted aqueous solution and the mixture was electrospun directly into GO/PVA NFs. This method is simple and effective to cause uniform distribution of GO in the fabricated polymer NFs. In another case, Ghobadi et al. prepared PVA/PAN/RGO ternary nanofibrous mats by electrospinning mixed PVA, PAN, and RGO together [35]. The created PVA/PAN/RGO ternary mats exhibited improved performance for metal-free antibacterial effects.

Metal nanoparticles could be added to the electrospinning to enhance the catalytical activity of the created GO—polymer hybrid NFs. In a typical study, Li and coworkers reported the electrospinning PVA NFs doped with GO—AgNP hybrid nanosheets for the fabrication of functional three-dimensional membrane electrode materials [36]. In their study, $AgNO_3$ was firstly added into GO solution, and then the GO—AgNP hybrids were formed via a green chemical synthesis. Then, PVA was added to the GO—AgNP hybrid solution at 90°C under stirring to obtain mixed solution with good dispersity, as shown in Fig. 5.3. After that, the mixed solution was electrospun to form PVA—GO—AgNP hybrid NFs on glassy carbon electrode (GCE) to produce three-dimensional membrane, which revealed great advantages for highly sensitive electrochemical determination of H_2O_2. This kind of nanofibrous membrane electrode has wider applications for the fabrication of electrochemical sensors and biosensors, as well as the design of three-dimensional functional nanomaterials in the future.

Other kind of popular two-dimensional transition metal dichalcogenide and MXene materials have also been electrospun into polymer NFs to produce functional hybrid NFs. For instance, Yu and Park introduced the electrospinning synthesis of PAN/MoS_2 composite NFs, which reveals rough surface by a high loading of two-dimensional MoS_2 nanosheets [37]. In addition, it was found that MoS_2 nanosheets were uniformly distributed inside the PAN matrix, and an enhanced thermal stability of the composites NFs was found. In another case, Mayerberger et al. reported the electrospinning production of $Ti_3C_2T_X$-chitosan nanofibers, which can be further used for the in vitro antibacterial studies due to the low cost, biodegradability,

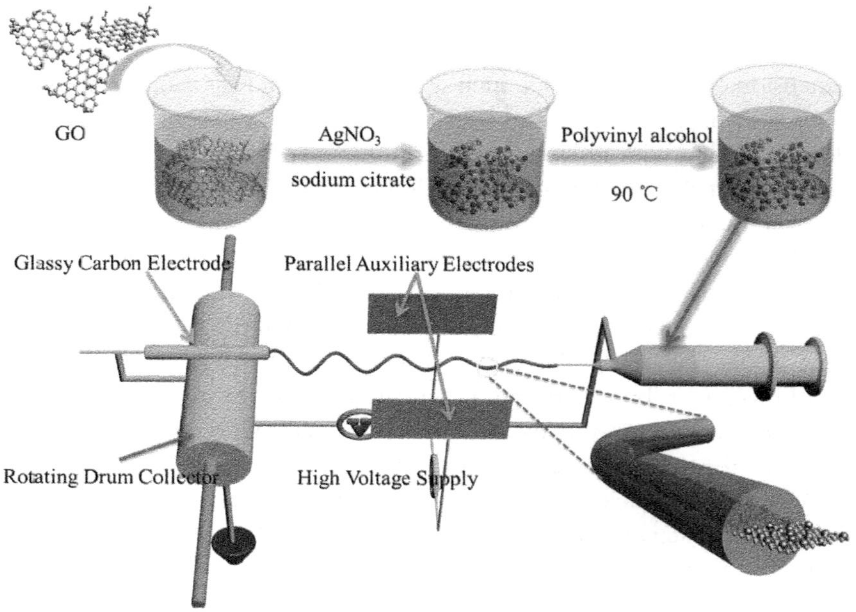

Figure 5.3 PVA–GO–AgNP hybrid nanofibrous membrane by electrospinning green synthesized GO–AgNP nanohybrids with PVA together. *Reprinted with permission from Y. Li, P.P. Zhang, Z.F. Ouyang, M.F. Zhang, Z.J. Lin, J.F. Li, Z.Q. Su, G. Wei, Nanoscale graphene doped with highly dispersed silver nanoparticles: quick synthesis, facile fabrication of 3D membrane-modified electrode, and super performance for electrochemical sensing, Adv. Funct. Mater. 26(13) (2016) 2122–2134. Copyright 2016, Wiley.*

nontoxicity, and antimicrobial properties of the fabricated hybrid NFs [38]. However, the above studies indicated that it is not easy to obtain fine NFs with good distribution of two-dimensional building blocks via electrospinning due to the interactions between two-dimensional materials and polymers. Therefore, appropriate chemical modification of two-dimensional building blocks and good dispersity in polymer solution are necessary to obtain ultrafine nanofibrous structure with electrospinning methods.

Recently, Chen et al. demonstrated the preparation of two-dimensional $Ni(OH)_2$ nanoplatelets on electrospun CNFs by the postmicrowave reaction [39]. The electrospun PAN NFs were removed by oxidizing the precursor NFs at 250°C for 3 h in air and then carbonized at 1100°C under N_2 atmosphere to form CNFs, which were then served as supports for the nucleation and growth of two-dimensional $Ni(OH)_2$ nanoplatelets using a microwave-assisted method. Due to the high catalytic activity of both $Ni(OH)_2$ nanoplatelets and CNFs, the produced $Ni(OH)_2$–CNF hybrid showed improved sensing properties as electrode materials.

5.3 Fabrication of biosensors

In this section, the fabrication of various biosensors including electrochemical, fluorescent, electrochemiluminescence, colorimetric, current–voltage (I–V), SPR, and microfluidic biosensors with the electrospun fibrous nanomaterials is presented and discussed.

5.3.1 Electrochemical biosensors

Due to the simple operation, quick response, high sensitivity and stability, as well good reproducibility, electrochemical biosensors have been widely used for bioanalysis and detection. Electrospinning nanofibrous materials have exhibited promising applications in electrochemical biosensing as it provided multipossibilities for producing various functional nanomaterials. Until now, a lot of studies have been reported by applying electrospinning electrochemical biosensors for determining small biomolecules, drugs, proteins, DNA, and others.

For the electrochemical detection of small biomolecules, such as glucose [26,33,40], dopamine [24,28], H_2O_2 [41], and ascorbic acid [32], functional building blocks were embedded or conjugated to electrospun NFs to form hybrid NFs for the modification of chemical electrodes. For instance, Liu et al. utilized a coaxial electrospinning route to prepare Au-modified SnO_2 hollow microtubes, which were further used to modify GCE to fabricate nonenzymatic electrochemical H_2O_2 biosensors [41]. In another case, Kim and coworkers demonstrated the fabrication of an electrochemical ascorbic acid biosensor by using electrospun RuO_2/TiO_2 NFs with high catalytic activity to modify the bare GCE [32]. The fabricated ascorbic acid biosensor could be used to real-time detect ascorbic acid over the rat liver tissues with high selectivity and sensitivity. A low detection limit of about 1.8 μM and a linear detection range of 10–1500 μM were achieved.

Recently, Tripathy et al. designed an electrochemical DNA nanobiosensor by using electrospun Mn_2O_3 NFs to modify a GCE, and then binding ssDNA probe onto the functionalized GCE [42], as shown in Fig. 5.4. The addition of ssDNA targets onto the GCE system caused DNA hybridization and the change of electrochemical signals, which can be used for the detection of DNA hybridization. In a further step, the designed biosensor was applied for the detection of Dengue consensus primer with a zeptomolar (120×10^{-21} M) detection limit. The very low detection limit was ascribed to the low bandgap of the electrospun Mn_2O_3 materials. The methodology

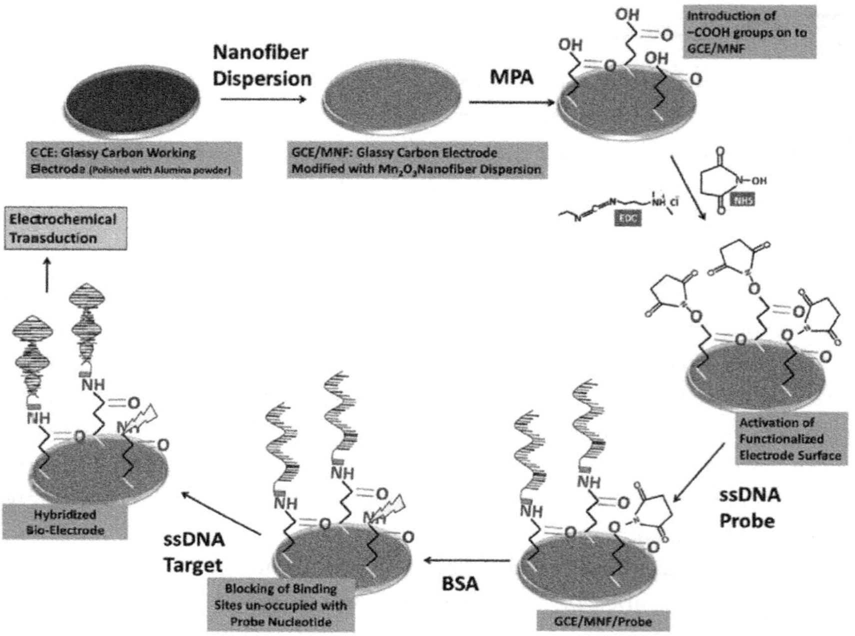

Figure 5.4 Fabrication of electrospun NF materials for electrochemical DNA biosensors. *Reprinted with permission from S. Tripathy, S.R.K. Vanjari, V. Singh, S. Swaminathan, S.G. Singh, Electrospun manganese (III) oxide nanofiber based electrochemical DNA-nanobiosensor for zeptomolar detection of dengue consensus primer, Biosens. Bioelectron. 90 (2017) 378–387. Copyright 2017, Elsevier BV.*

shown in this study can be easily modified by replacing the ssDNA probe with other probes to realize the high-performance detection of other DNA, RNA, and even virus. With the similar electrospinning and DNA hybridization, Kerr-Phillips et al. presented the fabrication of a highly sensitive, selective, label-free, electrochemical biosensor for the determination of non-Hodgkin lymphoma gene [43]. The obtained non-Hodgkin lymphoma gene biosensor showed a detection limit of 1×10^{-18} mol/L, which was more than 400-folds lower compared to a thin-film analogue.

The large amount of usage of drugs and pesticides caused serious effects on human living and natural environment, and therefore it is highly important for the detection of drugs and pesticides at trace levels. Previously, electrospun nanomaterials have been explored for the fabrication of electrochemical biosensors of levofloxacin [44], Idarubicin [45], 17α-ethinylestradiol [46], and atrazine [47], showing high potential as a simple tool for disease diagnostics and environmental analysis.

5.3.2 Fluorescent biosensors

To fabricate biosensors with fluorescent response toward bioanalytes, other components such as fluorescent molecules, quantum dots, rare-earth particles, metal nanoparticles, and polymers have been widely utilized.

Wang et al. for the first time demonstrated the fabrication of a fluorescent DNA biosensor by assembling DNA-functionalized AuNPs on electrospun polymer NFs [48]. In another case, Han and Koh demonstrated the fabrication of a fluorescent matrix metalloproteinases-9 (MMP-9) biosensor by integrating the electrospun hydrogel-framed NFs with a microfluidic device, in which the fluorescein isocyanate (FITC)-labeled MMP-9-specific peptides were firstly covalently immobilized on the electrospun NFs [49]. The addition of MMP-9 into the reaction chamber caused in the cleavage of the FITC-containing peptide fragments, generating fluorescent flow at the detection zone. With this strategy, a low detection limit of 10 pM with quick response of 30 min was achieved for the detection of MMP-9. It should be noted that this sensing technique can be used for creating other kinds of biosensors by replacing the peptides with other biomolecules and the integration with microfluidic system made the biosensors reusable.

Fluorescent quantum dots such as semiconductor and graphene quantum dots can be also bound onto electrospinning polymer NFs for the fabrication of highly sensitive biosensors. For instance, Tan and coworkers prepared polycaprolactone nanofibrous membranes doped with uniformly distributed oil-soluble cadmium selenide quantum dots, which could be directly employed as optical probe for H_2O_2 sensing [50]. It was found that the immersing of the electrospun cadmium selenide/polycaprolactone membranes into H_2O_2 solution quickly quenched the fluorescence of quantum dots, and in the presence of glucose oxidase, the fluorescent variation was linearly changed with the concentration of glucose. With the similar method, Zhang et al. reported a facile electrospinning to fabricate a nanofibrous PVA membrane doped with GQDs [23]. Ascribed to the three-dimensional structure, high surface area-to-volume ratio, and catalytic properties, the formed PVA/GQD membrane exhibited potential applications as dual-purpose electrochemical and fluorescent biosensors for detecting glucose and H_2O_2, as shown in Fig. 5.5. The fabricated fluorescent biosensors revealed linear detection ranges of 0.05—35 and 0.25—24 mM with corresponding detection limits of approximately 1.0 and 10.0 mM for the H_2O_2 and glucose, respectively. Besides, other rare-earth particles [51] and metal NPs [52] have also been used to conjugate with electrospun polymer NFs for biosensor applications.

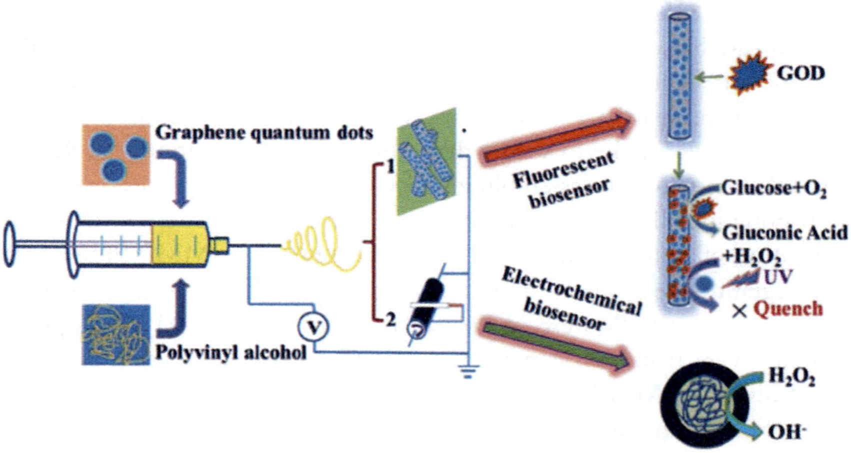

Figure 5.5 Electrospun fabrication of PVA/GQD NF-based dual-purpose fluorescent and electrochemical biosensors for biosensors of H_2O_2 and glucose. *Reprinted with permission from P. Zhang, X. Zhao, Y, Ji, Z. Ouyang, X. Wen, J. Li, Z. Su, G. Wei, Electrospinning graphene quantum dots into a nanofibrous membrane for dual-purpose fluorescent and electrochemical biosensors, J. Mater. Chem. B 3(12) (2014) 2487–2496. Copyright 2015, Royal Society of Chemistry.*

Due to the aggregation-induced emission of fluorescence, various polymers with aggregation-induced emission properties have been bound onto electrospun polymer NFs for the fabrication of fluorescent biosensors of *Escherichia coli* [53], alkaline phosphatase [54], and bacteria [55]. In a typical study, Zhao et al. reported the fabrication of a turn-on fluorescent biosensor by conjugating tetraphenylethylene mannose with electrospun polystyrene-co-maleic anhydride NFs [53], which exhibited rapid and sensitive detection for *Escherichia coli* with a range from 10^2 to 10^5 colony-forming unit (CFU)/mL and a detection limit of 10^2 CFU/mL. The strategies shown in their study provided a capacity to be expanded to exploit electrospun fibrous mats and other carbohydrate–cell interactions for bioanalysis and biosensing of pathogenic bacteria in the future.

5.3.3 Electrochemiluminescence biosensors

Electrochemiluminescence generated by an oxidation or reduction reaction on the electrode surface could be a useful tool to investigate the biorecognition reaction and can be utilized as a novel technique to fabricate label-free biosensors with high performance [56]. Electrospun nanofibrous materials could also be used as good supports for binding electroactive nanomaterials to prepare electrochemiluminescence sensors and biosensors [57,58].

Previously, Wang et al. reported a solid-state electrochemiluminescence biosensor of catechol based on the electrospinning-produced luminescent composite NFs [59]. To fabricate the biosensor, MWCNTs and $Ru(bpy)_3^{2+}$ were doped onto the electrospun nylon-6 NFs to form a composite Ru—MWCNTs—Nylon-6 NFs. Due to the unique three-dimensional structure, large specific surface area, and photoelectric properties of $Ru(bpy)_3^{2+}$, the fabricated composite NFs on GCE exhibited excellent electrochemiluminescence behaviors. With the fabricated biosensor, a detection limit for catechol of 1.0 nM was achieved successfully. In another case, Xu et al. developed a label-free electrochemiluminescence immunosensor for highly sensitive determination of aflatoxin B1 by immobilizing electrospun Fe_3O_4 NFs onto carbon horns [60]. It is clear that the carbon horns possessed good conductivity, biocompatibility, large specific surface area, and variable porosity, and the Fe_3O_4 NFs promoted the tight immobilization onto a magnetic electrode. Therefore, the synergistic effects made the fabricated aflatoxin B1 biosensor with a detection limit of 0.02 ng/mL and a linear detection range from 0.05 to 200 ng/mL.

Dai and coworkers produced a three-dimensional electrode by using electrospun polymer NFs functionalized with CNTs [61] and found that the formed CNTs/polymer NF materials exhibited highly strong electrochemiluminescence of peroxydisulfate $\left(S_2O_8{}^{2-}\right)$. Based on this finding, for the first time they demonstrated the fabrication of an immunosensor for the highly sensitive and label-free detection of α-fetoprotein. As shown in Fig. 5.6, CNTs and poly(methyl methacrylate) (PMMA) were first electrospun CNTs/PMMA NFs, and then chitosan was used with CNTs/PMMA together to form a 3D structure on an electrode through the electrodeposition. Due to the unique properties of the network-like interface of the electrode surface, strong electrochemiluminescence of $\left(S_2O_8{}^{2-}\right)$ was obtained. Afterward, the antibody of α-fetoprotein was applied to bind to the hybrid film, and the addition of α-fetoprotein to react with the antibody caused in decreasing of electrochemiluminescence signal. Therefore, a quantitative electrochemiluminescence immunosensor was prepared. Based on the change of electrochemiluminescence signal from the specific immune reaction, the fabricated immunosensor exhibited a wide dynamic response in the range of 0.1 pg/mL to 160 ng/mL with a detection limit of 0.09 pg/mL. Their study proved that the electrospinning is a facile technique to produce biocompatible, low-cost, and high-performance electrochemiluminescence biosensors for bioanalysis applications. In another study, Wang et al. fabricated an electrochemiluminescence biosensor for

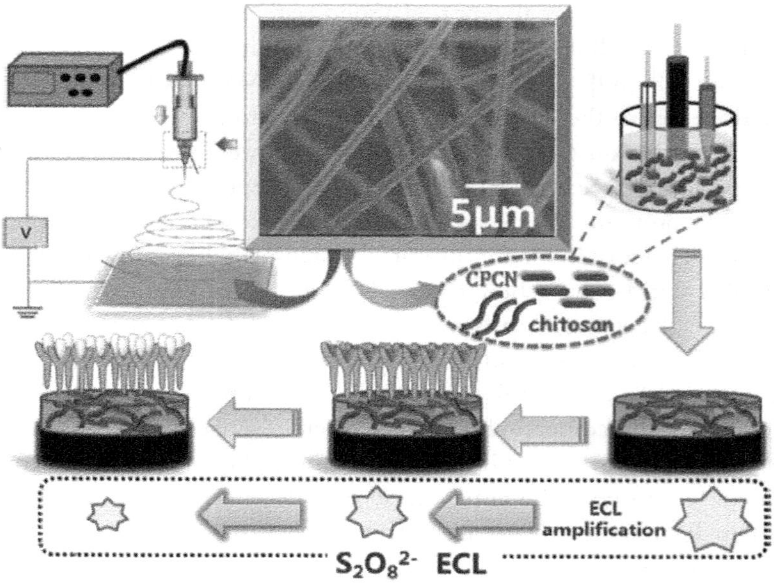

Figure 5.6 The production of electrospun CNTs/PMMA-based electrode for label-free electrochemiluminescence immunosensor of α-fetoprotein. *Reprinted with permission from H. Dai, G.F. Xu, S.P. Zhang, L.S. Gong, X.H. Li, C.P. Yang, Y.Y. Lin, J.H. Chen, G.N. Chen, Carbon nanotubes functionalized electrospun nanofibers formed 3D electrode enables highly strong ECL of peroxydisulfate and its application in immunoassay, Biosens. Bioelectron. 61 (2014) 575–578. Copyright 2014, Elsevier BV.*

detecting CdkN2A/p16 antioncogene based on the electrospun polymer NFs/CNTs doped with core–shell luminescent RuAg@AuNPs composite nanoparticles [62]. In a further study recently, they developed another protein P53 (TSP_{53}) immunosensor by using the electrospun MWCNTs–chitosan–AuNPs NFs as supports and the core–shell RuAg/SiO_2NPs-labeled TSP_{53} antibody as signal enhancer [63]. It was found that the increasing of TSP_{53} concentration was linearly related to the increasing of electrochemiluminescence signal in the range of 1 pg/mL to 1 ng/mL with a detection limit of 0.5 pg/mL. The excellent sensitivity and selectivity made it possible to use this electrochemiluminescence immunosensor as a promising tool for detecting tumor biomarkers.

5.3.4 Colorimetric biosensors

The electrospinning technique allowed rapid and cost-effective production of nanofibrous membranes that doped with nanoscale building blocks with optical signals for colorimetric biosensing. After the addition of bioanalytes onto the surface of electrospun functional membranes, the color changes could be easily observed by naked eyes, which promoted quick, direct, and highly sensitive determination of samples [64,65].

Yoo et al. for the first time demonstrated the fabrication of a colorimetric sensor of volatile organic compounds by using electrospun PEO/TEOS NFs and polydiacetylenes (PDAs) [65]. Their study indicated that the PDA-modified polymer NF mats exhibited organic solvent-dependent color change property, allowing for a straightforward "color pattern" procedure to differentiate between several common organic solvents.

Li and coworkers developed a colorimetric biosensor for detecting Pb^{2+} by immobilizing bovine serum albumin (BSA)-decorated AuNPs onto electrospun polyamide-6/nitrocellulose (PA-6/NC) NF mats [66]. Firstly, PA-6/NC NF mats were produced by the dual-component alternate distribution multifluidic electrospinning technique, and then BSA–AuNPs were bound onto the NF mats (Fig. 5.7). After immersing to the Pb^{2+} solution, the stability of BSA–AuNPs was increased and presented a significant absorbance decreasing band at 546 nm, which induced the visual color changes from pink to white. With this colorimetric assay, Pb^{2+} solution with a

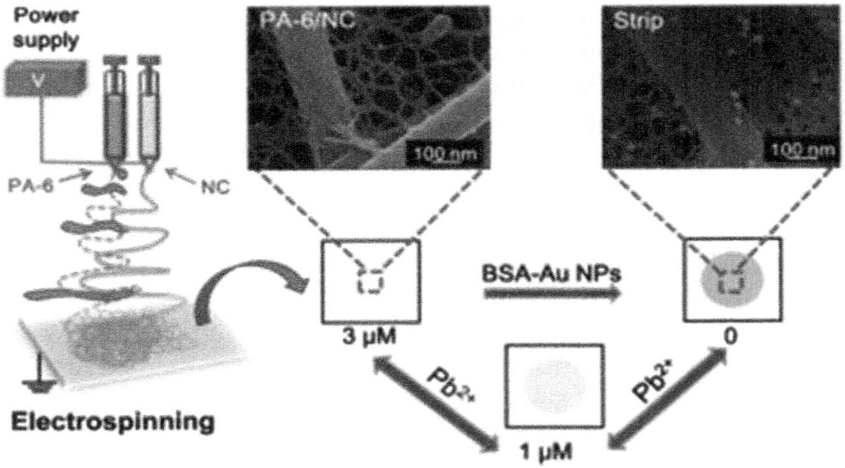

Figure 5.7 Schematic mode for the electrospinning fabrication of colorimetric biosensor by using BSA–AuNPs as an optical probe. *Reprinted with permission from Y. Li, Y. Si, X.Q. Wang, B. Ding, G. Sun, G. Zheng, W.J. Luo, J.Y. Yu, Colorimetric sensor strips for lead (II) assay utilizing nanogold probes immobilized polyamide-6/nitrocellulose nanofibers/nets, Biosens. Bioelectron. 48 (2013) 244–250. Copyright 2013, Elsevier BV.*

concentration as low as 0.2 μM could be detected. In another similar study, Mudabuka et al. reported the fabrication of a colorimetric ascorbic acid sensor based on bimetallic Cu—AuNPs in electrospun nylon NFs [67].

Sometime, the colorimetric biosensing can also be achieved by using fluorescent microscope. For instance, Senthamizhan and coworkers developed a colorimetric H_2O_2 biosensor by decorating electrospun fluorescent nanofibrous membrane with fluorescent gold nanoclusters [68]. It was found that the color variation from red to blue was dependent on the concentration of H_2O_2, and can be recognized visually by the help of the confocal laser scanning microscope. The produced H_2O_2 biosensor exhibited a detection limit of 500 nM with good accuracy and stability. This study paved a new way for the detection of bioanalytes with rapid readout, good sensitivity, and high selectivity.

5.3.5 Other biosensors (current—voltage, surface plasmon resonance, and microfluidic)

Besides the abovementioned biosensors, electrospun nanofibrous materials have revealed potential applications as other types of biosensors, including I—V electric, SPR, microfluidic, surface-enhanced Raman scattering (SERS) sensing.

Previously, Stafiniak et al. developed a novel I—V biosensor for detecting BSA by using the electrospun ZnO NFs [69]. After the production of ZnO NFs, an amorphous thin film of AlNx was deposited and used as a protective layer for the photolithography to fabricate ZnO NF sensor architecture. With the wet etching of AlNx layer, Ti/Au ohmic contacted ZnO NFs to finish the design of the I—V biosensor. In another case, Baranowska-Korczyc and coworkers described the design of an I—V protein sensor for the detection of horseradish peroxidase by using electrospun core—shell ZnO/ZnS NFs [27]. As shown in Fig. 5.8a, the ZnO NF-based biosensor platform was first prepared as the method that is similar to that by Stafiniak et al. [69], and then the fabricated biosensor was put into H_2S gas environment to promote the formation of ZnS on the surface of ZnO through gas-phase sulfidation (Fig. 5.8b). Finally, the ZnO/ZnS NFs-based I—V horseradish peroxidase sensor was produced, which can be used in various biological, highly ionic, acidic, and alkaline environments effectively.

SPR is a facile spectroscopic label-free technique for the detection of analytes on a metallic surface [72]. Luo et al. demonstrated a lateral-flow immunosensor based on electrospun cellulose nitrate nanofibrous membrane doped with magnetic nanoparticles for the highly sensitive detection

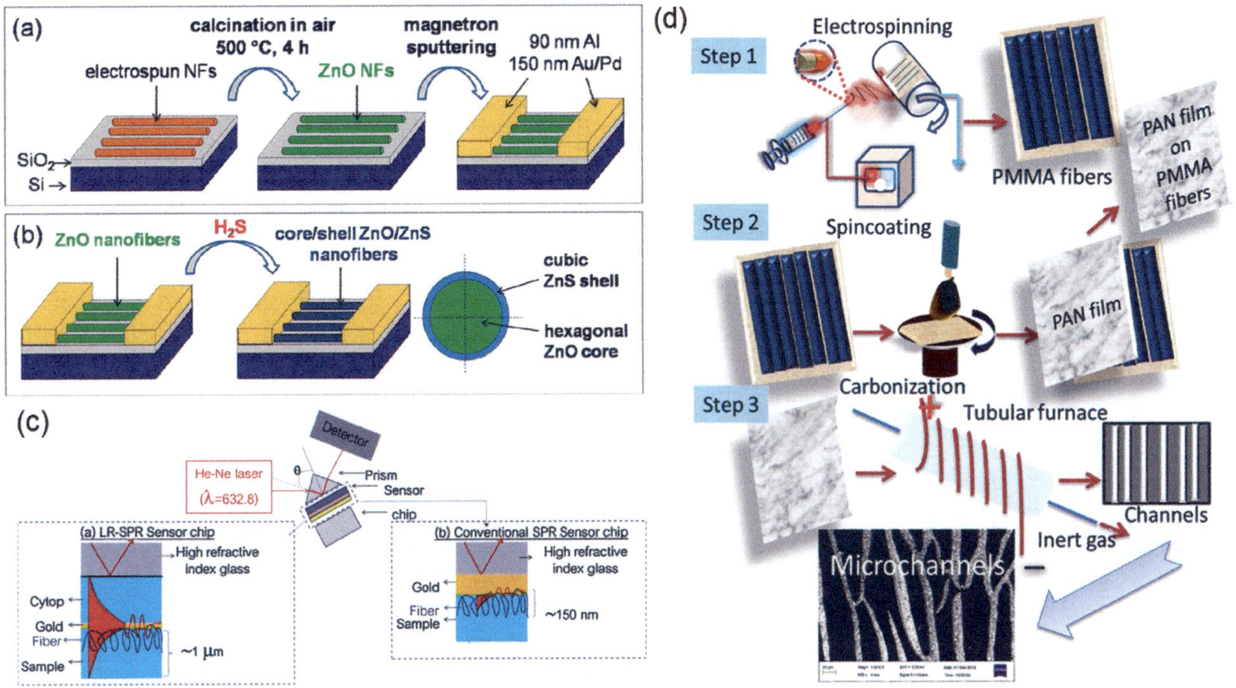

Figure 5.8 Fabrication of electrospun nanofiber–based materials for (a,b) I–V, (c) SPR, and (d) microfluidic biosensors. *(a,b) Reprinted with permission from A. Baranowska-Korczyc, K. Sobczak, P. Dluzewski, A. Reszka, B.J. Kowalski, L. Klopotowski, D. Elbaum, K. Fronc, Facile synthesis of core/shell ZnO/ZnS nanofibers by electrospinning and gas-phase sulfidation for biosensor applications, Phys. Chem. Chem. Phys. 17(37) (2015) 24029–24037. Copyright 2015, Royal Society of Chemistry; (c) Reprinted with permission from P. Netsuwan, H. Mimiya, A. Baba, S. Sriwichai, K. Shinbo, K. Kato, F. Kaneko, S. Phanichphant, Long-range surface plasmon resonance immunosensor based on water-stable electrospun poly(-acrylic acid) fibers, Sens. Actuators, B 204 (2014) 770–776. Copyright 2014, Elsevier BV; (d) Reprinted with permission from K. Mondal, M.A. Ali, S. Srivastava, B.D. Malhotra, A. Sharma, Electrospun functional micro/nanochannels embedded in porous carbon electrodes for microfluidic biosensing, Sens. Actuators, B 229 (2016) 82–91. Copyright 2016, Elsevier BV.*

of *E. coli* O157:H7 bacteria [73]. The fabricated biosensor exhibited a detection limit of 67 CFU/mL with a linear detection range from 10 to 10^4 CFU/mL. In addition, the detection could be finished within 8 min with high stability and reproducibility. In another study, Netsuwan and coworkers reported the fabrication of a long-range SPR immunosensor based on water-stable electrospun PAA NFs [70]. To increase the water solubility, poly(diallyldimethylammonium chloride) and PAA ultrathin films were layer-by-layer deposited onto the electrospun PAA NFs. This long-range SPR immunosensor has been utilized for the detection of human IgG by modifying the NFs with antihuman IgG. Compared to the conventional SPR spectroscopy, the long-range SPR has greater evanescent field intensity and penetration depth, and therefore has higher sensitivity, as shown in Fig. 5.8c.

Microfluidic chips based on electrospun nanomaterials can also be used for biosensing. For instance, previously, Liu et al. demonstrated the production of a microfluidic chip on the electrospun PVDF membrane, and the fabricated microfluidic biosensor enabled the detection of multiple pairs of protein—protein interactions in one experiment [74]. In another study, Jin et al. introduced a capillary flow microfluidic on-chip immunosensor by electrospinning HRP-tagged antibody with water-soluble PVP NFs and storing in a microfluidic PMMA chip [75]. The fabricated immunosensor exhibited a detection limit of 166 CFU/mL for sensing *E. coli* O157. In a very interesting work reported by Mondal et al. [71], microfluidic biosensing with electrospun functional micro-/nanochannels that embedded in porous carbon electrodes was demonstrated, as shown in Fig. 5.8d. In their study, PMMA NFs were firstly electrospun onto a Si wafer and then a PAN film was prepared on the NFs by spin coating. The high-temperature carbonization of the hybrid film produced micro-/nanochannels in the carbon electrode by adjusting the diameter of electrospun PMMA NFs. After the biofunctionalization of surface of materials with anti-aflatoxin B1, the fabricated immunosensor could be applied for detecting aflatoxin B1 with a detection limit of 1 pg/mL and a linear detection range of 10^{-12}—10^{-7} g/mL. This kind of microfluidic channels could also have potential applications in electrocatalysis, photocatalysis, drug delivery, and biological diagnostics in the future.

In addition, electrospinning provides a simple and effective way to prepare functional active substrates for SERS applications through conjugating metallic nanoparticles such as AuNPs, AgNPs, PtNPs, and bimetallic noble nanoparticles onto the electrospun material surface [76,77]. However, it is hard to realize the selective and sensitive detection of biological analytes. To solve this problem, the biofunctionalization of nanofibrous membranes and active NPs with antibodies for the fabrication of SERS-based immunosensors could be applied.

5.3.6 Summary on electrospun biosensors

Based on the above introduction and discussion, it can be found that electrospinning is a facile technique for the fabrication of various biosensors with high sensitivity and selectivity; however, current studies are mainly focused on the laboratory testing with the fabricated biosensors. There are some challenges, such as how to achieve in the high-throughput analysis, low production cost, and reliable testing, that should be overcome to promote the practical applications of electrospun biosensors. Here, we provide a table (Table 5.1) to summarize the materials, synthesis methods, fabrication, and applications of electrospun biosensors.

5.4 Summary and future prospects

In this chapter, we summarized recent advances in the electrospinning production and biosensor applications of various nanofibrous materials. Firstly, we introduced the methods and techniques to conjugate zero-dimensional nanoparticles/quantum dots, one-dimensional CNTs/nanowires/nanoneedles, and two-dimensional nanosheets/nanoplates to electrospun polymer NFs or CNFs, which can be realized usually by premixing electrospinning and posttreating after electrospinning. The formed electrospun nanofibrous nanomaterials exhibited unique structure and multifunctional properties. Secondly, we presented and discussed the fabrication of electrospun material–based biosensor platforms for the electrochemical, fluorescent, electrochemiluminescence, colorimetric, IV, SPR, microfluidic, and SERS detection of various analytes. The strategies shown in the electrospinning synthesis and the biosensor design are valuable and inspirable for readers in the fields of disease diagnostic, biomedicine, tissue engineering, and beyond.

In the last years, great achievements have been obtained on the fabrication of various biosensor platforms via electrospinning; still more efforts could be performed in the further. For instance, it is necessary to fabricate functional hybrid nanomaterials by electrospinning the composites of bio-nanomaterials and carbon-based nanomaterials, which will be beneficial for biosensors with higher selectivity and sensitivity. In addition, the

Table 5.1 Summary of the applied materials, synthesis methods, fabrication, and applications of electrospun biosensors.

Biosensor type	Materials	Analyte	Detection limit	Detection range	Reference
Electrochemical biosensors	Ag–Pt NPs	DA	0.11 μM	10–500 μM	[24]
	Ag/CuO NFs	Glucose	51.7 nM	0.50–500 μM	[26]
	MWCNTs	DA	0.15 μmol/L	1–70 μM	[28]
	RuO_2/TiO_2 nanofibers	Ascorbic acid	1.8 μM	10–1500 μM	[32]
	$NiCo_2O_4$/ECF	Glucose	1.5 μM	5–19.175 mM	[33]
	Mt	Glucose	0.7 μM	0.005–0.25 mM	[40]
	SnO_2 hollow microtubes	H_2O_2	0.60 μM	10 μM–1 mM	[41]
	GCE/Mn_2O_3 nanofibers	Dengue consensus primer	120×10^{-21} M	1 aM–1 μM	[42]
	CP	Lymphoma gene	1×10^{-18} M	1 aM–100 pM	[43]
	Ag/CeO_2	Levofloxacin	0.01 μM	0.03–10 μM	[44]
	TiO_2 NPs	IDA	3 nM	0.012–10 μM	[45]
	PVP/Chi/rGO	EE2	1.5×10^{-13} M	0.25–20.0 pM	[46]
	SnO_2 nanofibers	Atrazine	0.9 zM	1 zM–1 μM	[47]
Fluorescent biosensors	AuNPs	DNA	0.08 nM	0.1–10 nM	[48]
	MMP-9-specific peptides	MMP-9	10 pM	0–100 pM	[49]
	CdSe QDs	H_2O_2	–	–	[50]
	GQDs	Glucose	10.0 mM	0.25–24 mM	[23]
	GQDs	H_2O_2	1.0 mM	0.05–35 mM	[23]
	AgNPs	IgG	1.5 ng/mL	–	[52]
	TPE	*Escherichia coli*	102 CFU/mL	102–105 CFU/mL	[53]
	Fluorescein	Alkaline phosphatase	–	0–80 mU/mL	[54]

ECL biosensors	$Ru(bpy)_3^{2+}$	Phenol	1.0 nM	0–10 μM	[58]
	MWCNTs/$Ru(bpy)3^{2+}$	Catechol	1.0 nM	2 nM–2 μM	[59]
	Fe_3O_4 nanofibers	Aflatoxin B1	0.02 ng/mL	0.05–200 ng/mL	[60]
	CNTs	α-fetoprotein	0.09 pg/mL	0.1 pg/mL–160 ng/mL	[61]
	RuAg@AuNPs	CdkN2A/p16 antioncogene	0.5 fM	1.0×10^{-15}–1.0×10^{-12} M	[62]
	MWCNTs/Chitosan/ AuNPs nanofibers	TSP53	0.5 pg/mL	1 pg/mL–1 ng/mL	[63]
Colorimetric biosensors	PDA	VOCs	–	–	[65]
	BSA–AuNPs	Pb^{2+}	0.2 μM	0.2–1 μM	[66]
	Cu–AuNPs	Ascorbic acid	1.76×10^{-2} mg/L	1.76×10^{-2} –1.76×10^{5} mg/L	[67]
	AuNC	H_2O_2	500 nM	–	[68]
Others (IV, SPR, SERS)	ZnO nanofibers	BSA	10 mg/mL	34–50 mg/mL	[69]
	ZnO/ZnS nanofibers	HRP	–	–	[27]
	Magnetic nanoparticles	*E. coli* O157:H7 bacteria	67 CFU/mL	10–104 CFU/mL	[71]
	PAA nanofibers	IgG	–	–	[72]
	PVDF	Protein	20 μg/mL	–	[73]
	PVP	*E. coli* O157	166 CFU/mL	–	[74]
	PMMA nanofibers	Aflatoxin B1	1 pg/mL	10^{-12}–10^{-7} g/mL	[75]

addition of antibodies, enzymes, aptamers, and other target-recognized biomolecules onto the electrospun nanomaterials will be useful for viral, bacterial, gene, and drug biosensing. Another highly potential aspect is the fabrication of electrospun biosensors for point-of-care devices toward biomedical diagnosis. Electrospinning could be utilized to create functional nanomaterials on paper substrates to form paper-based point-of-care biosensors for colorimetric, fluorescent, and SERS detection of various diseases. Meanwhile, electrospinning could be utilized to fabricate biosensors that integrated with various optical, electronic, and electrochemical techniques or instruments to create multifunctional biosensors with easier operation, quick detection, higher sensitivity, and better stability.

References

[1] D.H. Reneker, I. Chun, Nanometre diameter fibres of polymer, produced by electrospinning, Nanotechnology 7 (3) (1996) 216–223.
[2] J.J. Xue, T. Wu, Y.Q. Dai, Y.N. Xia, Electrospinning and electrospun nanofibers: methods, materials, and applications, Chem. Rev. 119 (8) (2019) 5298–5415.
[3] Q. Liu, J.H. Zhu, L.W. Zhang, Y.J. Qiu, Recent advances in energy materials by electrospinning, Renew. Sustain. Energy Rev. 81 (2018) 1825–1858.
[4] W.H. Li, L.C. Zeng, Y. Wu, Y. Yu, Nanostructured electrode materials for lithium-ion and sodium-ion batteries via electrospinning, Sci. China Mater. 59 (4) (2016) 287–321.
[5] B. Sun, Y.Z. Long, H.D. Zhang, M.M. Li, J.L. Duvail, X.Y. Jiang, H.L. Yin, Advances in three-dimensional nanofibrous macrostructures via electrospinning, Prog. Polym. Sci. 39 (5) (2014) 862–890.
[6] M.F. Zhang, X.N. Zhao, G.H. Zhang, G. Wei, Z.Q. Su, Electrospinning design of functional nanostructures for biosensor applications, J. Mater. Chem. B 5 (9) (2017) 1699–1711.
[7] S. Zhang, Z.X. Jia, T.J. Liu, G. Wei, Z.Q. Su, Electrospinning nanoparticles-based materials interfaces for sensor applications, Sensors 19 (18) (2019) 3977.
[8] L. Wang, A.G. Wu, G. Wei, Graphene-based aptasensors: from molecule-interface interactions to sensor design and biomedical diagnostics, Analyst 143 (7) (2018) 1526–1543.
[9] L. Wang, Y.J. Zhang, A.G. Wu, G. Wei, Designed graphene-peptide nanocomposites for biosensor applications: a review, Anal. Chim. Acta 985 (2017) 24–40.
[10] F. Akbar, M. Kolahdouz, S. Larimian, B. Radfar, H.H. Radamson, Graphene synthesis, characterization and its applications in nanophotonics, nanoelectronics, and nanosensing, J. Mater. Sci. 26 (7) (2015) 4347–4379.
[11] F.R. Baptista, S.A. Belhout, S. Giordani, S.J. Quinn, Recent developments in carbon nanomaterial sensors, Chem. Soc. Rev. 44 (13) (2015) 4433–4453.
[12] X.J. Li, J.F. Ping, Y.B. Ying, Recent developments in carbon nanomaterial-enabled electrochemical sensors for nitrite detection, Trac. Trends Anal. Chem. 113 (2019) 1–12.
[13] Z.Q. Wang, S.S. Wu, J. Wang, A.L. Yu, G. Wei, Carbon nanofiber-based functional nanomaterials for sensor applications, Nanomaterials 9 (7) (2019) 1045.
[14] J.S. Huang, Y. Liu, T.Y. You, Carbon nanofiber based electrochemical biosensors: a review, Anal. Methods 2 (3) (2010) 202–211.

[15] J. Wang, Y.H. Lin, Functionalized carbon nanotubes and nanofibers for biosensing applications, Trac. Trends Anal. Chem. 27 (7) (2008) 619–626.
[16] G. Yang, K.L. Kampstra, M.R. Abidian, High-performance conducting polymer nanofiber biosensors for detection of biomolecules, Adv. Mater. 26 (29) (2014) 4954–4960.
[17] Z.Q. Su, J.W. Ding, G. Wei, Electrospinning: a facile technique for fabricating polymeric nanofibers doped with carbon nanotubes and metallic nanoparticles for sensor applications, RSC Adv. 4 (94) (2014) 52598–52610.
[18] M. Scampicchio, A. Bulbarello, A. Arecchi, M.S. Cosio, S. Benedetti, S. Mannino, Electrospun nonwoven nanofibrous membranes for sensors and biosensors, Electroanalysis 24 (4) (2012) 719–725.
[19] A. Senthamizhan, B. Balusamy, T. Uyar, Glucose sensors based on electrospun nanofibers: a review, Anal. Bioanal. Chem. 408 (5) (2016) 1285–1306.
[20] A. Celebioglu, F. Topuz, Z.I. Yildiz, T. Uyar, One-step green synthesis of antibacterial silver nanoparticles embedded in electrospun cyclodextrin nanofibers, Carbohydr. Polym. 207 (2019) 471–479.
[21] P. Li, M.F. Zhang, X.Y. Liu, Z.Q. Su, G. Wei, Electrostatic assembly of platinum nanoparticles along electrospun polymeric nanofibers for high performance electrochemical sensors, Nanomaterials 7 (9) (2017) 236.
[22] Z.C. Liu, Z.D. Yan, L. Jia, P. Song, L.Y. Mei, L. Bai, Y.Q. Liu, Gold nanoparticle decorated electrospun nanofibers: a 3D reproducible and sensitive SERS substrate, Appl. Surf. Sci. 403 (2017) 29–34.
[23] P. Zhang, X. Zhao, Y. Ji, Z. Ouyang, X. Wen, J. Li, Z. Su, G. Wei, Electrospinning graphene quantum dots into a nanofibrous membrane for dual-purpose fluorescent and electrochemical biosensors, J. Mater. Chem. B 3 (12) (2014) 2487–2496.
[24] Y.P. Huang, Y.E. Miao, S.S. Ji, W.W. Tjiu, T.X. Liu, Electrospun carbon nanofibers decorated with Ag-Pt bimetallic nanoparticles for selective detection of dopamine, ACS Appl. Mater. Interfaces 6 (15) (2014) 12449–12456.
[25] T. Xu, W. Jin, Z.Z. Wang, H.Y. Cheng, X.H. Huang, X.Y. Guo, Y. Ying, Y.P. Wu, F. Wang, Y. Wen, H.F. Yang, Electrospun CuO-Nanoparticles-Modified polycaprolactone @polypyrrole fibers: an application to sensing glucose in saliva, Nanomaterials 8 (3) (2018) 133.
[26] B.Z. Zheng, G.Y. Liu, A.W. Yao, Y.L. Xiao, J. Du, Y. Guo, D. Xiao, Q. Hu, M.M.F. Choi, A sensitive AgNPs/CuO nanofibers non-enzymatic glucose sensor based on electrospinning technology, Sens. Actuators, B 195 (2014) 431–438.
[27] A. Baranowska-Korczyc, K. Sobczak, P. Dluzewski, A. Reszka, B.J. Kowalski, L. Klopotowski, D. Elbaum, K. Fronc, Facile synthesis of core/shell ZnO/ZnS nanofibers by electrospinning and gas-phase sulfidation for biosensor applications, Phys. Chem. Chem. Phys. 17 (37) (2015) 24029–24037.
[28] L.A. Mercante, A. Pavinatto, L.E.O. Iwaki, V.P. Scagion, V. Zucolotto, O.N. Oliveira, L.H.C. Mattoso, D.S. Correa, Electrospun polyamide 6/Poly(allylamine hydrochloride) nanofibers functionalized with carbon nanotubes for electrochemical detection of dopamine, ACS Appl. Mater. Interfaces 7 (8) (2015) 4784–4790.
[29] Z.Q. Su, J.F. Li, Q. Li, T.Y. Ni, G. Wei, Chain conformation, crystallization behavior, electrical and mechanical properties of electrospun polymer-carbon nanotube hybrid nanofibers with different orientations, Carbon 50 (15) (2012) 5605–5617.
[30] P.P. Zhang, X.N. Zhao, X. Zhang, Y. Lai, X.T. Wang, J.F. Li, G. Wei, Z.Q. Su, Electrospun doping of carbon nanotubes and platinum nanoparticles into the beta-phase polyvinylidene difluoride nanofibrous membrane for biosensor and catalysis applications, ACS Appl. Mater. Interfaces 6 (10) (2014) 7563–7571.

[31] K.B. Paul, V. Singh, S.R.K. Vanjari, S.G. Singh, One step biofunctionalized electrospun multiwalled carbon nanotubes embedded zinc oxide nanowire interface for highly sensitive detection of carcinoma antigen-125, Biosens. Bioelectron. 88 (2017) 144–152.
[32] S.J. Kim, Y.K. Cho, C. Lee, M.H. Kim, Y. Lee, Real-time direct electrochemical sensing of ascorbic acid over rat liver tissues using RuO_2 nanowires on electrospun TiO_2 nanofibers, Biosens. Bioelectron. 77 (2016) 1144–1152.
[33] L.J. Liu, Z.H. Wang, J.H. Yang, G.L. Liu, J.J. Li, L. Guo, S.L. Chen, Q.H. Guo, $NiCo_2O_4$ nanoneedle-decorated electrospun carbon nanofiber nanohybrids for sensitive non-enzymatic glucose sensors, Sens. Actuators, B 258 (2018) 920–928.
[34] R.K. Mishra, M.H. Nawaz, A. Hayat, M.A.H. Nawaz, V. Sharma, J.L. Marty, Electrospinning of graphene-oxide onto screen printed electrodes for heavy metal biosensor, Sens. Actuators, B 247 (2017) 366–373.
[35] S. Ghobadi, S. Mehraeen, R. Bakhtiari, B. Shamloo, V. Sadhu, M. Papila, F.C. Cebeci, S.A. Gursel, PVA/PANI/rGO ternary electrospun mats as metal-free anti-bacterial substrates, RSC Adv. 6 (95) (2016) 92434–92442.
[36] Y. Li, P.P. Zhang, Z.F. Ouyang, M.F. Zhang, Z.J. Lin, J.F. Li, Z.Q. Su, G. Wei, Nanoscale graphene doped with highly dispersed silver nanoparticles: quick synthesis, facile fabrication of 3D membrane-modified electrode, and super performance for electrochemical sensing, Adv. Funct. Mater. 26 (13) (2016) 2122–2134.
[37] X. Yu, H.S. Park, Synthesis and characterization of electrospun PAN/2D MoS_2 composite nanofibers, J. Ind. Eng. Chem. 34 (2016) 61–65.
[38] E.A. Mayerberger, R.M. Street, R.M. McDaniel, M.W. Barsoum, C.L. Schauer, Antibacterial properties of electrospun Ti_3C_2Tz (MXene)/chitosan nanofibers, RSC Adv. 8 (62) (2018) 35386–35394.
[39] L.L. Chen, L.J. Liu, Q.H. Guo, Z.H. Wang, G.L. Liu, S.L. Chen, H.Q. Hou, Preparation of $Ni(OH)_{(2)}$ nanoplatelet/electrospun carbon nanofiber hybrids for highly sensitive nonenzymatic glucose sensors, RSC Adv. 7 (31) (2017) 19345–19352.
[40] B. Unal, E.E. Yalcinkaya, D.O. Demirkol, S. Timur, An electrospun nanofiber matrix based on organo-clay for biosensors: PVA/PAMAM-Montmorillonite, Appl. Surf. Sci. 444 (2018) 542–551.
[41] S. Liu, B. Yu, F. Li, Y. Ji, T. Zhang, Coaxial electrospinning route to prepare Au-loading SnO_2 hollow microtubes for non-enzymatic detection of H_2O_2, Electrochim. Acta 141 (2014) 161–166.
[42] S. Tripathy, S.R.K. Vanjari, V. Singh, S. Swaminathan, S.G. Singh, Electrospun manganese (III) oxide nanofiber based electrochemical DNA-nanobiosensor for zeptomolar detection of dengue consensus primer, Biosens. Bioelectron. 90 (2017) 378–387.
[43] T.E. Kerr-Phillips, N. Aydemir, E.W.C. Chan, D. Barker, J. Malmstrom, C. Plesse, J. Travas-Sejdic, Conducting electrospun fibres with polyanionic grafts as highly selective, label-free, electrochemical biosensor with a low detection limit for non-Hodgkin lymphoma gene, Biosens. Bioelectron. 100 (2018) 549–555.
[44] L. Tang, Y. Tong, R.F. Zheng, W.L. Liu, Y. Gu, C. Li, R.X. Chen, Z.Q. Zhang, Ag nanoparticles and electrospun CeO_2-Au composite nanofibers modified glassy carbon electrode for determination of levofloxacin, Sens. Actuators, B 203 (2014) 95–101.
[45] E. Arkan, G. Paimard, K. Moradi, A novel electrochemical sensor based on electrospun TiO_2 nanoparticles/carbon nanofibers for determination of Idarubicin in biological samples, J. Electroanal. Chem. 801 (2017) 480–487.
[46] A. Pavinatto, L.A. Mercante, M.H.M. Facure, R.B. Pena, R.C. Sanfelice, L.H.C. Mattoso, D.S. Correa, Ultrasensitive biosensor based on polyvinylpyrrolidone/chitosan/reduced graphene oxide electrospun nanofibers for 17 alpha - ethinylestradiol electrochemical detection, Appl. Surf. Sci. 458 (2018) 431–437.

[47] P. Supraja, S. Tripathy, S.R.K. Vanjari, V. Singh, S.G. Singh, Electrospun tin (IV) oxide nanofiber based electrochemical sensor for ultra-sensitive and selective detection of atrazine in water at trace levels, Biosens. Bioelectron. 141 (2019).

[48] H.M. Wang, D.Z. Wang, Z. Peng, W. Tang, N. Li, F. Liu, Assembly of DNA-functionalized gold nanoparticles on electrospun nanofibers as a fluorescent sensor for nucleic acids, Chem. Commun. 49 (49) (2013) 5568–5570.

[49] S.W. Han, W.G. Koh, Hydrogel-framed nanofiber matrix integrated with a microfluidic device for fluorescence detection of matrix metalloproteinases-9, Anal. Chem. 88 (12) (2016) 6247–6253.

[50] L.F. Tan, X.L. He, D. Chen, X.L. Wu, H.B. Li, X.L. Ren, X.W. Meng, F.Q. Tang, Highly H_2O_2-sensitive electrospun quantum dots nanocomposite films for fluorescent biosensor, J. Biomed. Nanotechnol. 9 (1) (2013) 53–60.

[51] Y.K. Fu, T. Chen, G. Wang, T.X. Gu, C.K. Xie, J. Huang, X. Li, S. Best, G.R. Han, Production of a fluorescence resonance energy transfer (FRET) biosensor membrane for microRNA detection, J. Mater. Chem. B 5 (34) (2017) 7133–7139.

[52] B.J. Yun, J.E. Kwon, K. Lee, W.G. Koh, Highly sensitive metal-enhanced fluorescence biosensor prepared on electrospun fibers decorated with silica-coated silver nanoparticles, Sensor. Actuator. B Chem. 284 (2019) 140–147.

[53] L. Zhao, Y.F. Chen, J. Yuan, M.H. Chen, H. Zhang, X.H. Li, Electrospun fibrous mats with conjugated tetraphenylethylene and mannose for sensitive turn-on fluorescent sensing of *Escherichia coli*, ACS Appl. Mater. Interfaces 7 (9) (2015) 5177–5186.

[54] L. Zhao, S.Z. Xie, X.J. Song, J.J. Wei, Z. Zhang, X.H. Li, Ratiometric fluorescent response of electrospun fibrous strips for real-time sensing of alkaline phosphatase in serum, Biosens. Bioelectron. 91 (2017) 217–224.

[55] J. Quiros, A.J.R. Amaral, G. Pasparakis, G.R. Williams, R. Rosal, Electrospun boronic acid-containing polymer membranes as fluorescent sensors for bacteria detection, React. Funct. Polym. 121 (2017) 23–31.

[56] Z.Y. Liu, W.J. Qi, G.B. Xu, Recent advances in electrochemiluminescence, Chem. Soc. Rev. 44 (10) (2015) 3117–3142.

[57] D. Shan, B. Qian, S.N. Ding, W. Zhu, S. Cosnier, H.G. Xue, Enhanced solid-state electrochemiluminescence of Tris(2,2 '-bipyridyl)ruthenium(II) incorporated into electrospun nanofibrous mat, Anal. Chem. 82 (13) (2010) 5892–5896.

[58] C.S. Zhou, Z. Liu, J.Y. Dai, D. Xiao, Electrospun Ru(bpy)(3)(2+)-doped nafion nanofibers for electrochemiluminescence sensing, Analyst 135 (5) (2010) 1004–1009.

[59] X.Y. Wang, X.B. Wang, S.M. Gao, Y. Zheng, M. Tang, B.A. Chen, A solid-state electrochemiluminescence sensing platform for detection of catechol based on novel luminescent composite nanofibers, Talanta 107 (2013) 127–132.

[60] G.F. Xu, S.P. Zhang, Q.R. Zhang, L.S. Gong, H. Dai, Y.Y. Lin, Magnetic functionalized electrospun nanofibers for magnetically controlled ultrasensitive label-free electrochemiluminescent immune detection of aflatoxin B1, Sens. Actuators, B 222 (2016) 707–713.

[61] H. Dai, G.F. Xu, S.P. Zhang, L.S. Gong, X.H. Li, C.P. Yang, Y.Y. Lin, J.H. Chen, G.N. Chen, Carbon nanotubes functionalized electrospun nanofibers formed 3D electrode enables highly strong ECL of peroxydisulfate and its application in immunoassay, Biosens. Bioelectron. 61 (2014) 575–578.

[62] X.Y. Wang, Y.J. Wang, Y.Q. Shan, M. Jiang, M. Gong, X. Jin, X.N. Wang, J. Cheng, An electrochemiluminescence biosensor for detection of CdkN2A/p16 anti-oncogene based on functional electrospun nanofibers and core-shell luminescent composite nanoparticles, Talanta 187 (2018) 179–187.

[63] X.Y. Wang, Y. Wang, M. Jiang, Y.Q. Shan, X. Jin, M. Gong, X.N. Wang, Functional electrospun nanofibers-based electrochemiluminescence immunosensor for detection of the TSP_{53} using $RuAg/SiO_{(2)}NPs$ as signal enhancers, Anal. Biochem. 548 (2018) 15–22.

[64] X.F. Wang, Y. Si, J.L. Wang, B. Ding, J.Y. Yu, S.S. Al-Deyab, A facile and highly sensitive colorimetric sensor for the detection of formaldehyde based on electro-spinning/netting nano-fiber/nets, Sens. Actuators, B 163 (1) (2012) 186–193.

[65] J. Yoon, S.K. Chae, J.M. Kim, Colorimetric sensors for volatile organic compounds (VOCs) based on conjugated polymer-embedded electrospun fibers, J. Am. Chem. Soc. 129 (11) (2007) 3038.

[66] Y. Li, Y. Si, X.Q. Wang, B. Ding, G. Sun, G. Zheng, W.J. Luo, J.Y. Yu, Colorimetric sensor strips for lead (II) assay utilizing nanogold probes immobilized polyamide-6/nitrocellulose nano-fibers/nets, Biosens. Bioelectron. 48 (2013) 244–250.

[67] B. Mudabuka, D. Ondigo, S. Degni, S. Vilakazi, N. Torto, A colorimetric probe for ascorbic acid based on copper-gold nanoparticles in electrospun nylon, Microchim. Acta 181 (3–4) (2014) 395–401.

[68] A. Senthamizhan, B. Balusamy, Z. Aytac, T. Uyar, Ultrasensitive electrospun fluorescent nanofibrous membrane for rapid visual colorimetric detection of H_2O_2, Anal. Bioanal. Chem. 408 (5) (2016) 1347–1355.

[69] A. Stafiniak, B. Boratynski, A. Baranowska-Korczyc, A. Szyszka, M. Ramiaczek-Krasowska, J. Prazmowska, K. Fronc, D. Elbaum, R. Paszkiewicz, M. Tlaczala, A novel electrospun ZnO nanofibers biosensor fabrication, Sens. Actuators, B 160 (1) (2011) 1413–1418.

[70] P. Netsuwan, H. Mimiya, A. Baba, S. Sriwichai, K. Shinbo, K. Kato, F. Kaneko, S. Phanichphant, Long-range surface plasmon resonance immunosensor based on water-stable electrospun poly(acrylic acid) fibers, Sens. Actuators, B 204 (2014) 770–776.

[71] K. Mondal, M.A. Ali, S. Srivastava, B.D. Malhotra, A. Sharma, Electrospun functional micro/nanochannels embedded in porous carbon electrodes for microfluidic biosensing, Sens. Actuators, B 229 (2016) 82–91.

[72] Z.B. Rezaei, S. Rastegarzadeh, A. Kiasat, In-situ decorated silver nanoparticles on electrospun poly (vinyl alcohol)/chitosan nanofibers as a plasmonic sensor for azathioprine determination, Colloid. Surface. 559 (2018) 266–274.

[73] Y.L. Luo, S. Nartker, M. Wiederoder, H. Miller, D. Hochhalter, L.T. Drzal, E.C. Alocilja, Novel biosensor based on electrospun nanofiber and magnetic nanoparticles for the detection of *E. coli* O157:H7, IEEE Trans. Nanotechnol. 11 (4) (2012) 676–681.

[74] Y.Y. Liu, D.Y. Yang, T. Yu, X.Y. Jiang, Incorporation of electrospun nanofibrous PVDF membranes into a microfluidic chip assembled by PDMS and scotch tape for immunoassays, Electrophoresis 30 (18) (2009) 3269–3275.

[75] S.Q. Jin, M.H. Dai, B.C. Ye, S.R. Nugen, Development of a capillary flow microfluidic *Escherichia coli* biosensor with on-chip reagent delivery using water-soluble nanofibers, Microsyst. Technol. 19 (12) (2013) 2011–2015.

[76] L.F. Zhang, X. Gong, Y. Bao, Y. Zhao, M. Xu, C.Y. Jiang, H. Fong, Electrospun nanofibrous membranes surface-decorated with silver nanoparticles as flexible and active/sensitive substrates for surface-enhanced Raman scattering, Langmuir 28 (40) (2012) 14433–14440.

[77] Y. Zhao, L. Sun, M. Xi, Q. Feng, C.Y. Jiang, H. Fong, Electrospun TiO_2 nanofelt surface-decorated with Ag nanoparticles as sensitive and UV-cleanable substrate for surface enhanced Raman scattering, ACS Appl. Mater. Interfaces 6 (8) (2014) 5759–5767.

PART TWO

Electrospraying

CHAPTER SIX

Fundamental concepts and insights into electrospraying for biomedical applications

Chih-Yao Chui, Hua Ye
Institute of Biomedical Engineering, Department of Engineering Science, University of Oxford, Oxford, United Kingdom

Abbreviations

Ca^{2+} Calcium ions
$CaCl_2$ Calcium chloride
DLS Dynamic light scattering
FTIR Fourier transport infrared spectroscopy
HFIP 1,1,1,3,3,3-hexafluoroiso-propanol
Oh Ohnesorge number
PCL Poly(caprolactone)
PLGA Poly(lactic-co-glycolic acid)
SEM Scanning electron microscopy

6.1 Introduction

Electrospraying is a unique technique which involves the spraying of fine liquid droplets following the application of an electric field [1]. It has been defined as the atomization of a liquid through Coulombic interaction of charges on the liquid and the applied electric field [2]. In other words, the electric force causes deformation of the liquid meniscus which leads to the formation of droplets. The advantages offered by electrospraying include the precise control over the size of the particles generated as well as the low shear stress levels and exposure time to strong organic solvents [3]. Electrospraying first became extensively utilized for fields such as mass spectroscopy and ink jet printing [3]. However, it has since attracted interest for several other applications such as cell therapy [4], drug delivery [3], food [5], painting [6], and several other industries. The various applications of electrospraying in biomedical engineering are very broad and in-depth review is beyond the scope of this chapter. However, very briefly, some of these

Biomedical Applications of Electrospinning and Electrospraying
ISBN: 978-0-12-822476-2
https://doi.org/10.1016/B978-0-12-822476-2.00001-7

applications are described that include cell encapsulation, where cells are suspended within a polymer solution and electrosprayed, for purposes of cellular delivery [7] or creating a stem cell differentiation environment [8]. Similarly, encapsulation of drug molecules within microbeads would allow more stable and controlled drug release [9]. Depending on the polymer solution used, droplets are sprayed either into a gelling bath where gelation occurs [10] or a volatile solvent is used which evaporates from the droplets in flight leaving solidified particles to be collected. Moreover, cell suspensions could also undergo electrospraying in order to directly "print" cells onto 3D scaffolds to create functional tissue constructs in tissue engineering [4].

The principals behind electrospraying were first developed by Lord Rayleigh in 1882 [11], who theoretically estimated that an electric field has the ability to deform liquid droplets at its interface. This led to the determination of the stability criteria on a charged droplet, called the Rayleigh limit, which is defined by the maximum charge a droplet could carry prior to breakup [11]. Following this work, several other studies, both theoretical and experimental, have been conducted on electrospraying. In 1917, Zeleny further investigated the concept of electrospraying by conducting an experiment demonstrating the breakup of glycerol droplets [12]. Through photography, this study successfully identified the parameters required for jet disruption. Despite this, the droplet diameters could only be estimated. Furthermore, Zeleny's predictions regarding the mechanics of droplet breakup are based on the assumption that droplet instability occurs when the internal pressure is equal to the external pressure of the droplet. In 1964, Taylor demonstrated theoretically that the said assumption was false and that the breakup mechanism would only occur if a pressure difference is present [13]. Taylor's study showed that conical points develop during droplet instability in the presence of an electric field, which axial jets project from. Additionally, the semivertical angle of the cone at the capillary outlet reaches equilibrium at 49.3 degrees [13,14]. This phenomenon is later known as the Taylor cone and the electrospraying mode, cone-jet electrospraying, the latter would be covered further later this chapter. Since then several researchers have investigated the mechanisms of electrospraying and explored it within multiple disciplines.

Here we present a comprehensive understanding on the fundamental aspects of electrospraying. We will explore the theory behind droplet generation and the various forces that play in role during this process. Moreover, the several parameters that would allow users to optimize the final particle size will be discussed. Although there is a large overlap in the particle generation process for all electrospraying applications, the focus on this chapter will be directed toward electrospraying for the biomedical engineering field.

6.2 Overview of electrospraying setup

Several studies have used electrospraying to generate microdroplets and therefore there have been a variety of setups utilized in order to optimize the diameter of the microdroplet required for each application. Typically a solution is pumped using a syringe pump exiting a nozzle or blunted needle, which also acts as the positive electrode [15,16]. The flight trajectory of the droplet moves toward the ground electrode and is collected on a collector. There are some varieties of the ground electrode, the simplest setup consists of a grounded metal plate (Fig. 6.1) either acting as the collector itself [10,17,18] or placed just below the Petri dish collector [4,19]. On the other hand, some setups utilize a ring electrode, located above the collector [20,21] (Fig. 6.1). It has been reported that the presence of the ring electrode would stabilize the size of the microdroplets generated [22]. Finally, parallel plate setups have also been investigated, where the needle itself is not charged but placed at 90 degrees to the positive plate (Fig. 6.1). It has been shown that in a parallel plate setup the average bead diameter was found to be much larger compared to the other setups [18].

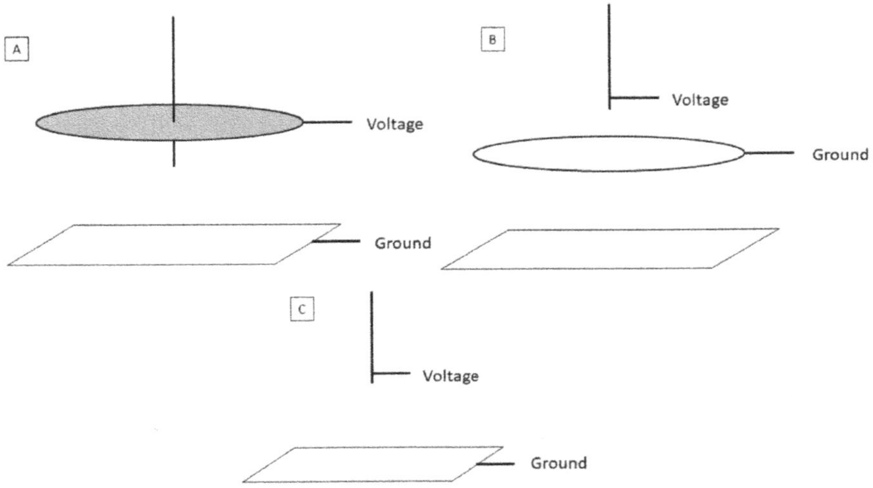

Figure 6.1 ***Various setups of electrospraying.*** (A) Charged needle setup with grounded metal plate. (B) Charged needle with grounded ring. (C) Parallel plate setup. *No Permissions Required.*

The droplet collector differs depending on the solution sprayed. In the case of a volatile organic solvent, the solvent evaporates during the flight path of the droplets. These leave microbeads of the solute which could be typically collected on a sheet of aluminum foil at the surface of the grounded metal plate [23]. In other setups, a Petri dish or a beaker is placed on top of the metal plate to collect particles [24]. The use of a conductive material for the collector restricts the deposition of particles in the charge area and limits potential loss of particles [23].

Electrospraying could also be used for solvents which do not evaporate during the spraying process but rather the droplets are sprayed into a gelling bath where the solvent gels to form microbeads. This has become a powerful technique for creating hydrogel-based microbeads, hydrophilic networks which absorb up to 1000 times their dry weight in water, which are used extensively in the biomedical field [25]. One of the most commonly used polymers is alginate, which could be ionically cross-linked by divalent ions, typically Ca^{2+}, transforming the aqueous solution into a hydrogel. One advantage of this is that the gels could be formed under mild conditions without requiring heating or strong organic chemicals [26]. Due to this, the collector is typically a $CaCl_2$ bath where alginate droplets would instantaneously gel upon contact [27–29].

Cell electrospraying or bioelectrospraying involves the direct spraying of a cell solution generating single cell suspensions. These setups typically utilize a Petri dish containing cell culture media as the collector [4]. One of the major issues during droplet collection is particle aggregation or binding [30]. This would lead to inconsistent particle sizes. In order to tackle this phenomenon, some studies have installed a rotating barrel as the collector, enabling continuous collection of microparticles or cell suspensions [31,32]. Similarly constant stirring of the gelling collection bath would also prevent particle aggregation [3].

A popular modification of the standard electrospraying setup is the coaxial setup. The system consists of two syringe pumps connected to a coaxial needle/nozzle which are concentrically located needles consisting of the outer shell and the inner core (Fig. 6.2). Hence, this would allow the delivery for two liquids independently and simultaneously [30]. This setup was first introduced by Loscertales et al. who demonstrated the production of nano-/microdroplets using two immiscible liquids [33]. Since then, several applications have been developed for coaxial electrospraying such as the encapsulation of drugs or cell suspensions within the core of the bead which are surrounded by a protective shell [34]. This differs from the standard solid

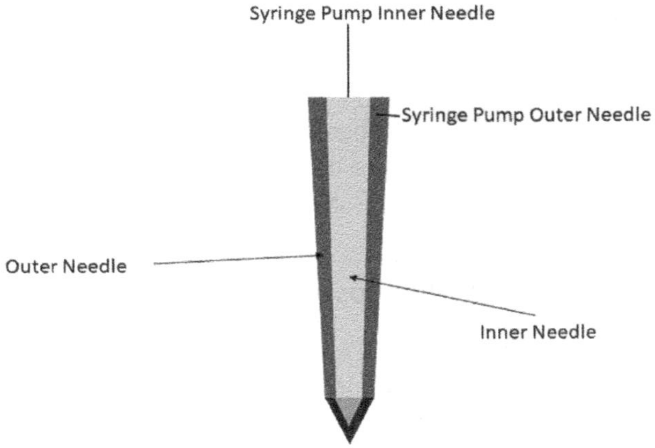

Figure 6.2 ***Coaxial Electrospraying.*** Coaxial electrospraying setup consisting of two needles, an outer shell and an inner core. *No Permissions Required.*

bead in standard electrospraying. Compared to the emulsion technique, a well-studied method for drug encapsulation, which involves rapid stirring to create an emulsion, coaxial electrospraying exerts a lower shear stress onto the particles keeping the drug cargo intact [24]. In some variants of coaxial electrospraying, the outer shell does not dispense fluid but rather compressed air flow. The gas flow increases air turbulence and generates a shear force which in addition to the electric field also disrupts the droplet formation at the meniscus. This hence leads to even smaller droplets being generated [16].

6.3 Insights into balance of forces during electrospraying

Typically, when a solution is pumped through a nozzle, even in the absence of an electric field, several forces act at the meniscus. The droplets gradually increase in size until its own weight or gravitational force overcomes the surface tension force present at the meniscus. During electrospraying, the presence of an electric field would induce a charge within the droplet. This leads to mutual charge repulsion to build up generating an outwardly directed force, which causes an apparent drop in surface tension generating an electrostatic pressure opposite to the capillary pressure [35]. Surplus charge then causes the breakup of the droplet into several microdroplets from the liquid tip, causing the droplet to leave the needle before the point where it falls off due to its own weight [36]. Several studies have investigated theoretically and experimentally the various forces acting on the droplet [13,16,37,38]. These forces are dependent on the electrospraying parameters applied, leading to various electrospraying modes, the most popular among them would be further discussed in the next section. This ultimately determines the size and the shape of the droplets generated.

6.4 Overview of electrospraying modes

The different process parameters applied during electrospraying lead to several electrospraying regimes or modes, which generate microdroplets in different ways [39]. This chapter would describe in detail the four most commonly seen modes of electrospraying: the dripping mode, the micro-dripping mode, the cone-jet mode, and the simple jet mode.

6.4.1 Dripping mode

The most basic mode of electrospraying is dripping mode which operates at low flow rates and electric fields [16,40]. In this mode, the liquid flows drop by drop through the capillary outlet, similar to that in the absence of an electric field. However, the presence of an electric field generates smaller droplets as well as increases the frequency of droplets as the electric force overcomes the surface tension faster than the weight of the droplet alone [15,35]. It should also be noted that at no voltage, the liquid slowly rises along the outer walls of the capillary as the droplet builds up before leaving the capillary tip. The wetting height gradually decreases as the voltage is increased, eventually becoming negligible [39].

A study by Cloupeau states that the maximum number of droplets emitted per second in dripping mode is 500, above this level the emission becomes irregular [39]. This phenomenon was demonstrated by Xie et al. using an alginate solution under dripping mode electrospraying. The droplet behavior and size were captured using a high-speed camera. As the voltage increases, the increasing electric field leads to a decrease in droplet size as well as increasing droplet frequencies (Fig. 6.3). However, the increase in voltage causes the mutual repulsive charges to suppress the surface tension creating a long neck between the primary droplet and needle tip. This would form satellite droplets after the main droplet breaks off. Further increase of the voltage causes the droplet to become unstable leading to a whipping behavior [22].

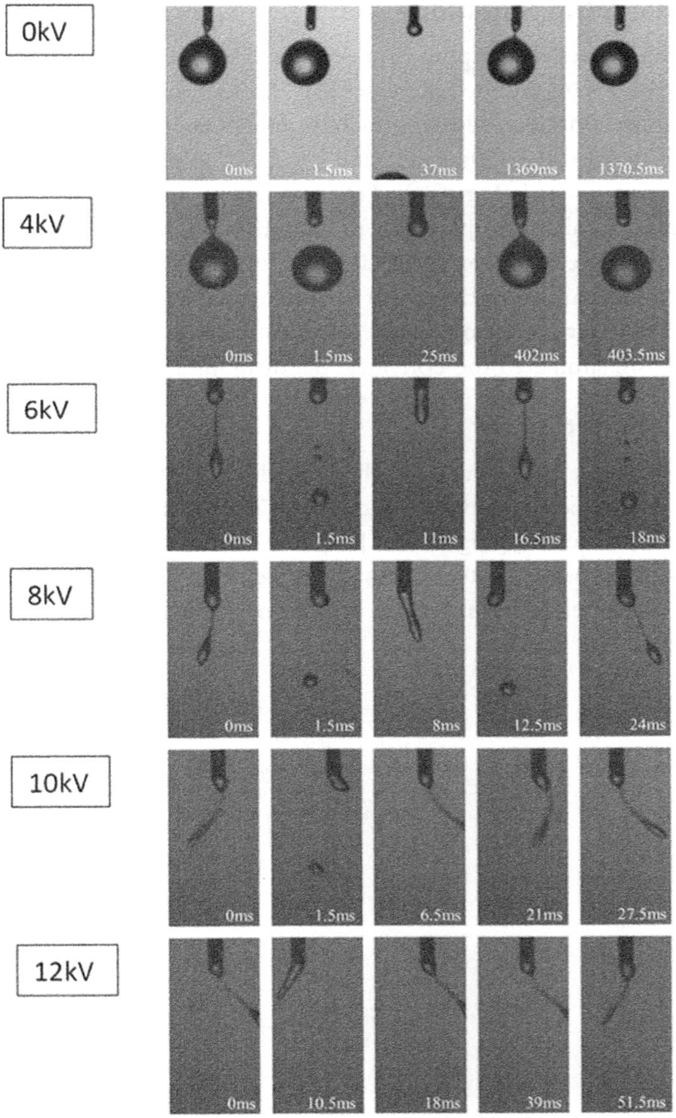

Figure 6.3 ***Dripping mode electrospraying.*** Dripping mode electrospraying with increasing voltage (0, 4, 6, 8, 10, 12 kV). Dripping frequency increases as voltage is increased. Satellite droplets were seen at 6 kV, created when the main droplet breaks off from the meniscus. At higher voltages (10 and 12 kV) nozzle vibration created jet instability and a whipping behavior was observed which made it difficult to observe droplets. *From J.W. Xie, C. Wang, C. Electrospray in the dripping mode for cell microencapsulation. Journal of Colloid and Interface Science 312 (2) (2007) 247–55. https://doi.org/10.1016/j.jcis.2007.04.023 249.*

6.4.2 Microdripping mode

At low flow rates the dripping mode would transition to a microdripping mode as the voltage applied increases [41]. Unlike the dripping mode where the meniscus contracts following each droplet detachment, a stable meniscus is formed in microdripping mode and a small droplet detaches from the end of the meniscus [15] (Fig. 6.4). The droplets produced via this mode are significantly smaller compared to the capillary outlet. Moreover, the frequency of droplet emission is significantly higher compared to the conventional dripping mode, normally up by one or two orders of magnitude [39]. Despite the faster emission rate, the emission still takes place on a droplet by droplet basis, similar to the conventional dripping mode [35].

6.4.3 Cone-jet mode

Cone-jet mode electrospraying is the most developed mode of electrospraying and is utilized in several studies [3,42,43]. At higher electric fields compared to the dripping mode [40], the electric field causes the liquid meniscus to transform into an axisymmetric cone [15]. This phenomenon was first observed experimentally by Zeleny [12]; however, the structure

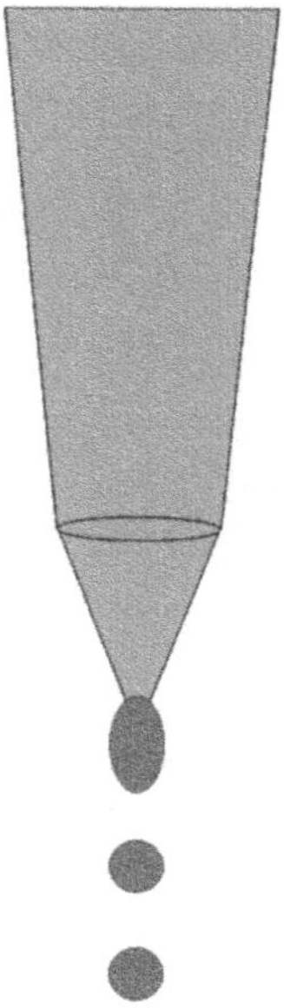

Figure 6.4 ***Microdripping mode electrospraying.*** A constant meniscus is present with small droplets detaching from the end of the meniscus. *No Permissions Required.*

is known to be first defined theoretically by Taylor in 1964 and hence is known as the Taylor cone [13]. A permanent jet can be seen extending from the apex of the cone [35]. As the electric field is increased, there is an acceleration of liquid in the cone creating a liquid jet at the apex of the cone. Excess charges eventually dissipate due to mutual repulsion causing breakup of the jet into droplets [38,43] (Fig. 6.5).

Within the cone-jet mode, the diameter of the jet narrows and the length shortens with increasing electric fields [15]. Additionally, the shape of the cone jet also varies with the conductivity of the liquid. In liquids with high conductivities, the jet formation zone is limited to the apex of the meniscus (Fig. 6.6). On the other hand, the acceleration zone would extend further for liquids with lower conductivity (Fig. 6.6) [35].

In order for the cone-jet mode to occur, the flow rate must be above a minimum flow rate. This rates depend on the type of liquid used. At this minimum flow rate, the jet breaks up due to asymmetric instabilities known as varicose instabilities [43]. During this, the liquid contracts and the jet disintegrates into uniform droplets, however, sometimes satellite droplets could also be formed [39]. Furthermore, the droplet uniformity in cone-jet mode is never as good compared to dripping or microdripping mode

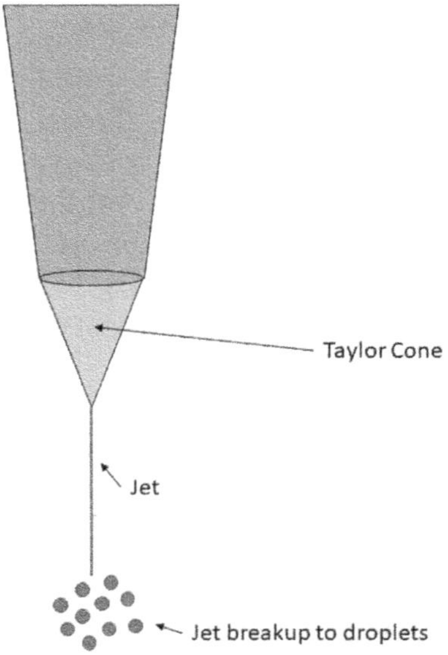

Figure 6.5 ***Cone-jet mode electrospraying.*** This mode is characterized by the presence of the Taylor cone with a liquid jet extending from the apex of the cone. Excess charges cause the jet to breakup into droplets. *No Permissions Required.*

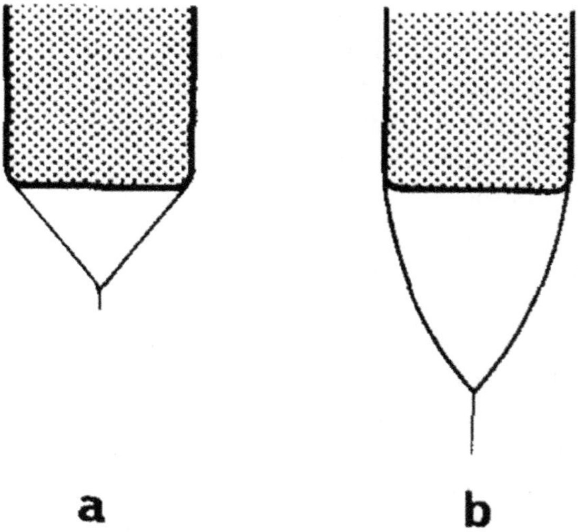

Figure 6.6 ***Taylor cone during cone-jet mode.*** The meniscus transforms into a Taylor cone during cone-jet mode. The excess charges cause a jet to accelerate from the Taylor cone. This acceleration is based on the conductivity of the liquid. (A) At high conductivities, the jet formation is limited to the apex of the Taylor cone before breaking into droplets. (B) On the other hand, at low conductivities, the acceleration zone would extend further away from the apex. *From M. Cloupeau, B. Prunet-Foch, B. Electrostatic spraying of liquids in cone-jet mode, Journal of Electrostatics 22 (1989) 135–139. https://doi.org/10.1016/0304-3886(89)90081-8.*

[44]. For slightly higher electric fields, kink instabilities could occur which are characterized by disordered winding threads thinning out regularly [39]. These occur due to the lateral or azimuthal instabilities of the jet [43]. As charges continue to increase beyond the permanent part of the jet, this leads to producing droplets of various sizes [38]. A study by Cloupeau and Prunet-Foch demonstrated that a certain flow rate must be achieved for kink stabilities to occur, the value of this flow rate is determined by the conductivity of the solution [39].

The popularity of the cone-jet mode is due to its ability to create microdroplets significantly smaller compared to the inner diameter of the capillary [45], with droplet sizes as low as 20 μm being generated [38]. As long as kink instabilities do not occur, the droplets generated in cone-jet mode are stable with a low standard deviation [46]. In addition to the small bead size formed, the cone-jet mode could generate a very large range of droplet sizes through the modification of the electrospraying parameters [35]. Hence, this mode allows suitable sized microbeads to be created for several bioprocess applications such as drug delivery, cell encapsulation, and microcarriers.

6.4.4 Simple jet mode

The main draw back of both the cone-jet mode and dripping mode is the low operating flow rates [38]. This limits the application of electrospraying in industry, as the flow rates for the aforementioned modes are too low for processes such as cooling towers, thermal desalination, and spray drying [45]. In order to overcome this limitation, another electrospraying mode, the simple jet mode which operates at a higher flow rate compared to cone-jet and dripping modes, has recently been explored [47]. Under the simple jet mode, the flow rate through the nozzle is increased so a constant stream of liquid jet is formed prior to the application of an electric field (Fig. 2.15) [39,45]. This occurs when the kinetic energy of the liquid exceeds the surface energy required for jet formation [48]. Due to the higher inertia within the liquid jet compared to the droplets in dripping mode or the cone in cone-jet mode, the electric field would only have a minor influence on the jet and hence creating droplet sizes significantly larger compared to those created using cone-jet mode [47].

The high flow rates applied would increase the rate of droplet formation overcoming the drawbacks of the cone-jet and dripping modes. This mode is far less understood and examined compared to the cone-jet mode. However, several studies have investigated the behavior of water while operating under simple jet mode, where uniform water droplets were generated under high throughput [45,47]. More recently, the trajectory pathways of water droplets under simple jet electrospraying have been successfully modeled [49] (Fig. 6.7). On the other hand, some studies have examined the behavior or alginate, a non-Newtonian liquid, under simple jet mode electrospraying and demonstrated the ability to create alginate microbeads with diameters of a few hundred micrometers [20,40]. The higher flow rate scales up the microdroplet production rate compared to cone-jet and dripping modes. Despite this, other production techniques such as the emulsion methods still possess superior scalability compared to simple jet electrospraying [50].

Despite the high production rate, the disadvantage of simple jet mode electrospraying is the limited effect of the electric field on the liquid jet leading to a limited range of bead sizes produced as well as significant larger beads compared to those generated by the cone-jet mode [47]. This limitation can be observed in a previous study of alginate bead production where the microbead diameter produced was limited to roughly between 200 and 300 μm [20]. Although the bead size is suitable for some applications, the

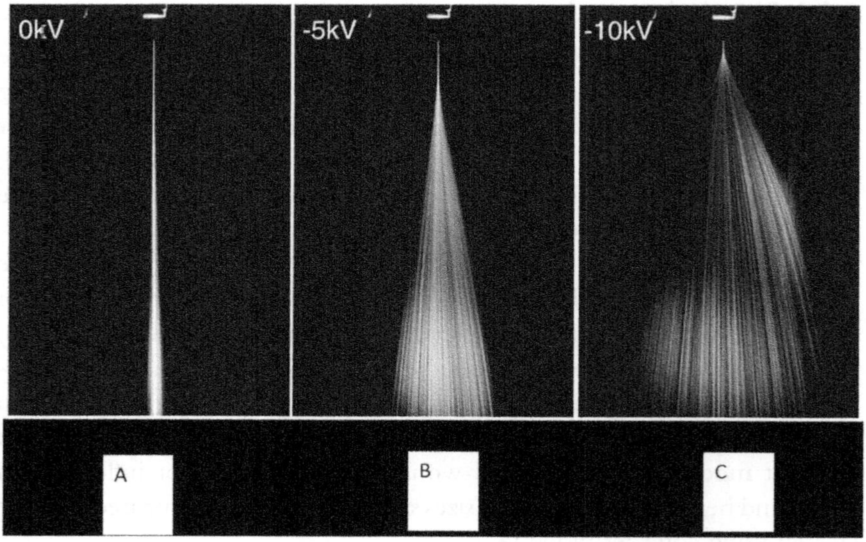

Figure 6.7 ***Electrospraying of deionized water at increasing voltages in simple jet mode.*** (A) Under no voltage, the flow rate is increased until a constant liquid jet is observed. (B) and (C) As an electric field is applied, the jet breaks up into charged droplets, generating microdroplets with high throughput. *From L.L.F. Agostinho, G. Tamminga, C.U. Yurteri, S.P. Brouwer, E.C. Fuchs, J.C.M. Marijnissen. Morphology of water electrosprays in the simple-jet mode. Physical Review E 86 (6) (2012). https://doi.org/10.1063/1.4729021.*

dripping or cone-jet mode produces a much larger range of bead diameter, several studies have demonstrated through the variation of voltage, flow rate, and several other parameters that alginate beads ranging 100 μm to a few mm could be produced [10,19,40].

6.5 Insights into electrospraying parameters

The size of the droplets produced during electrospraying is determined by several parameters, including voltage applied, electrode distance, the conductivity, and viscosity of the polymer solution [37,38]. Burgaski et al. have previously analyzed the various factors that affect the droplet size for the electrospraying of alginate. In a charged needle arrangement, where the needle acts as the positive electrode, the effect on the droplet relationship to electrospraying parameters is represented by Eq. (6.1), where r is radius of the droplet, r_0 is internal radius of the needle, ρ is relative density of the polymer, g is acceleration constant, Υ is surface tension, V is voltage applied, and H is electrode distance [51].

$$r = \left(\left[\frac{3}{2\rho g} \right] \left[r_0 \Upsilon - 2\varepsilon_0 \left(\frac{V}{\ln\left(\frac{4H}{r_0}\right)} \right)^2 \right] \right)^{\frac{1}{3}} \tag{6.1}$$

Voltage is the most commonly investigated parameter as it has the most direct effect on the electrostatic force on the droplets [3,10,19]. A higher voltage would generate smaller droplets [18,19,21] due to an increase in accumulated charge and hence a greater electrostatic force within the liquid, overcoming the droplet surface tension at a faster rate compared to lower voltages [16]. However, upon increasing voltage above a certain threshold, no further decrease has been observed, as the apparent drop in surface tension reaches its minimum [36]. Additionally, it has been reported in studies that at high voltages, the standard deviation of the droplets generated increases significantly, this is possibly due to sparking caused by ionization of air in the space between electrodes [18,52]. As mentioned, voltage plays an important role in determining the mode of electrospraying which occurs, for example cone-jet mode requires a higher electric field presence compared to the dripping mode. Several studies have demonstrated this and an increase in voltage causes the electrospraying mode to gradually shift from dripping mode into jetting mode following an unstable transition phase [19,53].

Electrospraying exhibits high electric potential to the cells about 2–4 kV/cm and the voltages applied could go up to 30 kV [23,36]. Some studies have shown that high electric charges applied during electrospraying are shown to cause significant membrane damage in cells [4,54]. This damage is most likely caused by irreversible electroporation. An electric field causes pores to open within the lipid bilayer of the cell as the electric field reaches a certain threshold, these pores would expand irreversibly causing cell rupture and death [55]. Despite this, it is widely reported that voltages up to several kV applied during electrospraying do not affect cell viability or growth up to several kV [4,19,51,56]. This is due to the fact that despite the high voltages applied, the current is typically low, which plays a key role in cell viability [57]. Hence, the high viability of cells undergoing electrospraying contributes to the popularity of the method for applications such as cell spraying or encapsulation.

In addition to voltage, the electrode distance also affects the overall electrostatic force applied to the liquid. A lower electrode distance would generate higher electric field strength lowering droplet diameter [16]. With the voltage being equal, smaller droplets would form in the presence of a lower electrode distance. It has been previously observed that even if the voltage limit is reached and droplet size no longer decreases with increasing voltage, decreasing the electrode distance would lead to further decrease in droplet diameter [20]. However, similarly to voltage, there would be a point where decreasing the electrode distance would not result in smaller droplets due to a result of air ionization in the space between electrodes which is accompanied by sparking due to the discharge between the electrodes [51]. Typically, the needle tip acts as the positive electrode [9,19], while the ground electrode is typically connected to the collector [42,58,59]. However, a conductive ring or disk, attached above the collecting dish, has also been utilized as a ground electrode [40]. Moreover, in some studies two parallel plates are used as positive and negative electrodes [51].

Aside from voltage and electrode distance, the solution properties of the polymer such as viscosity and conductivity also effect the rate at which the droplets leave the needle tip. Viscosity of the solution affects the jet breakup [3]. It should be noted that viscosity is related to several other parameters, for example, polymer concentration, molecular weight, and conductivity [3,36]. For electrospraying to occur, the viscosity of the solution is required to be below a certain threshold. Above said threshold, the jet would elongate into fibers rather than droplets in a process called electrospinning [60]. For certain polymers, a beaded fiber structure would occur in the transition period of electrospraying and electrospinning [61]. Within electrospraying regime, it has been shown in alginate solutions that a more viscous solution would generate larger droplets. This is due to less viscous solutions leaving the needle tip faster compared to higher viscosity solutions [36]. Higher viscosity is also associated with lower conductivity of the solution. Hence, a previous study demonstrated that a more viscous polycaprolactone solution requires a higher voltage in order to achieve a stable cone jet during electrospraying, which requires a stronger electric field to overcome the surface tension effects on the needle tip [62].Conductivity affects the charge build-up within the droplets. A polymer with higher conductivity would allow a faster charge build-up within the droplet compared to polymers of lower conductivity [3]. However, a higher conductivity would also favor the production of elongated particles rather than spherical [63]. This is due to the fact that high charge build-ups lead to instability within the liquid jet [64].

Flow rate is a very important parameter as it has a significant effect on both the shape and sizes of the beads produced [3]. While using organic solvents, it is vital that a flow rate is selected which ensures the fully evaporation of the solvent. Undissolved solvent could lead to disfigured particles upon contact with the collector as well as biocompatibility issues in biomedical applications [3,23]. As discussed above, there are several modes of electrospraying. Similarly to voltage, flow rate plays an important role during the transition between modes, in particular dripping mode and the cone-jet mode [16,39]. In a study by Moghadam el al, the authors found that an increase in flow rate shifts the transition range to lower voltages [40]. Moreover, studies have shown that the diameter of droplets increases with increasing flow rates this is due to more solution accumulating at the needle tip prior to droplet detachment [10,36].

The falling distance, the distance between the needle tip and the collector, plays a key role in the final droplet shape [65]. In electrospraying setups where the collecting plate acts as the ground electrode, the falling distance is also the electrode distance and hence could affect the electric field as descried above. The effects of falling distance on alginate microbeads produced by dripping mode electrospraying has been characterized empirically by Chan et al. Liquid properties of the solution including the surface tension, viscosity, droplet diameter, and density could be expressed using the Ohnesorge number (Oh) defined by Eq. (6.2), where v is kinematic viscosity of the electrosprayed solution, ρ is density of the electrosprayed solution, dp is diameter of the electrosprayed droplets, and γ is surface tension of the electrosprayed solution [66]:

$$\mathrm{Oh} = \frac{V\rho}{(\rho d_P \gamma)^{0.5}} \tag{6.2}$$

Below a critical Oh number, the viscous and surface tension forces within the droplet could not counteract the drag effect leading to droplet elongation and pear- or tear-shaped beads. Above this value the viscous and surface tension forces within the droplet would cause the droplet to transition into a more spherical shape. Hence, authors found that spherical beads could only be generated given an adequate falling distance to allow for this transition [66]. During collection of solidified microbeads, where a gelling bath is not present, the falling distance needs to be sufficiently high to ensure the total evaporation of the solvent. Similarly to flow rate, particles which are partially solvated while colliding with the collecting plate will be deformed and have a nonconsistent morphology [23].

Table 6.1 Summary of how particle size changes with electrospraying operating parameters.

Operating parameter	Effect on droplets
Voltage	Increase in voltage leads to decrease in microdroplet diameter due to charge increase
Electrode distance	Decrease in electrode distance leads to decrease in microdroplet diameter due to increase of electric field strength
Viscosity	Viscosity affects jet breakup, above a certain threshold electrospinning would form fibers
Conductivity	Polymers with a higher conductivity would lead to a higher charge build-up and smaller droplet size. However, too high conductivity can lead to unstable jets
Flow rate	Increase in flow rate increases droplet diameter due to increased liquid build-up prior to detachment
Falling distance	Plays a role in the droplet shape if surface tension and viscous forces have sufficient time during falling to counteract the drag effect Also ensures solvent has enough time to fully evaporate prior to droplet collection

A summary of how electrospraying operating parameters affect particle size is shown in Table 6.1.

6.6 Other notes

6.6.1 Choice of materials for electrospraying

There have been a wide variety of materials that have been electrosprayed for biomedical engineering applications. A few of them will be briefly mentioned here as it is not the main focus of this chapter. As mentioned previously, one of the most commonly electrosprayed materials is alginate. The instantaneous gelation with Ca^{2+} [67], as well as alginates biocompatibility [68], makes it a popular choice for electrospraying. Aside from alginate, poly(lactic-co-glycolic acid) (PLGA) microbeads have also been produced via electrospraying by using 1,1,1,3,3,3- hexafluoroisopropanol (HFIP) as a solvent [69]. Porous chitosan microbeads used as microcarriers were created by electrospraying a chitosan solution into a collection of liquid nitrogen for freeze-drying to occur [70]. Polycaprolactone (PCL)-based microcapsules have been created using coaxial electrospraying [46].

6.6.2 Methods to characterize electrosprayed particles

Following the production of electrosprayed particles, researchers have utilized several methods to characterize them. For biomedical applications containing living cells, an optical microscope is typically used to visualize the particles and they are characterized via image processing software such as Image J [20]. In order to overcome the resolution limit of an optical microscope, several studies have utilized scanning electron microscopy in order to investigate the morphology and the surface roughness of electrosprayed particles [71,72]. Subsequently, the chemical composition of electrosprayed particles is typically analyzed using Fourier transform infrared spectroscopy (FTIR). This is particularly useful for investigating the successful encapsulation of a drug following electrospraying where the FTIR spectrum of the final particles is compared to the spectrum of the drug and the electrosprayed polymer [73]. Particle size and distribution could easily be measured through image processing. However, another method that has been used is dynamic light scattering. This method detects the Brownian motion of particles in suspension and measures the intensity fluctuation due to Brownian motion which could be translated to particle diameter [30].

6.7 Summary and outlook

Electrospraying overcomes several drawbacks of other droplet producing methods allowing easily controllable droplet sizes under relatively mild conditions. The technique has emerged as a highly explored technology in the biomedical engineering field. This chapter provided an overview of the basics of the electrospraying process. We reviewed the various electrospraying setup deployed in various studies. Furthermore, we have summarized the most popular modes of electrospraying and highlighted the advantages and shortfalls of each. Importantly, we have also highlighted the various processing parameters that play a key effect in the final droplet size and morphology.

The development of electrospraying will continue to explore more materials that could be electrosprayed. This will lead to more applications within the biomedical field utilizing electrospraying. Additionally, more electrospraying setups especially handheld electrospraying devices or multinozzle devices will continually be developed and improved. Although there are several advantages to electrospraying, there remain challenges in the field. One of the biggest issues is the low throughput of electrospraying compared to other methods such as the emulsion method. This will create challenges in upscaling for applications such as creating microcarriers for large-scale stem cell expansion. However, with several advancements in the field, electrospraying is anticipated to expand its horizons in various fields of biomedical engineering.

References

[1] H. Watanabe, T. Matsuyama, H. Yamamoto, Preparation of immobilized enzyme gel particles using an electrostatic atomization technique, Biochem. Eng. J. 8 (2) (2001) 171–174, https://doi.org/10.1016/S1369-703X(01)00121-8.

[2] J.M. Grace, J.C.M. Marijnissen, A review of liquid atomization by electrical means, J. Aerosol Sci. 25 (6) (1994) 1005–1019, https://doi.org/10.1016/0021-8502(94)90198-8.

[3] N. Bock, T.R. Dargaville, M.a. Woodruff, Electrospraying of polymers with therapeutic molecules: state of the art, Prog. Polym. Sci. 37 (11) (2012) 1510–1551, https://doi.org/10.1016/j.progpolymsci.2012.03.002.

[4] S. Sahoo, W.C. Lee, J.C.H. Goh, S.L. Toh, Bio-electrospraying: a potentially safe technique for delivering progenitor cells, Biotechnol. Bioeng. 106 (4) (2010) 690–698, https://doi.org/10.1002/bit.22734.

[5] a Groboillot, D.K. Boadi, D. Poncelet, R.J. Neufeld, Immobilization of cells for application in the food industry, Crit. Rev. Biotechnol. 14 (2) (1994) 75–107, https://doi.org/10.3109/07388559409086963.

[6] D. Grafahrend, P. Jungbecker, G. Seide, H. Leonards, T. Gries, M. Möller, D. Klee, Development and Optimization of an Electrospraying Device for the Continuous Collection of Nano- and Microparticles, vols. 1–9, 2010.

[7] P. de Vos, M.M. Faas, B. Strand, R. Calafiore, Alginate-based microcapsules for immunoisolation of pancreatic islets, Biomaterials 27 (32) (2006) 5603–5617, https://doi.org/10.1016/j.biomaterials.2006.07.010.

[8] X. Li, T. Liu, K. Song, L. Yao, D. Ge, C. Bao, X. Ma, Z. Cui, Culture of neural stem cells in calcium alginate beads, Biotechnol. Prog. 22 (6) (2006) 1683–1689, https://doi.org/10.1021/bp060185z.

[9] Y. Wu, A. Duong, L.J. Lee, B.E. Wyslouzil, Electrospray Production of Nanoparticles for Drug/Nucleic Acid Delivery, 2007.

[10] W. Zhang, X. He, Encapsulation of living cells in small (approximately 100 μm) alginate microcapsules by electrostatic spraying: a parametric study, J. Biomech. Eng. 131 (7) (2009), https://doi.org/10.1115/1.3153326, 074515–074515.

[11] L. Rayleigh, On the equilibrium of liquid conducting masses charged with electricity, Philos. Mag. Series 5 14 (87) (1882) 184–186, https://doi.org/10.1080/14786448208628425.

[12] J. Zeleny, Instability of electrified liquid surfaces, Phys. Rev. 10 (1) (1917) 1–6, https://doi.org/10.1103/PhysRev.10.1.

[13] G. Taylor, Disintegration of Water Drops in an Electric Field, 1964.

[14] G. Taylor, Electrically driven jets, Proc. Royal Soc. London. A. Math. Phys. Sci. 313 (1515) (1969) 453–475, https://doi.org/10.1098/rspa.1969.0205.

[15] A. Jaworek, A. Krupa, Main modes of electrohydrodynamic spraying of liquids, in: Third International Conference on Multiphase Flow, 1998.

[16] J. Zhang, X. Li, D. Zhang, Z. Xiu, Theoretical and experimental investigations on the size of alginate microspheres prepared by dropping and spraying, J. Microencapsul. 24 (4) (2007) 303–322, https://doi.org/10.1080/02652040701339098.

[17] A. Alehosseini, B. Ghorani, M. Sarabi-Jamab, N. Tucker, Principles of electrospraying: a new approach in protection of bioactive compounds in foods, Crit. Rev. Food Sci. Nutr. 58 (14) (2018) 2346–2363, https://doi.org/10.1080/10408398.2017.1323723.
[18] B. Bugarski, Q. Li, M. F. a Goosen, D. Poncelet, R.J. Neufeld, Electrostatic droplet generation: mechanism, AIChE J. 40 (6) (1994), https://doi.org/10.1002/aic.690400613.
[19] L. Gasperini, D. Maniglio, C. Migliaresi, Microencapsulation of cells in alginate through an electrohydrodynamic process, J. Bioact. Compat Polym. 28 (5) (2013) 413–425, https://doi.org/10.1177/0883911513501599.
[20] C.Y. Chui, A. Odeleye, L. Nguyen, N. Kasoju, E. Soliman, H. Ye, Electrosprayed genipin cross-linked alginate–chitosan microcarriers for ex vivo expansion of mesenchymal stem cells, J. Biomed. Mater. Res. (2018) 122–133, https://doi.org/10.1002/jbm.a.36539.
[21] H. Moghadam, M. Samimi, A. Samimi, M. Khorram, Electrospray modeling of highly viscous and non-Newtonian liquids, Polym. Polym. Compos. 21 (7) (2013) 449–456, https://doi.org/10.1002/app.
[22] J. Xie, C.-H. Wang, Electrospray in the dripping mode for cell microencapsulation, J. Colloid Interface Sci. 312 (2) (2007) 247–255, https://doi.org/10.1016/j.jcis.2007.04.023.
[23] N. Bock, M.a. Woodruff, D.W. Hutmacher, T.R. Dargaville, Electrospraying, a reproducible method for production of polymeric microspheres for biomedical applications, Polymers 3 (4) (2011) 131–149, https://doi.org/10.3390/polym3010131.
[24] H. Nie, Z. Dong, D.Y. Arifin, Y. Hu, C.-H. Wang, Core/shell microspheres via co-axial electrohydrodynamic atomization for sequential and parallel release of drugs, J. Biomed. Mater. Res. 95 (3) (2010) 709–716, https://doi.org/10.1002/jbm.a.32867.
[25] A.S. Hoffman, Hydrogels for biomedical applications, Adv. Drug Deliv. Rev. 43 (2012) 3–12, https://doi.org/10.1016/j.addr.2012.09.010.
[26] P.R. Hari, T. Chandy, C.P. Sharma, Chitosan/calcium—alginate beads for oral delivery of insulin, J. Appl. Polym. Sci. 59 (11) (1996) 1795–1801, https://doi.org/10.1002/(SICI)1097-4628(19960314)59:11<1795::AID-APP16>3.3.CO;2-F.
[27] B. Bugarski, J. Smith, J. Wu, M. Goosen, Methods for animal cell immobilization using electrostatic droplet generation, Biotechnol. Tech. 7 (9) (1993) 677–682.
[28] C.-Y. Chui, A. Bonilla-Brunner, J. Seifert, S. Contera, H. Ye, Atomic force microscopy-indentation demonstrates that alginate beads are mechanically stable under cell culture conditions, J.e Mech. Beh. Biomed. Mater. 93 (2019) 61–69, https://doi.org/10.1016/j.jmbbm.2019.01.019. December 2018.
[29] NovaMatrix, Immobilization/Encapsulation of Cells in Alginate Beads, 2011.
[30] L. Zhang, J. Huang, T. Si, R. Xu, Coaxial electrospray of microparticles and nanoparticles for biomedical applications, Expert Rev. Med. Dev. 9 (11002139) (2013) 595–612, https://doi.org/10.1586/erd.12.58.Coaxial.
[31] J.J. Stankus, L. Soletti, K. Fujimoto, Y. Hong, D.A. Vorp, W.R. Wagner, Fabrication of cell microintegrated blood vessel constructs through electrohydrodynamic atomization, Biomaterials 28 (17) (2007) 2738–2746, https://doi.org/10.1016/j.biomaterials.2007.02.012.
[32] F. Wang, Z. Li, K. Tamama, C.K. Sen, J. Guan, Fabrication and characterization of prosurvival growth factor releasing, anisotropic scaffolds for enhanced mesenchymal stem cell survival/growth and orientation, Biomacromolecules 10 (9) (2009) 2609–2618, https://doi.org/10.1021/bm900541u.
[33] I.G. Loscertales, A. Barrero, I. Guerrero, R. Cortijo, Micro/Nano Encapsulation via Electrified Coaxial Liquid Jets, vol. 295, 2002, pp. 1695–1699 (March).

[34] S. Zhao, P. Agarwal, W. Rao, H. Huang, R. Zhang, Z. Liu, J. Yu, N. Weisleder, W. Zhang, X. He, Integrative Biology 3D culture of pluripotent stem cells †, Integ. Biol. 6 (2014) 874–884, https://doi.org/10.1039/C4IB00100A.
[35] M. Cloupeau, B. Prunet-Foch, Electrohydrodynamic spraying functioning modes: a critical review, J. Aerosol Sci. 25 (6) (1994) 1021–1036, https://doi.org/10.1016/0021-8502(94)90199-6.
[36] T.I. Klokk, J.E. Melvik, Controlling the size of alginate gel beads by use of a high electrostatic potential, J. Microencapsul. 19 (4) (2002) 415–424, https://doi.org/10.1080/02652040210144234.
[37] B.K. Ku, S.S. Kim, Electrospray characteristics of highly viscous liquids, J. Aerosol Sci. 33 (10) (2002) 1361–1378, https://doi.org/10.1016/S0021-8502(02)00075-7.
[38] M. Cloupeau, B. Prunet-Foch, Electrostatic spraying of liquids in cone-jet mode, J. Electrost. (1989) 135–159, https://doi.org/10.1016/0304-3886(89)90081-8.
[39] M. Cloupeau, B. Prunet-Foch, Electrostatic spraying of liquids: main functioning modes, J. Electrost. 25 (2) (1990) 165–184, https://doi.org/10.1016/0304-3886(90)90025-Q.
[40] H. Moghadam, M. Samimi, A. Samimi, M. Khorram, Electro-spray of high viscous liquids for producing mono-sized spherical alginate beads, Particuology 6 (4) (2008) 271–275, https://doi.org/10.1016/j.partic.2008.04.005.
[41] Y.-S. Hwang, J. Cho, F. Tay, J.Y.Y. Heng, R. Ho, S.G. Kazarian, D.R. Williams, A.R. Boccaccini, J.M. Polak, A. Mantalaris, The use of murine embryonic stem cells, alginate encapsulation, and rotary microgravity bioreactor in bone tissue engineering, Biomaterials 30 (4) (2009) 499–507, https://doi.org/10.1016/j.biomaterials.2008.07.028.
[42] M.F.A. Goosen, E.S.E. Mahmud, A.S. Al-ghafri, H.A. Al-hajri, Y.S. Al-sinani, B. Bugarski, Immobilization of Cells Using Electrostatic Droplet Generation, 2000, pp. 167–174, https://doi.org/10.1385/0-89603-386-4:167.
[43] R.P.a. Hartman, D.J. Brunner, D.M.a. Camelot, J.C.M. Marijnissen, B. Scarlett, Jet break-up in electrohydrodynamic atomization in the cone-jet mode, J. Aerosol Sci. 31 (1) (2000) 65–95, https://doi.org/10.1016/S0021-8502(99)00034-8.
[44] M. Cloupeau, B. Prunet-Foch, Research on electrohydrodynamic spraying, in: 4th International Conference of Liquid Atomization and Spray Systems, 1988, pp. 125–131.
[45] L.L.F. Agostinho, C.U. Yurteri, E.C. Fuchs, J.C.M. Marijnissen, Monodisperse water microdroplets generated by electrohydrodynamic atomization in the simple-jet mode, Appl. Phys. Lett. 100 (24) (2012) 1–5, https://doi.org/10.1063/1.4729021.
[46] Y.K. Hwang, U. Jeong, E.C. Cho, Production of uniform-sized polymer core-shell microcapsules by coaxial electrospraying, Langmuir 24 (6) (2008) 2446–2451, https://doi.org/10.1021/la703546f.
[47] L.L.F. Agostinho, G. Tamminga, C.U. Yurteri, S.P. Brouwer, E.C. Fuchs, J.C.M. Marijnissen, Morphology of water electrosprays in the simple-jet mode, Phys. Rev. 86 (6) (2012), https://doi.org/10.1103/PhysRevE.86.066317, 066317–066317.
[48] N.R. Lindblad, J. Schneider, Production of uniform-sized liquid droplets, J. Sci. Instrum. 42 (8) (1965) 635–638, https://doi.org/10.1088/0950-7671/42/8/338.
[49] O.M. Ondimu, V.A. Ganesan, M.J. Gatari, J.C.M. Marijnissen, L.L.F. Agostinho, Modeling simple-jet mode electrohydrodynamic-atomization droplets' trajectories and spray pattern for a single nozzle system, J. Electrost. 89 (2017) 77–87, https://doi.org/10.1016/j.elstat.2017.08.001.
[50] A.K.A.S. Brun-Graeppi, C. Richard, M. Bessodes, D. Scherman, O.-W. Merten, Cell microcarriers and microcapsules of stimuli-responsive polymers, J. Contr. Rel. 149 (3) (2011) 209–224, https://doi.org/10.1016/j.jconrel.2010.09.023.

[51] B. Bugarski, B. Amsden, M.F.A. Goosen, R.J. Neufeld, D. Poncelet, Effect of electrode geometry and charge on the production of polymer microbeads by electrostatics, Can. J. Chem. Eng. 72 (3) (1994) 517–521, https://doi.org/10.1002/cjce.5450720318.
[52] Y. Zhou, T. Sun, M. Chan, J. Zhang, Z. Han, X. Wang, Y. Toh, J.P. Chen, H. Yu, Scalable encapsulation of hepatocytes by electrostatic spraying, J. Biotechnol. 117 (1) (2005) 99–109, https://doi.org/10.1016/j.jbiotec.2004.11.004.
[53] H. Moghadam, M. Samimi, A. Samimi, M. Khorram, Study of parameters affecting size distribution of beads produced from electro-spray of high viscous liquids, Iranian J. Chem. Eng. 6 (3) (2009).
[54] M. Szumski, E. Kłodzińska, E. Dziubakiewicz, K. Hrynkiewicz, B. Buszewski, Effect of applied voltage on viability of bacteria during separation under electrophoretic conditions, J. Liq. Chromatogr. Relat. Technol. 34 (20) (2011) 2689–2698, https://doi.org/10.1080/10826076.2011.593223.
[55] R.P. Joshi, K.H. Schoenbach, Electroporation dynamics in biological cells subjected to ultrafast electrical pulses: a numerical simulation study, Phys. Rev. E: Stat. Phys., Plasmas, Fluids, Relat. Interdiscip. Top. 62 (1 Pt B) (2000) 1025–1033, https://doi.org/10.1103/PhysRevE.62.1025.
[56] S.N. Jayasinghe, Bio-electrosprays: the development of a promising tool for regenerative and therapeutic medicine, Biotechnol. J. 2 (8) (2007) 934–937, https://doi.org/10.1002/biot.200700063.
[57] S.N. Jayasinghe, Cell electrospinning: a novel tool for functionalising fibres, scaffolds and membranes with living cells and other advanced materials for regenerative biology and medicine, Analyst 138 (8) (2013), https://doi.org/10.1039/c3an36599a, 2215–2215.
[58] H. Kim, A. Ogata, J. Kim, High speed camera observation of electrospray, in: Electrostatics Joint Conference, 2009.
[59] V. Manojlovic, J. Djonlagic, B. Obradovic, V. Nedovic, B. Bugarski, Immobilization of cells by electrostatic droplet generation: a model system for potential application in medicine, Int. J. Nanomed. 1 (2) (2006) 163–171, https://doi.org/10.2147/nano.2006.1.2.163.
[60] O. Husain, W. Lau, M. Edirisinghe, M. Parhizkar, Investigating the particle to fibre transition threshold during electrohydrodynamic atomization of a polymer solution, Mater. Sci. Eng. C 65 (2016) 240–250, https://doi.org/10.1016/j.msec.2016.03.076.
[61] H. Fong, I. Chun, D.H. Reneker, Beaded nanofibers formed during electrospinning, Polymer 40 (16) (1999) 4585–4592, https://doi.org/10.1016/S0032-3861(99)00068-3.
[62] M. Enayati, Z. Ahmad, E. Stride, M. Edirisinghe, Size mapping of electric field-assisted production of polycaprolactone particles, J. R. Soc. Interface 7 (Suppl. 4) (2010), https://doi.org/10.1098/rsif.2010.0099.focus.
[63] S. Ramakrishna, K. Fujihara, W.E. Teo, T.-C. Lim, Z. Ma, An introduction to electrospinning and nanofibers, in: World Scientific: Singapore, vol. 3, 2005.
[64] F. Meng, Y. Jiang, Z. Sun, Y. Yin, Y. Li, Electrohydrodynamic liquid atomization of biodegradable polymer microparticles: effect of electrohydrodynamic liquid atomization variables on microparticles, J. Appl. Polym. Sci. 113 (2009) 526–534, https://doi.org/10.1002/app.30107.
[65] B.-B. Lee, P. Ravindra, E.-S. Chan, Size and shape of calcium alginate beads produced by extrusion dripping, Chem. Eng. Technol. 10 (2013), https://doi.org/10.1002/ceat.201300230 n/a-n/a.
[66] E.-S. Chan, B.-B. Lee, P. Ravindra, D. Poncelet, Prediction models for shape and size of ca-alginate macrobeads produced through extrusion-dripping method, J. Colloid Interface Sci. 338 (1) (2009) 63–72, https://doi.org/10.1016/j.jcis.2009.05.027.

[67] E.A. Nunamaker, E.K. Purcell, D.R. Kipke, In vivo stability and biocompatibility of implanted calcium alginate disks, J. Biomed. Mater. Res. 83 (4) (2007) 1128–1137.
[68] S. Mandal, S. Kumar, B. Krishnamoorthy, S.K. Basu, Development and evaluation of calcium alginate beads prepared by sequential and simultaneous methods, Brazilian J. Pharma. Sci. 46 (4) (2010) 785–793.
[69] P.-A. Mouthuy, L. Groszkowski, H. Ye, Performances of a portable electrospinning apparatus, Biotechnol. Lett. 37 (5) (2015) 1107–1116, https://doi.org/10.1007/s10529-014-1760-6.
[70] Y.-J. Maeng, S.-W. Choi, H.O. Kim, J.-H. Kim, Culture of human mesenchymal stem cells using electrosprayed porous chitosan microbeads, J. Biomed. Mater. Res. 92 (3) (2010) 869–876, https://doi.org/10.1002/jbm.a.32417.
[71] C. Luo, T. Okubo, M. Nangrejo, M. Edirisinghe, Preparation of polymeric nanoparticles by novel electrospray nanoprecipitation, Polym. Int. 64 (2) (2015) 183–187.
[72] A. Zarrabi, M. Vossoughi, ELECTROSPRAY: novel fabrication method for biodegradable polymeric nanoparticles for further applications IN drug delivery systems, in: Nanocon, 2009, 2009.
[73] M.K. Moghaddam, S.M. Mortazavia, T. Khayamian, Preparation of calcium alginate microcapsules containing n-nonadecane by a melt coaxial electrospray method, J. Electrost. 73 (2015) 56–64.

CHAPTER SEVEN

Innovations and advances in electrospraying technology

Deng-Guang Yu[1], Fenglei Zhou[2,3] Geoff J.M. Parker[2,4] Aiva Simaite[5], Matej Buzgo[5], Gareth R. Williams[3]

[1]School of Materials Science and Engineering, University of Shanghai for Science and Technology, Shanghai, China
[2]Centre for Medical Image Computing, Department of Computer Science, University College London, London, United Kingdom
[3]UCL School of Pharmacy, University College London, London, United Kingdom
[4]Bioxydyn Limited, Manchester, United Kingdom
[5]InoCure s.r.o., Prague, Czech Republic

Abbreviations

EHDA Electrohydrodynamic atomization
FDA Food and Drug Administration
MCE Modified coaxial electrospraying
MFE Multifluid electrospraying
PCL Poly(ε-caprolactone)
PEG Poly(ethylene glycol)
PLGA Poly(lactide-co-glycolide)
PMSQ Polymethylsilsesquioxane
PVP Polyvinylpyrrolidone
TAM Tamoxifen citrate

7.1 Introduction

The standard laboratory electrospraying experiment involves preparing a solution of a polymer in a volatile solvent, often with a functional component present too, and then extruding this through a needle (spinneret) toward a collector. The application of a high voltage between the spinneret and collector causes the formation of a solid product in the form of particles on the nano- to microscale. The process of electrospraying is detailed in Chapter 6. This is usually a low-throughput (<10 mL/h) process, and the use of a single solution results in a monolithic product with a homogeneous distribution of the particle components. These materials have a number of potential uses in the biomedical field (see Chapters 8–10), but there are some limitations which come with the monolithic structure.

Biomedical Applications of Electrospinning and Electrospraying
ISBN: 978-0-12-822476-2
https://doi.org/10.1016/B978-0-12-822476-2.00006-6

For instance, if electrosprayed particles are used for drug delivery, the high surface area of the particles means that a substantial proportion of the drug cargo is present near the surface of the material. This generally results in an initial "burst" of drug release. In a fast-dissolving formulation such a burst is not problematic, but where delayed or extended release formulations are required the burst can severely hamper performance. The low throughput of the standard electrospraying experiment also presents an issue for the translation of the product to the clinic. In this chapter, we will discuss recent technological advances in the electrospraying technology that allow these twin challenges to be overcome. First, we will consider multifluid electrospraying, and how it can be used to design products with complex micro- and nanoscale architectures. This enables issues of initial burst release to be overcome, as well as offering other advantages. Second, the scaling up of electrospraying will be explored and methods highlighted by which the process can be taken to industrial-level throughput. We will further consider how the commonly encountered problem of particle aggregation in the collected products can be overcome.

7.2 Multifluid electrospraying

Complex micro- and nanostructures have attracted increasing attention in recent years, resulting in a range of fabrication technologies being developed [1]. These can be either "top-down" or "bottom-up," and multifluid electrohydrodynamic atomization (EHDA) methods (mainly electrospraying and electrospinning) have a number of advantages over alternate routes. EHDA is a one-step and straightforward process, whereas many "bottom-up" methods are complex and hard to control (e.g., molecular self-assembly). The rapid drying in EHDA means that the structure of the macroscale spinneret is propagated into the solid product and thus, if the processing conditions are well optimized, it is possible to prepare a range of complex shapes including core/shell, Janus, or trilayer systems, and even combinations of core–shell and Janus features. A wide range of liquids (solutions, emulsions, suspensions, etc.) can be processed. This means that a very broad family of functional products can be conceived.

Compared with multifluid electrospinning (see Chapter 2), the analogous electrospraying process has developed more slowly, despite the fact that the first publication on coaxial EHDA reported electrosprayed core–shell particles [2]. In this study, the core fluid comprised an oil, which is on its own not processable by electrospraying. This is one of the many benefits of the

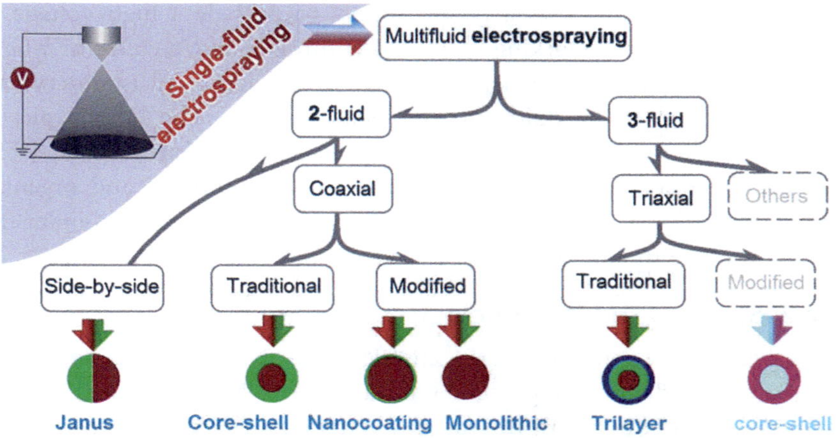

Figure 7.1 The currently reported multifluid electrospraying processes. A "traditional" process is one where either the shell fluid is independently processable into particles or both fluids can be processed alone; a "modified" process is one where the core fluid can be independently processed but the shell fluid cannot.

multifluid process: so as long as at least one of the liquids being used can be solidified by electrospraying, it is possible to generate solid products. This significantly increases the range of materials which can be processed.

There are a number of different multifluid electrospraying (MFE) processes which can be conceived (see Fig. 7.1). MFE processes are to date confined to the processing of two or three fluids. Two-fluid experiments can be coaxial (in which the spinneret comprises two concentric needles, one nested inside the other), which result in a core/shell product, or side by side (two fluids arranged parallel, yielding Janus particles). Three-fluid triaxial MFE (three concentric needles) has also been reported [3,4]; however, at the time of writing, the processing of four or more working fluids simultaneously in MFE has not been described. In contrast, four-fluid electrospinning is known [5], as are complex three-fluid experiments where core/shell fibers with a Janus core have been generated [6].

7.2.1 Experimental apparatus

The apparatus for conducting MFE is essentially the same as that used for the single-fluid experiment (Chapters 6 and 14) or multifluid electrospinning (Chapters 2 and 14). The key difference between single fluid and MFE is the need to consider carefully the compatibility and behavior of the different solutions in the latter experiment. As is shown in Fig. 7.1, the electrospraying system uses a power supply to provide a high voltage, a pump to dispense the working liquid at a controlled rate, a collector where the final solid particles are deposited, and a spraying head (spinneret) to introduce the working fluid into the electrical field. The latter typically comprises a simple flat-tipped needle in the single-fluid process. In MFE, however, the spraying head is structured to accommodate and organize the working fluids. Multiple pumps are typically also required to independently dispense the different liquids at varied rates.

7.2.2 Standard multifluid electrospraying

As discussed in Chapters 8—10, the single-fluid electrospray process has been widely explored for a range of applications [7,8]. MFE has attracted less attention to date, but with the surge in exploration of nanomaterials over the past two decades increasing efforts have been applied to the preparation of polymer micro- and nanoparticles via electrospraying [9—12]. Similarly to electrospinning, electrospraying is developing to prepare complex multiple-chamber particles using MFE. Correspondingly, the main concern of researchers has gradually shifted from "how can I achieve high-quality solid particles through electrospraying" to "how can I manipulate the structures of the electrosprayed particles produced."

For a successful single-fluid electrospraying process, the key experimental parameters to be considered are threefold: the working fluids (e.g., concentrations of solutes, selection of solvent(s), surface tension, viscosity, and so forth); the operational conditions (e.g., applied voltage, spinneret-to-collector distance, the fluid flow rate); and the environmental situation (temperature and relative humidity). Among these, the most important are the applied voltage, the concentration of the solutes in the working fluids, and the compatibility between the liquids. Often there is an optimal value of the solute concentration which allows high-quality solid particles to be generated. If the solute concentration is too low, the resultant products may comprise "wet" particles (with residual solvent still present in them) or even films resulting from the merging of wet particles on the collector plate. If the solute concentration is too high, the resultant products will be large particles, or beads-on-a-string or spindles-on-a-string fiber—particle hybrids. The latter result from a combination of electrospraying and electrospinning taking place; a continued increase in solute concentration will lead to electrospinning and fiber products. Thus, for a given working fluid, there is always a sprayable concentration range, just as there is a spinnable window for generating electrospun nanofibers.

In comparison with single-fluid electrospraying, MFE is much more powerful in terms of the range of structures that it can generate. However, its implementation is more complicated and there are additional parameters that must be balanced during the process. The simultaneous treatment of multiple working fluids in MFE requires at least that these fluids are compatible with minimal interfacial tension between them. The process will fail if one solution coagulates or precipitates when it comes into contact with another fluid. The relative flow rates of the two fluids need to be carefully matched, and the amount of solution dispensed per unit time needs to be harmonized with the applied voltage for a continuous MFE process (that is, one where the Taylor cone is stable and there is no deposition of solid material on the spinneret) which yields dry products.

The most widely explored MFE process is coaxial electrospraying, producing core/shell particles using a concentric spinneret. This has a number of advantages for biomedical applications. For instance, the initial burst of release often observed with monolithic particles from single-fluid electrospraying can be prevented or delayed by generating core/shell particles with a blank polymer shell and drug present in the core alone [13,14]. If the shell is made of a pH-sensitive polymer, then drug release can be prevented in e.g. the stomach and targeted to the small intestine for enhanced absorption [15,16]. Multiple drugs can be incorporated into different compartments of the particles for multifunctionality. Fragile protein-active ingredients (which are often degraded by the organic solvents used in electrospraying) may more easily be processed in the coaxial experiment since an aqueous protein solution can be used as the core fluid, minimizing contact with the organic solvent/polymer shell [17]. Side-by-side spraying to prepare Janus particles has also received some attention in the biomedical field, for instance, to prepare formulations with different active ingredients in the two sides of the particle [18], and there are also a handful of papers using triaxial spinnerets to prepare three-layer particles [13]. These applications are discussed in more detail in Chapters 8–10.

7.2.3 Modified multifluid electrospraying

In standard coaxial electrospraying, either both fluids can be independently sprayed to yield a dry product or the shell solution can be processed alone. So-called "modified" coaxial electrospraying (MCE) is a variant of MFE which is characterized by the use of a shell-working fluid which, when sprayed alone, does not yield solid particles. That is, the shell solution is "unsprayable" in MCE, while the core fluid is sprayable. The MCE process has been shown to have a number of benefits. The presence of a shell solvent or solution in MCE means that there is an air–solvent-working fluid interface in the initial stages of electrospraying, instead of an air-working fluid interface (as in conventional single-fluid electrospraying). This affects the evaporation behavior of the core solvent, and in turn the solidification behavior. For instance, in standard single-fluid electrospraying, it is common to observe the accumulation of solid products on the spinneret as the experiment proceeds. This arises because of attractive interactions between the working fluid and the (typically metal) spinneret head [19]. The use of a pure solvent as the shell fluid in MCE can help to overcome this issue. It has also been noted that in some cases the applied voltage in traditional single-fluid electrospraying is not sufficient to form solid particles, and some additional energy is required to achieve this [20]. This problem too can be resolved with the use of a pure solvent as the shell fluid in MCE. As a result of these considerations, the MCE process is generally simple to run for a prolonged period of time, and the fabricated particles tend to be more reproducible and controllable in their properties.

Compared with single-fluid and traditional coaxial electrospraying, MCE allows the creation of composite particles with higher quality (in terms of particle diameter, size distribution, shape, and internal homogeneity), permits the overall particle shape (e.g., spherical, disc shaped) to be adjusted to enhance functional performance, and may be employed to generate nanoparticles with a thin coating at the exterior [21–23]. Exemplar data showing drug-loaded zein nanoparticles generated by single-fluid and MCE are depicted in Fig. 7.2. In this example, a solvent was used as the shell

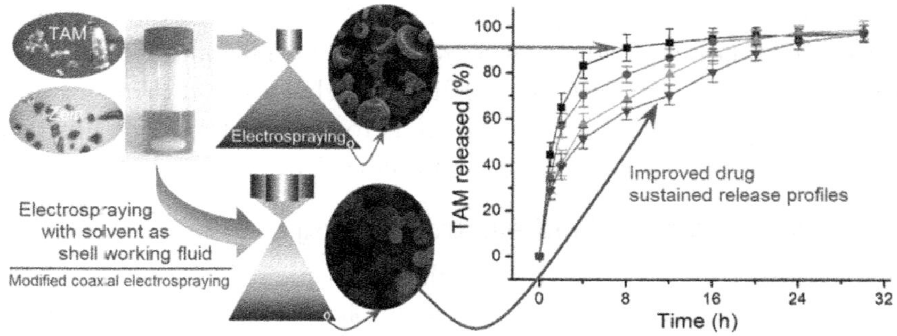

Figure 7.2 A comparison between tamoxifen citrate (TAM)–loaded zein nanoparticles prepared by single-fluid electrospraying and MCE. The latter have more regular spherical morphologies and extend the drug release time. *Adapted with permission from Z.-P. Liu, Y.-Y. Zhang, D.-G. Yu, D. Wu, H.-L. Li, Fabrication of sustained-release zein nanoparticles via modified coaxial electrospraying, Chem. Eng. J. 334 (2018b) 807–816. Copyright Elsevier 2018.*

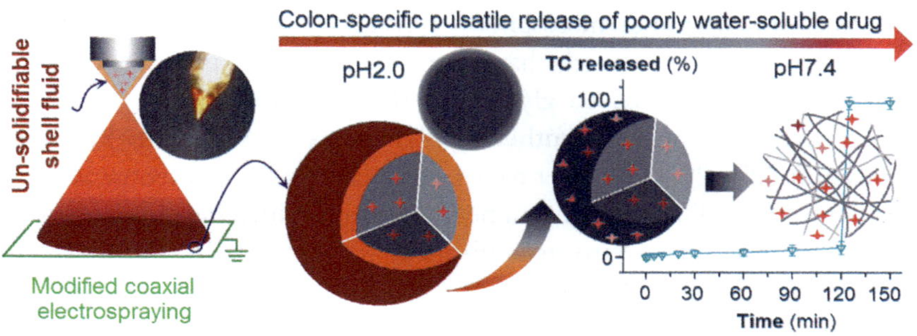

Figure 7.3 Schematic representation illustrating the use of MCE to deposit a thin layer of shellac on a tamoxifen citrate/PVP core for potential colon-targeted pulsatile release. *Reproduced with permission from K. Wang, H.-F. Wen, D.-G. Yu, Y. Yang, D.-F. Zhang, Electrosprayed hydrophilic nanocomposites coated with shellac for colon-specific delayed drug delivery, Mater. Des. 143 (2018) 248–255. Copyright Elsevier 2018.*

fluid. The MCE process yields spherical particles able to extend drug release over a prolonged period of time. Analogous materials prepared with single-fluid spraying had concave shapes and led to faster release [22].

In addition to a pure solvent or solvent blend, other unsprayable solutions can also be employed as shell-working fluids, resulting in new nanostructures for functional applications. For instance, MCE has been employed to coat a thin layer of shellac on drug (tamoxifen citrate)–polymer (polyvinylpyrrolidone; PVP) composite particles (Fig. 7.3) [23]. The resultant core–shell nanoparticles give delayed colon-targeted release when exposed to pH conditions representative of oral drug delivery. In another example, a dilute solution containing 5% (w/v) of the drug helicid and 10% (w/v) PVP K10 was employed as the shell-working fluid in MCE. A very thin helicid–PVP layer with a thickness of 7 nm could be deposited on a blank shellac core [24]. In vitro dissolution tests demonstrated that all the poorly water-soluble helicid was freed immediately upon the formulation being added to an aqueous medium, despite the insolubility of the core shellac.

7.2.4 Hollow structures

One of the major benefits of MFE is the ability to generate hollow structures. These can be applied, for instance, as cell mimics or to provide increased surface areas for sensor applications. Coaxial electrospraying was first demonstrated to be capable of producing hollow structures in 2010 when polymethylsilsesquioxane (PMSQ) microspheres with a hole in the surface were reported after electrospraying a PMSQ shell solution and a volatile liquid core [25]. It was subsequently shown that it is possible to tune the wall thickness of these microspheres through variation of the processing parameters [26]. This work has been extended to poly(-caprolactone) (PCL) and poly(lactide-co-glycolide) (PLGA), two Food and Drug Administration—approved synthetic polymers widely used in biomedical applications [27—29]. The latter have been shown to have potential as "phantoms" for the calibration of magnetic resonance imaging equipment and validation of the measurements performed.

7.3 Collector considerations

The compartmental structure of the products of MFE is largely governed by the spinneret and the fluids fed into it, as discussed above. However, the collector used also merits discussion. Collecting dispersed particles efficiently is a major challenge in electrospraying. In pharmaceutical and biomedical applications, having well-dispersed particles is particularly important so that they can be delivered via oral or parenteral routes (e.g., as intravenous or subcutaneous injections) with good dose reproducibility [7,11,30]. All the processing parameters, including the working distance between the nozzle tip and collector, have to be optimized to ensure sufficient evaporation of solvent from the particles, thus preventing them merging and enhancing collection efficiency. Even with this optimization, a significant loss of particles (>60% of theoretical yields) to the surroundings can occur inside the electrospraying device; that is, particles deposit in places other than the desired collector as they travel to the nearest grounded object in order to discharge [31].

Single-fluid electrosprayed particles are often collected on glass slides, grounded aluminum foil, or in a liquid bath collector (Fig. 7.4a), where they tend to aggregate or stick to each other (Fig. 7.4b—c) and even form thin films (Fig. 7.4d), especially after lengthy operation times [32]. It is very challenging to disperse these aggregates or films into individual particles. The problem of aggregation can however be addressed by appropriate selection of the liquid in a bath collector. The liquid should be miscible with the particle and solvent used for electrospraying, because a completely immiscible interface between the liquid and the particle/solvent (e.g., electrospraying PCL/$CHCl_3$ into a water bath) could result in thin film formation. Various liquid media have been explored in efforts to collect separated particles, including water-based (water, water—ethanol mixtures, aqueous buffers) or organic antisolvent-based collecting systems [8,11].

It is well accepted that the method of collecting electrosprayed particles can influence their final shape and morphology. For example, in one study

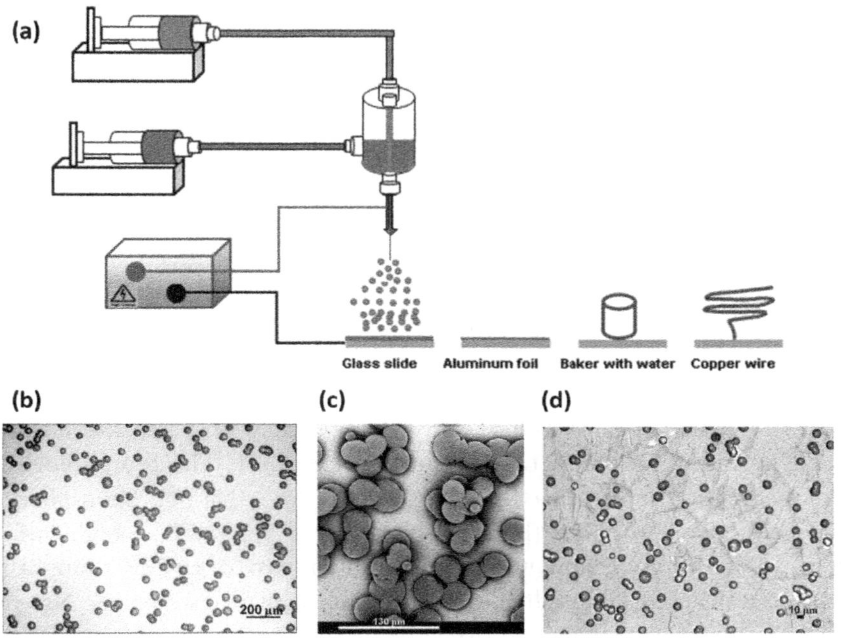

Figure 7.4 (a) schematic illustration of electrospraying using various collecting systems and (b–d) optical/scanning electron micrographs of PCL particles collected on different substrates: (b) on a glass slide; (c) on aluminum foil; (d) in a water bath. *Reproduced with from F.-L. Zhou, P. L. Hubbard Cristinacce, S. J. Eichhorn, G. J. M. Parker, Preparation and characterization of polycaprolactone microspheres by electrospraying, Aerosol. Sci. Technol. 50 (2016) 1201–1215; an open access article published under a CC BY 4.0 license.*

[33], a water bath was used to collect particles electrosprayed from PCL/chloroform, resulting in the particles having a porous surface. In other studies, the electrospraying of PCL/methylene chloride or PCL/chloroform into water without stirring led to the formation of a thin film on the water surface [32,34], while electrospraying of poly(methyl methacrylate)/methylene chloride gave particles [34]. In a cyclohexane collecting bath, PCL particles on the surface of the collecting bath were found to be much smaller than those collected in the bath [34]. When a solution of poly(vinyl alcohol) in deionized water was used to collect particles in the multijet electrospraying of PLGA, it was found to stabilize the products and prevent aggregation [35,36]. A grounded spring-shaped metal wire, placed in the spraying zone between the spinneret and the grounded plate, increased the efficiency of particle capture, and resulted in the formation of a 3D tubular aggregate structure on the wire after an extended operation time. These results

demonstrate that the interactions between the particle and collection media are critical for obtaining well-dispersed products. By careful selection of the liquid medium used for collection in single-fluid electrospray, it is possible to obtain good control of particle size, shape, and morphology while ensuring the products are well dispersed.

To date, there is no well-established method for collecting well-dispersed particles in MFE, though the approaches described above have been demonstrated to be suitable here. Most often, particles are collected either on a grounded electrode or in a container underneath the electrode. Various fit-for-purpose collecting systems have been developed to collect core—shell particles and were also found to affect the particle morphology. Gao et al. used liquid media (ethanol, water/ethanol, and phosphate buffered saline (PBS)) to collect core—shell particles in the coaxial electrospraying of silicon oil/PCL core/shell particles [37]. The morphology of the particles formed varied from spherical (in ethanol), hemispherical (water/ethanol) to oblate (PBS) in shape (Fig. 7.5) [37]. The high surface tension of the collection media in the latter two cases was thought to compress the particles into hemispheres or oblate-shaped structures. Nguyen and coworkers have suggested that aqueous systems are better suited for the collection of particles with a water-soluble core and lipophilic shell, and vice versa [30].

Zhou et al. conducted a systematic exploration of coaxial electrospraying, using aluminum foil and ethanol collectors to produce hollow microspheres with a PCL shell [28]. Particles deposited on aluminum foil tended to form small clumps, within which neighboring microspheres merged with one other, and in the ethanol bath hollow microspheres

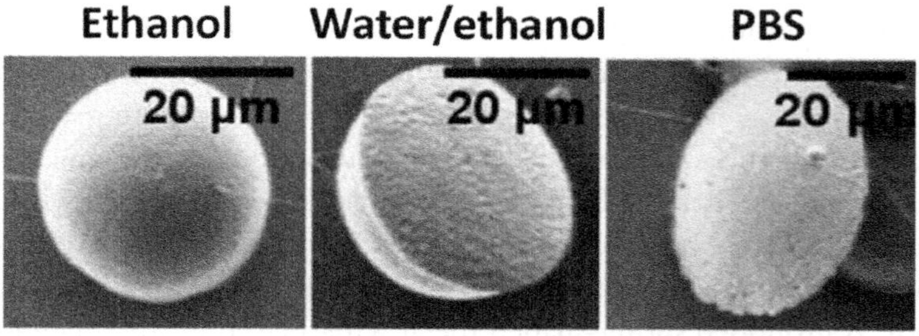

Figure 7.5 PCL—silicone oil particles electrosprayed into different solvents. *Reproduced with permission from Y. Gao, D. Zhao, M.-W. Chang, Z. Ahmad, X. Li, H. Suo, J.-S. Li, Morphology control of electrosprayed core—shell particles via collection media variation, Mater. Lett. 146 (2015) 59—64. Copyright Elsevier 2015.*

with a single hole on the surface were generated when the core fluid comprised a solution of poly(ethylene glycol) (PEG) in chloroform. The porosity and the presence of the surface hole were dependent on the core solutions and the flow rates. Porous particles were obtained when using a PEG/water or PEG/water–ethanol core. The microspheres deposited on aluminum foil did not have porous surfaces and had much smaller sizes than those deposited in ethanol. Similar findings have also been obtained during the coaxial electrospraying of PEG/PLGA core/shell particles [29].

7.4 Scale-up

The main obstacle to the industrial use of EHDA techniques, both electrospraying and electrospinning, is their low throughput and relatively low yield. The low throughput originates from the fact that in an electrospraying experiment the particle size depends on the flow rate (via the size of the dispensed droplets), with increasing flow rates causing particle sizes to rise. To generate small particles ($<10\ \mu m$) extremely low flow rates are needed. The low yield stems from the difficulties in efficient particle collection (see Section 7.3 above), and particularly the adhesion of the particles to the walls of the collecting chamber. A range of strategies to up-scale the production of electrosprayed particles have been developed and will be discussed below. Many of these are adapted from high-throughput techniques for the production of nanofibers (electrospinning).

7.4.1 Upscaling strategies

The strategies for upscaling electrospinning can be grouped into two main groups: needle multiplexing (multineedle approaches) and needleless electrospinning (multijet approaches). These are illustrated in Fig. 7.6. Both have been intensively investigated [38–41] and several high-throughput

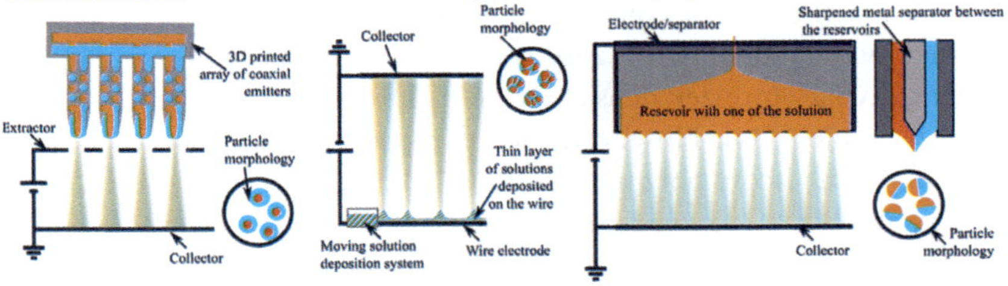

Figure 7.6 The main approaches to scale-up of electrospraying.

electrospinning devices have been commercialized. These same principal upscaling strategies are being considered for electrospraying.

The main advantage of the multineedle approach is that the processing parameters can be relatively easily transferred from needle-based benchtop experiments, though reoptimization will likely be necessary owing to the increased complexity of the electric fields in multinozzle systems. In addition, the particle size and morphology can be easily controlled. Therefore, all the approaches used for generation of multimaterial particles in the lab (coaxial and triaxial electrospraying, Janus electrospraying, etc.) can be upscaled. An array of dispensing capillaries can be used as an emitter, and since each individual needle can be supplied at a relatively low throughput, large amounts of material can be produced without increasing the product particle size. It has been shown that, at a given solution flow rate, particles produced with a single-needle electrospray system have similar sizes to those produced with multineedle electrospraying systems [42]. Through adjustment of the flow rate, applied voltage, and deposition distance, the size of the particles produced can be varied [43].

Despite the clear promise of the multineedle approach, a major issue arises from the fact that the electric field around each needle has a significant effect on its neighbors. Thus, if the packing density of needles is too high, there will be an inhomogeneous electric field. As a result, variability in the products collected can be expected. These effects are especially significant at the edges of the multiplex array, leading to production of larger particles. There is also electrostatic shielding between the spinnerets and the collector, which means that the closer together the dispensing capillaries are, the higher the voltage which needs to be applied to achieve a given electrostatic potential. This phenomenon is caused by the space charge of the solution and particle cloud, which creates an insulating layer between the electrodes and the collector. The most common strategy to eliminate the space charge effects is to use an additional extractor electrode, which is located between the emitter and collector.

Using such extractor collectors, multiplexed emitters have been manufactured with a density of 250 sources/cm^2. Even higher multiplexed electrospraying atomizer density of 460 sources/cm^2 was achieved using micromachining [44]. However, such dense arrays cannot be used for the atomization of viscous polymer solutions. To date, only multiplexed devices with an array of 19 sources spaced >500 μm apart have been validated for the electrospraying of PLGA particles [45]. Such an array was also employed for generating core/shell particles with encapsulated drug in a two-step process. A blend of PLGA and the active ingredient was used to make monodisperse particles by electrospraying, and the particles were then coated with poly(vinyl alcohol) in a liquid bath collector [35]. In the latter case, a distance greater than 2.5 mm between the emitters was implemented to prevent jet deformation.

7.4.2 Scaling up multifluid electrospraying

Multineedle MFE is also possible, but has only been demonstrated on a smaller scale. For example, a simple multinozzle coaxial electrospray system has been explored with two side-by-side coaxial nozzles at varied distances [46]. Multiphysics simulation showed that optimized needle spacing could lead to a packing density of up to 3000 needles/m^2. Scaling up coaxial electrospraying to that level would require advanced multichannel and multipump devices that are difficult to manufacture. Proof of concept of such multiplexed coaxial emitters was produced by 3D printing by Olvera-Trejo et al. These authors fabricated 25 coaxial emitters and used them for manufacturing core/shell droplets of oil in water [47]. However, the flow rates which could be achieved here were modest, at up to 2 mL/h, and the droplet size was limited to 20 μm in diameter. When increasing the production rate of multicompartment particles by multiplexing, significant limitations remain in device manufacturability. In Olvera-Trejo's study, the emitters were produced using 3D printing, and could only be used to spray water-based solvents. More advanced and expensive manufacturing technologies (e.g. direct metal laser sintering) are needed to manufacture similar devices for drug-delivery applications.

The issue of interference between the electric fields around adjacent needles is particularly acute in MFE. It has been shown that if the density of needles is too high, this will cause jet bending and may compromise the spherical shape and the core–shell structure of the particles. Some solutions to this problem have been suggested. For example, multiphysics simulations of multineedle coaxial electrospraying showed that particle homogeneity can be improved by adjusting the nozzle alignment (higher and lower nozzles), and the electric field distribution can be improved and jet bending avoided by using "dummy" nozzles (which do not dispense fluid) at the edges of the array [48]. Alternatively, needle interference can also be avoided by using hydrophobic orifices (that is, a plate made of a hydrophobic material with holes in it) or multipore arrays to dispense the working fluids in place of needles. Orifices as emitters were demonstrated to be effective at high densities of up to 115 holes/cm^2 [49] or 213 emitters/cm^2 [50]. High-throughput production of polymer microparticles by electrospraying has also been reported [51], but with a much lower density of orifices. Such systems are easier to fabricate using microelectromechanical systems technologies than protruding needles with high aspect ratio geometries, making it cheaper and easier to upscale with orifice spraying. However, such systems are yet to be demonstrated in MFE.

Another challenge in upscaling MFE is the manufacturability of the dispensing system. Organizing a series of stand-alone coaxial nozzles into a parallel array is not a convenient solution, as the inner and outer channel of every nozzle would need to be connected to a syringe pump. While this is feasible for a few needles (at the moment it has only been demonstrated with two coaxial needles), further upscaling is limited by the bulkiness and control of such systems. It is much more efficient if one pump can supply all the core channels and another all outer channels via a construction of divergent tubes. However, in this case, each channel must be supplied evenly at a constant feed flow, which poses additional manufacturing challenges [52]. For example, in the 25-nozzle 3D printed emitter for coaxial spinning discussed above [47], ensuring a homogeneous flow in all nozzles required helical channels that create a large hydraulic impedance per liquid feed. While complex geometries can be easily implemented in 3D printed devices, their scalability is limited by the cost of 3D printing (relatively high costs of resin), resolution (channels with diameters lower than 450 μm cannot currently be fabricated), and material (3D printing resins such as epoxy resin are not resistant to many of the solvents used for electrospraying). Moreover, 3D printed emitters are nonconductive, and to initiate EHDA, an electric field was instead applied between the extractor electrode and the collector. This leads to a lower electric field strength at the nozzle and limits the throughput of the process. Manufacturing of similar systems from metals (or solvent-resistant polymers) could be achieved using direct metal sintering and fused filament formation methods. However, in both cases the resolution of the features on the emitter plate would be decreased, which would limit the achievable particle size and the packing density of the emitters.

7.4.3 Needleless electrospraying

Needleless electrospraying is an alternative approach to upscale the production of micro-/nanoparticles. Rather than using a spinneret or emitter plate, this applies an electric field directly to a solution, and at a certain critical voltage Taylor cones are generated and jets emitted. However, despite continuous advancements in needleless electrospinning techniques, few high-throughput electrodes have been validated for electrospraying. Noteworthy examples of proven approaches are electrospraying from stationary wire electrodes [53], multijet field-injection electrospraying [54], and slit electrospraying [55]. The main advantage of needleless technology is that jets are initiated through the formation of a static wave on the polymer solution surface, which leads to the generation of emitting jets with an optimal distribution. This allows for a more robust process that is less sensitive to the processing conditions (e.g., the polymer solutions used) than multineedle approaches. To obtain multimaterial particles using needleless EHDA, three strategies could be used: blend electrospraying, emulsion electrospraying, and MFE.

Blend electrospraying. Needleless blend electrospraying of a polymer mixture has been demonstrated on wire-based needleless electrospinning devices, for instance, using a blend of poloxamer 188 and dextran to deposit particles on an electrospun fiber mat [56]. Needleless electrospraying of aerogel-mixed polymers was also achieved using the multijet field-injection electrospraying (wire in a nozzle)-based technique. In this case too, microdroplets were deposited on electrospun fabrics [57]. These proof of concept experiments demonstrate that needleless electrospinning systems can in principle be used for electrospraying. However, in order to produce core—shell particles, emulsion electrospraying or MFE from needleless systems will have to be realized.

Emulsion electrospraying. Emulsion electrospraying is an alternative route to coaxial electrospraying for the production of core—shell nanoparticles. The applications of emulsion electrospraying have been demonstrated with protein [58] and drug encapsulation [59]. Needleless emulsion electrospinning has been shown to be a promising technique for upscaling the production of core—shell nanofibers [60]. However, emulsion electrospraying from needleless electrodes has not yet been demonstrated.

Needleless multiliquid slit electrospraying. Another approach for producing multicompartment particles at high throughput is upscaling needleless coaxial electrospraying. This can be achieved by using slit electrodes with two or more liquids supplied separately in a side-by-side manner (see Fig. 7.6). Slit electrodes, weir electrodes, and cylindrical coaxial spinnerets can all be used to produce electrospun core—shell or Janus nanofibers [61] at scale. For example, slit electrodes have been used to produce core—shell nanofibers at rates of up to 1 L/h [62,63]. Similar electrodes could be used for high-throughput MFE. However, to date, only the needleless electrospraying of two component Janus particles has been reported [55]. In this study, a microchannel cojetting device (a 7-cm plate with optimized curvature) with a sharp metal separator was used to simultaneously dispense the two liquids. Electrospraying at 2−26 mL/h was achieved. However, at higher flow rates nonspherical disk-shaped particles were produced; this was thought to be a result of incomplete solvent evaporation in the resulting high-solvent environment.

Challenges of needleless EHDA. The key limitation to the more widespread investigation of needleless electrospraying is the lack of dedicated commercially available equipment and/or the possibility to customize commercial equipment to optimize the process. For instance, the most commonly used high-throughput electrospinning apparatus does not allow changes in spinneret-to-collector distance and only supports collection on textiles in a roll-to-roll process. Compared to electrospinning, electrospraying requires much longer drying times, and these can only be achieved at reduced flow rates. Drying in a high-throughput setting is even slower because of the larger emitted droplet size and the surrounding solvent cloud, which both hinder effective drying. Thus, high-throughput electrospraying requires air-assisted drying. Several methods explored to enable this are discussed in the next section. In addition, the challenge of implementing a particle collection system to ensure well-dispersed products are generated is even more of a problem in the high-throughput setting than it is on benchtop devices.

7.4.4 Particle collection

For industrial applications, particle collection must be automated in such a way that continuous manufacturing becomes possible. This is problematic for two key reasons. First, it is difficult to achieve complete particle drying in this setting. Second, it is difficult to collect isolated particles, as they tend to agglomerate on the collector. To solve the first challenge, drying can be assisted by an air flow in specially designed cyclone chambers [31,58]. Two of the designs for collection chambers in continuous particle collection are depicted in Fig. 7.7. Air stream collection also prevents damage to particles, which can arise when they impact with the collector. To reduce the loss of small particles after electrospraying, electrostatic precipitators have also been tested [64,65]. However, even with continuous collection implemented, in one study only 300 mg of particles was collected in 24 h [31]. Combinations of high-throughput emitters and advanced collection systems are needed to increase the particle production yield and bring electrospraying, particularly MFE, closer to industrial applications. One such system was developed by

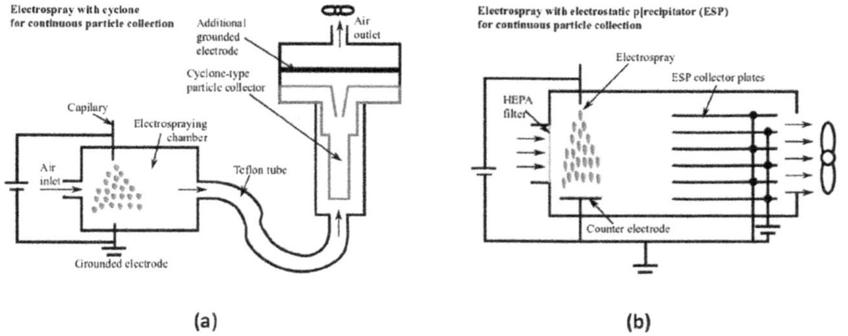

Figure 7.7 Schematic illustrations of electrospraying combined with air-assisted drying and (a) a cyclone collector as developed by Ref. [31], (b) the electrostatic precipitator devised by Ref. [64].

the company Bioinicia (the Fluidnatek LE500 Capsultek pilot-plant). This uses a drying chamber and a cyclonic detector, and has been shown to generate high-quality individual particles comprising zein and a fish oil solution with a throughput of 600 mL/h [66].

7.5 Conclusions and future perspectives

This chapter has sought to provide an overview of key recent developments in the electrospraying technology. We first discuss advances allowing multiple fluids to be processed simultaneously to yield complex multicompartment architectures. This has resulted in a range of core/shell and Janus particles having been prepared, with improved functional performance where systems are fully optimized. Hollow materials can be fabricated, and the use of modified coaxial electrospraying (MCE) has been shown to improve the quality of monolithic particles generated (by using a blank solvent as the shell-working fluid) and to be able to apply a thin coating to particle cores. Attention has also been paid to particle collection, and routes to avoid aggregation are discussed. Scale-up of the electrospraying process is considered, and an overview of the routes to generate industrial quantities of materials is provided.

It is the authors' view that there are many more exciting developments in electrospraying technology to follow in the future. Coaxial electrospraying and MCE are now well established in the literature, but beyond this, there are a range of alterative processes waiting to be developed, particularly modified triaxial electrospraying and three-fluid side-by-side electrospraying. These will lead to particles with increasingly complex multiple chamber structures, and thus greater and more advanced functional performance.

There remains much work to be done in developing electrospraying collectors, both for lab-scale and high-throughput processes, and challenges in ensuring a sufficient drying time and avoiding aggregation are still to be overcome. In terms of scale-up, there is significant scope to adapt the technologies implemented for high-throughput electrospinning to the electrospraying setting, particularly to process multiple fluids simultaneously. Progress here has been rather slow. However, the field has advanced very rapidly in recent years, and we are confident that if this rate of progress continues, then electrosprayed biomedical products have an excellent chance of making it into the clinic in the next decade or so.

References

[1] B.P. Isaacoff, K.A. Brown, Progress in top-down control of bottom-up assembly, Nano Lett. 17 (2017) 6508–6510.

[2] I.G. Loscertales, A. Barrero, I. Guerrero, R. Cortijo, M. Marquez, A.M. Gañán-Calvo, Micro/nano encapsulation via electrified coaxial liquid jets, Science 295 (2002) 1695.

[3] Z.-C. Yao, C. Zhang, Z. Ahmad, Y. Peng, M.-W. Chang, Microparticle formation via tri-needle coaxial electrospray at stable jetting modes, Ind. Eng. Chem. Res. 59 (2020) 14423–14432.

[4] M.F. Pina, W. Lau, K. Scherer, M. Parhizkar, M. Edirisinghe, D. Craig, The generation of compartmentalized nanoparticles containing siRNA and cisplatin using a multi-needle electrohydrodynamic strategy, Nanoscale 9 (2017) 5975–5985.

[5] S. Labbaf, H. Ghanbar, E. Stride, M. Edirisinghe, Preparation of multilayered polymeric structures using a novel four-needle coaxial electrohydrodynamic device, Macromol. Rapid Commun. 35 (2014) 618–623.

[6] S. Chang, M. Wang, F. Zhang, Y. Liu, X. Liu, D.-G. Yu, H. Shen, Sheath-separate-core nanocomposites fabricated using a trifluid electrospinning, Mater. Des. 192 (2020) 108782.

[7] J. Wang, J.A. Jansen, F. Yang, Electrospraying: possibilities and challenges of engineering carriers for biomedical applications—a mini review, Front. Chem. 7 (2019).

[8] J. Xie, J. Jiang, P. Davoodi, M.P. Srinivasan, C.-H. Wang, Electrohydrodynamic atomization: a two-decade effort to produce and process micro-/nanoparticulate materials, Chem. Eng. Sci. 125 (2015) 32–57.

[9] X.-Y. Li, Z.-B. Zheng, D.-G. Yu, X.-K. Liu, Y.-L. Qu, H.-L. Li, Electrosprayed sperical ethylcellulose nanoparticles for an improved sustained-release profile of anticancer drug, Cellulose 24 (2017) 5551–5564.

[10] Y.-Y. Yang, M. Zhang, Z.-P. Liu, K. Wang, D.-G. Yu, Meletin sustained-release gliadin nanoparticles prepared via solvent surface modification on blending electrospraying, Appl. Surf. Sci. 434 (2018) 1040–1047.

[11] S.K. Boda, X. Li, J. Xie, Electrospraying an enabling technology for pharmaceutical and biomedical applications: a review, J. Aerosol Sci. 125 (2018) 164–181.

[12] B. Niu, P. Shao, Y. Luo, P. Sun, Recent advances of electrosprayed particles as encapsulation systems of bioactives for food application, Food Hydrocolloids 99 (2020) 105376.

[13] Y.-H. Lee, M.-Y. Bai, D.-R. Chen, Multidrug encapsulation by coaxial tri-capillary electrospray, Colloids Surf. B Biointerfaces 82 (2011) 104–110.

[14] H.-W. Yeh, D.-R. Chen, In vitro release profiles of PLGA core-shell composite particles loaded with theophylline and budesonide, Int. J. Pharm. 528 (2017) 637–645.
[15] A. Smeets, R. Koekoekx, W. Ruelens, M. Smet, C. Clasen, G. Van Den Mooter, Gastro-resistant encapsulation of amorphous solid dispersions containing darunavir by coaxial electrospraying, Int. J. Pharm. 574 (2020) 118885.
[16] S. Hao, B. Wang, Y. Wang, Y. Xu, Enteric-coated sustained-release nanoparticles by coaxial electrospray: preparation, characterization, and in vitro evaluation, J. Nanoparticle Res. 16 (2014) 2204.
[17] M. Zamani, M.P. Prabhakaran, E.S. Thian, S. Ramakrishna, Protein encapsulated core–shell structured particles prepared by coaxial electrospraying: investigation on material and processing variables, Int. J. Pharm. 473 (2014) 134–143.
[18] B. Sanchez-Vazquez, A.J.R. Amaral, D.G. Yu, G. Pasparakis, G.R. Williams, Electrosprayed Janus particles for combined photo-chemotherapy, AAPS PharmSciTech 18 (2017) 1460–1468.
[19] W. Li, D.-G. Yu, K. Chen, G. Wang, G.R. Williams, Smooth preparation of ibuprofen/zein microcomposites using an epoxy-coated electrospraying head, Mater. Lett. 93 (2013) 125–128.
[20] L. Ding, T. Lee, C.-H. Wang, Fabrication of monodispersed Taxol-loaded particles using electrohydrodynamic atomization, J. Contr. Release 102 (2005) 395–413.
[21] Z.-P. Liu, L.-L. Zhang, Y.-Y. Yang, D. Wu, G. Jiang, D.-G. Yu, Preparing composite nanoparticles for immediate drug release by modifying electrohydrodynamic interfaces during electrospraying, Powder Technol. 327 (2018a) 179–187.
[22] Z.-P. Liu, Y.-Y. Zhang, D.-G. Yu, D. Wu, H.-L. Li, Fabrication of sustained-release zein nanoparticles via modified coaxial electrospraying, Chem. Eng. J. 334 (2018b) 807–816.
[23] K. Wang, H.-F. Wen, D.-G. Yu, Y. Yang, D.-F. Zhang, Electrosprayed hydrophilic nanocomposites coated with shellac for colon-specific delayed drug delivery, Mater. Des. 143 (2018) 248–255.
[24] D.-G. Yu, X.-L. Zheng, Y. Yang, X.-Y. Li, G.R. Williams, M. Zhao, Immediate release of helicid from nanoparticles produced by modified coaxial electrospraying, Appl. Surf. Sci. 473 (2019) 148–155.
[25] M.-W. Chang, E. Stride, M. Edirisinghe, A new method for the preparation of monoporous hollow microspheres, Langmuir 26 (2010b) 5115–5121.
[26] M.-W. Chang, E. Stride, M. Edirisinghe, Controlling the thickness of hollow polymeric microspheres prepared by electrohydrodynamic atomization, J. R. Soc. Interface 7 (2010a) S451–S460.
[27] L. Zhang, J. Huang, T. Si, R.X. Xu, Coaxial electrospray of microparticles and nanoparticles for biomedical applications, Expet Rev. Med. Dev. 9 (2012) 595–612.
[28] F.-L. Zhou, A. Chirazi, J.E. Gough, P.L. Hubbard Cristinacce, G.J.M. Parker, Hollow polycaprolactone microspheres with/without a single surface hole by co-electrospraying, Langmuir 33 (2017) 13262–13271.
[29] F.-L. Zhou, H. Wu, D.J. Mchugh, I. Wimpenny, X. Zhang, J.E. Gough, P.L. Hubbard Cristinacce, G.J.M. Parker, Co-electrospraying of tumour cell mimicking hollow polymeric microspheres for diffusion magnetic resonance imaging, Mater. Sci. Eng. C 101 (2019) 217–227.
[30] D.N. Nguyen, C. clasen, G. Van Den Mooter, Pharmaceutical applications of electrospraying, J. Pharmaceut. Sci. 105 (2016) 2601–2620.
[31] D. Grafahrend, P. Jungbecker, G. Seide, H. Leonards, T. Gries, M. Möller, D. Klee, Development and optimization of an electrospraying device for the continuous collection of nano- and microparticles, Open Chem. Biomed. Methods J. 3 (2010) 1–9.

[32] F.-L. Zhou, P.L. Hubbard Cristinacce, S.J. Eichhorn, G.J.M. Parker, Preparation and characterization of polycaprolactone microspheres by electrospraying, Aerosol. Sci. Technol. 50 (2016) 1201−1215.

[33] Y. Wu, R.L. Clark, Controllable porous polymer particles generated by electrospraying, J. Colloid Interface Sci. 310 (2007) 529−535.

[34] C.H. Park, M.Y. Kim, J.Y. Yoo, K.-H. Kim, J.-C. Lee, J. Lee, Preparation of polymer/drug nano- and micro-particles by electrospraying, Macromol. Symp. 249−250 (2007) 116−119.

[35] B. Almería, T.M. Fahmy, A. Gomez, A multiplexed electrospray process for single-step synthesis of stabilized polymer particles for drug delivery, J. Contr. Release 154 (2011) 203−210.

[36] B. Furtmann, J. Tang, S. Kramer, T. Eickner, F. Luderer, G. Fricker, A. Gomez, B. Heemskerk, P.S. Jähn, Electrospray synthesis of poly(lactide-co-glycolide) nanoparticles encapsulating peptides to enhance proliferation of antigen-specific $CD8^+$ T cells, J. Pharmaceut. Sci. 106 (2017) 3316−3327.

[37] Y. Gao, D. Zhao, M.-W. Chang, Z. Ahmad, X. Li, H. Suo, J.-S. Li, Morphology control of electrosprayed core−shell particles via collection media variation, Mater. Lett. 146 (2015) 59−64.

[38] P. Vass, E. Szabó, A. Domokos, E. Hirsch, D. Galata, B. Farkas, B. Démuth, S.K. Andersen, T. Vigh, G. Verreck, G. Marosi, Z.K. Nagy, Scale-up of electrospinning technology: applications in the pharmaceutical industry, WIREs Nanomed. Nanobiotechnol. 12 (2019).

[39] M. Yu, R.-H. Dong, X. Yan, G.-F. Yu, M.-H. You, X. Ning, Y.-Z. Long, Recent advances in needleless electrospinning of ultrathin fibers: from academia to industrial production, Macromol. Mater. Eng. 302 (2017) 1700002.

[40] L. Persano, A. Camposeo, C. Tekmen, D. Pisignano, Industrial upscaling of electrospinning and applications of polymer nanofibers: a review, Macromol. Mater. Eng. 298 (2013) 504−520.

[41] H.S. Salehhudin, E.N. Mohamad, W.N.L. Mahadi, A. Muhammad Afifi, Multiple-jet electrospinning methods for nanofiber processing: a review, Mater. Manuf. Process. 33 (2018) 479−498.

[42] M. Parhizkar, P.J.T. Reardon, J.C. Knowles, R.J. Browning, E. Stride, R.B. Pedley, T. Grego, M. Edirisinghe, Performance of novel high throughput multi electrospray systems for forming of polymeric micro/nanoparticles, Mater. Des. 126 (2017) 73−84.

[43] J.D. Regele, M.J. Papac, M.J.A. Rickard, D. Dunn-Rankin, Effects of capillary spacing on EHD spraying from an array of cone jets, J. Aerosol Sci. 33 (2002) 1471−1479.

[44] B. Lojewski, W. Yang, H. Duan, C. Xu, W. Deng, Design, fabrication, and characterization of linear multiplexed electrospray atomizers micro-machined from metal and polymers, Aerosol. Sci. Technol. 47 (2013) 146−152.

[45] B. Almería, W. Deng, T.M. Fahmy, A. Gomez, Controlling the morphology of electrospray-generated PLGA microparticles for drug delivery, J. Colloid Interface Sci. 343 (2010) 125−133.

[46] W.-C. Yan, Y.W. Tong, C.-H. Wang, Coaxial electrohydrodynamic atomization toward large scale production of core-shell structured microparticles, AIChE J. 63 (2017) 5303−5319.

[47] D. Olvera-Trejo, L.F. Velásquez-García, Additively manufactured MEMS multiplexed coaxial electrospray sources for high-throughput, uniform generation of core−shell microparticles, Lab Chip 16 (2016) 4121−4132.

[48] W.-C. Yan, P. Davoodi, Y.W. Tong, C.-H. Wang, Computational study of core-shell droplet formation in coaxial electrohydrodynamic atomization process, AIChE J. 62 (2016) 4259−4276.

[49] R. Bocanegra, A.G. Gaonkar, A. Barrero, I.G. Loscertales, D. Pechack, M. Marquez, Production of cocoa butter microcapsules using an electrospray process, J. Food Sci. 70 (2005) e492–e497.
[50] S. Dandavino, C. Ataman, C.N. Ryan, S. Chakraborty, D. Courtney, J.P.W. Stark, H. Shea, Microfabricated electrospray emitter arrays with integrated extractor and accelerator electrodes for the propulsion of small spacecraft, J. Micromech. Microeng. 24 (2014) 075011.
[51] C. Zhang, M.-W. Chang, Z. Ahmad, W. Hu, D. Zhao, J.-S. Li, Stable single device multi-pore electrospraying of polymeric microparticles via controlled electrostatic interactions, RSC Adv. 5 (2015) 87919–87923.
[52] M.S. Lhernould, P. Lambert, Compact polymer multi-nozzles electrospray device with integrated microfluidic feeding system, J. Electrost. 69 (2011) 313–319.
[53] M. Loepfe, A. Duss, K.A. Zafeiropoulou, O. Bjorgvinsdottir, M. D'este, D. Eglin, G. Fortunato, J. Klasen, S.J. Ferguson, K. Wuertz-Kozak, O. Krupkova, Electrospray-based microencapsulation of epigallocatechin 3-gallate for local delivery into the intervertebral disc, Pharmaceutics 11 (2019) 435.
[54] C. Berkland, D.W. Pack, K. Kim, Controlling surface nano-structure using flow-limited field-injection electrostatic spraying (FFESS) of poly(d,l-lactide-co-glycolide), Biomaterials 25 (2004) 5649–5658.
[55] J.H. Jordahl, S. Ramcharan, J.V. Gregory, J. Lahann, Needleless electrohydrodynamic cojetting of bicompartmental particles and fibers from an extended fluid interface, Macromol. Rapid Commun. 38 (2017) 1600437.
[56] R. Böttjer, T. Grothe, D. Wehlage, A. Ehrmann, Electrospraying poloxamer/(bio-) polymer blends using a needleless electrospinning machine, J. Text. Fibrous Mater. 1 (2018), 2515221117743079.
[57] A. Shaid, L. Wang, R. Padhye, A. Jadhav, Needleless electrospinning and electrospraying of mixture of polymer and aerogel particles on textile, Adv. Mater. Sci. Eng. 2018 (2018) 1–7.
[58] J. Xie, C.-H. Wang, Encapsulation of proteins in biodegradable polymeric microparticles using electrospray in the Taylor cone-jet mode, Biotechnol. Bioeng. 97 (2007) 1278–1290.
[59] S.R. Prasad, A. Jayakrishnan, T.S.S. Kumar, Combinational delivery of anticancer drugs for osteosarcoma treatment using electrosprayed core shell nanocarriers, J. Mater. Sci. Mater. Med. 31 (2020) 44.
[60] M. Buzgo, E. Filova, A.M. Staffa, M. Rampichova, M. Doupnik, K. Vocetkova, V. Lukasova, R. Kolcun, D. Lukas, A. Necas, E. Amler, Needleless emulsion electrospinning for the regulated delivery of susceptible proteins, J. Tissue Eng. Regen. Med. 12 (2018) 583–597.
[61] L. Vysloužilová, J. Valtera, K. Pejchar, J. Beran, D. Lukáš, Design of coaxial needleless electrospinning electrode with respect to the distribution of electric field, Appl. Mech. Mater. 693 (2014) 394–399.
[62] L. Vyslouzilova, M. Buzgo, P. Pokorny, J. Chvojka, A. Mickova, M. Rampichova, J. Kula, K. Pejchar, M. Bilek, D. Lukas, E. Amler, Needleless coaxial electrospinning: a novel approach to mass production of coaxial nanofibers, Int. J. Pharm. 516 (2017) 293–300.
[63] X. Yan, J. Marini, R. Mulligan, A. Deleault, U. Sharma, M.P. Brenner, G.C. Rutledge, T. Freyman, Q.P. Pham, Slit-surface electrospinning: a novel process developed for high-throughput fabrication of core-sheath fibers, PLoS One 10 (2015) e0125407.

[64] J.-H. Kim, H.-S. Lee, H.-H. Kim, A. Ogata, Electrospray with electrostatic precipitator enhances fine particles collection efficiency, J. Electrost. 68 (2010) 305–310.
[65] G. Tepper, R. Kessick, A study of ionization and collection efficiencies in electrospray-based electrostatic precipitators, J. Aerosol Sci. 39 (2008) 609–617.
[66] M.A. Busolo, S. Torres-Giner, C. Prieto, J.M. Lagaron, Electrospraying assisted by pressurized gas as an innovative high-throughput process for the microencapsulation and stabilization of docosahexaenoic acid-enriched fish oil in zein prolamine, Innovat. Food Sci. Emerg. Technol. 51 (2019) 12–19.

CHAPTER EIGHT

Applications of electrospraying in tissue engineering and beyond

Poornima Dubey[1], P. Gopinath[2], Duncan Q.M. Craig[3], Vinita Takiar[1,4]

[1]Department of Radiation Oncology, University of Cincinnati College of Medicine Cincinnati, Cincinnati, OH, United States
[2]Department of Biotechnology, Joint Faculty in Centre for Nanotechnology, Indian Institute of Technology Roorkee, Roorkee, Uttarakhand, India
[3]UCL School of Pharmacy, London, United Kingdom
[4]Cincinnati Department of Veterans Affairs (VA) Medical Center, Cincinnati, OH, United States

8.1 Introduction

Electrospraying (E-spray), using electrohydrodynamic atomization method, has been widely explored for the production and formulation of micro- and nanostructures for various biomedical applications, including drug delivery, theranostics, implant coatings, and tissue engineering (TE) [1,2]. E-spray is analogous to electrospinning; however, it is distinct as an approach in that, despite using the same experimental setup as electrospinning, it can typically achieve nano- or microparticles using more dilute polymeric solutions. This setup includes a syringe pump, a syringe, a high-voltage power supply, and a grounded conductive surface. E-spray technology also has the flexibility to produce a wide variety of particles, including blending polymers, metal particles, microbubbles, polyplexes, amphiphilic natural and synthetic polymers, silica, and lipids [1,2]. E-spray—generated nano- and microparticles have been exploited for the incorporation of small chemical molecules such as drugs, proteins, nucleic acids, cells, and other bioactive therapeutics [3,4].

Electrosprayed polymeric particles are also widely used to encapsulate several elements as well as integrate many polymers to form multiple layered (di, tri, etc.) coaxial polymeric particles [4]. Hence, alongside the development of electrospinning for the synthesis of nanofibrous scaffolds that mimics the fibrous structure of the native extracellular matrix, lately, E-spray has garnered attention for tissue repair and regenerative medicines [5]. TE comprises technologies for engineering human tissues in a precise manner that may enable the repair and substitution of injured or diseased organs [6]. Successful TE necessitates specific chemistry between distinct scaffolds,

Biomedical Applications of Electrospinning and Electrospraying
ISBN: 978-0-12-822476-2
https://doi.org/10.1016/B978-0-12-822476-2.00009-1

cells, and growth factors (GFs), ensuing a new functional tissue. For body tissue regeneration, TE approaches can be scaffold, GF, or cell based [6].

Typically, the E-spray process comprises the production of a vaporized spray of the polymeric carrier (cargo) and encapsulant matrix. The process involves a low flow rate (in mL/hr) by a syringe pump, which leads to a volatile solution of the blended polymeric matrix and encapsulates payload sprayed with a needle of different gauze size onto a ground collector into a solid or liquid substrate. An electrical potential difference will be generated by the opposite charges applied to the needle and collection substrate for the generation of tens of kilovolts, which results in the generation of a Taylor cone. Generally, in a monoaxial spray setup, all of the sprayed constituents get blended during the process; though in a multiaxial spray setting, the discrete solutions (e.g., drug molecules in the aqueous phase and polymers in an organic solvent) do not blend till they dispense from their respective conduits within the syringe needle before entering the Taylor cone as an outlet. This design of discrete mixing leads to the formation of core—shell particles wherein an inner core contains drug molecules with an outer polymeric layer as a shell. With high polymeric concentrations, the polymer chain entanglement led to the formation of a higher viscosity solution; instead of forming particles, the Taylor cone-jet ejects a continuous fiber which travels to the collection substrate, in a process known as *electrospinning*. Though at the lower polymeric concentrations the solution viscosity remains relatively low, it leads to the ejection of liquid droplets owing to the repulsive forces that occur due to the nature of like charges controlling the cohesive forces of viscosity and surface tension; this phenomenon is called *electrospraying (ES)* [7]. In the context of TE approaches, E-spray technology—mediated nano-/microparticles might be explored to deliver bioactive materials either to the cell vicinity or directly into the interior of the cells after cellular internalization. The proteins released (including GFs or low molecular weight cell differentiation agents) can target and regulate the performance and the fate of the cells for tissue repair and regeneration.

8.2 Electrospray particulate systems as scaffolds in tissue engineering and beyond

Microparticle and microcapsule formulations are not only commonly explored for biomedical studies and biological applications, with functions including payload delivery, but also to facilitate 3D cell culture in TE [8,9]. Microparticle scaffolds essentially work as the building blocks for the delivery of soluble factors, directing the fabrication of TE scaffolds, giving rise to injectable systems for in situ scaffold formation or either by fusion giving rise to porous scaffolds, evading complicated surgery procedures. The role of microparticles in TE serves various purposes, including (i) the integration into the hydrogels or porous scaffolds directing formation of the pores [10], (ii) serving as the multifaceted delivery systems for macromolecules, for instance, dual release profile systems [11,12]. The microparticles loaded with bioactive molecules could also be injected targeting for controlled delivery, relying on polymer degradation, diffusion [13], or by means of stimuli-responsive polymeric properties mediated triggering the release of the bioactive molecules [14—17].

Microspheres are the three-dimensional (3D) porous scaffoldings leading to the tissue regeneration and drug delivery [15]. It offers added advantages over 3D scaffolds. 3D scaffolds can be difficult to construct for filling irregularly shaped defects, while microspheres can be easily injected into any defect irrespective of the shape and geometry [18]. Further, the injectability of microspheres is considered to be minimally invasive treatments, while gross surgical procedures are necessary for the implantation of 3D porous scaffolds. The increased use of injectable microspheres also coincides with advancements in biomedical imaging technologies for tracking them in the body postinjection.

In conjunction with the self-assembling/ionically cross-linked hydrogels, microspheres present the brilliant class of injectable biomaterials. Though injectable microspheres work similarly to other 3D scaffolds, they can deliver GFs/drugs and cells to the site of injury for tissue regeneration. Natural polymers, for instance, chitosan, gelatin, and alginate, along with synthetic polymers such as poly-lactic-co-glycolic acid and polycaprolactone, have been widely explored for the fabrication of microspheres for numerous applications [19]. The choice of the scaffolding material for microsphere fabrication is marked by its biodegradability, as essential for drug delivery, as well as tissue repair and growth [19]. Also, the fabrication technique can chiefly alter the texture, morphology, and particle size of the microspheres [19]. A study showed the fabrication of aerogel microspheres using high-pressure spraying of cellulose nanofibrils by using the steel nozzle into liquid nitrogen. E-spray presents a great process to improve control of both particle size and distribution associated with nano-/microparticles for a wide range of morphologies [20].

Different methods have been explored for the fabrication of a wide range of microsphere morphologies, including solid, hollow, porous, and nanofiber microspheres. Lately, nanofiber microspheres have captivated noteworthy consideration for biomedical applications because of their injectable and biomimetic properties. An ES of aqueous dispersions of electrospun fiber segments into a cryo coolant was recently done as an innovative way for the exploration of nanofiber microsphere fabrication to determine their possible applications for cell delivery (Fig. 8.1). Cryo cutting or homogenization led to ES of aqueous dispersions of electrospun nanofiber segments of the desired length collected either into liquid nitrogen by freeze-drying and by thermal treatment resulted in the nanofiber microspheres. A wide range of morphologies can be attained, such as the solid, nanofibrous, porous nanofibrous microspheres, or hollow nanofibrous microspheres (Fig. 8.2). Furthermore, this combination approach offers the fabrication of a wide range of inorganic bioactive glass and polymeric nanofiber—based microspheres with their small nanofiber distributions, indicating the broad applicability of this system. The approach results in higher cellular carrier efficiency of nanofibrous microspheres compared to only solid microsphere assemblies with a rat bone marrow—derived mesenchymal

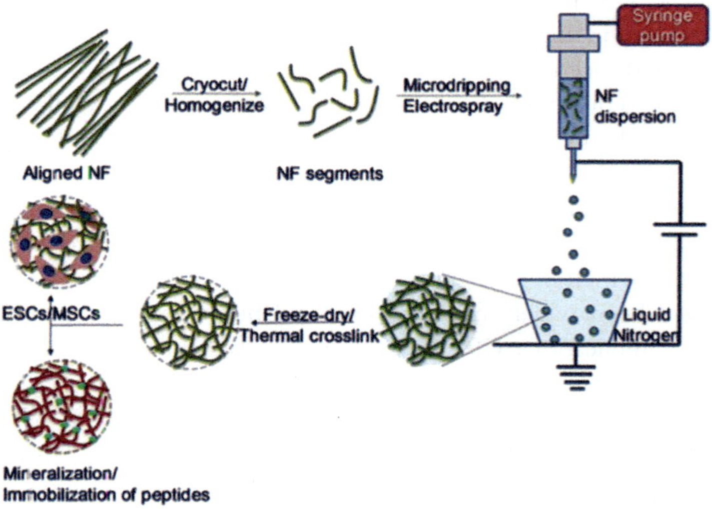

Figure 8.1 Schematic overview of the fabrication of NF microspheres from segmented/homogenized electrospun NFs and their applications for stem cell and drug/peptide delivery. *Reprinted with permission from ref. S.K. Boda, S. Chen, K. Chu, H.J. Kim, J. Xie. Electrospraying electrospun nanofiber segments into injectable microspheres for potential cell delivery. ACS Appl. Mater. Interfaces 10 (2018) 25069–25079 Copyright © 2018, American Chemical Society.*

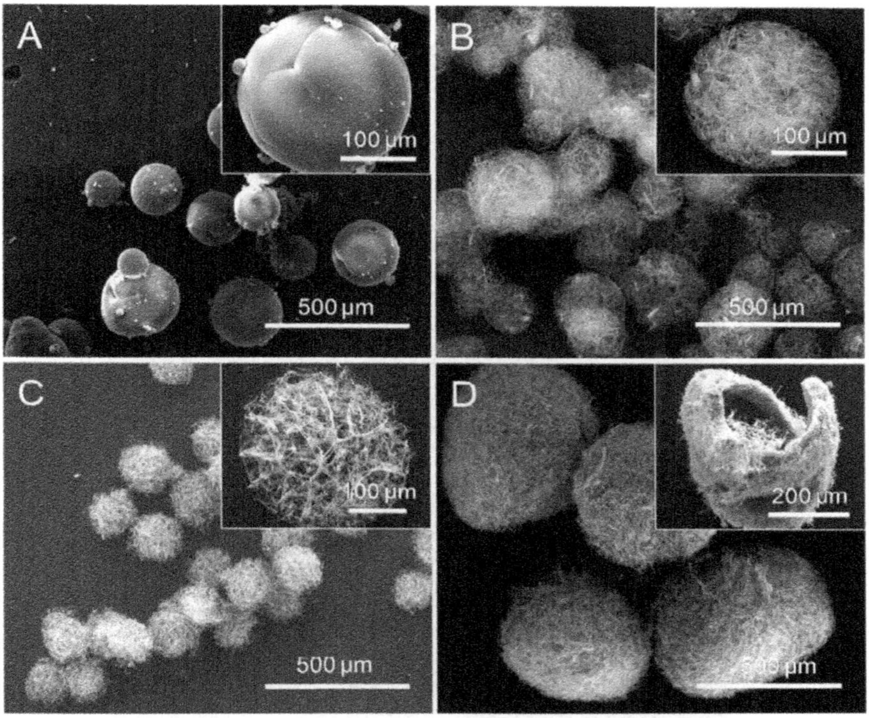

Figure 8.2 Different morphologies of PCL—gelatin (1:1) microspheres fabricated by electrospray microdripping—solid (a), nanofiber (b), porous nanofiber (c), and hollow nanofiber microspheres (d). *Reprinted with permission from ref. S.K. Boda, S. Chen, K. Chu, H.J. Kim, J. Xie. Electrospraying electrospun nanofiber segments into injectable microspheres for potential cell delivery. ACS Appl. Mater. Interfaces 10 (2018) 25069—25079, Copyright © 2018, American Chemical Society.*

stem cells, together with the development of microtissue-like structure assemblies in situ, when injected into microchannel devices. Notably, mouse embryonic stem cells experienced neural differentiation grown on the nanofiber microspheres, indicated by positive staining of β—III—tubulin and neurite outgrowth (Fig. 8.3). Hence, this lately established method for producing injectable nanofiber microspheres with enhanced viability and maintenance of stem cells presents a significant potential for cell therapy applications [21].

It is well established that among current advancements in the field of cancer therapy, immunotherapy has gathered significant attention, where tumor cell—directed immunotherapy has been recognized for precise

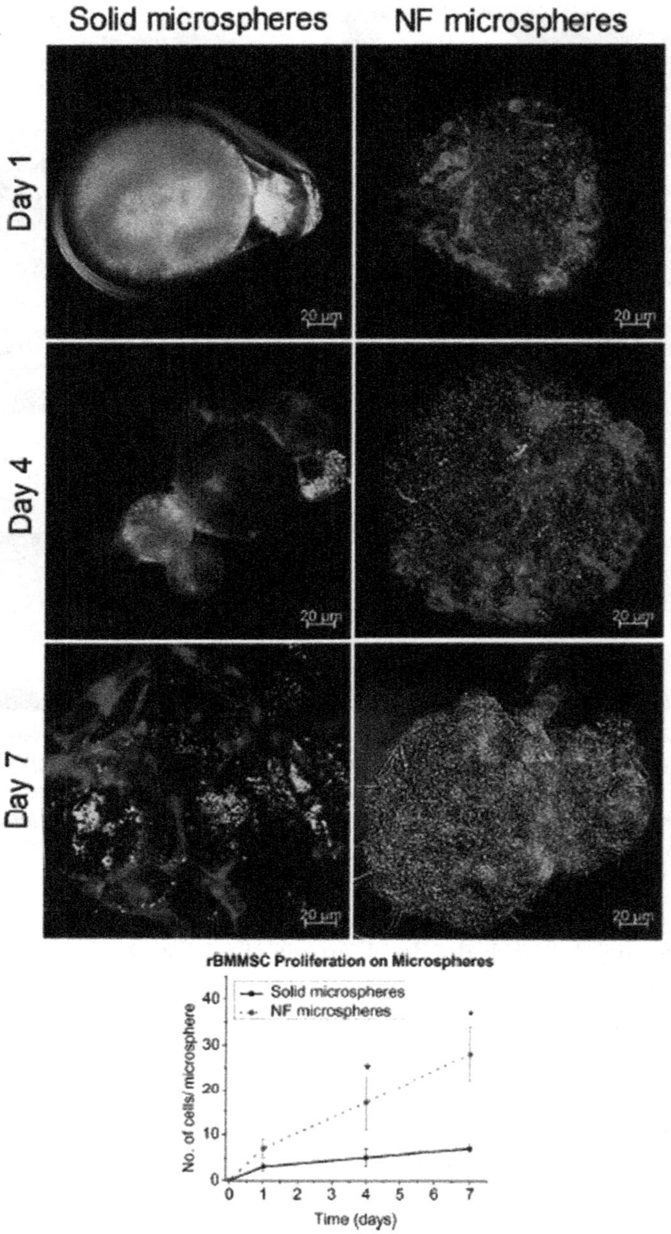

Figure 8.3 Comparative proliferation of rat bone marrow–derived mesenchymal stem cells (rBMMSCs) on PCL–gelatin (1:1) solid and nanofiber (NF) microspheres. Confocal images show cell cytoskeleton in red due to the staining of F-actin with Alexa Fluor Phalloidin 546, nuclei in blue due to DAPI, and the microspheres in the bright-field

targeting of a diversity of tumor tissues, both in vivo and in vitro conditions, attaining extraordinary therapeutic benefits. Remarkably, encouraged by the stem cell niche, a very recently done study had discovered a scale-up method for the generation of porous microspheres with encapsulated natural killer (NK) cells through the microfluidic electrospray technology for in situ tumor immunotherapy (Figs. 8.4 and 8.5) [22]. The electrospray microspheres were generated with porous and tailorable microstructures morphologies due to the multipurpose, but precise, fluid control in the microfluidic electrospray system. This combined technology-led generated porous microspheres protected encapsulated NK-92MI cells from the outer multifaceted milieu permitted for boosted proliferation and functionality (Fig. 8.6). Interestingly, it was found that granzymes and perforin were secreted from the encapsulated NK-92MI cells in a controlled manner, which displayed robust killing effects on tumors both in vitro and in vivo. Notably, with constant growth and proliferation, the NK-92MI cells grow from the exterior of porous microspheres and travel into the neighboring remaining tumor tissues, with further killing of tumor cells. Importantly, not any side effects were experienced due to the innate host immune system after injecting the NK-92MI cell–encapsulated microspheres into tumors in vivo. Hence, the development of porous microspheres developed in combination with electrospray technology encapsulating the NK cells presents a great possibility for tumor immunotherapy, offering a promising therapeutic choice for cancer management [22].

8.3 Bioelectrospraying for tissue engineering applications

Electrospinning materials together with cells does not present ideal to attain sufficient cellular tissue constructs as the tensile force, shear force, and other physical effects in the electrospinning process, which are detrimental

transmitted light. The cell proliferation data shown are mean $\pm$ sd of cell nuclei counted from $\geq$15 microspheres per group per time point. *Indicates statistically significant difference between the two groups with $P < .05$, where P denotes there is no significant difference between the compared means. *Reprinted with permission from ref. D. Wu, Y. Yu, C. Zhao, X. Shou, Y. Piao, X. Zhao, Y. Zhao, S. Wang. NK-Cell-Encapsulated porous microspheres via microfluidic electrospray for tumor immunotherapy, ACS Appl. Mater. Interfaces 11 (2019) 33716–33724, Copyright © 2018, American Chemical Society.*

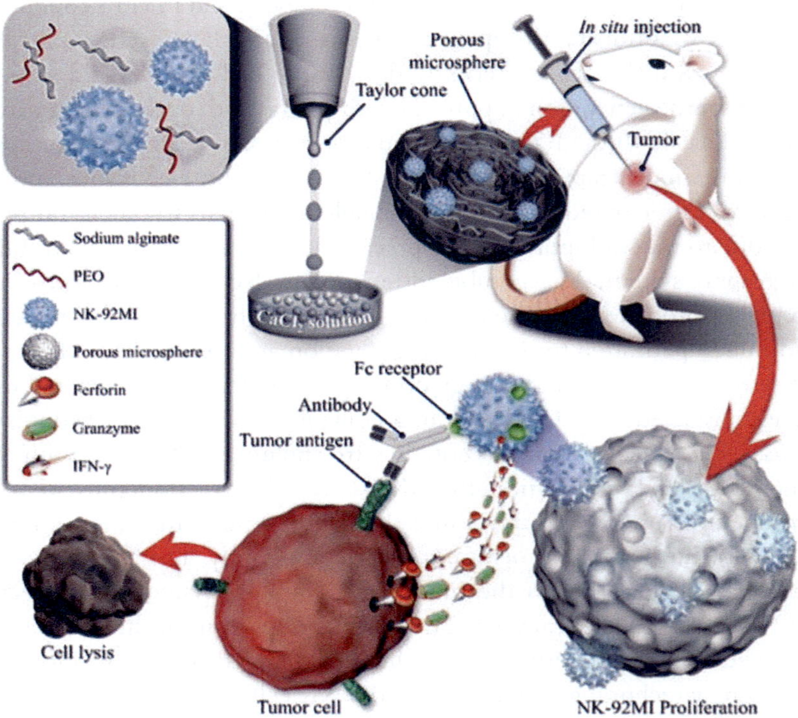

Figure 8.4 Schematic diagram of the fabrication and in situ injection of NK-92MI-laden poly (ethylene oxide) (PEO)/alginate solution (ALG) porous microspheres for tumor immunotherapy. *Reprinted with permission from ref. D. Wu, Y. Yu, C. Zhao, X. Shou, Y. Piao, X. Zhao, Y. Zhao, S. Wang. NK-Cell-Encapsulated porous microspheres via microfluidic electrospray for tumor immunotherapy, ACS Appl. Mater. Interfaces 11 (2019) 33716–33724, Copyright © 2019, American Chemical Society.*

to cellular differentiation, growth, and function [23]. To address these issues, bioelectrospraying technology was investigated. As an extension of ES technology, bioelectrospraying allows for the synthesis of matrices of cells-embedded scaffolds that lead to engineered tissues and organs [24,25]. Bioelectrospraying encompasses the spraying of living cells in the presence of an electrical potential difference and is pioneered by the Jayasinghe research group, which electrosprayed two types of cells, human blood and Jurkat cells, with the demonstration of cells viability with trypan blue staining [24,25].

Bioelectrospraying offers a unique method with the capacity to handle highly concentrated suspensions (>106 cells/mL) [25]; furthermore, this

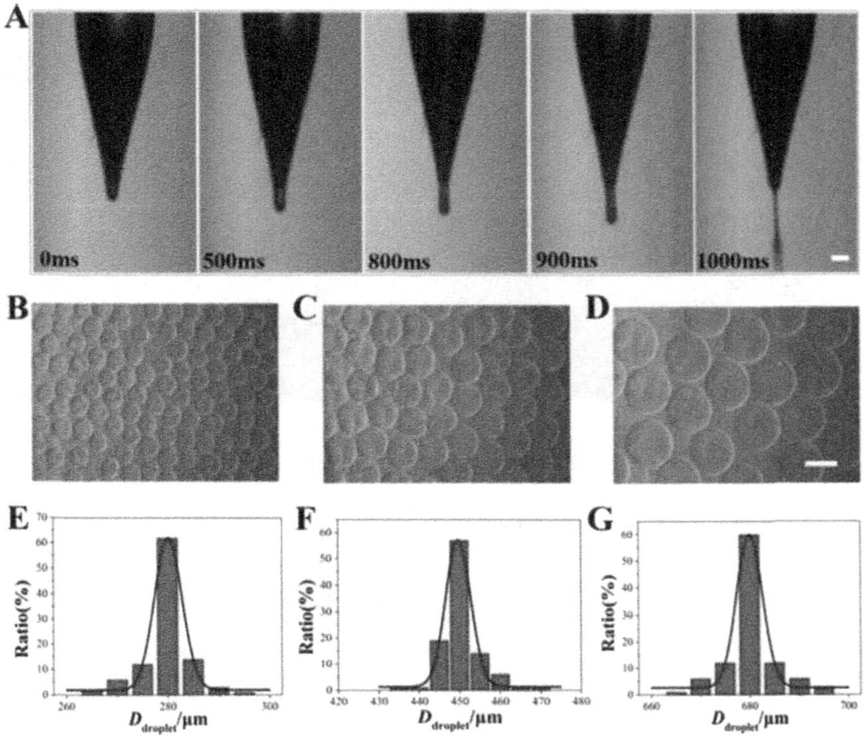

Figure 8.5 Generation of PEO/ALG microspheres via microfluidic electrospray. (a) The formation of PEO/ALG droplets during the process of microfluidic electrospray. Scale bar is 200 μm. (b–d) Bright-field microscopic images of PEO/ALG porous microspheres. Scale bar is 500 μm. (e–g) Diameter distribution of PEO/ALG porous microspheres, 100 microspheres were measured for each map. *Reprinted with permission from ref. D. Wu, Y. Yu, C. Zhao, X. Shou, Y. Piao, X. Zhao, Y. Zhao, S. Wang. NK-Cell-Encapsulated porous microspheres via microfluidic electrospray for tumor immunotherapy, ACS Appl. Mater. Interfaces 11 (2019) 33716–33724, Copyright © 2019, American Chemical Society.*

technique also offers the possibility of forming nano-/microstructures encapsulating cells by using large gauge needles, thus limiting any cell damage caused by shear forces on the cells. The benefit of bioelectrospraying over other methods, such as aerosol delivery and ink-jet printing, includes processing of denser cell suspensions with finer droplets generations. Hence, bioelectrospraying offers a wide range of applications, from bioanalytics to diagnostics, with notably demonstrating its potential from tissue regeneration and repair.

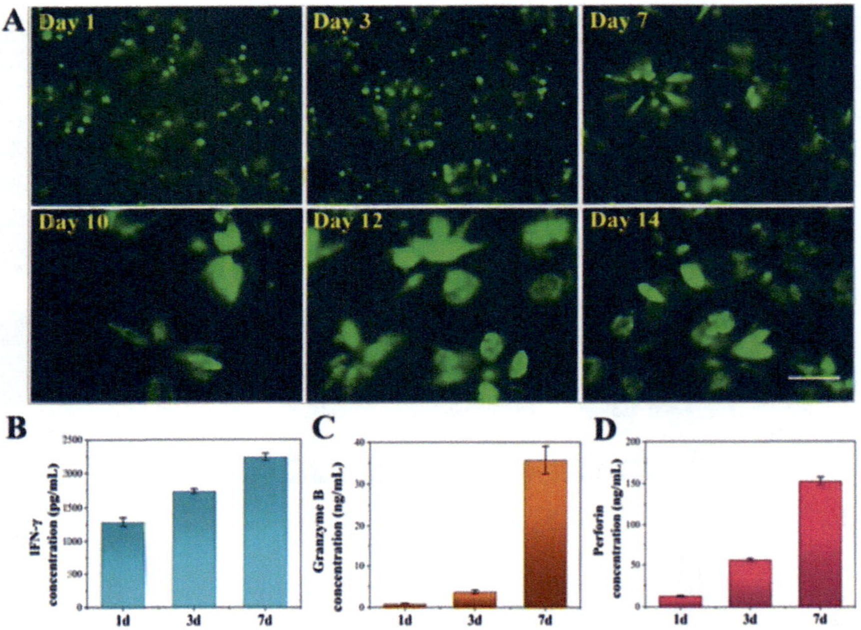

Figure 8.6 Proliferation of NK-92MI encapsulated in porous microspheres. (a) Representative images of NK-92MI cells in porous microspheres at day 1, 3, 7, 10, 12, and 14. Scale bar is 200 μm. (b–d) The secretion ability of NK-92MI microspheres at day 1, 3, and 7. IFN-γ, granzyme B, and perforin were measured using enzyme-linked immunosorbent assay (ELISA) kits according to the manufacturers' instructions. *Reprinted with permission from ref. D. Wu, Y. Yu, C. Zhao, X. Shou, Y. Piao, X. Zhao, Y. Zhao, S. Wang. NK-Cell-Encapsulated porous microspheres via microfluidic electrospray for tumor immunotherapy, ACS Appl. Mater. Interfaces 11 (2019) 33716–33724, Copyright © 2019, American Chemical Society.*

It permits the design of synthetic constructs with a requirement for significantly reduced bioreactor time. Furthermore, the combination of conventional electrospinning with bioelectrospraying process offers the possibility of generation of nanofibrous scaffolds with a uniform distribution of cells for TE and regenerative medicine [26]. A study undertaken showed that a microintegration method of combining electrospinning and electrospray technology would promote even distribution and cell infiltration within the scaffolding structure. The combination of electrospinning with spraying would not only stop the cell damage from conventional electrospinning but also allow the straight incorporation of living cells into the scaffolding. Moreover, researchers are also investigating ways to deposit a single cell into the droplet by optimizing different parameters of bioelectrospraying and the droplet sizes of cellular suspension [27].

8.4 Protein delivery for tissue engineering applications

E-spray was used for encapsulation of BSA protein into chitosan particles, cross-linked by tripolyphosphate [28]. The advantages of the technique were lack of organic solvent, presence of chitosan dispersion, and absence of an emulsifier. The potential of emulsion ES was explored for microencapsulation of proteins using food-grade emulsions with improved safety of a thermosensitive hydrophobic bioactive molecules. Precisely, a whey protein concentrate, the gelatin, and a soy protein isolate were compared as emulsion matrices for encapsulation of α-linolenic acid. Soybean oil was explored as the hydrophobic component for the emulsion ES method, exploring the effect of protein type and emulsion protocol used on colloidal stability. ES and spray drying were compared and oil was then substituted by the ω-3 fatty acid as an emulsifier. While spray drying resulted in massive bioactive degradation, ES demonstrated to be an appropriate substitute, attaining microencapsulation efficiencies of around ~70% [29].

8.5 Nucleic acid delivery for tissue engineering applications

E-spray can be used to achieve high-efficiency nonviral transfection of bacteria and cell lines with the plasmid of interest in high conductivity culture medium onto a monolayer of cells [1]. The mixture of pET30a-green fluorescent protein (GFP) plasmid and gold nanoparticles was electrosprayed as a thin layer over the *Escherichia coli*, where the bacterial transformation was noticed by the uptake of gold nanoparticles detected under transmission electron microscope and the construction of GFP expressing bacterial colonies over the agar plate [30]. In another study, the stability of plasmid DNA or protein molecule in the E-spray buffer with the solution conductivity and processing parameters was investigated for maximum transfection efficiency. The bioelectrospraying-based combinatorial method and cell line transduction were established in human cell lines by using recombinant self-inactivating lentiviral vectors expressing GFP [31]. Along with gene delivery into cell monolayers, E-spray is similarly effective for the delivery of other plasmids into cell tissues or into the whole organism. For instance, by focusing E-spray of GFP plasmid onto chick embryo, localized GFP expression was attained. Pertaining to siRNA delivery, bicompartmental particles were formed by cojetting of ES liquid solutions of poly(lactide-co-glycolide)—polyethyleneimine (PLGA—PEI) combined with dyes and siRNA for imaging and pH-responsive siRNA delivery, respectively. Though cationic lipid or cationic polymeric formulations are prevalent methods for gene and siRNA delivery, E-spray of the plasmid into a suitable buffer is a reasonable substitute for bacterial/cell transformation [32]. Recently nucleic acid—based therapies using E-spray have been investigated in lung disease. A study has recognized the possibility of using electrospray to deliver nucleic acids to both individually in porcine tracheal tissue sections and whole lung ex vivo and with effective bronchoscopic electrospray delivery [33].

8.6 Conclusions and future outlook

EHD techniques, especially ES, have been used for the production of various scaffoldings from nano-/microparticles for various applications. The host template or matrices used for the creation of nano-/microparticles scaffolds for TE can range from natural to synthetic polymers to inorganic and metallic composites nano-/micromaterials. The ability to yield particles of different diameters with distinct dimensions is a distinctive feature of the ES methods. The scaffolding materials morphology can be altered by the solution parameters, including the molecular weight, viscosity, temperature, and the concentration of the polymeric solution, along with controlling the processing parameters, including conductivity, tip-to-collector distance, applied voltage, among others. The specific ES techniques permit the manufacturing of a variety of nanostructured materials with necessary properties for the regeneration and repair of tissue and organs. TE encompasses the amalgamation of medicine, biology, engineering, and life science. Numerous studies have explored this rapidly emerging field, aiming for developing scaffolding materials supporting cellular growth and expansion. Though E-spray offers advantage over existing methods from conventional microparticle-producing methods such as solvent casting, coacervation, emulsification, and spray drying, by supporting growth of the 3D structures along and sufficient porosity for cell proliferation and growth within the scaffoldings, delivery of GFs and bioactive remained a key for cell growth and expansion within the scaffolds. Though E-spray offers delivery of bioactive, including gene and protein molecules, the systems need further improvement in safeguarding to achieve the suitable quantity and delivery to the precise location. There is a need for more studies offering realistic solutions to these existing limitations by developing a high-standard platform for delivering molecules in highly efficient and small doses needed by the target tissues for significant growth and repair tissue with minimum undesired side effects.

Acknowledgments

PD would like to thank IMODE grant for support to carry out E-spray-related research at UCL, and PD is also thankful to VA and the Gromada grant for her current research support.

References

[1] S.K. Boda, X. Li, J. Xie, Electrospraying an enabling technology for pharmaceutical and biomedical applications: a review, J. Aerosol Sci. 125 (2018) 164–181.
[2] S. Radhakrishnan, R. Seeram, Electrosprayed nanoparticles for drug delivery and pharmaceutical applications, Biomatter 3 (2013) e24281.
[3] J. Wang, J.A. Jansen, Y.F. Electrospraying, Possibilities and challenges of engineering carriers for biomedical applications—a mini review, Front. Chem. 7 (2019) 258.
[4] R.T. Steipel, M.D. Gallovic, C.J. Batty, E.M. Bachelder, K.M. Ainslie, Electrospray for generation of drug delivery and vaccine particles applied in vitro and in vivo, Mater. Sci. Eng. C Mater. Biol. Appl. 105 (2019) 110070.
[5] N. Maurmann, L.E. Sperling, P. Pranke, Electrospun and electrosprayed scaffolds for tissue engineering, Adv. Exp. Med. Biol. 1078 (2018) 79–100.
[6] K. Dzobo, N.E. Thomford, D.A. Senthebane, H. Shipanga, A. Rowe, C. Dandara, M. Pillay, K.S.C.M. Motaung, Advances in regenerative medicine and tissue engineering: innovation and transformation of medicine, Stem Cell. Int. 2018 (2018) 2495848.
[7] C. Syandan, I.-C. Liao, A. Andrew, W.L.K. Electrohydrodynamics, A facile technique to fabricate drug delivery systems, Adv. Drug Deliv. Rev. 61 (2009) 1043–1054.
[8] W. Li, L. Zhang, X. Ge, B. Xu, W. Zhang, L. Qu, C.-H. Choi, J. Xu, A. Zhang, H. Lee, D.A. Weitz, Microfluidic fabrication of microparticles for biomedical applications, Chem. Soc. Rev. 47 (2018) 5646–5683.
[9] A. Vossoughi, H.W.T. Matthew, Encapsulation of mesenchymal stem cells in glycosaminoglycans-chitosan polyelectrolyte microcapsules using electrospraying technique: investigating capsule morphology and cell viability, Bioeng. Transl. Med. 3 (2018) 265–274.
[10] G. Acharya, C.S. Shin, M. McDermott, H. Mishra, H. Park, I.C. Kwon, K. Park, The hydrogel template method for fabrication of homogeneous nano/microparticles, J. Contr. Release 141 (2010) 314–319.
[11] Q. Liu, H. Huang, H. Chen, J. Lin, Q. Wang, Food-grade nanoemulsions: preparation, stability and application in encapsulation of bioactive compounds, Molecules 24 (2019) 4242.
[12] M. Iqbal, Y. Tao, S. Xie, Y. Zhu, D. Chen, X. Wang, L. Huang, D. Peng, A. Sattar, M.A.B. Shabbir, H.I. Hussain, S. Ahmed, Z. Yuan, Aqueous two-phase system (ATPS): an overview and advances in its applilk, Mcations. Biol. Proced. 2016 18 (2016) 1–18.
[13] Y. Zou, J. Song, X. You, J. Yao, S. Xie, M. Jin, X. Wang, Z. Yan, G. Zhou, L. Shui, Interfacial complexation induced controllable fabrication of stable polyelectrolyte microcapsules using all-aqueous droplet microfluidics for enzyme release, ACS Appl. Mater. Interfaces 11 (2019) 21227–21238.

[14] Y. Chao, S.Y. Mak, Q. Ma, J. Wu, Z. Ding, L. Xu, H.C. Shum, Emergence of droplets at the nonequilibrium all-aqueous interface in a vertical hele-shaw cell, Langmuir 34 (2018) 3030–3036.

[15] A.Í.S. Morais, E.G. Vieira, S. Afewerki, R.B. Sousa, L.M.C. Honorio, A.N.C.O. Cambrussi, J.A. Santos, R.D.S. Bezerra, J.A.O. Furtini, E.C. Silva-Filho, T.J. Webster, A.O. Lobo, Fabrication of polymeric microparticles by electrospray: the impact of experimental parameters, J. Funct. Biomater. 1 (2020) 4.

[16] H. Lee, S. An, S. Kim, et al., Readily functionalizable and stabilizable polymeric particles with controlled size and morphology by electrospray, Sci. Rep. 8 (2018) 15725.

[17] E. Boel, R. Koekoekx, S. Dedroog, I. Babkin, M.R. Vetrano, C. Clasen, G.V. Mooter, Unraveling particle formation: from single droplet drying to spray drying and electrospraying, Pharmaceutics 7 (2020) 625.

[18] M. Singh, C.P. Morris, R.J. Ellis, M.S. Detamore, C. Berkland, Microsphere-based seamless scaffolds containing macroscopic gradients of encapsulated factors for tissue engineering, Tissue Eng. C Methods 14 (2008) 299–309.

[19] S. Pina, V.P. Ribeiro, C.F. Marques, F.R. Maia, T.H. Silva, R.L. Reis, J.M. Oliveira, Scaffolding strategies for tissue engineering and regenerative medicine applications, Materials 12 (2019) 1824.

[20] J. Xie, C.-H. Wang, Electrospray in the dripping mode for cell microencapsulation, J. Colloid Interface Sci. 312 (2007) 247–255.

[21] S.K. Boda, S. Chen, K. Chu, H.J. Kim, J. Xie, Electrospraying electrospun nanofiber segments into injectable microspheres for potential cell delivery, ACS Appl. Mater. Interfaces 10 (2018) 25069–25079.

[22] D. Wu, Y. Yu, C. Zhao, X. Shou, Y. Piao, X. Zhao, Y. Zhao, S. Wang, NK-Cell-Encapsulated porous microspheres via microfluidic electrospray for tumor immunotherapy, ACS Appl. Mater. Interfaces 11 (2019) 33716–33724.

[23] Y. Ma, Y. Liu, H. Chen, Q. Hu, Application and analysis of biological electrospray in tissue engineering, Open Biomed. Eng. J. 9 (2015) 133–137.

[24] S.N. Jayasinghe, A. Townsend-Nicholson, Stable electric-field driven cone–jetting of concentrated biosuspensions, Lab Chip 6 (8) (2006) 1086–1090.

[25] S.N. Jayasinghe, Cell electrospinning: a novel tool for functionalising fibres, scaffolds and membranes with living cells and other advanced materials for regenerative biology and medicine, Analyst 138 (8) (2013) 2215–2223.

[26] R.D. Juliana, R. Nilza, B.-S. Sara, A.R. Costa-Pinto, N. Alves, L. Ana, Oliveira in situ enabling approaches for tissue regeneration: current challenges and new developments, Front. Bioeng. Biotechnol. 8 (2020) 85.

[27] A.S. Bongiovanni, F. Montini Ballarin, G.A. Abraham, Combination of electrospinning with other techniques for the fabrication of 3D polymeric and composite nanofibrous scaffolds with improved cellular interactions, Nanotechnology 31 (2020) 172002.

[28] Y. Xu, M.A. Hanna, Electrosprayed bovine serum albumin-loaded tripolyphosphate cross-linked chitosan capsules: synthesis and characterization, J. Microencapsul. 24 (2007) 143–151.

[29] L.G. Gómez-Mascaraque, A. López-Rubio, Protein-based emulsion electrosprayed micro- and submicroparticles for the encapsulation and stabilization of thermosensitive hydrophobic bioactives, J. Colloid Interface Sci. 465 (2016) 259–270, https://doi.org/10.1016/j.jcis.2015.11.061.

[30] Y.-H. Lee, B. Wu, W.-Q. Zhuang, D.-R. Chen, Y.J. Tang, Nanoparticles facilitate gene delivery to microorganisms via an electrospray process, J. Microbiol. Methods 84 (2) (2011) 228–233.

[31] E. Ward, E. Chan, K. Gustafsson, S.N. Jayasinghe, Combining bio-electrospraying with gene therapy: a novel biotechnique for the delivery of genetic material via living cells, Analyst 135 (5) (2010) 1042–1049.
[32] A.C. Misra, S. Bhaskar, N. Clay, J. Lahann, Multicompartmental particles for combined imaging and siRNA delivery, Adv. Mater. 24 (28) (2012) 3850–3856.
[33] P. Riddell, J.L. Gilbert, E.L. Molloy, S. Finnegan, J.J. Egan, S. O'Dea, Delivery of nucleic acids to ex vivo porcine airways using electrospray, Exp. Lung Res. 44 (2018) 405–416.

CHAPTER NINE

Electrospray particles as drug delivery systems: concepts, strategies, and applications

Shreya Thakkar[1], **Manju Misra**[2]
[1]Department of Pharmaceutics, National Institute of Pharmaceutical Education and Research (NIPER), Ahmedabad, Gujarat, India
[2]Graduate School of Pharmacy, Gujarat Technological University Gandhinagar Campus Nr. Government Polytechnic K-6 Circle, Gandhinagar, Gujarat, India

List of abbreviations

BCS Biopharmaceutics classification system
CYP3A Cytochrome P450 3A
HIV Human immunodeficiency virus
MDROs Multidrug-resistant organisms
NIRF Near-infrared fluorescence
PCL Polycaprolactone
PEG Polyethylene glycol
PLA Polylactic acid
PLGA Poly(lactic-co-glycolic acid)
PVA Polyvinyl alcohol
PVP Polyvinyl pyrrolidone
SEM Scanning electron microscopy
STZ Streptozotocin

9.1 Introduction

The prime objective of any drug delivery system is to ensure that the pharmaceutical agent reaches the site of action and produces desired pharmacological effect. This has necessitated the need to focus on the developability of a drug candidate from the drug delivery perspective during drug development program itself. Several advancements in technology, especially nanotechnology, have facilitated the process of drug delivery in a biological system, by effectively countering the physiological arrangement and the chemical and biochemical barriers associated with the physiological structures, which forms the first line of defense. A drug delivered by any route is likely to encounter these barriers before reaching at the site of action and this very

Biomedical Applications of Electrospinning and Electrospraying
ISBN: 978-0-12-822476-2
https://doi.org/10.1016/B978-0-12-822476-2.00013-3

much depends on the physicochemical and biochemical characteristics of the molecule. Conventional methods of micro-/nanoparticle preparation like solvent evaporation, single and double emulsion, spray-drying, coacervation, etc., have some disadvantages, such as low drug-loading efficiency, limitations in scaling up, lack of particle-size monodispersity, reduced capacity to fabricate small particles (below 100 nm), and difficulty in incorporating hydrophilic drugs. Besides, most of these techniques necessitate the need for particle separation from dispersing solution or surfactants used in formulation process, which may pose additional problems. The possibility of inactivation or degradation of drug cannot be also ruled out, considering organic solvent exposure, high shear stress, elevated temperature, and aqueous organic interfaces, when using conventional methods [1]. In past few years, electrohydrodynamic processes viz. electrospinning and electrospraying have been effectively explored to customize the physicochemical properties of drug for biomedical and drug delivery applications, especially in the area of tissue engineering, diagnostics, therapeutics, etc.

Electrohydrodynamic processes like electrospinning and electrospraying utilize electrical and hydrodynamic forces to regulate the operation as well as material properties. It was reportedly used way back in 1902, when the first patent entitled "Apparatus for Electrical Dispersion of Fluids" was registered. Though the conceptual findings were known to the scientific community since 1882 when Rayleigh proposed the theory of "Rayleigh limit," this technique remained almost anonymous for years. However, recent revelations by the researchers working in the field of biomedical and drug delivery applications have made this technique more popular by exploring several heterogeneous scaffolds and nanomedicine-based applications. Electrospinning has been extensively used for preparing fibers of the submicron size range by exploring variety of polymers, metals, composites, etc., offering unique two-dimensional applications. The amalgamation of drug nanoparticles or drug as such with the polymer has been also used to produce several electrospun scaffolds with specific alignment of nanoparticles alongside nanofibers for better stability.

Electrospraying, also referred to as sister technology to electrospinning, is one of the most efficient techniques for the preparation of nanoparticles/nanospheres. The basic principle of electrospraying is to apply a high voltage to a polymeric solution which results in emission of the polymer from the syringe in the form of nanoparticles. As these nanoparticles exhibit zero-dimensional nature, and self-dispersing nature due to columbic repulsion, they can be used in numerous biological, medicinal, or pharmaceutical applications. The process of electrospraying also offers several advantages like scalable synthesis, reproducibility, and high encapsulation efficiency over conventional methods of nano-/microparticle preparation. It also allows processing at ambient temperature/pressure thereby facilitating the incorporation of sensitive drug molecules including living cells, enzymes, and proteins in a single-step process. Electrospraying has been explored as a novel method for preparation of not only various synthetic polymeric nanoparticles but also for natural polymer nanoparticles (protein or carbohydrate) for drug delivery applications without any loss of bioactivity of either the drug or encapsulating biomolecules. By variations in operating conditions nanocarriers with different morphologies have been reported including microspheres [2], core—shell type [3], multilayer [4], porous [5], etc. Electrosprayed nanoparticles can encapsulate drugs and can be specific drug carriers because of their active surface absorption, binding or complexation with drug. Thus, the electrosprayed nanoparticle technology opens a new domain for drug delivery applications and its therapeutic use. A series of reviews have been written to highlight the importance of electrospraying in drug delivery [1,6—9].

This book chapter will provide insights into the basic principle of electrospraying with specific emphasis on its utility in the field of drug delivery. Parameters affecting the process and its impact on the output of the electrosprayed particles will be also discussed. Further application of electrosprayed micro-/nanoparticles in new domains of drug delivery applications and therapeutic use will be also highlighted.

9.2 Electrohydrodynamic technique: the basic principle

The electrospraying assembly consists of four basic elements; viz. electrical power (for high-voltage supply), metal needle (works as spraying nozzle), metal collector (to collect particles generated), and pump (works as flow controller) (Fig. 9.1). All these can be enclosed within a chamber to achieve desirable output within defined working ranges of temperature and humidity [10]. The process works by applying high electrical voltage to the needle tip containing solution to be processed. In absence of the electrical field, liquid is held at the needle tip in the hemispherical shape owing to the surface tension. As the electrical field is applied, it starts to elongate forming a conical shape termed as "Taylor cone." Further increase in the electrical field results in increasing the repulsive forces in drop and at the

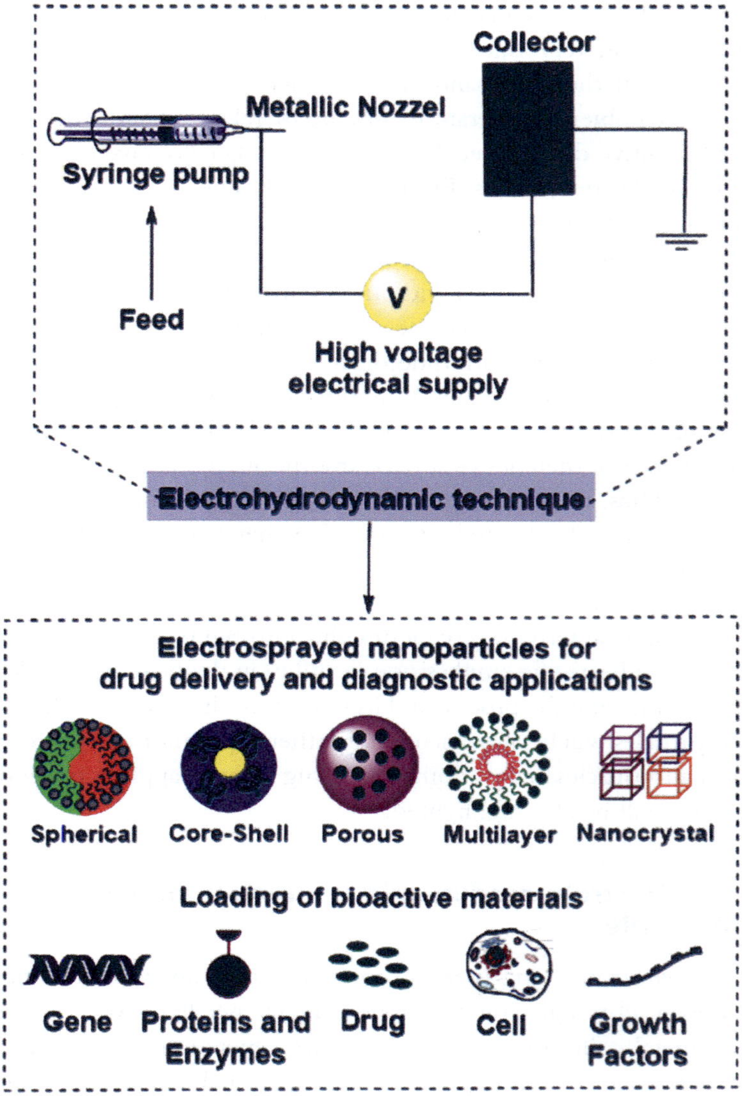

Figure 9.1 Basic setup of the electrohydrodynamic processes and their applications in biomedical and pharmaceutical field.

point where these repulsive forces overcome surface tension of the liquid, a charged jet is ejected from the apex of conical meniscus and the product is collected at collector on the opposite side. At this juncture, the processing parameters and properties of solution/suspension/melt to be processed decide the output in terms of whether the process is electrospinning or electrospraying. However, the obtained size may depend on needle gauge diameter, applied voltage, flow rate, and working distance for different drug delivery systems. In general, higher polymer concentration in the solution leads to whipping instability in jet ejected, forming fibers in the submicron range with random orientation. The eventual chain entanglement plays a crucial role in defining the process to be electrospinning or electrospraying [11].

The process of electrospraying is more or less similar to that of electrospinning except that the polymer concentration is either low or absent and higher electrical voltage is required to cause atomization than electrospinning, resulting in smaller particles at the collector instead of the fibers. These primary droplets are then subjected to the phenomenon of Rayleigh disintegration or Coulomb fission. During their flight to the collector, the solvent from these primary droplets evaporates causing them to shrink leading to the increase in the charge concentration and thus further subdivision of the primary droplets into smaller offspring. However, the prerequisite to obtain monodisperse particles is to further prevent the Coulomb fission and further disruption of charged droplets. This could be achieved by changing nozzle and needle configuration. Also based on the increase in the intensity of applied voltage, the electrospraying mode changes from initial dripping to microdripping, spindle, Taylor cone-jet mode, and multijet mode that is mostly described by the spraying geometry. Among all these modes, the Taylor cone-jet mode is the most preferred one as it produces the most stable, reproducible, and easily controllable highly monodisperse microparticles or nanoparticles [12]. As described previously, nanoparticles having different morphologies ranging from hollow, cup-shaped, porous, cell shaped, spherical, core shell, multilayered, to Janus have been reported by the several authors for varied applications using electrospraying [9]. Fig. 9.1 depicts schematic flow of electrohydrodynamic technique, surface morphology of the particles formed, and its various applications in biomedical and pharmaceutical field.

9.3 Process–property relationship in electrospraying

Precise monitoring of the operational parameters and properties of solution to be processed governs the size and morphology of final product in electrospraying. In fact, in order to get the desired output of monodispersed micro- or nanoparticles, a critical balance of interplay between

Table 9.1 Impact of operational parameters and solution properties on nature of electrosprayed product.

Parameter	Effect	Reference
Operational parameters affecting properties of final product		
Applied voltage	Increase in voltage results in decreased particles size (till an optimum value)	[15]
Flow rate	Increased flow rates are associated with larger particle size	[16–18]
Tip-to-collector distance	Decrease in tip-to-collector distance enhances possibility of getting larger particles	[17,19]
Temperature	Higher operating temperatures are known for more uniform particles	[20,21]
Humidity	Higher humidity results in increased tendency of forming more and more circular pores in particles	[22]
Formulation-related properties affecting process and final product		
Polymer concentration	Higher polymer concentration leads to increased particle size, depending on the voltage applied	[23]
Surface tension	Higher surface tension results in higher particle size, while reduced surface tension results in lesser morphological defects	[24]
Solvent conductivity	Solvent with higher conductivity results in fine particles	[25]
Solvent volatility	Higher solvent volatility leads to higher chances of surface defects and increased numbers of pores	[24,26]
Viscosity	Higher viscosity of solution increases the particle size	[23]

formulation-related (polymer, solvent) and process-related parameters (operating voltage, liquid flow rate, needle/nozzle diameter, working distance, temperature, humidity, etc.) is very essential, and the same had been highlighted in the reviews by Pawar et al. [6] and N. Bock et al. [13,14]. Table 9.1 enlists some of these important parameters affecting the final product obtained from electrospraying.

9.3.1 Operational parameters affecting electrospraying

Although effect of operational parameters on final product is interdependent, in general, increasing the applied voltage till an optimum range results in decrease in the particle size of interest. Abyadeh et al. have reported decrease in the particle size as well as size distribution of chitosan nanoparticles at higher voltages produced by electrospraying [27]. Decreased particle size could be attributed to the higher repulsive forces that would have resulted in better atomization. Cao et al. in the similar way have reported decrease in the particle size of polyvinyl alcohol/silk fibroin nanofibers when voltage was increased from 16 to 20 kV (Fig. 9.2) [28].

Another group of researchers have evaluated the effect of applied voltage on morphology and particle size of the poly (lactide) (PLA) nanoparticles loaded with bovine serum albumin. It was reported that at a constant polymer concentration of 3% and flow rates of 0.5 mL/h, increasing the voltage from 10 to 15 kV resulted in the disappearance of tails from the particles and resulted in more spherical particles. Authors mentioned that this specific observation was dependent on the voltage, as at lower voltage, electrical forces were not sufficient to overcome surface tension resulting in particles with tails. Further it was found that, at constant flow rates, increasing the applied voltage resulted in decreasing the particle size [29].

Another important parameter affecting final product is flow rate of the solution to be processed. In general, higher flow rates are associated with increased particle size. This phenomenon could be attributed to the fact that increased flow rates at constant voltage could result in uneven liquid

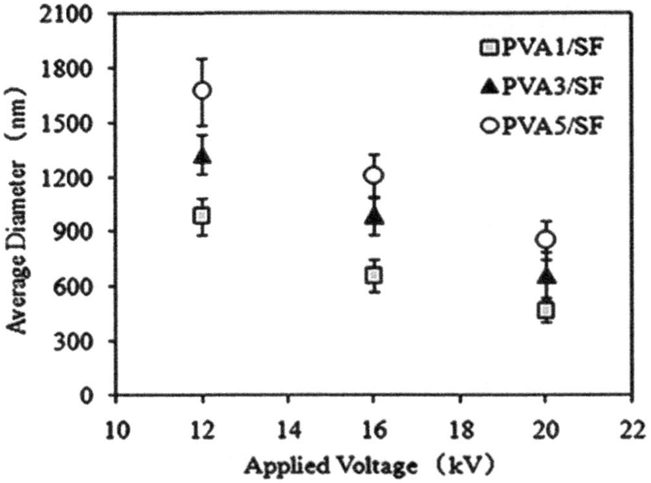

Figure 9.2 Average diameters of the PVA/SF nanoparticles at different concentrations of PVA. *PVA*, polyvinyl alcohol; *SF*, silk fibroin. *Reprinted/adapted with permission from Cao et al., Sci. Rep. 7 (2017), 1–9.*

distribution at the needle tip and/or insufficient time for solvent evaporation [30–32]. Lee et al. have nicely reported importance of flow rates while preparing nano-/microparticles of functionalized poly(styrene-random-glycidyl methacrylate) copolymers. Particle sizes of 1.98 ± 0.29 and 4.67 ± 0.64 μm were reported by authors at flow rates of 0.6 mL/h and 9 mL/h, respectively, as shown in Fig. 9.3 [33].

Vapor pressure of the solvent plays important role in size of the particle obtained as shown in Fig. 9.4. For the solvents having higher vapor pressure, higher flow rates are advised and vice-versa. Tip-to-collector distance not only governs the solvent evaporation time but is also responsible for the formation of stable Taylor cone. It is advisable to use shorter distances for low conductivity solvent with higher volatility and the opposite is true as well. Similarly temperature and humidity may also impact the electrosprayed

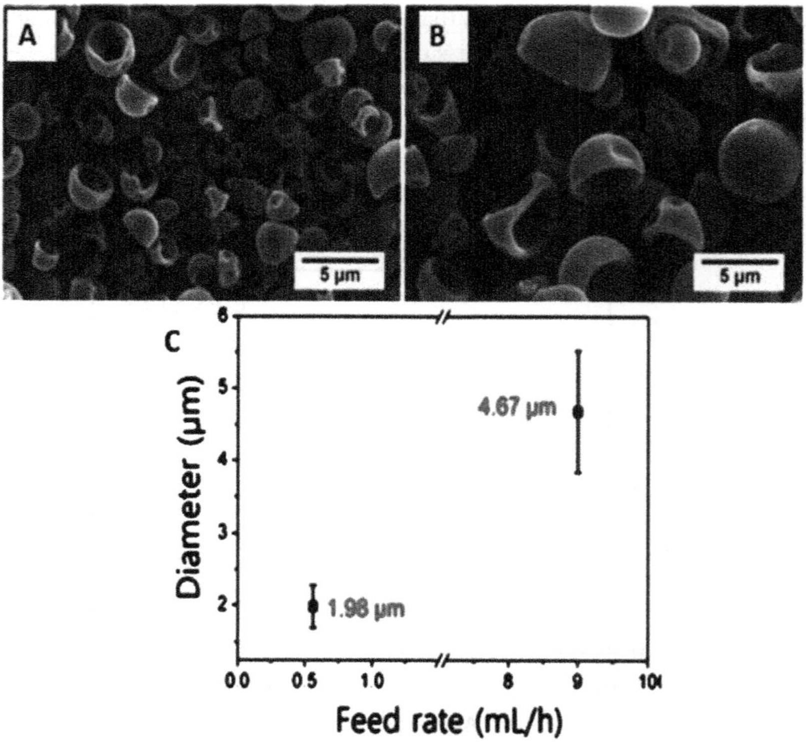

Figure 9.3 ***Scanning electron microscopy images of electrosprayed particles formed at different feed rate.*** A: 0.6 mL/h, and B: 9 mL/h. C: Particle size as a function of flow rate. *Reprinted/Adapted with permission from, Lee et al. Sci. Rep. 8 (1) (2018) 1–10.*

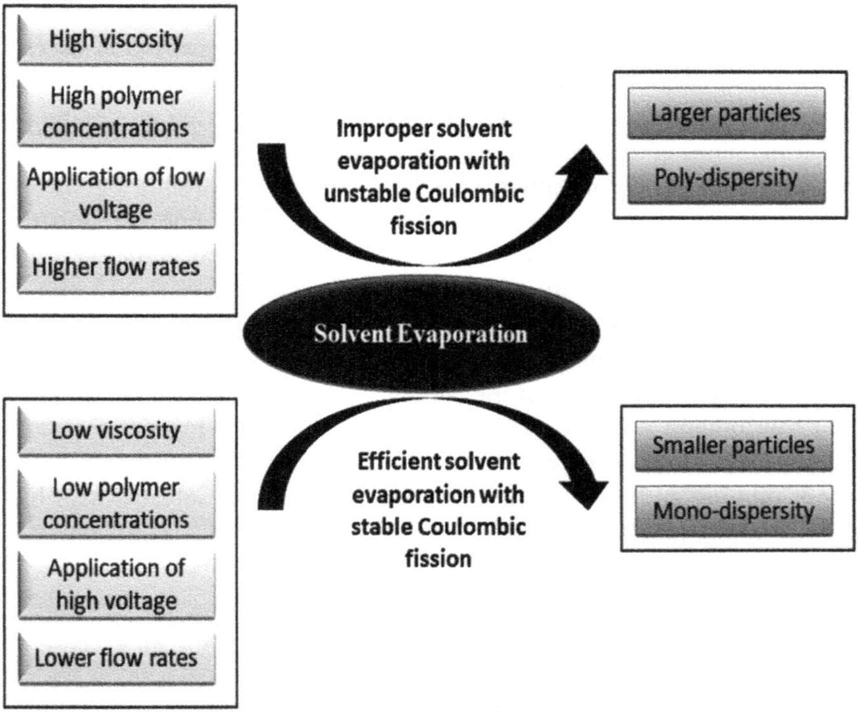

Figure 9.4 ***Effect of various parameters on solvent evaporation and final size of particles produced.*** *Reprinted/Adapted with permission from, Pawar et al. J. Controlled Release 286 (2018) 179–200.*

particle formed. Increase in temperature is reported to result in smaller more uniform particles, while an increase in humidity is known to produce hollow pores on the surface of the particles [34].

9.3.2 Formulation-related factors affecting electrospraying

Properties of solution to be processed through electrohydrodynamic technique are equally important as it governs the process and subsequently the end product. Liquid droplet is held at the nozzle tip by virtue of surface tension. When applied voltage is sufficient to overcome surface tension and to generate Coulombic repulsion, jet formation takes place. If the solution has a very high electrical conductivity, it disturbs balance between viscoelastic, electrostatic, frictional forces, and surface tension leading to unstable jet. Contrary to this, if the electrical conductivity is too low, it hinders the formation of Taylor cone and whole process. Jaworek and group have suggested the values of 10^{-11} to 10^{-1} S/m for electrical conductivity of solution to be processed [34].

Viscosity of a solution which depends upon polymer concentration is important parameter affecting process and product. Increases in the viscosity of the solution interrupt involvement of surface tension as the driving force in the process and are also responsible for difficulties during processing viz. clogging of nozzle and many more. An optimum range is required for better processing. Polymer concentration in the solution is responsible for converting one variant to the other at some point. Lee et al. have reported formation of particles out of electrospraying at lower polymer concentration, while higher polymer concentrations resulted in shifting process to electrospinning resulting in formation of fibers instead of particles as is shown in Fig. 9.5.

Similarly, the solvents used in the process, based on their boiling point, may also affect the texture of the particle formed. In general, it is reported that low boiling solvents when used alone may result in pore formation on surface of dried particle and frequent clogging of needle, due to higher vapor pressure and low boiling point in comparison to solvents with high boiling point [6,24]. In specific cases, the addition of a cosolvent with

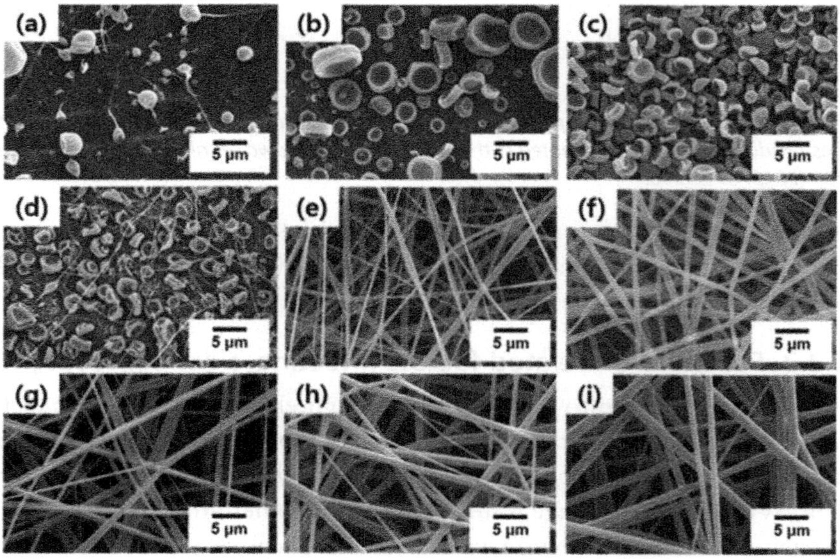

Figure 9.5 ***Scanning electron microscopy images of electrosprayed/electrospun particles/nanofibers with varying polymer solution concentrations.*** (a) 1 wt%, (b) 3 wt%, (c) 5 wt%, (d) 10 wt%, (e) 14 wt%, (f) 15 wt%, (g) 16 wt%, (h) 17 wt%, and (i) 18 wt%. *Reprinted/Adapted with permission from, Lee et al. Sci. Rep. 8 (1) (2018) 1–10.*

different properties than the solvent is needed to cosolubilize the drug and the polymer or to adjust the viscosity and/or the conductivity of the liquid; however, this may not be universally applied in all cases. Moreover, solvents with higher boiling point lead to slower drying rates and demand a greater nozzle—collector distance to ensure the formation of the particles [35].

9.4 Electrospraying in drug delivery: strategies and applications

Electrospraying owing to its unique advantage of producing monodispered particles in nano-/microrange has been of tremendous use in the field of drug delivery. Nanoparticles prepared in this way are known for providing anticipated release profile viz. faster/sustained/stimuli responsive by virtue of selecting adequate base polymer. Selection of the base polymer is generally based on the desired drug release profile and electrospraying can be easily controlled to generate nanoparticles with prerequisite morphologies.

For example, nanoparticles produced using hydrophilic polymers having large number of pores can provide faster dissolution rates for poorly water-soluble drug candidates owing to the enhanced surface area and porous structure. Most of the published studies related to application of electrospraying in drug delivery can be majorly classified into two categories; firstly, studies wherein physicochemical properties of the drug have been modified with the end objective of surface area, solubility, and dissolution enhancement and the second, studies wherein electrospraying process was used to encapsulate or serve as cargo to deliver drug to the desired site of action to target disease. The following section will discuss these applications in detail.

9.4.1 Strategies in developing electrosprayed drug delivery systems

Electrospraying has been used extensively to modify physicochemical properties of drug candidates by formulating them as solid dispersion, drug nanocrystals, amorphous solid dispersion, inclusion complex, etc. In general, the development of drug nanocarriers for poorly soluble pharmaceuticals represents a special task and still faces some unresolved issues. The therapeutic application of hydrophobic, poorly water-soluble agents is associated with some serious problems, since low water-solubility results in poor absorption and low bioavailability. Particulate level properties are often modified during the process of electrospraying resulting in size reduction, often up to nanoscale or even induction of amorphization.

These modifications are extremely beneficial considering the fact that most of the recently discovered active pharmaceutical ingredient suffers from poor aqueous solubility and any solid-state modification process like nanocrystallization requires solidification of nanosuspension as final step [36]. Processes like lyophilization and spray drying which are routinely used for such drying process often suffer from limitations like tedious, lengthy process, sensitivity of product to stress of heat/cool, etc., which is not the case in electrospraying.

9.4.1.1 Solid dispersions

In addition, drying can be also induced by electrospraying, resulting in production of nanocrystalline solid dispersion, which can be considered as a promising alternative for poorly aqueous soluble compounds. In a study by Thakkar et al., Erlotinib nanocrystals were prepared and dried using both lyophilization and electrospraying process to compare the nature of dried product. The results revealed significant improvement in solubility of both lyophilized and electrosprayed nanocrystals and were attributed to change in crystals size along with partial amorphization of the drug [37].

Similar studies were reported for olanzapine nanosuspension, which also exhibited changes in crystallinity upon electrospraying with particle size distribution in the range of 270–275 nm offering enhanced solubility than pristine drug. Powder X-ray diffraction though clearly revealed that drug was present in crystalline form in electrosprayed particles [38].

9.4.1.2 Nanocomposites

Depending upon the final crystal state of the processed drug (crystalline/amorphous), electrosprayed nanocrystals can be thermodynamically stable although polymorphic modifications may appear during the process. These nanocrystals owing to their small size and high surface to volume ratio will significantly improve the solubility and dissolution rate of the poorly soluble drug. Due to the higher free energy of active pharmaceutical ingredients in the amorphous state and larger surface area derived from submicron particles, electrosprayed formulation is expected to improve the dissolution of poorly water-soluble drugs.

Bohr et al. demonstrated the use of electrospraying in fabricating poly(lactic-co-glycolic acid) (PLGA) microspheres containing large amounts of celecoxib, a biopharmaceutics classification system (BCS) Class II compound, in amorphous form, which were stable for close to 8 months upon storage, resulting in much faster release compared to pure drug [39].

9.4.1.3 Aerosols

Electrospraying has been also explored for production of aerosols because monodisperse particles with controllable size and shape can be produced which are amenable for administration by inhalation route. Ijsebaert et al. [40] developed an aerosol generator of beclomethasone dipropionate by using electrospraying. In the study, a configuration of nozzle-discharge needle was used for atomizing beclomethasone dipropionate solution in ethanol into fine highly charged droplets which were neutralized by a direct-current corona discharge. This avoided uncontrolled disruption resulting in easy aerosol production with narrow-sized particle distribution. During electrospraying, quick solvent evaporation often leads to the formation of porous, wrinkled, or shell-like particles with low mass density and such particle morphologies are beneficial for pulmonary drug delivery.

9.4.1.4 Inclusion complexes

In one such novel application of electrospraying crystalline inclusion complexes were prepared for finasteride by Katrajkar et al. [41] with the objective to improve its solubility. Finasteride inclusion complexes were formed with biodegradable hydrophilic polymer polyethylene glycol (PEG). Compared with pure drug crystals the inclusion complex showed higher solubility and faster dissolution rates.

Similarly Cylcodextrin and linalool inclusion complexes were made using electrospinning to improve the solubility of Linalool. Three types of modified cyclodextrin (HPβCD, MβCD, and HPγCD) were used to electro spin Cyclodextrin/linalool inclusion complexes to obtain nanofibrous webs which dissolved in water within 2 seconds [42]. Asli et al. reported eugenol cyclodextrin inclusion complexes for enhanced water solubility, high temperature stability, and improved antioxidant activity. An important concern, however, which remains here while using this technique mainly for forming inclusion complexes is the likelihood of change in polymorphic form of drug which could not be ruled out [43].

9.4.1.5 Other strategies

Similarly electrospraying has been extensively explored for formulating various types of sustained/controlled release drug delivery formulation and the same has been discussed exhaustively in the review by Nguyen et al.

[44]. As reported by Lee et al. [45] coaxial dual-capillary electrospray is capable of producing monodisperse drug-loaded particles with high encapsulation efficiency.

Coaxial tricapillary electrospraying is another technique for fabrication of particles with core—middle—shell structure, which can be used for the production of multidrug-loaded particles. Using this method, different drugs can be easily incorporated into core, middle, and outer layers of particles, separately, producing multidrug-loaded particles in one step with customize release profile of drug from one formulated particle. This can drastically reduce frequency of drug administration especially involving complex prescription [46]. Although several attempts have been made to combine particle fabrication and surface modification by electrospraying, there is still great scope for creating immobilized functional groups on the surface to facilitate drug delivery, cell uptake, and impart particle—tissue interactions.

9.4.2 Applications of electrosprayed drug delivery systems in medicine

Formation of drug nanoparticles to achieve targeted drug delivery has drastically impacted the way therapeutics are delivered. Electrospraying technology answers the potential needs of nanoparticle production with added benefits of particle size customization, surface morphology modulation, scalability, reproducibility, effective encapsulation, etc. Owing to these advantages, many drugs have been electrosprayed with and without polymer carriers to improve their physicochemical properties and to enhance drug delivery aspects. Electrosprayed particles prepared by incorporation of biodegradable polymer carriers have also shown potential of sustained release of encapsulated drugs. Thus, it could be used as one of the promising techniques for the preparation of nanoparticles for varied pharmaceutical applications. Table 9.2 summarizes leading examples for use of electrosprayed products in drug delivery field for effective treatment of various ailments.

9.4.2.1 Application of electrosprayed drug delivery system in the management of diabetes

Diabetes is a metabolic disorder characterized by hyperglycemic condition and is associated with various microvascular and macrovascular complications. The prevalence of diabetes is higher in developing countries and it is in fact one of the most common noncommunicable lifestyle diseases. Various synthetic and natural molecules have been reported to prevent diabetic complications by different groups of researchers including electrosprayed insulin.

Table 9.2 Drug delivery applications of electrosprayed material.

Polymer/base utilized	Form of electrosprayed material	Drug loaded	Key findings	Reference
Electrospun material in effective management of diabetes				
Pectin–arabinoxylans	Microbeads	Insulin	Optimized voltage and flow rates reported to obtain beads of 1.02 ± 0.24 μm were 11 KV and 0.972 mL/h, respectively; authors used semiautomated technique and reported it to be suitable for industrial applications as well	[47]
Ethyl cellulose/Pluronic F-127	Microspheres	Insulin	No modifications in secondary structure of the insulin was observed by far-ultraviolet circular dichroism analysis; authors reported electrospraying to be a single-step technique for incorporation of bioactive cargos and obtaining it in a solid powder form	[48]
Maize bran arabinoxylans/maize wastewater arabinoxylans	Core–shell particles	Insulin	Particles of 2.9 mm suggested smooth surface with ability of maintaining integrity in stomach and intestine; authors claim 76% of the insulin to be released in colon part only	[49]
Electrospun material in effective management of cancer				
PLGA/chitosan	Composite microparticles	Paclitaxel + Topotecan	Composite particles were found to be maintaining delayed release for drug Topotecan providing sequential combination therapy against lung cancer	[50]

(Continued)

Table 9.2 Drug delivery applications of electrosprayed material.—cont'd

Polymer/base utilized	Form of electrosprayed material	Drug loaded	Key findings	Reference
Poly(tetramethylene succinate)	Microparticles	Gramicidin	A sustained release profile of drug was observed with retention of its activity	[51]
PLGA	Porous microspheres	Oridonin	Electrosprayed porous microspheres exhibited efficient lung deposition in vitro and in vivo and showed higher antitumor activity against lung cancer as confirmed by the CT images	[52]
Polyvinyl alcohol (PVA)/silk fibroin	Core—shell nanoparticles	Doxorubicin	The apoptotic activity of prepared nanoparticles when incubated with MDA-MB-231 cells was found to be increased with time	[28]
Poly(butylene adipate-co-butylene terephthalate)	Nanoparticles	Docetaxel	Fluorescent microscopy revealed prepared nanoparticles to be successfully up-taken by ovarian cancer cells. *In vitro* cytotoxicity studies suggested cell viability of the drug-loaded nanoparticles was significantly lower than the free drug. Nanoparticles significantly enhanced antitumor efficacy of the drug in nude mice	[53]
Biocompatible diblock and triblock polymers	Microparticles	Doxorubicin	The results revealed electrospraying to be a new potential method to fabricate drug-loaded polymer vesicles with controllable size for effective drug delivery of anticancer molecules	[54]
Electrospraying in encapsulating drug molecules for neurological disorders				
Without any polymer	Nanocrystals	Carbamazepine	Study showed preparation of drug nanocrystals and collection in solid form following single-step preparation. Drug nanocrystals were found to be significantly enhancing the dissolution rates and solubility of the drug candidate showing potential of electrospraying technique to process drug nanoparticles devoid of polymers as well	[55]

Electrospraying in encapsulating antiviral, antibacterial drug molecules				
Polyvinyl pyrrolidone (PVP) and Eudragit L100	Core–shell particles	Lopinavir + Ritonavir	Coaxial electrospray deposition of drug Lopinavir along with another molecule Ritonavir in enteric coated particles resulted in higher oral absorption of drug Lopinavir	[56]
Eudragit L100	Core–shell particles	Darunavir	Core–shell nanoparticles resulted in an entrapment efficiency of almost 90%. Use of enteric polymer as a core polymer reduced drug release in acidic medium as shown in the *in vitro* dissolution test	[57]
PVP	Core–shell microparticles	Acyclovir	Authors reported nearly eightfold increase in permeation rates across the sublingual mucosa compared with pristine form of drug	[58]
PLGA	Core–shell microparticles	Curcumin	Coaxial electrospraying was utilized for higher encapsulation efficiencies and better control of drug release over single axial electrospray process	[59]
Gelatin	Microspheres	Curcumin	Enhanced water solubility and bioaccessibility of curcumin was reported	[60]
Electrospraying in encapsulating antiinflammatory molecules				
PLGA	Nanobeads	Triamcinolone acetonide	Authors prepared nanobeads with an intention to obtain prolonged antiinflammatory activity. *In vitro* drug release suggested sustained release for drug after preparing it via simple, one-step, and cost-effective electrospraying process	[61]
Eudragit L100-55	Microparticles	Prednisolone	Authors used pH-sensitive polymer to achieve site-specific delivery of the drug. Drug release studies suggested reduced drug release at acidic stomach pH, whereas a rapid release of drug was observed when pH was increased to 6.8 showing potential to be used in inflammatory bowel disease	[62]

(*Continued*)

Table 9.2 Drug delivery applications of electrosprayed material.—cont'd

Polymer/base utilized	Form of electrosprayed material	Drug loaded	Key findings	Reference
Zein and glycerol	Micro-/nanoencapsules	β-Carotene	β-Carotene has potential as antiinflammatory compound still poor stability, sensitivity toward light, temperature, oxygen, and its poor water solubility results in low bioaccessibility and bioavailability. Authors reported ~1.7-fold increased permeability of drug resulting in enhanced bioavailability	[63]
Glutaraldehyde-crosslinked gelatin	Microparticles	Epigallocatechin 3-gallate	Rapid degradation and/or depletion of this compound makes delivery challenging. Localized controlled delivery of compound to the intervertebral disc resulted in reduced localized inflammation	[64]
Sodium alginate and chitosan	Microparticles	Chlorella protothecoides oil	Authors reported electrospraying to be suitable for obtaining smaller nanoparticles with homogeneous distribution, along with higher loading efficiency as compared to the conventional method of microencapsulation	[65]
PLGA	Microparticles	11H-indeno[1,2-b] quinoxalin-11-one oxime (IQ-1)	Polymer matrix was found to be having controlled release of compound following non-Fickian kinetics	[66]
Electrospraying in encapsulating drug molecules against asthma				
Polycaprolactone (PCL)	Nanobeads	Budesonide	Rapid elimination of the drug from body is major obstacle for this drug. Authors reported preparation of aqueous suspensions of nearly monodispersed, nano-sized PCL particles showing controlled drug release	[67]

- Data not reported.

Chu et al. have reported pectin-arabinoxylans—based electrosprayed composite microbeads for effective entrapment of insulin. Coaxial electrospraying technique resulted in faster formation of insulin-loaded beads without aggregation. Optimized voltage and flow rates resulted in beads of 1.02 ± 0.24 μm using 11 KV and 0.972 mL/h, respectively. Authors used semiautomated technique and reported it to be suitable for industrial applications as well [47]. Another group of authors reported preparation of insulin-loaded microspheres of palmitic/stearic acid and ethyl cellulose/Pluronic F-127. Particles of size approximately 1 μm were obtained using electric field of 30 kV and propanol as solvent of interest. When incorporating proteins using electrospraying technique many a times question has been raised regarding degradation of protein structure with subsequent loss of functionality. Authors ruled out the probability showing no modifications in secondary structure of the insulin using far-ultraviolet circular dichroism spectroscopy. Authors reported electrospraying to be a single-step technique for incorporation of bioactive cargos and obtaining it in a solid powder form [48].

Another important study was reported by Trinh et al. who has reported electrosprayed chitosan—insulin nanospheres to be delivered in the form of a novel injectable pH-temperature—sensitive hydrogel for effective insulin delivery in type-I diabetes as depicted in Fig. 9.6. The chitosan—insulin

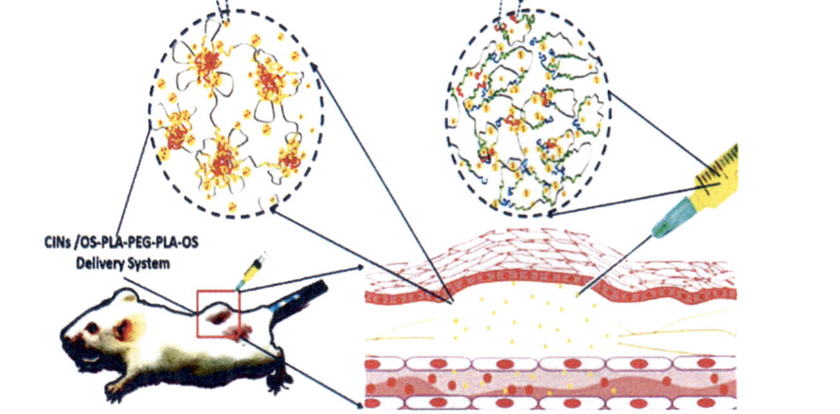

Figure 9.6 Schematic illustration of hydrogels loaded with chitosan—insulin composite injection and the release of insulin thereof. *Reprinted/Adapted with permission from, Trinh et al. Biomater. Sci. 14 (2020) 1—32.*

nanospheres were developed using electrospraying technique and were incorporated in pH- and temperature-sensitive hydrogel, made up with oligomer serin-b-poly(lactide)-bpoly(ethylene glycol)-b-poly(lactide)-b-oligomer serin (OS-PLA-PEG-PLA-OS) pentablock copolymer. Authors reported biological properties of insulin to be maintained and a blood glucose reducing effect was found for 60 h when injected in streptozotocin (STZ)-induced diabetic mouse model showing the potential of developed strategy [68].

9.4.2.2 Application of electrosprayed drug delivery systems in the management of cancer

Cancer is a complex series of disease condition characterized by uncontrolled cell growth leading to malignancies. Very high mortality and recurrence rates have been reported for various types of cancers showing urgent need for effective therapy and early diagnosis. Advancement in the field of electrosprayed nanoparticles has rendered this technique useful in formulating anticancer drugs as an effective treatment strategy.

Arya et al. have reported electrosprayed composite micro-/nanoparticles for combination therapy of drugs Paclitaxel and Topotecan. Chitosan—PLGA composite particles maintained delayed release of drug Topotecan to provide sequential exposure of these drugs. Combination was found to be providing synergistic effect in NCI—H460 cellular aggregates (nonsmall cell lung cancer cell line) generated *in-vitro* [50]. Study clearly indicates capability of electrospraying technique to encapsulate multiple drugs in single carrier with properties of modulating their release profile. Interesting findings were reported by Lee et al. while using electrosprayed nanocomposites for targeted delivery to the tumor site. Nanocomposites of hyaluronic acid—ceramide and soluplus were developed for encapsulating and targeting drug resveratrol at the tumor site (Fig. 9.7). Stringent control over electrospraying parameters resulted in formation of nanocomposites with mean particle size of 230 nm, while entrapment efficiency for drug was found to be more than 80%. *In vitro* drug release studies suggested pH-dependent sustained drug release profile [69].

Hyaluronic acid was utilized in the nanocomposite with the goal of achieving targeting effect by virtue of its interaction with CD44 receptor. Targetability of prepared nanocomposites was accessed in MDA-MB-231 tumor-xenograft mouse model using near-infrared fluorescence imaging. Results suggested better accumulation of hyaluronic acid containing nanocomposites at tumor site in 24 h showing effective tumor targeting [69].

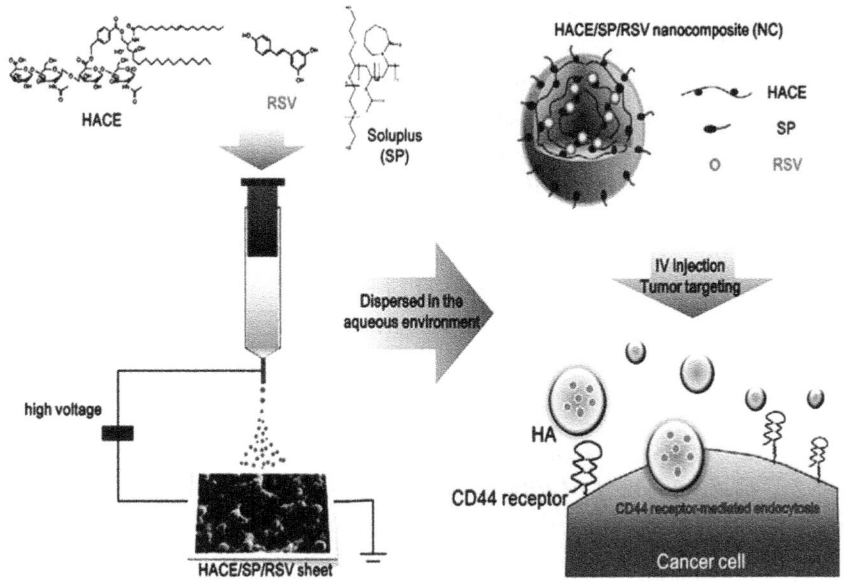

Figure 9.7 Schematic illustration of hyaluronic acid–ceramide/soluplus nanocomposites fabricated using electrospraying technique for targeted delivery to the tumor site. *Reprinted/Adapted with permission from, Lee et al. Colloids Surf., B Biointerfaces 145 (2016) 267–274.*

Study revealed potential of electrospraying technique in generating materials with desired properties thus opening a new arena in the drug delivery field. Apart from all these aforementioned leading examples, there are numerous studies reported by various research groups showing potential of electrospraying technique to generate material that can effectively incorporate anticancer drugs for effective treatment of different cancer types. Some such other examples have been enlisted in Table 9.2.

9.4.2.3 Application of electrosprayed drug delivery systems in the management of infections

Infectious diseases are the leading cause of mortality worldwide, with viruses in particular making major impact on healthcare and socioeconomic development, more so in the present pandemic of COVID-19. Electrosprayed nanoparticles owing to their surface and size could be customized to penetrate the cell membrane of pathogenic microorganisms and interfere with important molecular pathways. In combination with optimal antibiotics, nanoparticles have demonstrated synergy and may aid in limiting the global crisis of emerging bacterial resistance [70,71]. Lopinavir, a human immunodeficiency virus (HIV) protease inhibitor, has widespread use as antiviral molecule and is used in the treatment of HIV infection and is known to be cytochrome P450 3A (CYP3A) substrate presenting challenges in its oral delivery. Sakuma et al. have reported coaxial electrospray deposition of drug Lopinavir along with another molecule Ritonavir in enteric coated particles. Results revealed higher oral absorption of drug Lopinavir when delivered with Ritonavir in enteric coated electrosprayed particles [56]. Some other examples for encapsulation of antiviral agents have been enlisted in Table 9.2. Yuan et al. have reported curcumin-loaded microparticles for controlled release of drug. Coaxial electrospraying was utilized for higher encapsulation efficiencies and better control of drug release over single axial electrospray process [59].

9.4.2.4 Application of electrosprayed drug delivery systems in the management of inflammation

Several antiinflammatory drugs have been encapsulated as nanoparticles to achieve targeted delivery, to reduce adverse effects, and to improve administration of drugs. Some of the recently developed stimuli-responsive nanoparticles are especially interesting as they could enhance the drug delivery specificity for biomedical applications too. Furthermore, chronic inflammation due to autoimmune processes and infectious diseases which needs carriers precisely delivering the therapeutic compounds to the target sites could be achieved using nanonization approach [72].

Jahangiri et al. have reported triamcinolone acetonide–loaded nanobeads of PLGA to obtain prolonged antiinflammatory activity of drug. *In vitro* drug release studies suggested sustained release of drug after preparing it via simple, one-step, and cost-effective electrospraying process [61]. Apart from the synthetic drug molecules, various natural compounds viz. β-carotene, ellagic acid, and some other flavanols are frequently used as an antiinflammatory agent. Numerous reports have mentioned electrospraying of such molecules to provide antiinflammatory response. Table 9.2 compiles all such examples of electrosprayed particles containing natural antiinflammatory molecules. Another group of authors have reported electrosprayed microparticles of drug prednisolone for effective intestinal delivery.

In this study, authors used pH-sensitive polymer to achieve site-specific delivery of the drug. Drug release studies suggested reduced drug release at acidic stomach pH, whereas a rapid release of drug was observed when pH was increased to 6.8 showing potential to be used in inflammatory bowel disease [62].

9.4.2.5 Application of electrosprayed drug delivery systems in the management of other ailments

Polymeric micro- and nanoparticles are capable of being administered as oral, injectable, inhalable, topical, and local drug-delivery systems and could be formulated using electrospraying method. There is limited literature on the use of electrosprayed particles to manage other ailments such as neurological disorders and thus clearly shows that there is a room for further exploration. Wang et al. have reported production of carbamazepine nanocrystals by electrospraying technique for enhancement of its dissolution rates. This was an interesting study showing preparation of drug nanocrystals and collection in solid form following single-step preparation. Drug nanocrystals were found to be significantly enhancing the dissolution rates and solubility of the drug candidate showing potential of electrospraying technique to process drug nanoparticles devoid of polymers as well [55].

Similarly Zhu et al. have developed a novel, simple, and quick method for preparing inhalable oridonin-loaded PLGA porous microspheres using the electrospraying technique. The electrosprayed porous microspheres obtained were porous, rough, and were suitable for pulmonary delivery because of their ideal aerodynamic diameters. These desirable attributes facilitated delivery via inhalation route and efficient lung deposition. Most of the oridonin was released from the electrosprayed particles within 20 h based on drug diffusion and via PLGA erosion [52].

9.5 Trends in electrospraying

In past few years, electrospraying has been explored for delivery of bioactive cargoes like genes, living cell, plasmid DNA, growth factors, enzymes, etc. The fragile nature of these cargoes especially due to the high sensitivity toward fluctuation in surrounding ambience makes the process very difficult and challenging.

Often the process of loading living cells and whole organisms is called "bioelectrospraying" [73]. It has become an appealing tool for cell delivery in scaffolds for tissue engineering applications and is considered to be safe for cells due to the low current (usually in the nanoampere range), albeit the high voltage up to several kilovolts. Few such papers report a variety of cells being subjected to electrospraying, including fibroblasts, adipose-derived stem cells, periodontal ligament cells, retinal pigment epithelial cells, umbilical vascular endothelial cells, gastric epithelial cells [74], bone marrow–derived mesenchymal stem cells [75], etc. The results revealed no distinct adverse effect of the electrospraying process on cell vitality, morphology, and proliferation. Further, Boda et al. [76] has suggested electrospraying of DNA plasmid in a suitable buffer preferably a high-conductivity culture medium as an alternative for bacterial/cell transformation with high efficiency. Abyadeh et al. illustrated a rapid transformation method for electrospraying chitosan/pDNA into a bacterial culture, for increasing the penetration of plasmid into bacteria [77].

Growth factor delivery with good efficiency and efficacy is still a challenge for tissue regeneration therapies, despite several advancements. Electrospraying was effectively used to prevent denaturation of growth factor by limiting the exposure to organic solvents. Further to assist growth factor bioactivity, stabilizers like PEG and trehalose were added to PLGA to prepare vascular endothelial growth factor or bone morphogenetic protein-loaded carriers via electrospraying [13]. A few studies explored the possibility of using electrospraying to encapsulate coenzyme Q10 in copovidone using acetone as the solvent. Characterization studies using both in vitro and in vivo evaluation showed enhanced bioavailability of the electrosprayed microparticles [78]. The field is still evolving and there is scope for more technological advancements particularly in exploring electrospray particles for growth factor delivery in tissue engineering and other allied fields.

9.6 Challenges and future opportunities

Electrospraying is a simple, versatile technique offering numerous advantages viz. reproducibility, better control over particle size, morphology, size distribution, shape, and many more for a wide range of base compounds that are used in pharmaceutical and biomedical field. Easy alterations in drug release profiles including fast release, controlled release, targeted release, and many more can readily be achieved by cautious selection of the base material as well as the altering particle morphologies. Apart from the benefits of working with single drug molecules, many-a-times authors have reported incorporation of multiple drugs and some have even specifically utilized it for sequential drug delivery (delivery of drug one after another) for achieving synergism. It is beneficial in terms of being a single-step method for producing particles with desired size in solid form. Besides drug molecules, electrospraying technique has been found useful in formulating proteins without altering their secondary structure and functionality. Researchers working in the area of bioelectrospraying have even reported effective embedding of stem cells [79] using electrospraying technique which clearly indicate adaptability of technique in cell delivery field.

Nevertheless, despite such prolific use, there are no commercially available products for drug delivery in the market based on this technique. This could be attributed to the fact that although stringent control over processing parameters renders achieving particles with desired characteristics quite easy, but still optimization of these parameters makes this process much more complex. With so many process-related and formulation-related variables to be optimized in order to get desired output, the technique has its own set of problems, which may need newer perspective to tackle on commercial scale. Parameters like solution viscosity, solvent volatility, solvent conductivity, tip-to-collector distance, flow rate, applied voltage, operating temperature, pressure in the processing chamber, and so forth drastically influence particle size, shape, morphology, size distribution as all these are interdependent.

Another major bottleneck for the scale-up of this process is low throughput as at many instances lower flow rates are preferred making the process more and more tedious. Although researchers have worked in this direction and numerous advances have been made in the technique, still these are not up to the mark. One of such advancements in technique includes use of multi-nozzle spray system to expedite the process. Kang et al. have reported novel kind of a nozzle with array of holes at the side providing multiple jet emission to yield smaller particles with narrower size distribution [80]. Continuous manufacturing is one of the processes gaining more and more attention by pharmaceutical industries these days. Also authors have reported continuous production technique to obtain higher yields. Despite all these advancements, with the present machine which are used for electrospraying, the output in terms of quantity probably will be very difficult to match with already existing techniques like spray-drying, lyophilization, etc.

9.7 Conclusion

Electrospraying is a simple, versatile technique based on the principle of electrohydrodynamic atomization and is reported to have tremendous use in the drug delivery by not only altering the physicochemical aspects of the drug but by also helping in controlled/sustained or targeted delivery. With host of different morphologies offered by electrosprayed particles ranging from hollow to Janus type, the possibility of loading different type and different size of cargo is also tremendous. In comparison to conventional methods, it offers better control over size, size distribution, surface morphology, shape, etc. Owing to these advantages it has been widely explored to formulate solid dispersion, amorphous dispersion, crystalline inclusion complexes for enhancing particulate level properties of several BCS class II drugs. The porosity and surface roughness of electrosprayed particles offer huge potential for its use in inhalation products. Electrosprayed particles have been also used to deliver drugs belonging to different therapeutic categories like anticancer, antibiotics, antiretrovirals, and many others. Due to unique surface properties, these electrosprayed particles can be layered with more than one active with possibility of achieving sustained, targeted delivery. There are small limitations though in terms of output and mass production which is less in electrospraying technique than in conventional methods. Despite these limitations, electrospraying offers huge expanse for further exploration especially in terms of delivery of biological cargoes, having low dose, stability concerns with conventional techniques. Electrospraying represents a nanotechnology that is gradually maturing and its use will grow as companies implement this technology as a platform drug-delivery technique in near future.

Acknowledgments

The authors want to thank the Ministry of Chemicals and Fertilizers for providing the funding and the Department of Science and Technology and SERB for providing the funding to authors in the form of INSPIRE faculty award (Grant number LSBM-13) and SERB EMR/2016/007966).

References

[1] M. Zamani, M.P. Prabhakaran, S. Ramakrishna, Advances in drug delivery via electrospun and electrosprayed nanomaterials, Int. J. Nanomed. 8 (2013) 2997.

[2] M. Jafari-Nodoushan, J. Barzin, H. Mobedi, Size and morphology controlling of PLGA microparticles produced by electro hydrodynamic atomization, Polym. Adv. Technol. 26 (2015) 502–513.

[3] H.N. Ho, I. Laidmäe, K. Kogermann, A. Lust, A. Meos, C.N. Nguyen, J. Heinämäki, Development of electrosprayed artesunate-loaded core–shell nanoparticles, Drug Dev. Ind. Pharm. 43 (2017) 1134–1142.

[4] M. Rasekh, C. Young, M. Roldo, F. Lancien, J.-C. Le Mével, S. Hafizi, Z. Ahmad, E. Barbu, D. Gorecki, Hollow-layered nanoparticles for therapeutic delivery of peptide prepared using electrospraying, J. Mater. Sci. Mater. Med. 26 (2015) 256.

[5] C. Zhang, Y. Li, Y. Hu, Y. Peng, Z. Ahmad, J.-S. Li, M.-W. Chang, Porous yolk–shell particle engineering via nonsolvent-assisted trineedle coaxial electrospraying for burn-related wound healing, ACS Appl. Mater. Interfaces 11 (2019) 7823–7835.

[6] A. Pawar, S. Thakkar, M. Misra, A bird's eye view of nanoparticles prepared by electrospraying: advancements in drug delivery field, J. Contr. Release 286 (2018) 179–200.
[7] C.U. Yurteri, R.P. Hartman, J.C. Marijnissen, Producing pharmaceutical particles via electrospraying with an emphasis on nano and nano structured particles-a review, KONA Powder Part. J. 28 (2010) 91–115.
[8] R. Sridhar, S. Ramakrishna, Electrosprayed nanoparticles for drug delivery and pharmaceutical applications, Biomatter 3 (2013) e24281.
[9] J. Wang, J.A. Jansen, F. Yang, Electrospraying: possibilities and challenges of engineering carriers for biomedical applications—a mini review, Front. Chem. 7 (2019) 258.
[10] J.D. Schiffman, C.L. Schauer, A review: electrospinning of biopolymer nanofibers and their applications, Polym. Rev. 48 (2008) 317–352.
[11] J.A. Bhushani, C. Anandharamakrishnan, Electrospinning and electrospraying techniques: potential food based applications, Trends Food Sci. Technol. 38 (2014) 21–33.
[12] A. Alehosseini, B. Ghorani, M. Sarabi-Jamab, N. Tucker, Principles of electrospraying: a new approach in protection of bioactive compounds in foods, Crit. Rev. Food Sci. Nutr. 58 (4) (2018) 2346–2363.
[13] N. Bock, T.R. Dargaville, M.A. Woodruff, Electrospraying of polymers with therapeutic molecules: state of the art, Prog. Polym. Sci. 37 (2012) 1510–1551.
[14] L. Peltonen, H. Valo, R. Kolakovic, T. Laaksonen, J. Hirvonen, Electrospraying, spray drying and related techniques for production and formulation of drug nanoparticles, Expet Opin. Drug Deliv. 7 (2010) 705–719.
[15] D.S. Katti, K.W. Robinson, F.K. Ko, C.T. Laurencin, Bioresorbable nanofiber-based systems for wound healing and drug delivery: optimization of fabrication parameters, J. Biomed. Mater. Res. B Appl. Biomater. 70 (2004) 286–296.
[16] H.F. Guo, B.G. Xu, Numerical Study of Taylor Cone Dynamics in Electrospinning of Nanofibers, I. K. E. Materials, Trans Tech Publisher, 2017, pp. 1–40.
[17] S. Megelski, J.S. Stephens, D.B. Chase, J.F. Rabolt, Micro-and nanostructured surface morphology on electrospun polymer fibers, Macromolecules 35 (2002) 8456–8466.
[18] T.J. Sill, H.A. von Recum, Electrospinning: applications in drug delivery and tissue engineering, Biomaterials 29 (2008) 1989–2006.
[19] J. Doshi, D.H. Reneker, Electrospinning process and applications of electrospun fibers, J. Electrost. 35 (1995) 151–160.
[20] F. Huang, Q. Wei, J. Wang, Y. Cai, Y. Huang, Effect of temperature on structure, morphology and crystallinity of PVDF nanofibers via electrospinning, E-Polymers 8 (2008) 1758–1765.
[21] C. Wang, H.-S. Chien, C.-H. Hsu, Y.-C. Wang, C.-T. Wang, H.-A. Lu, Electrospinning of polyacrylonitrile solutions at elevated temperatures, Macromolecules 40 (2007) 7973–7983.
[22] C.L. Casper, J.S. Stephens, N.G. Tassi, D.B. Chase, J.F. Rabolt, Controlling surface morphology of electrospun polystyrene fibers: effect of humidity and molecular weight in the electrospinning process, Macromolecules 37 (2004) 573–578.
[23] H. Shao, J. Fang, H. Wang, T. Lin, Effect of electrospinning parameters and polymer concentrations on mechanical-to-electrical energy conversion of randomly-oriented electrospun poly (vinylidene fluoride) nanofiber mats, RSC Adv. 5 (2015) 14345–14350.
[24] W. Liu, C. Huang, X. Jin, Electrospinning of grooved polystyrene fibers: effect of solvent systems, Nanoscale Res. Lett. 10 (2015) 237.
[25] C.H. Park, Preparation of Polymer/Drug Nano-and Micro-Particles by Electrospraying, I. M. Wiley Symposia,Online Library, Wiley Online Library, 2007.

[26] S. Chakraborty, I.-C. Liao, A. Adler, K.W. Leong, Electrohydrodynamics: a facile technique to fabricate drug delivery systems, Adv. Drug Deliv. Rev. 61 (2009) 1043–1054.

[27] M. Abyadeh, A.A.K. Zarchi, M.A. Faramarzi, A. Amani, Evaluation of factors affecting size and size distribution of chitosan-electrosprayed nanoparticles, Avicenna J. Med. Biotechnol. 9 (2017) 126.

[28] Y. Cao, F. Liu, Y. Chen, T. Yu, D. Lou, Y. Guo, P. Li, Z. Wang, H. Ran, Drug release from core-shell PVA/silk fibroin nanoparticles fabricated by one-step electrospraying, Sci. Rep. 7 (2017) 1–9.

[29] Y. Xu, M. Skotak, M. Hanna, Electrospray encapsulation of water-soluble protein with polylactide. I. Effects of formulations and process on morphology and particle size, J. Microencapsul. 23 (2006) 69–78.

[30] S. Freitas, H.P. Merkle, B. Gander, Ultrasonic atomisation into reduced pressure atmosphere—envisaging aseptic spray-drying for microencapsulation, J. Contr. Release 95 (2004) 185–195.

[31] N. Arya, S. Chakraborty, N. Dube, D.S. Katti, Electrospraying: a facile technique for synthesis of chitosan-based micro/nanospheres for drug delivery applications, J. Biomed. Mater. Res. B Appl. Biomater. 88 (2009) 17–31.

[32] A. Gholami, H. Tavanai, A. Moradi, Production of fibroin nanopowder through electrospraying, J. Nanoparticle Res. 13 (2011) 2089–2098.

[33] H. Lee, S. An, S. Kim, B. Jeon, M. Kim, I.S. Kim, Readily functionalizable and stabilizable polymeric particles with controlled size and morphology by electrospray, Sci. Rep. 8 (2018) 1–10.

[34] A. Jaworek, Micro-and nanoparticle production by electrospraying, Powder Technol. 176 (2007) 18–35.

[35] A. Sosnik, Production of drug-loaded polymeric nanoparticles by electrospraying technology, J. Biomed. Nanotechnol. 10 (2014) 2200–2217.

[36] E. Ahire, S. Thakkar, M. Darshanwad, M. Misra, Parenteral nanosuspensions: a brief review from solubility enhancement to more novel and specific applications, Acta Pharm. Sin. B 8 (2018) 733–755.

[37] S. Thakkar, D. Sharma, M. Misra, Comparative evaluation of electrospraying and lyophilization techniques on solid state properties of erlotinib nanocrystals: assessment of in-vitro cytotoxicity, Eur. J. Pharmaceut. Sci. 111 (2018) 257–269.

[38] N. Anup, S. Thakkar, M. Misra, Formulation of olanzapine nanosuspension based orally disintegrating tablets (ODT); comparative evaluation of lyophilization and electrospraying process as solidification techniques, Adv. Powder Technol. 29 (2018) 1913–1924.

[39] A. Bohr, J. Kristensen, M. Dyas, M. Edirisinghe, E. Stride, Release profile and characteristics of electrosprayed particles for oral delivery of a practically insoluble drug, J. R. Soc. Interface 9 (2012) 2437–2449.

[40] J.C. Ijsebaert, K.B. Geerse, J.C. Marijnissen, J.-W.J. Lammers, P. Zanen, Electrohydrodynamic atomization of drug solutions for inhalation purposes, J. Appl. Physiol. 91 (2001) 2735–2741.

[41] K. Katrajkar, S. Thakkar, B. Kshirsagar, B. Sirsikar, S. Polaka, M. Misra, Development and evaluation of crystalline inclusion complex of finasteride using electrospraying as a novel approach, J. Drug Deliv. Sci. Technol. (2020) 101887.

[42] Z. Aytac, Z.I. Yildiz, F. Kayaci-Senirmak, T. Tekinay, T. Uyar, Electrospinning of cyclodextrin/linalool-inclusion complex nanofibers: fast-dissolving nanofibrous web with prolonged release and antibacterial activity, Food Chem. 231 (2017) 192–201.

[43] A. Celebioglu, Z.I. Yildiz, T. Uyar, Fabrication of electrospun eugenol/cyclodextrin inclusion complex nanofibrous webs for enhanced antioxidant property, water solubility, and high temperature stability, J. Agric. Food Chem. 66 (2018) 457–466.

[44] D.N. Nguyen, C. Clasen, G. Van den Mooter, Pharmaceutical applications of electrospraying, J. Pharmaceut. Sci. 105 (2016) 2601–2620.
[45] Y.-H. Lee, M.-Y. Bai, D.-R. Chen, Multidrug encapsulation by coaxial tri-capillary electrospray, Colloids Surf. B Biointerfaces 82 (2011) 104–110.
[46] W. Kim, S.S. Kim, Synthesis of biodegradable triple-layered capsules using a triaxial electrospray method, Polymer 52 (2011) 3325–3336.
[47] A. Rascón-Chu, J.A. Díaz-Baca, E. Carvajal-Millan, E. Pérez-López, A.T. Hotchkiss, H. González-Ríos, R. Balandrán-Quintana, A.C. Campa-Mada, Electrosprayed core–shell composite microbeads based on pectin-arabinoxylans for insulin carrying: aggregation and size dispersion control, Polymers 10 (2018) 108.
[48] R. Bussano, D. Chirio, L. Costa, F. Turci, M. Trotta, Preparation and characterization of insulin-loaded lipid-based microspheres generated by electrospray, J. Dispersion Sci. Technol. 32 (2011) 1524–1530.
[49] R. Paz-Samaniego, A. Rascón-Chu, F. Brown-Bojorquez, E. Carvajal-Millan, M. Pedroza-Montero, E. Silva-Campa, N. Sotelo-Cruz, Y.L. López-Franco, J. Lizardi-Mendoza, Electrospray-assisted fabrication of core-shell arabinoxylan gel particles for insulin and probiotics entrapment, J. Appl. Polym. Sci. 135 (2018) 46411.
[50] N. Arya, D.S. Katti, Poly (d, l-lactide-co-glycolide)–chitosan composite particles for the treatment of lung cancer, Int. J. Nanomed. 10 (2015) 2997.
[51] S. Maione, L.J. del Valle, M.M. Pérez-Madrigal, C. Cativiela, J. Puiggalí, C. Alemán, Electrospray loading and release of hydrophobic gramicidin in polyester microparticles, RSC Adv. 6 (2016) 73045–73055.
[52] L. Zhu, M. Li, X. Liu, Y. Jin, Drug-loaded PLGA electrospraying porous microspheres for the local therapy of primary lung cancer via pulmonary delivery, ACS Omega 2 (2017) 2273–2279.
[53] J. Varshosaz, E. Ghassami, A. Noorbakhsh, A. Jahanian-Najafabadi, M. Minaiyan, R. Behzadi, Poly (butylene adipate-co-butylene terephthalate) nanoparticles prepared by electrospraying technique for docetaxel delivery in ovarian cancer induced mice, Drug Dev. Ind. Pharm. 44 (2018) 1012–1022.
[54] W. Li, S. Liu, H. Yao, G. Liao, Z. Si, X. Gong, L. Ren, L. Wang, Microparticle templating as a route to nanoscale polymer vesicles with controlled size distribution for anticancer drug delivery, J. Colloid Interface Sci. 508 (2017) 145–153.
[55] M. Wang, G.C. Rutledge, A.S. Myerson, B.L. Trout, Production and characterization of carbamazepine nanocrystals by electrospraying for continuous pharmaceutical manufacturing, J. Pharmaceut. Sci. 101 (2012) 1178–1188.
[56] S. Sakuma, S. Matsumoto, N. Ishizuka, K. Mohri, M. Fukushima, C. Ohba, K. Kawakami, Enhanced boosting of oral absorption of lopinavir through electrospray coencapsulation with ritonavir, J. Pharmaceut. Sci. 104 (2015) 2977–2985.
[57] D.N. Nguyen, C. Clasen, G. Van den Mooter, Encapsulating darunavir nanocrystals within Eudragit L100 using coaxial electrospraying, Eur. J. Pharm. Biopharm. 113 (2017) 50–59.
[58] Z.-P. Liu, L. Cui, D.-G. Yu, Z.-X. Zhao, L. Chen, Electrosprayed core–shell solid dispersions of acyclovir fabricated using an epoxy-coated concentric spray head, Int. J. Nanomed. 9 (2014) 1967.
[59] S. Yuan, F. Lei, Z. Liu, Q. Tong, T. Si, R.X. Xu, Coaxial electrospray of curcumin-loaded microparticles for sustained drug release, PloS One 10 (2015) e0132609.
[60] J. Gómez-Estaca, R. Gavara, P. Hernández-Muñoz, Encapsulation of curcumin in electrosprayed gelatin microspheres enhances its bioaccessibility and widens its uses in food applications, Innovat. Food Sci. Emerg. Technol. 29 (2015) 302–307.
[61] A. Jahangiri, S. Davaran, B. Fayyazi, A. Tanhaei, S. Payab, K. Adibkia, Application of electrospraying as a one-step method for the fabrication of triamcinolone acetonide-PLGA nanofibers and nanobeads, Colloids Surf. B Biointerfaces 123 (2014) 219–224.

[62] T. Shams, U. Illangakoon, M. Parhizkar, A. Harker, S. Edirisinghe, M. Orlu, M. Edirisinghe, Electrosprayed microparticles for intestinal delivery of prednisolone, J. R. Soc. Interface 15 (2018) 20180491.
[63] L. Mahalakshmi, M.M. Leena, J. Moses, C. Anandharamakrishnan, Micro-and nano-encapsulation of β-carotene in zein protein: size-dependent release and absorption behavior, Food Func. 11 (2020) 1647−1660.
[64] M. Loepfe, A. Duss, K.-A. Zafeiropoulou, O. Björgvinsdóttir, M. D'Este, D. Eglin, G. Fortunato, J. Klasen, S.J. Ferguson, K. Wuertz-Kozak, Electrospray-based microencapsulation of epigallocatechin 3-gallate for local delivery into the intervertebral disc, Pharmaceutics 11 (2019) 435.
[65] C.Y. Karakaş, D. Özçimen, A novel approach to production of Chlorella protothecoides oil loaded nanoparticles via electrospraying method: modelling of critical parameters for particle sizing, Biotechnol. Appl. Biochem. (2020), https://doi.org/10.1002/bab.1977.
[66] E. Kibler, A. Lavrinenko, I. Kolesnik, K. Stankevich, E. Bolbasov, V. Kudryavtseva, A. Leonov, I. Schepetkin, A. Khlebnikov, M.T. Quinn, Electrosprayed poly (lactic-co-glycolic acid) particles as a promising drug delivery system for the novel JNK inhibitor IQ-1, Eur. Polym. J. (2020) 109598.
[67] B. Midhun, K. Shalumon, K. Manzoor, R. Jayakumar, S. Nair, M. Deepthy, Preparation of budesonide-loaded polycaprolactone nanobeads by electrospraying for controlled drug release, J. Biomater. Sci., Polym. Ed. 22 (2011) 2431−2444.
[68] T.A. Trinh, D. Le, H.G.V. Ho, T.C.T. To, V.V.L. Nguyen, D. Huynh, D. Lee, A novel injectable pH-temperature sensitive hydrogel containing chitosan-insulin electrosprayed nanosphere composite for an insulin delivery system in type I diabetes treatment, Biomater. Sci. (2020).
[69] S.Y. Lee, J.-J. Lee, J.-H. Park, J.-Y. Lee, S.-H. Ko, J.-S. Shim, J. Lee, M.Y. Heo, D.-D. Kim, H.-J. Cho, Electrosprayed nanocomposites based on hyaluronic acid derivative and Soluplus for tumor-targeted drug delivery, Colloids Surf. B Biointerfaces 145 (2016) 267−274.
[70] N.-Y. Lee, P.-R. Hsueh, W.-C. Ko, Nanoparticles in the treatment of infections caused by multidrug-resistant organisms, Front. Pharmacol. 10 (2019) 1153.
[71] L. Singh, H.G. Kruger, G.E. Maguire, T. Govender, R. Parboosing, The role of nanotechnology in the treatment of viral infections, Ther. Adv. Infect. Dis. 4 (2017) 105−131.
[72] A. Mahdavi Gorabi, N. Kiaie, Ž. Reiner, F. Carbone, F. Montecucco, A. Sahebkar, The therapeutic potential of nanoparticles to reduce inflammation in atherosclerosis, Biomolecules 9 (2019) 416.
[73] S.N. Jayasinghe, J. Auguste, C.J. Scotton, Platform technologies for directly reconstructing 3D living biomaterials, Adv. Mater. 27 (2015) 7794−7799.
[74] Y. Xin, G. Chai, T. Zhang, X. Wang, M. Qu, A. Tan, M. Bogari, M. Zhu, L. Lin, Q. Hu, Analysis of multiple types of human cells subsequent to bioprinting with electrospraying technology, Biomed. Rep. 5 (2016) 723−730.
[75] Z. McCrea, Y. Arnanthigo, S.-A. Cryan, S. O'Dea, A novel methodology for bio-electrospraying mesenchymal stem cells that maintains differentiation, immunomodulatory and pro-reparative functions, J. Med. Biol. Eng. 38 (2018) 497−513.
[76] S.K. Boda, X. Li, J. Xie, Electrospraying an enabling technology for pharmaceutical and biomedical applications: a review, J. Aerosol Sci. 125 (2018) 164−181.
[77] M. Abyadeh, E. Sadroddiny, A. Ebrahimi, F. Esmaeili, F.S. Landi, A. Amani, Electrosprayed chitosan nanoparticles: facile and efficient approach for bacterial transformation, Int. Nano Lett. 7 (2017) 291−295.

[78] W.Y. Fung, M.T. Liong, K.H. Yuen, Preparation, in-vitro and in-vivo characterisation of CoQ10 microparticles: electrospraying-enhanced bioavailability, J. Pharm. Pharmacol. 68 (2016) 159–169.
[79] Y. Xu, J. Peng, G. Richards, S. Lu, D. Eglin, Optimization of electrospray fabrication of stem cell–embedded alginate–gelatin microspheres and their assembly in 3D-printed poly (ε-caprolactone) scaffold for cartilage tissue engineering, J. Orthop. Transl. 18 (2019) 128–141.
[80] J.S. Kang, I. Park, J.H. Jung, S.S. Kim, Free-surface electrospray technique using a multi-hole array, J. Aerosol Sci. 55 (2013) 25–30.

CHAPTER TEN

Applications of electrospraying in biosensing, diagnostics, and beyond

Chikim Nguyen, Fang Yang
Department of Dentistry - Regenerative Biomaterials, Radboud university medical center, Nijmegen, the Netherlands

Abbreviations

number
1D 1-dimensional
2D 2-dimensional
3D 3-dimensional
Abs antibodies
anti-HRP Horseradish peroxidase antibody
Au Gold
BaAlg Barium alginate
$BaCl_2$ Barium chloride
BSA Bovine serum albumin
CaAlg Calcium alginate
CFU Colony-forming unit
CGO Crumpled graphene oxide
CHO-ITO Aldehyde-modified indium-tin oxide
CNT(s) Carbon nanotube(s)
CO Carbon monoxide
CO_2 Carbon dioxide
COVID-19 Pandemic of coronavirus disease 2019
Cyt. c Cytochrome *c*
dMRI Diffusion magnetic resonance imaging
DNA Deoxyribonucleic acid
Dox Doxorubicin
E-spray Electrospray
E. coli *Escherichia coli*
EAG Electrospray aerosol generator
EHDA Electrohydrodynamic atomization
ESFDA Electrostatic force directed assembly
FET Field-effect transistor
FITC Fluorescein isothiocyanate
G/PVP/PANI Graphene, polyvinylpyrrolidone, and polyaniline

Biomedical Applications of Electrospinning and Electrospraying
ISBN: 978-0-12-822476-2
https://doi.org/10.1016/B978-0-12-822476-2.00007-8

H_2 Hydrogen
$H2O_2$ Hydrogen peroxide
H2S Hydrogen sulfide
HIV Human immunodeficiency viruses
IgG Immunoglobulin G
IgM Immunoglobulin M
MB(s) Microbubble(s)
MEMS Microelectromechanical systems
MERS-CoV Middle East respiratory syndrome—related coronavirus
MESDD Multiplexed E-spray deposition device
MP(s) Microparticle(s)
MRI Magnetic resonance imaging
Na_2SO_4 Sodium sulfate
NaAlg Sodium alginate
NP(s) Nanoparticle(s)
PCL Poly(ε-caprolactone)
PDMS Polydimethylsiloxane
PEG Polyethylene-glycol
PGNs Phosphate-based glass nanospheres
pH Power of hydrogen
PLGA Poly(lactic-co-glycolic acid)
ppb Parts per billion
PPG Poly(3,4-ethylenedioxythiophene), poly(styrene sulfonate), and graphene
ppm Parts per million
Pt Platinum
PVA Poly(vinyl alcohol)
PVDF Poly-vinylidene fluoride
QD Quantum dots
Ref. References
rGO Reduced graphene oxide
RSD Relative standard deviation
SARS-CoV Severe acute respiratory syndrome coronavirus
SAW-ED Surface acoustic wave atomization with electrostatic deposition
SERS Surface-enhanced Raman scattering
SF_6 Sulfur hexafluoride
SnO_2 Tin oxide
SPION(s) Superparamagnetic iron oxide nanoparticle(s)
SPs Spheres
Ta Tantalum
TGA Thioglycolic acid
tPA Tissue plasminogen activator
TRGO Thermally reduced graphene oxide
YSP(s) Yolk—shell particle(s)
α-LA α-Lactalbumin
ZnAc Zinc acetate dihydrate
ZnO Zinc oxide

10.1 Introduction

The outbursts of life-threatening diseases like cancers [1], viral infections [2,3], and heart diseases [4], to name a few, have continuously posed new challenges and requirements for developing effective diagnosis, prevention, and treatment strategies. Following the past epidemics, SARS-CoV in 2002 and MERS-CoV in 2012, a new coronavirus disease outbreak (COVID-19) caused by SARS-CoV-2 has rapidly spread across the world and affected a large percent of the population [5]. At this moment, when these words are being typed, humankind is still fighting with the serious COVID-19 pandemic that can dramatically disrupt the global economy, healthcare systems, and even more in the short run [6]. Therefore, tackling disease outbreaks, for instance, by searching and developing useful diagnostic tools, is of utmost priority. Indeed, accurate and fast detection assist in not only limiting the spread of the transmissible diseases but also allowing specific treatments and bettering the outcomes of patients with other diseases [1].

In the past 50 years, great achievements have been made in the field of nanoscience and technology, which overcomes various shortcomings in conventional medicine (e.g., lack of efficiency and specificity) and brings medical diagnostics to the next level of performance [7]. One such technological advancement is electrospraying or electrohydrodynamic atomization (EHDA). By maintaining the capillary needle and the grounded collector at a high voltage (a few kilovolts), sample solutions are forced to come out of the needle in the form of micro-/nanosized particles/droplets and are deposited onto the collector/substrate (Fig. 10.1a) [8]. By virtue of advantages mentioned in the previous chapter(s), E-spray has been widely used in various disciplines such as mass spectrometry, materials deposition (e.g., surface coating, thin-film production, micro-/nanopatterning), micro-/nanoparticle, and capsule fabrications, notably for biomedical applications including tissue engineering, advanced aerosol drug delivery, biosensing, and diagnostics [9,10].

Biosensor is defined as an analytical device where a specific biological interaction between a targeted analyte and its complementary receptor (e.g., enzymes, proteins/nucleotides, antibodies, cells) takes place, giving rise to a physicochemical response that is picked up by a transducer element (Fig. 10.1b). Examples of such response can be an alteration of an electrical signal (e.g., potential, current), an optical signal (e.g., light intensity, refractive index), a thermal signal (heat transfer), or a mechanical signal (mass

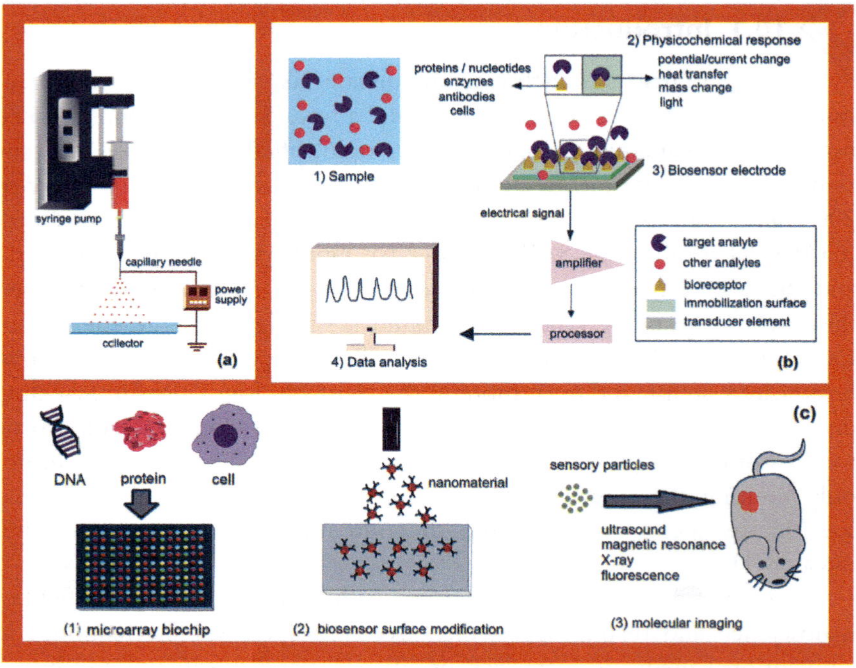

Figure 10.1 Schematic descriptions of (a) a typical setup of E-spray, (b) of a typical biosensor system, (c) three main applications of E-spray in biosensing and diagnostics (microarray biochip fabrication, biosensor surface modification, molecular imaging with sensory particles). *No Permission Required.*

change). The resulting transducer signal is typically in an electrical form that can be amplified, analyzed quantitatively, and processed into meaningful parameters for scientists to study the biological processes [11–13]. Biosensors have been widely used for numerous detection fields, ranging from biotechnological industries [14,15] to environmental [16], pharmaceutical [17], food researches [18], as well as clinical diagnostics. Following the first invention of the glucose enzyme electrode (glucometer for diabetes patients) by Clark and Lyon in 1962, several biosensing kits have been further developed for testing in pregnancy, infectious diseases (e.g., HIV, tuberculosis), metabolites (e.g., cholesterol, dopamine), whole cells, proteins, and nucleic acids. It is irrefutable that biosensors play important roles in life science researches and industries as well as human lives, therefore optimizing their performances are exceptionally crucial nowadays [19].

In this chapter, the focus will be put on the use of E-spray as a means of materials deposition to fabricate biochips and modify the biosensor surfaces along with its functions to produce sensory particles as well as other systems for biosensing and diagnostics purposes (Fig. 10.1c). Eventually, the limitations, challenges, conclusion, and outlook of ES in these topics will be discussed.

10.2 Fabrication of biosensors by electrospray

A biosensor typically contains a transducer element with a surface architecture where several important events such as immobilization, biorecognition, and sensing process occur (b). Deposition and immobilization of bioreceptors on the surface are challenging tasks in biosensor fabrication as they require preservation of the targeted biorecognition events as well as device stability for multiple usages with high reproducibility. Moreover, it is often necessary to functionalize the bare transducer surface by coating with proper materials to improve the sensitivity and biocompatibility of the biosensor. In both cases, the versatile assistance of E-spray may open a new door into high-performance biosensors and diagnostics [19–21].

10.2.1 Fabrication of biochips by electrospray depositions of bioreceptors

Among various deposition techniques (e.g., electrospraying, microspotting, ink-jet printing, microcontact printing), E-spray has arisen as a promising one due to its ability to simultaneously deposit a large amount as well as types of materials (e.g., DNA, proteins, polysaccharides, and biocompatible polymers) in a noncontact mode with retention of structures and activities [19,20] as well as high deposition efficiency [22], and cost-effectiveness [23]. Regarding these advantages, there have been several suggestions made for implementing E-spray to fabricate biosensor chips, particularly in micropatterning of proteins, DNA [24] and cells [23] for high throughput analyses (e.g., drug discovery, biochemical assays, biosensors, and disease diagnosis) [22]. While DNA microarrays provide a huge amount of valuable genomic information (e.g., gene expression profiling and DNA sequences) [25], protein microarrays reveal information at the protein level (e.g., post-translational modifications, protein–DNA interactions, or protein–protein interactions) [26]. Besides, cell-based sensors containing organized/patterned living cells immobilized on the transducer surfaces allow high-throughput monitoring of environmental perturbations such as the presence of toxic or pathogenic agents [23].

10.2.1.1 First attempts to develop DNA and protein biochips

The idea of using E-spray technique to fabricate DNA/protein microarray arose when Morozov et al. observed the complete activity preservation of alkaline phosphatase after being deposited by E-spray in the presence of disaccharides as protective substances [20]. Later, by using E-spray, they successfully generated mono- and multicomponent arrays with tiny spot sizes of 2–6 μm [24]. The patterns of multiple deposits were easily made by using a dielectric mask with holes on it. Several dots of diverse proteins (e.g., bovine serum albumin, human serum albumin, chicken ovalbumin, and human hemoglobin), DNA strands, and other organic substances (e.g., synthetic dyes) could be deposited concurrently under the control of electric field through an array of holes in the mask covering any moderately conductive substrate. After each deposition, the mask was shifted to another position for a new deposition. In the later step, by using different nozzles containing different solutions, multicomponent matrices and libraries could be created [22,24]. The deposited products could further be immobilized via different immobilization methods (e.g., covalently conjugating proteins to a dextran-grafted substrate) [27].

Additionally, under the dry condition of E-spray (less than 30% humidity), it was shown that the deposited proteins and DNA could reserve their potentials to specifically bind antibodies and complement with DNA probes, respectively [22,24,27,28]. This has enabled the further uses of E-spray to fabricate microarrays for qualitative and quantitative analyses of biological samples using, for instance, the protocols of DNA hybridization assay, dot-immunobinding assay, and enzyme-linked immunosorbent assay. Indeed, the protein arrays were successfully applied to rapidly detect West Nile virus-specific immunoglobulin M molecules in chicken serum [29] or *Mycobacterium tuberculosis*–specific immunoglobulins in human serum [30,31] with good sensitivity.

10.2.1.2 Further attempts to develop DNA and protein biochips

Following the study of Morozov et al. in 1999, there have been several attempts with some deviations in the E-spray setup and operation (e.g., different solutions, substrates, voltages, masks, and so on) to develop biochips. Most of them were summarized in Table 10.1 and the review [22]. Nonetheless, the use of a mask for patterning may lead to several drawbacks since highly charged E-spray particles can be unessentially deposited on the upper surface of the mask during electrospraying. Consequently, their accumulation creates electrostatic forces with the

Table 10.1 Biomolecular chips developed using E-spray technique.

Applications	E-Spray solutions	Substrates	Mask	Spot size; # of spots or wells	Some remarks	Reference
Protein film	Alkaline phosphatase	Quartz microbalance	Teflon or parafilm sheet	Film	Complete preservation of the enzyme activity at low current and humidity in the presence of disaccharides	[20]
Mono- and multicomponent microarrays	Lambda DNA, alkaline phosphatase (AP), horseradish peroxidase, HHb, human serum albumin (HSA), bovine serum albumin, ovalbumin, IgG fraction of a goat anti-HSA antiserum, mouse monoclonal antibiotin AP conjugate, some synthetic dyes	Gene screen membrane, metals (aluminum plating on a plastic film, gold on mica and silicon), semiconductors (SnO_2 layer on glass), nitrocellulose and PVDF membranes, Whatman paper, plasma-cleaned glass, and freshly cleaved mica	Inorganic (mica, glass), plastic (polypropylene, polyethylene, teflon, polystyrene, and others)	2–6 μm; varied number	Multiple dots can be deposited simultaneously; shifting the mask, followed by new substance deposition enabled multicomponent matrix formation	[24]
Protein microarray	Antichicken IgM antibody, West Nile virus antigens	Plasma-activated membrane made of regenerated cellulose	Nylon mesh	30–50 μm; spaced by 150 μm	Functionalized magnetic beads were used as active labels; fast assay time of 15 min	[29]
Protein microarray	*Mycobacterium tuberculosis*, polyclonal antibody, ovalbumin	Plasma-activated membrane made of regenerated cellulose	Polystyrene mesh, polyester mesh	7 spots	Functionalized magnetic beads were used as active labels; sensitivity of 10 fg/mL	[30,31]
Protein chip	Lactate dehydrogenase, glucose-6-phosphate dehydrogenase, pyruvate kinase	Silicon substrates (2 × 1 cm) with a 50-nm-thick silicon nitride top layer	n/a	130 and 350 μm at spray distance of 220 and 400 μm, respectively	Spots were generated by a computer-controlled x-y-z table system where deposition relied on electric field strength, which was characterized by the distance between substrate and capillary tip; E-spraying directly into wells	[32]
Protein chip	Enolase, lactate dehydrogenase, pyruvate kinase	Well (400 μm wide, 50 μm deep) in silicon substrate	n/a	250–350 μm; 25 wells	Quantitative analysis of enzymatic reactions in nanoliter volumes on-chip; E-spraying directly into wells; evaporation of assay liquid could be prevented using coverslip	[107]

(Continued)

Table 10.1 Biomolecular chips developed using E-spray technique.—cont'd

Applications	E-Spray solutions	Substrates	Mask	Spot size; # of spots or wells	Some remarks	Reference
Protein chip	Rhodamine B	Silicon wafer having 200, 300, 400 μm wide, 19.8–55 μm deep and 200–400 μm apart wells coated with a 50 nm-thick silicon nitride layer	n/a	Arrays of 25 and 100 wells	Suitable for quantitative analysis; E spraying directly in wells; evaporation could be prevented using coverslip	[33]
Protein microarray	Protein A, biotin	Substrate with microfabricated hydrogel features (1–10 μm)	n/a	n/a	Multiple needles for simultaneous spraying; delivery of picoliter volumes; one sharp edge on each tip to avoid the accumulation of charges at the corners, thereby preventing multiple flows and corona discharge; Schiff base chemistry followed by reductive amination was utilized for covalent immobilization	[34]
Protein microarray	Human cytokines	Aldehyde-modified indium-tin oxide (CHO-ITO) glass plate	Flat dielectric masks with holes of 150 μm in diameter or slit-like apertures of 300 μm in width	Stripe width of about 250 μm	The microarrays were also integrated into microfluidic chips with a PDMS microchannel; sensitivity of 100 pg/mL; allowed high-throughput detection	[26]
Protein and nanoparticle array; gas (CO, H_2) sensor	Collagen–FITC conjugate; silver, copper, zinc oxide, and polystyrene latex nanoparticles	200-Nm thick SiO_2-coated Si substrate; nonconducting glass substrates; 0.1-mm thick flexible poly(ethylene-terephthalate) film	Silicon nitride masks and flexible epoxy masks (opening size: 500 nm to 50 μm)	Varied	Ion-induced focusing mask to improve the array density; deposit distinct materials on the same substrate without contamination; no surface modifications needed	[35]
Protein film, calcium sensing	α-Lactalbumin	Poly(ethylene terephthalate) film coated with aluminum	n/a	Pore diameters of 40–600 nm	Rough and fine porous structure; cross-linking after deposition to become freestanding and insoluble to water	[36]
Cell patterning	Fibronectin	Silicon substrates with a polished {111} face	n/a	Droplets of 40–100 nm	Increasing the surface density of deposited fibronectin could improve fibroblast attachment	[37]

Cell patterning	PLGA particles	Hydrophobic substrate (plastic slides) coated with pluronic F127 (cell adhesion inhibitor); dielectric glass slides	Dielectric mask with hole size of 150 × 150 μm	Particle size ranging from 200 nm to several tens of microns	Various patterns including patterned dots, circles, squares, and bands; a high voltage could be applied directly to the mask to generate an "electrostatic focusing effect" that would improve the patterned precision deposition of particles	[23]
Cell patterning	PCL or PLGA particle	Hydrophobic PDMS—coated glass slides	Stainless steel mesh	Size gradient	Applying additional voltages to the mask and grounding point, bar, or line electrode positioned under the substrate allowed particle patterns with both uniform size and size gradients	[38]
Cell patterning	Bacterial cells (*Staphylococcus epidermidis*)	Silicon wafer	n/a	Around 10 μm diameter spots, containing a single cell	Drop-on-demand 1D and 2D patterning with E-spray pulsed jet; line pattern was possible; single bacterial cell could be manipulated in the solid and gas phase (beside liquid phase)	[39,40]
Cell patterning	Yeast cells	Silicon wafer with a diameter of 12 cm placed on a stainless-steel plate	n/a	Distances between spots of 30, 83, 158 μm	Multidimensional patterns; pulsed jet E-spray mode; the system showed high alcoholic fermentation rate; distance between the droplets could be varied by changing translation speed	[41]

forthcoming E-spray particles and hampers the precise shapes of the resulting patterns [42]. There are, indeed, alternative ways to generate patterns/arrays apart from the uses of masks. For example, Moerman et al. have early used E-spray to reproducibly dispense liquid volumes between 50 and 600 pL into wells of a microarray [43,107]. Further, E-spray was developed to deliver reagent solutions (e.g., enolase, lactate dehydrogenase, pyruvate kinase, glucose-6-phosphate dehydrogenase, rhodamine B) into nanosized wells (50 μm depth and 400 μm width) of microarrays to quantitatively monitor enzyme-based reactions with luminescence (Fig. 10.2a) [32,33]; n.d.). Notably, rows of spots were generated by a computer-controlled x-y-z table system. After each deposition, spraying was stopped immediately by shifting the substrate downward to increase the distance between the substrate and the capillary tip and decrease the electric field. The spraying could be resumed for the next deposition by quickly moving the substrate sideways to a new well and lifting it upward to restore the high electric field (Fig. 10.2b) [32,107].

Instead of using a single needle, a multiplexed E-spray deposition device (MESDD) comprising of multiple sprayings at the same time could significantly increase the speed of microarray production in a noncontact fashion. MESDD manufactured by the silicon micromachining technology contains four parallel E-spray source tips with only one sharp edge on each tip to avoid the accumulation of charges at the corners, thereby preventing occurrences of multiple flows and corona discharge during operation [34]. This approach excludes the uses of the capillary needle and dielectric mask, which introduce complexity for their precise alignments in the system. In addition, the hydrogel patterned substrate functionalized with aldehyde groups could allow protein molecules to covalently link through strong amide bonds for immobilization. The system made in this way would perfectly fit the planar microfabrication platform and the miniaturization approach of the lap-on-chip technology. Particularly, while microfluidics enables minimal consumption of analyte volumes, MESDD allows delivering of tiny volumes that can significantly improve the capacity of the integrated devices. Another approach with E-spray—based microarrays for high-throughput immunoassay on an aldehyde-modified indium-tin oxide (CHO-ITO) glass plate substrate was also introduced and further integrated into microfluidic chips with a polydimethylsiloxane (PDMS) microchannel for concurrent detection of human cytokines with appreciable sensitivity (100 pg/mL) [26]. The protein dots sprayed on the CHO-ITO substrate were uniform in size and remained highly active after deposition.

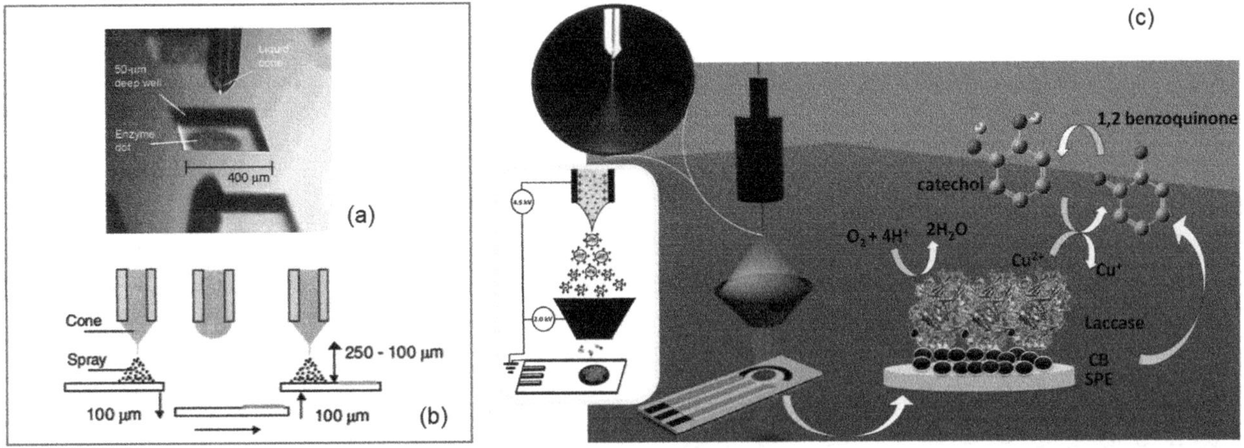

Figure 10.2 (a) Prefilling of nanoliter wells (180 × magnified) with 400-µm width and 50-µm depth. (b) Schematic view of controlled spraying: spraying stops by increasing the distance between the tip and substrate, spraying resumes by restoring the distance. (c) Schematic representation of the E-spray setup applied for laccase immobilization on carbon black-nanomodified screen-printed electrodes (left); the Taylor cone recorded by the camera during E-spray deposition (in the inset); the catalytic reaction of laccase leading to catechol oxidation and dioxygen reduction is indicated by the arrows (right). *(a) Reprinted with permission from R. Moerman, J. Knoll, C. Apetrei, L.R. Van Den Doel, G.W.K. Van Dedem. Quantitative analysis in nanoliter wells by prefilling of wells using electrospray deposition followed by sample introduction with a coverslip method, Anal. Chem. 77 (2005) 225–231. https://doi.org/10.1021/ac0400515. Copyright 2005, American Chemical Society; (b) Reprinted with permission from R. Moerman, J. Frank, J.C.M. Marijnissen, T.G.M. Schalkhammer, G.W.K. Van Dedem, Miniaturized electrospraying as a technique for the production of microarrays of reproducible micrometer-sized protein spots, Anal. Chem. 73 (10) (2001) 2183–2189. https://doi.org/10.1021/ac001041g. Copyright 2001, American Chemical Society; (c) Reprinted with permission from M.C. Castrovilli, P. Bolognesi, J. Chiarinelli, L. Avaldi, A. Cartoni, P. Calandra, E. Tempesta, M.T. Giardi, A. Antonacci, F. Arduini, V. Scognamiglio, Electrospray deposition as a smart technique for laccase immobilisation on carbon black-nanomodified screen-printed electrodes, Biosens. Bioelectron. 163 (2020) https://doi.org/10.1016/j.bios.2020.112299. Copyright 2020, Elsevier B.V.*

In another case, You et al. presented an ion-induced focusing mask that could be continually applied to improve the array density and/or deposit distinct materials on the same substrate without contamination [35]. Particularly, this mask was conducted under simultaneous deposition of ions and charged aerosols that gave rise to invisible electrostatic lenses surrounding each mask opening, through which E-spray particles were convergently guided into the opening center instead of landing and accumulating on the mask surface. This, therefore, has reduced the loss of deposited materials and generated a high-resolution parallel patterning, for instance, collagen and metal nanoparticles arrays for prospective sensing applications (e.g., zinc oxide nanoparticle patterns for effectively sensing CO and H_2 gas).

Besides protein arrays, protein thin films (e.g., α-Lactalbumin (α-LA) [36], iron-free cytochrome *c* (Cyt. *c*) [45]) could also be generated by versatile E-spray deposition method for biosensing purposes. After being deposited, the α-LA film could be cross-linked to become freestanding and insoluble to water. The surface morphologies of the cross-linked α-LA films were investigated and showed rough and fine porous structure with pore diameters varied from 40 to 600 nm, potentially increasing the active surface area, and thus improving the detection ability. Additionally, the mechanochemical measurements (isometric tensions) of the films based on the conformational changes of α-LA caused by calcium ions binding were studied. The deposited α-LA films could respond specifically to different concentrations of calcium ions, indicating high biological activity preservation of the film [36]. Moreover, a transparent iron-free Cyt. *c* protein film successfully made by ESD is also promising for protein microarray fabrication. However, in this study, E-spray conditions and cross-linking agent should be optimized to limit the interference on the protein tertiary structure [45]. Besides, Castrovilli et al. recently applied E-spray to immobilize laccase enzyme on carbon black-nanomodified screen-printed electrodes for selective amperometric detection of catechol in the presence of other interfering components (e.g., lead, atrazine, cadmium, paraoxon) with the linear range of 2.5—50 μM and the limit of detection of 2 μM (Fig. 10.2c) [44]. Moreover, laccase was shown to retain its activity up to 3 months at room temperature and allow up to 25 measurements with good stability in case of storing and working, respectively.

Apart from several efforts to adjust the setup and operation of E-spray, the performance and applications of biochips can also be improved by employing appropriate detection methods as well as specific biorecognition elements and analytes (e.g., electrophoretic capturing of charged analytes from the flow on an antibody array [46], applying micromagnetic beads coated with secondary antibodies as labels [31,46], coupling with high-resolution charged-coupled device detector, detecting different cytokines [26], using coverslip to completely avoid the evaporation of assay liquid during monitoring of enzyme-based reactions (n.d.) and so on). These approaches are involved in the later stage, after the deposition step of the microarray production, and thus will not be described in detail here.

10.2.1.3 Cell patterning in cell-based sensors

Cell patterning usually includes deposition of cell-adhesion molecules (e.g., fibronectin [37], collagen [47], polymers [23]) with designed patterns onto a substrate coated with a hydrophobic material [38] or cell adhesion inhibitor [23], followed by cell seeding and adhesion above the patterned molecules. For instance, Xie et al. generated a variety of cell patterns including dots, circles, squares, and bands by initially coating the substrate with a cell adhesion blocker (pluronic F127), followed by E-spray deposition of cell-adhesive poly(lactic-co-glycolic acid) (PLGA) particles through a mask that gave the patterns of interest. Subsequently, cells were cultured on the substrate and patterned correspondingly to the PLGA particle patterns. In addition, cell-adhesive materials like fibronectin and collagen could also be sprayed along with the polymers to enhance the cell adhesive capability. Especially, in this study, a high voltage could be applied directly to the mask to generate an electrostatic focusing effect that would improve the patterned precision deposition of particles [23].

In a related process, Yan et al. showed that cell patterns could be formed on the cell-adhesive poly(ε-caprolactone) (PCL) or PLGA particle patterns deposited on hydrophobic PDMS-coated glass slides [38]. While uniform patterns were typically observed in the previous studies with E-spray deposition through a mask, this study especially demonstrated the particle patterns with both uniform size and size gradients. This was made by applying additional voltages to the mask and grounding point, bar, or line electrode positioned under the substrate (Fig. 10.3a and b). Indeed, different configurations of the ground electrode caused different gradient patterns and the size of particle patterns determined the size of the cell patterns. Therefore, the thick PDMS coating (Fig. 10.3b) ($\sim$100 μm) resulted in uniform patterns of PLGA particles and cells (Fig. 10.3c), whereas without/thin PDMS coating ($\sim$10 μm) (Fig. 10.3a) gave both of them gradient patterns (Fig. 10.3d).

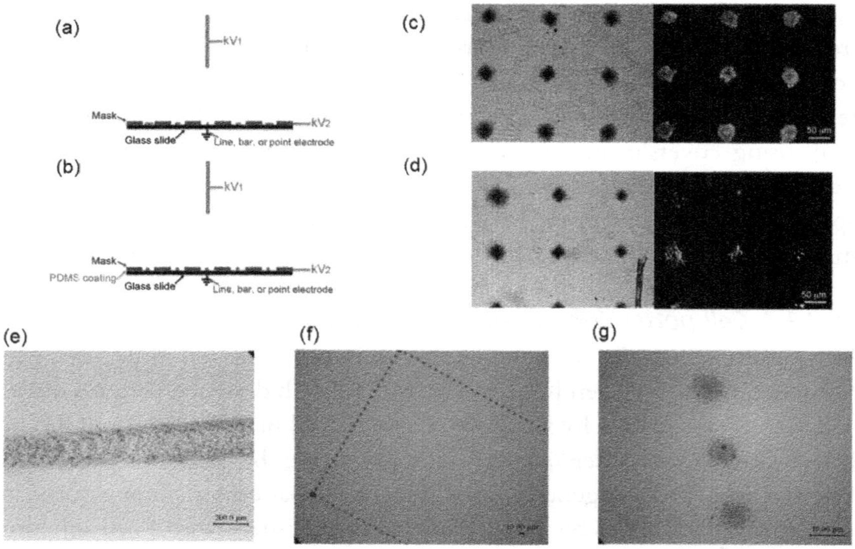

Figure 10.3 Schematic of electrical field–guided E-spray deposition with (a) glass slide substrate gives a gradient particle pattern, and (b) PDMS-coated glass slide substrate gives uniform particle pattern. Optical phase contrast (left) and fluorescence microscopy (right) images of living cell (stained in green) patterns formation on the PLGA particle patterns deposited on (c) thick PDMS–coated or (d) thin PDMS–coated glass slide substrate. (e) Line patterns of electrosprayed bacterial cells (*Staphylococcus epidermidis*) just after the deposition process; (f) Rectangular 2D pattern of bacterial suspension spots (average spot diameter of 7 μm); (g) Magnified picture of a 2D pattern with a scale bar of 10 μm. *(a,b,c,d) Reprinted with permission from W.C. Yan, J. Xie, C.H. Wang, Electrical field guided electrospray deposition for production of gradient particle patterns, ACS Appl. Mater. Interfaces 10 (22) (2018) 18499–18506. https://doi.org/10.1021/acsami.8b02914. Copyright 2018, American Chemical Society; (e,f,g) Reprinted with permission from K. Kim, B.U. Lee, G.B. Hwang, J.H. Lee, S. Kim, Drop-on-demand patterning of bacterial cells using pulsed jet electrospraying, Anal. Chem. 82 (5) (2010) 2109–2112. https://doi.org/10.1021/ac9027966. Copyright 2010, American Chemical Society.*

Interestingly, Kim et al. utilized pulsed-mode E-spray to produce 1D and 2D arrays of bacterial cells (one bacteria per spot) on a raw silicon wafer (Fig. 10.3f and g) [39]. This technology is often referred to as voltage-modulated E-spray, nano-E-spray, or drop-on-demand E-spray where a high voltage is applied to the glass capillary (tip diameter of 1–30 μm) in short pulses and results in a fixed and extremely small volume (on the order of pico- and femtoliters) of droplet ejects from the tip of a periodically formed short-lived (microseconds) Taylor cone in a stable frequency pulsation [48]. While the jet is formed, the ground plate of the E-spray is shifted horizontally at a speed of 0.4–2 mm/s, generating an array of spots. Besides, the line patterns (Fig. 10.3e) could also be generated by performing at the relatively higher flow rate and lower translation speed as compared to the spot patterning (Fig. 10.3f and g) [39]. Further improvements on drop-on-demand E-spray have enabled the production of more complex alphabetical patterns of bacterial cells. Additionally, the viability of the patterned cells was tested positively by staining methods [40]. Recently, a multidimensional patterning of viable yeast cells at cellular resolution was generated similarly by pulsed jet E-spray and showed promising applications in the microfermentation process as well as biochips [41].

10.2.2 Biosensor surface modifications by electrospray depositions of nanomaterials

Direct conjugation of bioreceptors to a bare transducer surface is often associated with negative feedbacks such as toxicity to the bioreceptors, reduction in the performance and lifespan of the biosensor [11,19,49]. Therefore, approaches to incorporate biocompatible nanomaterials with good electrical conductivity, mechanical, optical, and/or magnetic properties onto biosensor surfaces are considered to overcome these limitations. Indeed, nanomaterials can enhance the surface areas as well as the surface-to-volume ratios of the sensing systems, thereby enabling larger amounts of biological components to be captured on their surfaces along with improving the detection limits, sensitivity, and specificity. Furthermore, nanomaterials can function as effective immobilization layers for bioreceptors while maintaining their catalytic activities and innate features. Some nanomaterials may even support catalytically active centers, replacing enzymes in nonenzymatic-based biosensor [19,50]. Hereby in this part, depositions of nanomaterials (e.g., graphene, zinc oxide, gold nanoparticle) onto the electrode surface with E-spray were given as examples to improve the performance of biosensors (Table 10.2).

10.2.2.1 Deposition of graphene-based materials

Graphene displays fast electron transportation, outstanding mechanical strength, thermal conductivity, and biocompatibility [49,57]. Graphene is usually combined with other materials (e.g., metals, metal oxides, other carbon-based materials) to become useful nanocomposites for electronic devices, including biosensors [62]. For example, by using E-spray, Liu et al. deposited a nanocomposite composed of poly(3,4-ethylenedioxy thiophene), poly(styrene sulfonate), and graphene nanoplatelets (PPG

Table 10.2 Applications of E-spray in surface modifications of biosensors.

Application	E-Spray solution	Substrate	Some remarks	Reference
Detection of dopamine	PPG composite	Fluorine doped tin oxide electrode	Sulfuric acid treatment improved electrode–electrolyte interface, electrochemical activity, stability, and current response	[51]
Detection of cholesterol	G/PVP/PANI composite	Paper-based electrode	PVP enabled a large surface area and high conductivity; modified electrode gave a threefold improved current signal and a better cyclic voltammogram for standard ferri/ferrocyanide; performed supreme electrocatalytic oxidation of H_2O_2; amperometric detection of cholesterol (limit of detection of 1 μM)	[52]
Detecting Zn(II), Cd(II), and Pb(II)	G/PANI nanocomposite	Trimethylsilylated Nafion-coated electrodes	Detection limits equal to or lower than 1 ppb, good reproducibility (%RSD $<$ 11) and broad linear ranges (1–300 μg/L)	[53]
Detection of H_2O_2	G/Nafion nanocomposite film	ITO electrode	Assess the toxicity level of nanomaterials for biomedical and environmental applications	[54]

Detection of free chlorine	Crumpled graphene oxide (CGO)	Surface of tin oxide (SnO_2) nanocolumn electrode	High selectivity and sensitivity in PBS at pH 7.4 and real tap water with the sensitivity of 2.69 and 5.86 μA/μM/cm, respectively, within a broad linear range of 0.1 −10.08 ppm	[63]
Detection of H_2O_2	Graphene films	Patterned 3D structures (e.g., carbon micropillar electrodes)	Precise thickness and controlled morphology; 3D provides larger surface areas and enhanced chemical functionality compared to traditional 2D	[55]
Gas sensor	Precursor zinc acetate dihydrate (ZnAc)/glycerol solution	Space between two Au electrodes on a glass substrate	Alterations of resistance in alcohol vapors and air were measured to calculate the sensing response	[56]
Photodetectors and gas sensor	First, depositing graphene flakes and subsequently zinc oxide	Silicone substrate	The film showed satisfactory electrical performance and high transparency	[57]
Ultrasonic sensing underwater condition	Orderly piezoelectric ZnO nanorods	Au/chromium/silicon substrates	Hydrothermal process was needed in addition to E-spray	[58]
FET sensor to detect Hg(II)	Au NPs	rGO sheets	E-spray in combination with ESFDA technique; Au NPs were further functionalized with TGA containing a thiol group for anchoring Au NPs to the surface and a carboxylic group for chelation of Hg(II) ion; lowest detected Hg(II) concentration of 2.5×10^{-8} M and rapid response (<10 s)	[59]

(Continued)

Table 10.2 Applications of E-spray in surface modifications of biosensors.—cont'd

Application	E-Spray solution	Substrate	Some remarks	Reference
Protein sensor	Au NP—antibody conjugates	Thermally reduced graphene oxide (TRGO)	Low detection limit on the order of ng/mL and is promising for detecting numerous proteins by adjusting suitable antibodies	[60]
Protein sensor	Au NPs coated with horseradish peroxidase antibody (anti-HRP)	The outer surface of carbon nanotubes (CNTs)	E-spray and ESFDA technique	[60,61]

composite) onto a fluorine-doped tin oxide electrode for sensitive detection of dopamine in aqueous medium containing interfering species like ascorbic acid and uric acid [51]. Moreover, additional sulfuric acid treatment of the PPG composite has enabled ameliorations of electrode—electrolyte interface, electrochemical activity, stability, and current response.

Another nanocomposite of graphene, polyvinylpyrrolidone, and polyaniline (G/PVP/PANI) was successfully prepared by Ruecha et al. using ES technique to modify a paper-based electrode [52]. The droplet-like nanostructures (average size of 160 ± 1.02 nm) and the presence of PVP in the modified electrode had enabled a large surface area and high conductivity, respectively, which substantially enhanced the electrochemical sensitivity of the sensor. The modified electrode gave a threefold increased current signal and a better cyclic voltammogram for standard ferri/ferrocyanide as compared to the raw electrode. Besides, it also performed supreme electrocatalytic oxidation of hydrogen peroxide (H_2O_2) and amperometric detection of cholesterol with a limit of detection of 1 μM. Further study with trimethylsilylated Nafion-coated electrodes modified with G/PANI nanocomposite showed increased sensitivity for detecting Zn(II), Cd(II), and Pb(II) in the presence of common interfering metals (e.g., Mn(II), Cu(II), Fe(III), Fe(II), Co(III), and Ni(II)) with detection limits equal to or lower than 1 ppb, good reproducibility (%RSD < 11), and broad linear ranges (1—300 μg/L) [53]. The system could measure metals in human serum with high efficiency. Similarly, Yoon et al. developed a cell-based electrochemical sensing system for the detection of released H_2O_2 using the ITO electrode modified with a G/Nafion nanocomposite film by E-spray deposition [54]. The system is promising to assess the toxicity level of nanomaterials for biomedical and environmental applications. Additionally, a crumpled graphene oxide—tin oxide (CGO-SnO_2) composite electrode was produced by decorating the surface of SnO_2 nanocolumns with CGO using E-spray [63]. The electrodes displayed high selectivity and sensitivity for detection of free chlorine in phosphate buffer solution at pH 7.4 and real tap water with the sensitivity of 2.69 and 5.86 μA/μM/cm, respectively, within a broad linear range of 0.1—10.08 ppm.

Notably, the integration of graphene onto patterned 3D structures (e.g., carbon micropillar electrodes) with precise thickness and controlled morphology was achieved by Penmatsa et al. using E-spray deposition [55]. A 3D coating is advantageous because it provides larger surface areas and enhanced chemical functionality compared to traditional 2D designs.

The morphologies of the deposited graphene films were shown to be influenced by substrate temperature, deposition time, and nozzle to substrate distance. In addition, the amperometric response of graphene/carbon micropillar electrode arrays displayed excellent electrochemical activity, enhanced charge transfer, sensitive, rapid, and linear response toward the changes in hydrogen peroxide concentration, especially, in the range between 250 and 5.5 mM.

10.2.2.2 Deposition of zinc oxide—-based materials

Semiconductor ZnO-based materials exhibiting high electron transportation and supreme radiation hardness for numerous applications, including sensors, can also be deposited using E-spray. For example, precursor zinc acetate dihydrate (ZnAc)/glycerol solution was electrosprayed over the space between two Au electrodes on a glass substrate, followed by calcination process to create ZnO thin film of which resistance alterations in alcohol vapors (R_g) and air (R_0) were measured to calculate the sensing response defined as resistance ratio R_0/R_g. The ratio increased with the concentration of alcohol vapors and the deposition time of E-spray [56]. For another instance, graphene/zinc oxide composite thin film made by E-spray deposition may be promising for the fabrication of optoelectronic devices such as photodetectors and gas sensor devices. This composite thin film can be made by first coating the silicone substrate with graphene flakes and subsequently depositing zinc oxide [57]. The film showed satisfactory electrical performance and high transparency. For another example, Pan et al. applied E-spray and hydrothermal process to grow orderly piezoelectric ZnO nanorods, which generate electricity via external force-induced deformations, selectively on Au/chromium/silicon substrates for ultrasonic sensing underwater condition [58]. The ZnO nanorods were obtained with heights of 3—5 μm (aspect ratio from 10 to 16) and the electric field of 800 V/mm was determined to achieve uniform seed layers. Also, they observed that the more the E-spray times, the denser the coverage rates; nevertheless, the electrosprayed droplets and the uniformity became larger and poorer, respectively.

10.2.2.3 Deposition of gold nanoparticles

Decorating gold nanoparticles (Au NPs) prepared beforehand with well-known functionalization chemistry onto the sensor surfaces has been recognized as an effective indirect immobilization strategy, especially for biomolecules, with preservation in biological activities, increase in sensitivity, selectivity, and stability. For instance, Chen et al. reported a hybrid platform based on reduced graphene oxide (rGO) and thioglycolic acid (TGA)-functionalized Au NPs (rGO/TGA-AuNP) that could be used as a field-effect transistor (FET) sensor to detect Hg(II) in solutions (Fig. 10.4a) [59]. Notably, Au NPs were assembled on the rGO sheets by E-spray combining with electrostatic force directed assembly (ESFDA) technique. Au NPs were further functionalized with TGA containing a thiol group for anchoring Au NPs to the surface and a carboxylic group for chelation of Hg(II) ion. The system gave the lowest detected Hg(II) concentration of 2.5×10^{-8} M and rapid response (<10 s) after the addition of Hg(II)-containing solution to the active area of the sensors. In another case, they introduced a protein sensor using thermally reduced graphene oxide (TRGO) ES-decorated with Au NP—antibody conjugates (Fig. 10.4b) [64]. The system showed the lower detection limit on the order of ng/mL and is promising for detecting numerous proteins by adjusting suitable antibodies. Similarly, Au NPs coated with horseradish peroxidase antibody (anti-HRP) were deposited by E-spray and ESFDA onto the outer surface of carbon nanotubes (CNTs) (Fig. 10.4c) [60,61]. Upon the introduction of antigen HRP, the drain current was increased owing to the specific binding of HRP with anti-HRP detected by FET measurements. The schematic of Au NP-anti HRP conjugates deposition by E-spray and assembly by ESFDA is shown in Fig. 10.4d. Similar setups were applied to the two previous examples.

10.3 Fabrication of sensory micro-/nanoparticles for molecular imaging

Molecular imaging (e.g., magnetic resonance imaging (MRI), ultrasound, fluorescence imaging) allows investigating biological processes at the cellular and subcellular levels in intact organisms/cells. Besides being executed as a deposition method, E-spray has shown promising applications in several imaging modalities for biosensing and diagnostics. This is achieved by generating micro- and nanoparticles that act as molecular probes (e.g., fluorescent molecules/dyes), contrast agents (e.g., microbubble, magnetic particle), and/or theranostic platforms, which integrate diagnostic imaging capability with therapeutic functions (Table 10.3) [80,81]. The small-sized sensory particles are advantageous due to easy administration and potentially escaping the immune system responses, hence elongating their useful lives [50].

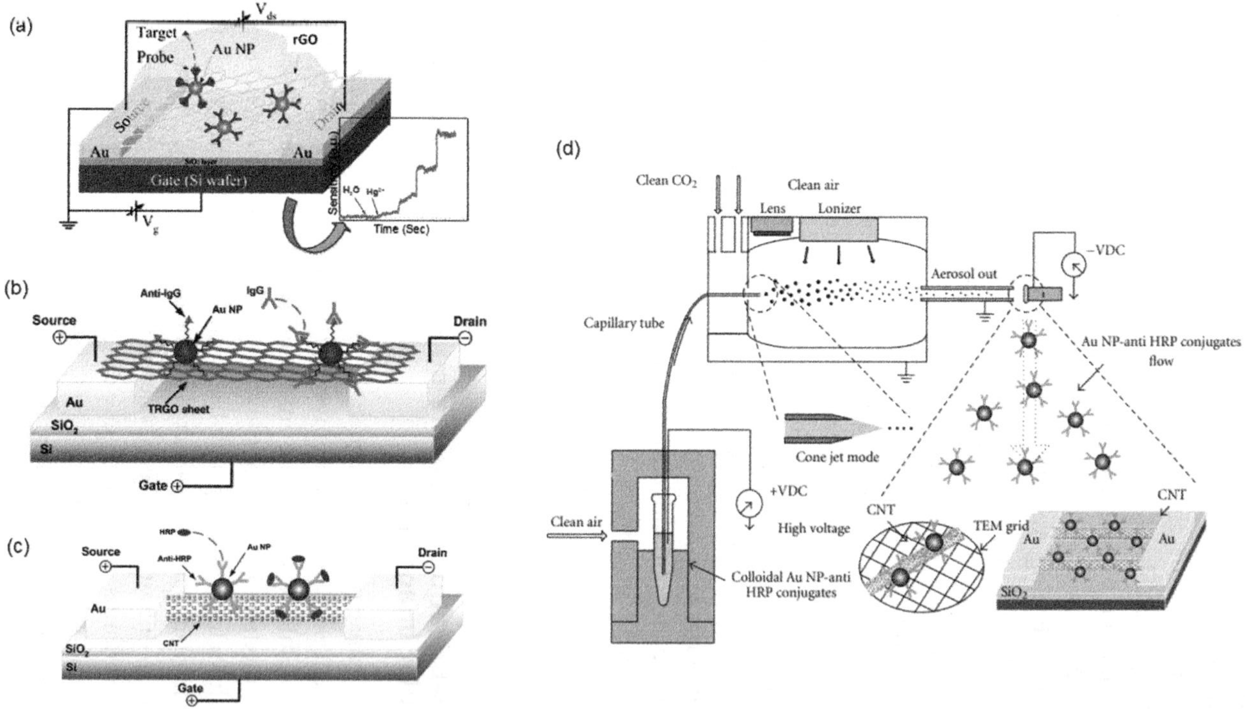

Figure 10.4 (a) Schematic of a rGO FET (TGA probe was anchored to the rGO surface through Au NPs and specifically recognized Hg(II)). (b) Schematic of a TRGO FET (Anti-IgG was anchored to the TRGO sheet surface through Au NPs and specifically recognized the complementary IgG). (c) Schematic of a CNTFET (Anti-HRP was anchored to the CNT surface through Au NPs and specifically recognized HRP). (d) Schematic of Au NP—anti HRP conjugates deposition by an E-spray and their subsequent assembly onto CNTs by ESFDA. *(a) Reprinted with permission from K. Chen, G. Lu, J. Chang, S. Mao, K. Yu, S. Cui, J, Chen, Hg(II) ion detection using thermally reduced graphene oxide decorated with*

functionalized gold nanoparticles, Anal. Chem. 84 (9) (2012) 4057–4062. https://doi.org/10.1021/ac3000336. Copyright 2012, American Chemical Society; (b) Reprinted with permission from S. Mao, G. Lu, K. Yu, Z. Bo, J. Chen, Specific protein detection using thermally reduced graphene oxide sheet decorated with gold nanoparticle-antibody conjugates, Adv. Mater. 22 (32) (2010). 3521–3526. https://doi.org/10.1002/adma.201000520. Copyright 2010, Wiley; (c) Reprinted with permission from S. Mao, G. Lu, K. Yu, Z. Bo, J. Chen, Specific biosensing using carbon nanotubes functionalized with gold nanoparticle-antibody conjugates, Carbon N. Y., vol. 48, no. 2, pp. 479–486, 2010, https://doi.org/10.1016/j.carbon.2009.09.065. Copyright 2009, Elsevier B.V.; (d) Reprinted with permission from J. Chen, S. Mao, G. Lu, K. Yu, Protein viability on Au nanoparticles during an electrospray and electrostatic-force-directed assembly process, J. Nanomater. 2010. https://doi.org/10.1155/2010/196393. Copyright 2010, Shun Mao et al.

Table 10.3 Applications of E-spray in producing sensory micro-/nanoparticles for molecular imaging.

Application	Particle type	Sizes	Some remarks	Reference
Ultrasound imaging	Phospholipid-coated air MBs	5.1 ± 2 μm	Hybrid electrospray/T-junction device; stability up to 2 h	[83]
Ultrasound imaging	Glycerol-coated air MBs	2–8 μm	The ratio between the liquid flow rate in the outer needle and the air-flow rate (set at 1.7 μL/s) in the inner needle was 1.5; addition of polyethylene glycol 400 to glycerol could improve the MBs stability, lifetime, and also minimize their sizes	[65,84]
Ultrasound imaging	Bovine serum albumin (BSA) MBs	40–800 μm	Enhancing the flow rate of the BSA solution could decrease the polydispersity of the MBs; uses of distilled water-glutaraldehyde, glycerol, and glycerol-Tween 80 collection media, instead of BSA, lead to remarkable stability improvement; also, increasing the concentration of BSA solution could improve the compression stiffness	[66]
Ultrasound theranostic	tPA-BSA MBs and tPA-lipid MBs	41% tPA-lipid MBs (3 and 6 μm), 36% tPA-lipid MBs(6–9 μm),	Well-dispersed and less bubble-aggregated properties; tPA-lipid MBs gave more promising sizes for medical applications	[67]

		tPA-BSA MBs (41 μm)	(e.g., ischemic stroke therapy); MBs could be traced at a low-intensity ultrasound, while ultrasound at high intensity could trigger their drug releases; utilizing sulfur hexafluoride gas (SF_6) as the core showed an enhancement in the stability of tPA-lipid bubbles	
Ultrasound imaging	Biodegradable $P_2O_5-CaO-Na_2O$ phosphate-based glass nanospheres (PGNs)	200−500 nm	E-spray of the sol−gel mixture into silicone oil; PGNs could label cells in vitro and in vivo with the detection limits of 5 and 9 μg/mL, respectively.; easily metabolized degraded products within the body	[68]
MRI theranostic	Magnetic polymer yolk−shell particles (YSPs)	Mean diameter of 13.5 ± 1.74 μm	Using a trineedle coaxial E-spray technique with the stable cone-jet mode; magnetic Fe_3O_4 NPs (20 nm) embedded in the PCL shell, an interfacing silicone oil layer, and a PCL core; multifunctional theranostic agents, magnetically controlled delivery, multiactive co-encapsulation with low cytotoxicity	[69]

(*Continued*)

Table 10.3 Applications of E-spray in producing sensory micro-/nanoparticles for molecular imaging.—cont'd

Application	Particle type	Sizes	Some remarks	Reference
MRI theranostic	Tristearin core–shell particle system that encapsulates superparamagnetic iron oxide nanoparticles (SPIONs) (10–15 nm) with genistein, a BODIPY fluorescent dye, and PEG	0.65–1.2 μm in diameter	Encapsulation in a single step under ambient conditions using a coaxial electrospray process; PEG was added to avoid particle aggregation and ensure water solubility, while BODIPY gave excellent optical properties; cellular internalization observed with only 4 h of incubation; high drug encapsulation efficiencies of 92%; low toxicity	[70]
MRI	Fe_3O_4-loaded polymeric particles	Varied, from 1300 to 2000 nm	Oleic acid–capped magnetite NPs were incorporated into biocompatible and biodegradable PLGA FPs; oleic acid prevented magnetite aggregation; elevating the voltage did not influence the particle size significantly; nonetheless, the particle size increased substantially as the flow rate increased; a wide range magnetite content could be obtained	[71]
X-ray imaging	BaS04@BaAlg microspheres	200–1800 mm in diameter	In vivo imaging gave real-time location, distribution, and stable embolization over 3 weeks with	[72]

			radiodensity fluctuation within 7% of the starting value over 52 days; angiographic and histological analyses on an embolized kidney confirmed the complete blood vessels occlusion of the targeted kidney, including peripheral vessels, by the microspheres	
X-ray theranostic	Calcium alginate (CaAlg) microspheres loaded with tantalum (Ta) nanoparticles (Ta@CaAlg microspheres)	150–1200 μm	Maintained good X-ray imaging of the embolized sites up to 4 weeks and showed an excellent embolic effect; Ta@CaAlg microspheres could be loaded with a model drug (e.g., Dox) with pH-dependent release profile for promising therapeutic effects	[73]
Fluorescence theranostic	Acetyl curcumin (AC)-loaded PLGA core/shell liposome NPs	650 ± 50 nm	For drug delivery as well as bioimaging and screening for anticancer purposes	[74]
Fluorescence theranostic	Lipoplexes: lipids encapsulated imaging reagent (quantum dots, QD605) and the therapeutic reagent (Cy5-labeled antisense oligodeoxynucleotides, Cy5-G3139)	194 ± 15 nm	Static micromixer-coaxial E-spray setup; polydispersity of 0.024 ± 0.006	[75]

(Continued)

Table 10.3 Applications of E-spray in producing sensory micro-/nanoparticles for molecular imaging.—cont'd

Application	Particle type	Sizes	Some remarks	Reference
Fluorescence imaging	Composite spheres of CsPbBr3 nanocrystals encapsulating green luminescence PVDF	614 nm	The products showed a full width at half maximum of 20 nm, remained stable in water, and could be used in cell membrane imaging with low toxicity; may enable a novel cell analysis in aqueous environments	[76]
SERS, fluorescence imaging	Anisotropic biohybrid microparticles (MPs)	1.19 ± 0.17 μm (dry) and 4.08 ± 0.58 μm (swollen)	Spatioselectively coupled with two different antibodies (Abs) for fluorescence-based multiplexing sensing of biomolecules using co-jetting E-spray system	[77,78]
Fluorescence theranostic	Red blood cell-like particles	Close to 5–8 μm	Concave morphology; a large surface area-to-volume ratio as carriers for drugs and imaging agents; avoided filtration in the spleen, prolonging their half-time in the body	[79]

10.3.1 Fabrication of contrast agents for ultrasound imaging

Microbubble (MB) consisting of a gas core stabilized by a shell made of proteins, phospholipids, or polymers have been widely used as contrast agents for real-time diagnostic ultrasound imaging [82]. A functional MB must be smaller than 8 μm in diameter, but larger than 1−2 μm and sufficiently stable to safely traverse the bloodstream and enable a resonance frequency within the medical imaging frequency range (usually 1−10 MHz). Besides several common approaches (e.g., sonication and high shear mixing) to prepare MBs, E-spray has promisingly emerged as a technique to produce stable, narrow size-distributed (1−10 μm) MBs with long lifetime. For instance, Pancholi et al. developed a hybrid electrospray/T-junction device comprised of three glass capillaries fused into a T-junction embedded in a plastic block and each of them was inserted into a steel tube (Fig. 10.5a) [83]. The top, horizontal, and bottom tube was connected to a pressure tank supplying gas, a stainless steel syringe, and a power supply to maintain the constant flow rate, to transfer the suspension, and to atomize the resulting bubble−liquid suspension in an E-spray process, respectively. By optimizing the gas and the flow rate of the continuous phase, as well as the E-spray voltage, monodisperse phospholipid-coated air MBs of 5.1 ± 2 μm were produced with stability up to 2 h.

Alternatively, Farook et al. applied a coaxial E-spray technique to directly prepare narrow size−distributed MBs by allowing glycerol solution flow in the outer needle and undergo a stable cone-jet mode, while the air flowed through the inner needle at the same time [65]. When the ratio between the liquid flow rate in the outer needle and the air-flow rate (set at 1.7 μL/s) in the inner needle was 1.5, MBs with the size range of 2−8 μm were obtained. Moreover, Li et al. noticed that the addition of polyethylene glycol 400 to glycerol could strongly improve the MBs stability, lifetime, and also minimize their sizes [84]. Similarly, Mahalingam et al. implemented coaxial E-spray to generate bovine serum albumin (BSA) MBs with sizes ranging from 40 to 800 μm [66]. They observed that enhancing the flow rate of the BSA solution could decrease the polydispersity of the MBs and the uses of distilled water−glutaraldehyde, glycerol, and glycerol−Tween 80 collection media, instead of BSA solution collection medium, lead to remarkable stability improvement. Also, increasing the concentration of BSA solution from 5 wt% to 15 wt% could improve the compression stiffness of the MBs from 8 to 20 N/m.

Recently, MBs were synthesized as theranostic agents, which incorporated drugs into the shell layers, via coaxial E-spray. For example, Yan

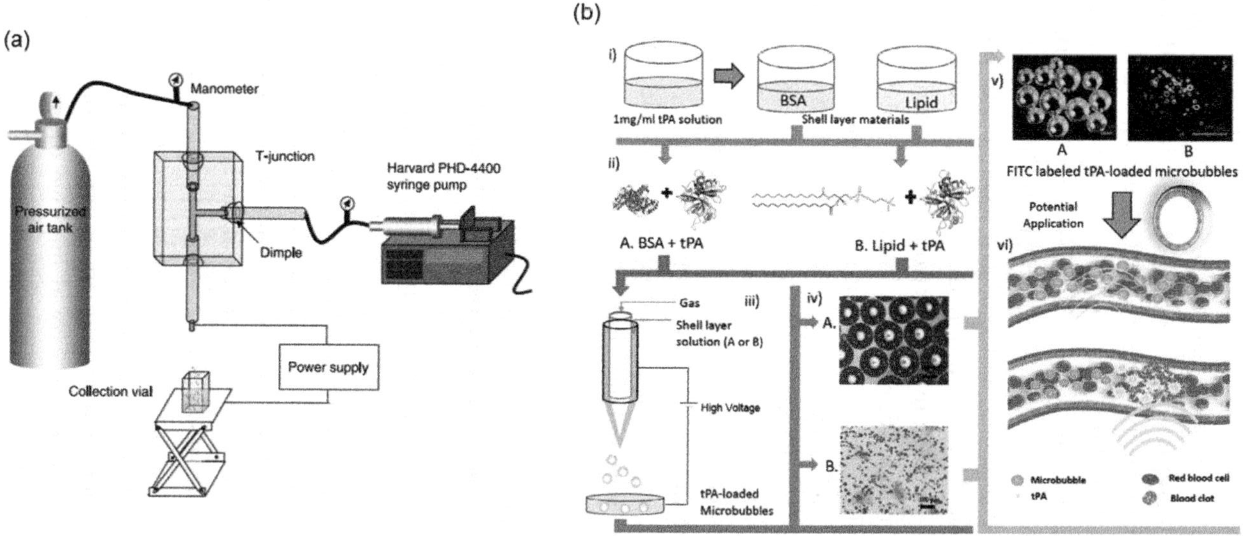

Figure 10.5 (a) Schematic showing hybrid electrospray/T-junction device. (b) Schematic of (i) preparation of shell layer solution, (ii) molecular structures of tPA, BSA, and lipid, (iii) coaxial E-spray method for the synthesis of tPA-loaded MBs, (iv) synthesized tPA-BSA MBs (A) and tPA-lipid MBs (B), (v) fluorescence images of FITC labeled tPA-BSA MBs (A) and tPA-lipid MBs (B) showed that tPA located at the shells, and (vi) potential diagnosis and therapeutic (by triggering release) applications of MBs at a low- and high-intensity ultrasound, respectively. *(a) Reprinted with permission from K. Pancholi, E. Stride, M. Edirisinghe, Generation of microbubbles for diagnostic and therapeutic applications using a novel device, J. Drug Target. 16 (6) (2008) 494–501. https://doi.org/10.1080/10611860802184884. Copyright 2008, Taylor & Francis Online Informa UK Limtied; (b) Reprinted with permission from W.C. Yan, Q.W. Chua, X.J. Ong, V.K. Sharma, Y.W. Tong, C.H. Wang, Fabrication of ultrasound-responsive microbubbles via coaxial electrohydrodynamic atomization for triggered release of tPA. J. Colloid Interface Sci. 501 (2017) 282–293. https://doi.org/10.1016/j.jcis.2017.04.073. Copyright 2017, Elsevier B.V.*

et al. successfully generated a model drug (tissue plasminogen activator, tPA)-entrapped BSA, and lipid MB with well-dispersed and less bubble-aggregated properties (Fig. 10.5b) [67,85]. Minimum sizes for tPA-BSA and tPA-lipid MBs were achieved by optimizing the operating conditions (e.g., voltage, core/shell flow rate ratio as well as tPA volume ratio). Specifically, about 41% of the tPA-lipid MBs had diameters varying between 3 and 6 μm and roughly 36% of them were in the range of 6−9 μm, whereas the size of tPA-BSA MBs was roughly 41 μm. Therefore, tPA-lipid MBs gave more promising sizes for medical applications (e.g., ischemic stroke therapy) than tPA-BSA MBs did. Additionally, the MBs could be traced at a low-intensity ultrasound, while ultrasound at high intensity could trigger their drug releases. Moreover, utilizing sulfur hexafluoride gas (SF_6) as the core showed an enhancement in the stability of tPA-lipid bubbles.

Besides that, biodegradable P_2O_5−CaO−Na_2O phosphate-based glass nanospheres (PGNs) were also produced as contrast agents for ultrasound imaging by E-spray of the sol−gel mixture into silicone oil [68]. These PGNs could label mouse mesenchymal stem cells in vitro and in vivo with the detection limits of 5 and 9 μg/mL, respectively. No toxicity of the imaging doses was found with cell counts down to 4000. Additionally, ion-release studies verified the degradation of these PGNs into aqueous media with easily metabolized degraded products within the body.

10.3.2 Fabrication of contrast agents for magnetic resonance imaging

Magnetic particles such as iron oxide nanoparticles with high magnetism have been broadly used as contrast agents in MRI due to their large surface area, improved relaxation properties, enhanced contrasting effect, and good biocompatibility [86]. Several reports have recently addressed the uses of E-spray to fabricate iron oxide NP-based contrast agents for MRI. For instance, Zhang et al. successfully synthesized near-uniform magnetic polymer yolk−shell particles (YSPs) (mean diameter of 13.5 ± 1.74 μm) using a trineedle coaxial E-spray technique with the stable cone-jet mode (Fig. 10.6a and b) [69]. The nozzle system consisted of three concentrically aligned stainless steel needles, three syringe pumps, a high-voltage power supply, and a metallic ground ring electrode. The solution injected to each needle corresponded with the layer order of YSPs: magnetic Fe_3O_4 nanoparticles (about 20 nm in diameter) embedded in the poly(ε-caprolactone) (PCL) shell, an interfacing silicone oil layer, and a PCL core (Fig. 10.6c). The MRI relaxation time was reduced by increasing the

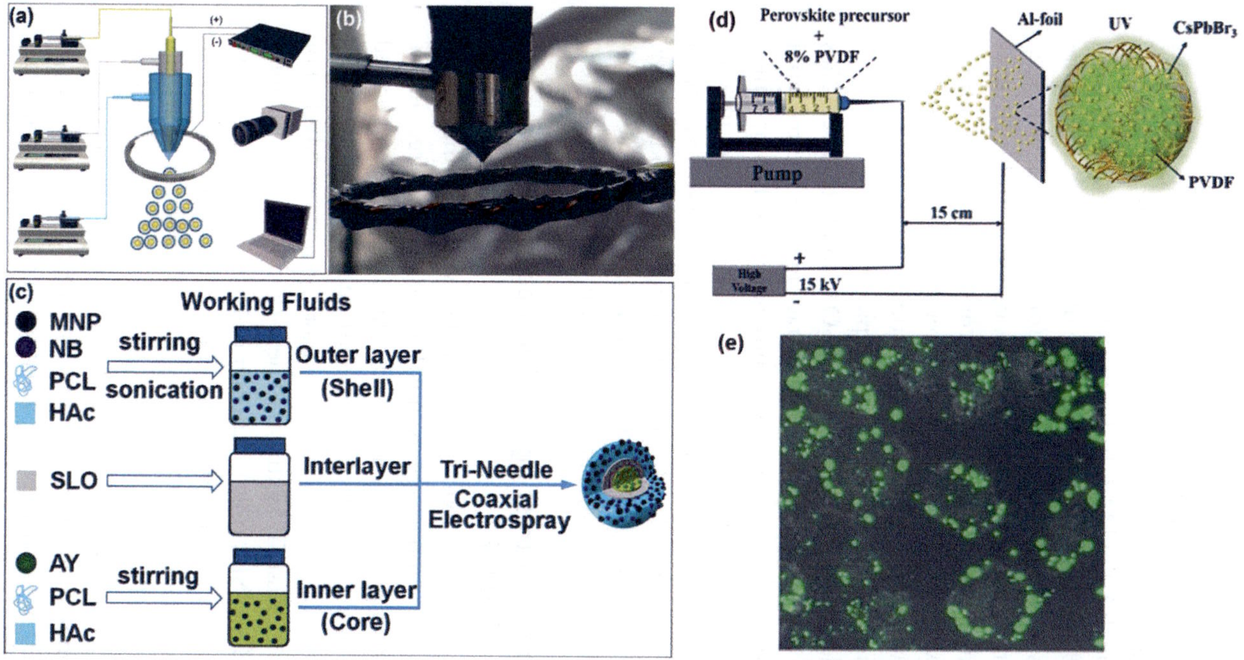

Figure 10.6 (a) Schematic illustration of the trineedle coaxial E-spray used to fabricate magnetic YSPs; (b) Image of the stable jetting behavior of the trineedle nozzle system; (c) Material formulation, production, and compartments of probe-loaded magnetic YSPs. The core and shell layers were stained with acridine yellow (AY) and Nile blue (NB), respectively, and the magnetic NP (MNP) was incorporated at the shell. (d) Schematic illustration of the preparation process of CsPbBr3 nanocrystals @ PVDF composite spheres via E-spray method. Perovskite precursor is N, N-dimethylformamide containing PbBr2 and CsBr; (e) The confocal microscope image of MCF-7 cells incubated with CsPbBr3@PVDF composites for 24 h at 37°C. *(a-c) Reprinted with permission from C. Zhang, Z.C. Yao, Q. Ding, J.J. Choi, Z. Ahmad, M.W. Chang, J.S. Li, Tri-needle coaxial electrospray engineering of magnetic polymer yolk-shell particles possessing dual-imaging modality, multiagent compartments, and trigger release potential, ACS Appl. Mater. Interfaces 9 (25) (2017) 21485–21495. https://doi.org/10.1021/acsami.7b05580 Copyright 2017, American Chemical Society; (d-e) Reprinted with permission from F. Wang, H. Wang, A. Ali, Y. Zhang, X. Cui, Y. Liu, In-situ one-step electrospray fabrication of polyvinylidene fluoride encapsulated CsPbBr3 spheres with high stability and cell imaging application, Inorg. Chem. Commun. 106 (2019) 99–103. https://doi.org/10.1016/j.inoche.2019.05.032. Copyright 2019, Elsevier B.V.*

magnetic nanoparticles content, and the frequency of the ultrasound backscatter signal could also be adjusted through the loading dosage of YSP. Interestingly, the magnetic YSPs exhibited not only potential as multifunctional theranostic agents for dual-imaging modality but also as magnetically controlled delivery, multiactive coencapsulation with low cytotoxicity at 5 mg/mL (Cell Counting Kit-8 assay, L929 murine cells).

For another example, Rasekh et al. introduced a tristearin core–shell particle system that encapsulates superparamagnetic iron oxide nanoparticles (SPIONs) (mean diameter of 10–15 nm) together with a model drug (genistein), a BODIPY fluorescent dye, and polyethylene-glycol (PEG) in a single step under ambient conditions using a coaxial E-spray process for theranostic purposes [70]. Tristearin developed into the shell layer was let flow through the outer needle, while SPIONs, PEG, genistein, and BODIPY dye were infused into the inner needle. Hydrophilic PEG excipient was added into the system to avoid particle aggregation and to ensure water solubility, while BODIPY gave excellent optical properties for cellular imaging. The resulting particles were of 0.65–1.2 μm in diameter with cellular internalization observed with only 4 h of incubation and drug encapsulation efficiencies reached as high as 92%. In addition, they were applicable for MRI and showed low toxicity at 0.5 mg/mL (MTT, HeLa cells). Additionally, Faramarzi et al. produced high magnetite (Fe_3O_4)-loaded polymeric particles by incorporating the oleic acid–capped magnetite nanoparticles into biocompatible and biodegradable fine particles of poly lactic-co-glycolic acid (PLGA) using conventional E-spray apparatus [71]. Oleic acid functioned in this system as a surface modifier to prevent magnetite aggregation and more particle uniformity was achieved in the voltage range of 14 kV. In addition, elevating the voltage was shown not to influence the particle size significantly; nonetheless, the particle size increased substantially as the flow rate increased. Magnetite loaded PLGA fine particles were produced in a wide range of magnetite to PLGA from 20% to 320% and resulted in a magnetite content of 16%–72%, respectively. However, increasing the magnetite ratios to 320% could reduce the particle sphericity and form heterogeneous structures.

10.3.3 Fabrication of contrast agents for X-ray imaging

Recently, E-spray has been developed to fabricate contrast agents for X-ray imaging. For example, the integrated system containing biocompatible barium alginate (BaAlg) microspheres as embolic agents loaded with $BaSO_4$ particles as contrast agents were synthesized by electrospraying the mixture of sodium alginate (NaAlg) and sodium sulfate (Na_2SO_4) into droplets and collecting them in a bath containing barium chloride ($BaCl_2$) [72]. This step enabled $BaSO_4$ particles formation simultaneously with the cross-linking of alginate droplet, resulting in $BaSO_4$@BaAlg microspheres varied from 200 to 1800 mm in diameter. Further in vivo imaging with digital radiography and computed tomography not only gave feedback of their real-time location and distribution but also their stable embolization over 3 weeks with radiodensity fluctuation within 7% of their starting value over 52 days. Moreover, angiographic and histological analyses on an embolized kidney confirmed the complete blood vessels occlusion of the targeted kidney, including peripheral vessels, by the microspheres. Similarly, calcium alginate (CaAlg) microspheres loaded with tantalum (Ta) nanoparticles (Ta@CaAlg microspheres) were also manufactured by E-spray [73]. The microspheres could maintain good X-ray imaging of the embolized sites up to 4 weeks and showed an excellent embolic effect. Besides functioning as embolic and contrast agents, Ta@CaAlg microspheres could be loaded with a model drug (e.g., Dox) with pH-dependent release profile for promising therapeutic effects.

10.3.4 Fabrication of particles for fluorescence imaging

Several MBs and magnetic particles described above could be labeled with fluorophores for imaging. Besides those, there are several other particles similarly manufactured using E-spray for fluorescence imaging modality. For instance, Reddy et al. prepared uniform acetyl curcumin–loaded PLGA core/shell liposome nanoparticles using E-spray for drug delivery as well as bioimaging and screening for anticancer purposes [74]. The AC chosen as the anticancer drug in this study also possessed fluorescent property. Therefore, when being incubated with cells, acetyl curcumin–loaded particles could be imaged with multicolor fluorescence, which is promising for cell imaging studies. In another case, Wu et al. reported a novel technique, called the static micromixer-coaxial E-spray, to synthesize theranostic lipoplexes in a single step with high reproducibility [75]. By using static micromixer in this setup, the imaging reagent (quantum dots, QD605) stream and the therapeutic reagent (Cy5-labeled antisense oligodeoxynucleotides, Cy5-G3139) stream were brought together at the microscaled stream width and subsequently reduced to nanoscale by the repeated stretching–folding activity of the static mixing units. The multilayered mixture then flew through the inner needle of the coaxial electrospray system, while dissolved lipids in ethanol flew through the outer needle.

The resulting lipoplexes exhibited high encapsulation efficiency, high uniformity (polydispersity of 0.024 ± 0.006), and the mean diameter by volume of 194 ± 15 nm. In addition, QD605 and Cy5 formed the Förster resonance energy transfer pair, and hence enabled visualization of the cellular uptake and intracellular fate of theranostic lipoplexes by flow cytometry and confocal microscopy. Moreover, through a one-pot ES process, Wang et al. successfully prepared composite spheres comprised of $CsPbBr_3$ nanocrystals encapsulating green luminescence poly-vinylidene fluoride (PVDF) (Fig. 10.6d) [76]. The products showed a full width at half maximum of 20 nm, remained stable in water, and could be used in MCF-7 cell membrane imaging with low toxicity (Fig. 10.6e). These advantages may enable a novel cell analysis in aqueous environments.

Interestingly, for the first time, Chan et al. developed anisotropic biohybrid microparticles (MPs) spatioselectively coupled with two different antibodies (Abs) for fluorescence-based multiplexing sensing of biomolecules using co-jetting E-spray system [77]. Particularly, poly(acrylamide-co-acrylic acid) was chemically modified with acetylene or maleimide groups to introduce different targeting biological elements into each compartment of the anisotropic MPs. Modified polymer solutions containing two distinct fluorescent dyes were separately injected into two needles aligned side-by-side in the co-jetting E-spray setup, which allowed parallel flows. The resulting anisotropic MPs were subsequently stabilized by thermal imidization, followed by bioconjugation with two types of polyclonal antibodies on two compartments of MPs via Huisgen 1,3-dipolar cycloaddition and maleimide-thiol coupling reaction. Eventually, the two compartments of the MPs could spatioselectively bind to their corresponding monoclonal Ab-immobilized substrates by recognizing their specific antigens and forming sandwich-type immunocomplexes. Such ordered orientation and direct binding established by the spatiospecific molecular interactions has brought about a novel fluorescence-based multiplexing biosensing system. Similarly, Jang et al. used co-jetting E-spray to synthesize a novel dual nanoprobe based on both surface-enhanced Raman scattering (SERS) and nondestructive fluorescence imaging [78]. The probe could immobilize two distinct types of monoclonal antibodies against two types of bacterial pathogens, *Escherichia coli* (*E. coli*) and *Francisella tularensis*, for multiplexed detection.

Furthermore, several attempts to synthesize red blood cell-like particles with a large surface area-to-volume ratio as carriers for drugs and imaging agents were achieved using E-spray [79]. Typically, the concave morphology of the particles can be tailored by careful control of the solvent evaporation and diffusion processes. Such favorable morphology not only allows incorporations of cargos (e.g., incorporating both magnetite nanoparticles and fluorescent dye for dual modality of MRI and fluorescence imaging [87]) but also avoids filtration in the spleen, thus prolonging their half-time in the body.

10.4 Fabrications of other biosensors

Besides the ones described above, E-spray also shows potential applications in manufactures of other biosensing systems such as SERS substrates, cantilever sensors, as well as functional hollow sphere structures and aerosols (Table 10.4).

In particular, E-spray allowed depositions of several preformed SERS-substrate NPs (e.g., silica NPs (SiNPs) [93], silver NPs (AgNPs) [88,89]) that bring about fast, effective, and sensitive detections. For instance, electrospraying AgNPs over analytes that had been formerly dropcast on conducting ITO glass slides has enabled rapid (4−6 min) nanomolar and micromolar SERS detection of p-mercaptobenzoic acid and 2,4-dinitrotoluene, respectively, with enhanced reproducibility and ~33 times less required amount of the AgNPs solution compared to that used in the conventional drop-casting methods. Low amount of AgNP, as well as short analysis or exposure time in E-Spray-SERS, allowed detection *E. coli* at its lowest concentration limit of 10^2 CFU/mL with low toxicity effect [88]. In another case, micropatterning of SiNPs by electrospraying through a stencil mask was conducted with high reproducibility and accuracy, followed by deposition of AgNPs via a modified silver mirror reaction. The Ag/SiNP combination prepared in this way resulted in SERS detection sites with significantly enhanced sensitivity and can be integrated with microfluidic units to develop high-performance micrototal analysis systems for both sample preparation and analysis [93]. Besides that, Chiu et al. applied coaxial ES to synthesize a new, freestanding, versatile, and large-scale core−shell microstructure substrate, which contained Ag@silicate nanohybrids of silver nanoparticles (AgNPs)/triblock copolymer surfactant (copolymer)/silicate nanoplatelets assembled outside poly(vinyl alcohol) (PVA) core for SERS sensing [94]. Particularly, PVA solution and the Ag@silicate hybrids were dispensed from the inner and outer needles, respectively. The core−shell Ag@silicate/PVA nanosphere substrate exhibited a significantly high SERS signal intensity, with values reached as high as 5.1×10^5 for adenine

Table 10.4 Applications of E-spray in other biosensors.

Application	Material solution	Substrate/Sizes	Some remarks	Reference
SERS sensing	Silver NPs (AgNPs)	ITO glass slides substrate	Rapid (4–6 min) nano-, micromolar SERS detection of p-mercaptobenzoic acid and 2,4-dinitrotoluene with enhanced reproducibility; ~33 times less amount of AgNPs; short analysis/exposure time; allowed detection of *E. coli* at its lowest concentration limit of 10^2 CFU/mL with low toxicity effect	[88,89]
SERS sensing	Ag@silicate nanohybrids	Around 100 nm in length and 1 nm in thickness	AgNPs/triblock copolymer surfactant (copolymer)/silicate nanoplatelets assembled outside poly(vinyl alcohol) (PVA) core was fabricated with co-E-	[94]

(Continued)

Table 10.4 Applications of E-spray in other biosensors.—cont'd

Application	Material solution	Substrate/Sizes	Some remarks	Reference
			spray; exhibited a significantly high SERS signal intensity (high as 5.1×10^5 for adenine molecules); additional antibacterial activity owing to Ag	
SU-8 photoresist cantilever sensors	Protein films	Cantilever; cell surface proteins; folate receptors	E-spray depositing protein films on the cantilever; depositing antibodies against cell surface proteins displayed by fungal and bacterial pathogens as well as folate receptors in cancer cells; mechanochemical interactions such as binding affinities between biomacromolecules (e.g., nucleic acids, proteins) and their ligands can be detected	[9]

H_2S gas sensing	Pt-functionalized meso-/macroporous SnO_2 hollow spheres	Stainless steel substrate	Core–shell structures were synthesized upon calcination of single-nozzle as E-sprayed spheres comprising of Sn and Si precursors, followed by etching and decorating with Pt NPs; gave excellent and selective responses to H_2S against interfering gas molecules at 250°C	[90]
Standard reference materials in dMRI	Hollow PLGA microspheres (ethylene glycol or PEG/chloroform core and PLGA/chloroform shell)	12.2–14.2 μm, close to the lower size limit of cancer cells that often have diameters larger than 10 μm	The bulk sample was structured as a hollow cylinder/3D tubule; developed as tumor cell–mimicking structures; microspheres with PEG/chloroform cores did not have surface opening and gave promising use in quantitative validation and	[91]

(*Continued*)

Table 10.4 Applications of E-spray in other biosensors.—cont'd

Application	Material solution	Substrate/Sizes	Some remarks	Reference
			calibration of dMRI; microspheres with ethylene glycol cores possessed one opening for encapsulation, gene/drug delivery, biomedical imaging, and theranostics	
Noninvasive disease diagnosis	Aerosol particles	Micrometer-sized particles	Produced by electrospray aerosol generator (EAG); allowed detection of airborne viruses; measured the regaining of nanoparticles in exhaled air for novel noninvasive chronic obstructive pulmonary disease diagnosis	[92]

molecules in DNA and potentially possessed additional antibacterial activity owing to Ag component.

Moreover, the mechanochemical interactions such as binding affinities between biomacromolecules (e.g., nucleic acids, proteins) and their ligands can be detected, for instance, by SU-8 photoresist cantilever sensors fabricated by depositing protein films on the cantilever using E-spray. A similar approach can be executed for pathogen sensing by depositing antibodies against cell surface proteins displayed by fungal and bacterial pathogens as well as folate receptors in cancer cells [9].

In addition, using E-spray, several hollow sphere structures can be generated not only for applications in drug delivery systems but also in biosensors (e.g., gas sensors, ion-sensors, pH sensors, and so on) with increased surface area and accessibility for target analytes [90,95,96]. For example, spherical $SiO_2@SnO_2$ core–shell structures were produced upon calcination of single-nozzle electrosprayed spheres (SPs) comprising of silicon and tin precursors. Subsequently, the SiO_2 core was etched away in NaOH solution to obtain meso-/macroporous SnO_2hollow SPs. Further functionalization of hollow SPs with platinum (Pt) nanoparticles yielded gas-sensing materials with excellent and selective responses to H_2S against interfering gas molecules [90]. Interestingly, hollow microspheres generated by co-E-spray can be used as phantom structures for medical diagnostics. For instance, Zhou et al. developed tumor cell–mimicking structures as standard reference materials in diffusion MRI (dMRI) by employing co-ES in the fabrication of hollow PLGA microspheres and their depositions on a copper wire positioned on a ground electrode [91]. Further removal of the wire allowed the bulk sample to structure as a hollow cylinder/3D tubule. The microspheres made with either ethylene glycol or PEG/chloroform core and PLGA/chloroform shell along with their miscible interface resulted in a stable jet formation and well-defined hollow structures. The hollow microspheres synthesized with PEG/chloroform cores did not show surface opening and their tubular structures were successfully constructed into a water-filled MR phantom, which could restrict water diffusion similarly as tumor cells, for promising use in quantitative validation and calibration of dMRI. On the other hand, the hollow microspheres generated with ethylene glycol cores possessed one opening on their surfaces and thus may be possible for encapsulation, gene/drug delivery, biomedical imaging, and theranostics.

Moreover, monodisperse, submicrometer aerosols can also be produced by E-spray in the so-called electrospray aerosol generator (EAG) (Model

3480, TSI Inc., St. Paul, MN, USA), where aerosols are emitted from the capillary tip under high-voltage electric field and further mixed with air and CO_2 to evaporate the liquid/solvent. The remaining parts are subsequently neutralized with an ionizer and transported to other integrated components, for instance, quartz crystal microbalance chamber for real-time mass-sensitive detection of airborne viruses such as Vaccinia viruses in the aerosols [97]. Also, AEG has been commonly used to produce aerosol particles for aerosol studies including airspace dimension assessment, which measures the regaining of nanoparticles in exhaled air after each single-breath inhalation followed by breath-hold, for novel noninvasive chronic obstructive pulmonary disease diagnosis [92,98].

10.5 Limitations of electrospray in biosensing and some recent technological developments of ES

Although E-spray is a versatile technique with numerous potential applications in biosensing and diagnostics, several inherent problems have narrowed its use to small, laboratory scale, especially in case of microarray biochips fabrication and/or micro-/nanopatterning. This may be due to limitations of conventional E-spray, for instance, in the choice of solution materials, substrates, additional use of a mask or a template, low patterning precision, relatively low throughput, and so on. Fortunately, E-spray has been continuously and actively advanced until recently to overcome these challenges.

As aforementioned, a mask or template commonly added to the basic configuration may disrupt the precise shape of the pattern. To improve this property, there are attempts to create a focused electric field on the electroconductive substrate to employ electrostatic forces to the electrosprayed particles for their depositions on the selective region of the substrate, for example, by employing a voltage directly to an electroconductive mask, using a patterned, grounded electrode [38], or applying an ion-induced electrostatic lens [35]. Nonetheless, these approaches are limited in that they are not suitable for nonconductive substrates such as PDMS. Therefore, Lee et al. have recently suggested a novel electrolyte solution—assisted electrospray deposition method, which promotes direct deposition of nano-/microparticles on various substrates including nonconductive PDMS substrate with significantly high efficiency [42]. This was done by first modifying the wettability of the nonconductive surface using oxygen plasma treatment with or without a mask, thus enabling the electrolyte solution to cover the selective or entire region of the substrate, respectively. Further ES deposition allowed the electrosprayed particles to be easily positioned on the surface of electrolyte solution, resulting in nano-/microparticle patterning on the substrate. By simply adjusting the operation parameters of the system including time, applied voltage, polymer concentration, and flow rate, the diameter of the particles and the thickness of the particle layer were controlled. Moreover, functionalizing the PDMS surface, for instance, with the line pattern of biocompatible polycaprolactone nanoparticles by ES has enabled selective cell patterning (e.g., NIH/3T3 fibroblasts and C2C12 myoblasts).

Besides that, the use of conventional E-spray is also restricted to diluted low conductive precursor materials (<5 mS/cm). In other words, for highly conductive solutions such as protein buffers, the spraying process is difficult and usually requires a desalting step that may perturb the protein activity or cause aggregation. To overcome this hurdle, an improved spraying method that combines high-frequency surface acoustic wave atomization with electrostatic deposition (SAW-ED) for manufacturing functionally active protein chips with a minimum required solution was introduced by Kim et al. [99,100]. Particularly, SAW-ED allows atomizing and spraying of highly concentrated and conductive protein solutions into microscale droplets by surface vibration with a rapid dehydration process, thereby limiting the loss of protein biological activity. Additionally, the deposition driven by electrostatic forces can be patterned with the use of an insulator mask for array and film formation purposes. However, SAW-ED requires being operated at a relatively high frequency, which is expensive, and the atomization is not a continuous process, thereby negatively influencing the deposition time, collection efficiency, and residual bioactivity [100,101]. Furthermore, most SAW atomizers are restricted to highly conductive low-density proteins, thus narrowing the material choices. Recently, a hybrid between SAW and E-spray (or EHDA) has increasingly become attractive for producing several conductive functional thin films and patterns with good morphological, mechanical, and electrical properties as it combines the benefits of SAW and EHDA and eliminates their drawbacks [101]. Particularly, EHDA is utilized as the first atomizer that constantly supplies small droplets (few microns) to the SAW atomizer, which subsequently breaks down the droplets into very uniform, submicron size. This approach reduces the active liquid volume to be atomized with SAW, therefore decreasing its required frequency and power consumption. Moreover, a wide range of conductive materials with different densities and molecular weights can be applied using SAW-EHDA. The technique has been successfully applied to fabricate several humidity sensors with good responses [101,102].

Alternatively, a near-field E-spray technology can be used to print droplets into minimal areas for micro-/nanopatterning by controlling the movement of the substrate, without any masks/templates. Different from the conventional E-spray where the spraying distance between the nozzle and collector is typically tens of centimeters, such parameter in the near-field E-spray technique is reduced to several millimeters [103]. Li et al. replaced the use of capillary nozzle with a stainless-steel probe in the near-field E-spray setup [104]. Additionally, by optimizing several parameters (e.g., applied voltage, deposition time, solution conductivity, flow rate) in the near-field E-spray, the precision of deposited patterning, which is usually low owing to the charge repulsion between E-spray droplets, can be improved [103]. Near-field E-spray displays an easy and promising way for on-demand deposition of micro-/nanopatterns with high resolution for applications in the fabrication of electronic and biosensor devices [104].

Moreover, to maintain the stable cone-jet mode of conventional E-spray, low flow rates are usually applied, which however may reduce the throughput of the technique [105]. Multiplexing enables cheap and mass production, which is promising for industrial applications of E-spray. Currently, several multiplexed E-spray deposition techniques have been proposed, in addition to the one created by Bhatnagar et al. [34], with significantly enhanced throughput as compared to the conventional single-emitter E-spray. For example, Olvera-Trejo et al. reported micron-sized microelectromechanical systems (MEMS) with multiplexed coaxial electrospray sources (up to 25 emitters/cm^2) for parallel production of uniform core—shell microparticles [106]. Parhizkar et al. designed high-throughput E-spray systems with four separate needles being attached to either a rectangular or a circular metallic plate and showed that circular plate configuration enabled easy control of the system and produced particles with higher uniformity, whereas required lower voltages under the same conditions as the rectangular plate configuration. Nonetheless, both geometries resulted in stable cone jets and roughly equal amounts of particles at the same collection time [105].

In this part, even though there have been several technical improvements suggested for conventional E-spray to overcome its limitations, most of them are quite recent and have not been widely translated for uses, especially in biosensing. Therefore, the next challenge for scientists and engineers is not only continuing improving E-spray performance but also bringing those advancements to massive productions and applications. This interesting phase will result in multiplexed E-spray that can hugely produce well-patterned and/or diverse, functional micro-/nanostructures to promisingly revolutionize the field of biosensing in the future, especially for effective diagnosis of diseases.

10.6 Conclusion and outlook

As highlighted in this chapter, over the past 20 years, there have been numerous updates on E-spray in terms of technical design and application range including fabrications of biochips, sensory micro-/nanoparticles, biosensor surface modifications, as well as manufactures of other biosensing systems. Even though the synthesis and deposition of micro-/nanostructures through conventional E-spray is an environmentally friendly, biocompatible, flexible, one-step procedure at ambient conditions, most of them are still restricted to laboratory scale and hence have not been further expanded for massive uses in biosensing industries and clinical diagnostics. Therefore, we hope that this chapter will inspire scientists and engineers to work on improving E-spray both in technical aspects as well as translating its recent technical advancements to large-scale, high-throughput productions with diverse applications in biosensing and diagnostics. Especially, in the midst of COVID-19 pandemic, we hope that E-spray technique will become useful in limiting the spread of the virus, saving numerous lives and bringing normal life back soon.

References

[1] D. Kalyane, N. Raval, R. Maheshwari, V. Tambe, K. Kalia, R.K. Tekade, Employment of enhanced permeability and retention effect (EPR): nanoparticle-based precision tools for targeting of therapeutic and diagnostic agent in cancer, Mater. Sci. Eng. C 98 (2019) 1252–1276, https://doi.org/10.1016/j.msec.2019.01.066.

[2] J. Grebely, G.J. Dore, S. Morin, J.K. Rockstroh, M.B. Klein, Elimination of HCV as a public health concern among people who inject drugs by 2030 - what will it take to get there, J. Int. AIDS Soc. 20 (1) (2017), https://doi.org/10.7448/IAS.20.1.22146.

[3] M.L. Nogueira, C.F. Estofolete, A.C.B. Terzian, E.P.B. Mascarin do Vale, R.C.M.A. da Silva, R.F. da Silva, H.J. Ramalho, I.M.M. Fernandes Charpiot, N. Vasilakis, M. Abbud-Filho, Zika virus infection and solid organ transplantation: a new challenge, Am. J. Transplant. 17 (3) (2017) 791–795, https://doi.org/10.1111/ajt.14047.

[4] D. Stewart, M.L. McPherson, Symptom management challenges in heart failure: pharmacotherapy considerations, Heart Fail. Rev. 22 (5) (2017) 525–534, https://doi.org/10.1007/s10741-017-9632-5.

[5] X. Li, W. Wang, X. Zhao, J. Zai, Q. Zhao, Y. Li, A. Chaillon, Transmission dynamics and evolutionary history of 2019-nCoV, J. Med. Virol. 92 (5) (2020) 501–511, https://doi.org/10.1002/jmv.25701.
[6] R. Anderson, K. Heesterbeek, T.D. Hollingsworth, How will country-based mitigation measures influence the course of the COVID-19 epidemic? Lancet 395 (2020) https://doi.org/10.1016/S0140-673620, 30567–5.
[7] R.K. Satvekar, B.M. Tiwale, S.H. Pawar, Emerging trends in medical diagnosis: a thrust on nanotechnology, Med. Chem. 4 (4) (2014) 407–416, https://doi.org/10.4172/2161-0444.1000172.
[8] K. Songsurang, N. Praphairaksit, K. Siraleartmukul, N. Muangsin, Electrospray fabrication of doxorubicin-chitosan-tripolyphosphate nanoparticles for delivery of doxorubicin, Arch Pharm. Res. (Seoul) 34 (4) (2011) 583–592, https://doi.org/10.1007/s12272-011-0408-5.
[9] S.K. Boda, X. Li, J. Xie, Electrospraying an enabling technology for pharmaceutical and biomedical applications: a review, J. Aerosol Sci. 125 (2018) 164–181, https://doi.org/10.1016/j.jaerosci.2018.04.002.
[10] P. Mehta, R. Haj-Ahmad, M. Rasekh, M.S. Arshad, A. Smith, S.M. van der Merwe, X. Li, M.W. Chang, Z. Ahmad, Pharmaceutical and biomaterial engineering via electrohydrodynamic atomization technologies, Drug Discov. Today 22 (1) (2017) 157–165, https://doi.org/10.1016/j.drudis.2016.09.021.
[11] J.A. Goode, J.V.H. Rushworth, P.A. Millner, Biosensor regeneration: a review of common techniques and outcomes, Langmuir 31 (23) (2015) 6267–6276, https://doi.org/10.1021/la503533g.
[12] D. Grieshaber, R. MacKenzie, J. Vörös, E. Reimhult, Electrochemical biosensors - sensor principles and architectures, Sensors 8 (3) (2008) 1400–1458, https://doi.org/10.3390/s8031400.
[13] S.K. Metkar, K. Girigoswami, Diagnostic biosensors in medicine — a review, Biocat. Agricul. Biotechnol. 17 (2019) 271–283, https://doi.org/10.1016/j.bcab.2018.11.029.
[14] M. Niculescu, T. Erichsen, V. Sukharev, Z. Kerenyi, E. Csöregi, W. Schuhmann, Quinohemoprotein alcohol dehydrogenase-based reagentless amperometric biosensor for ethanol monitoring during wine fermentation, Anal. Chim. Acta 463 (1) (2002) 39–51, https://doi.org/10.1016/S0003-2670(02)00344-6.
[15] A.C.d.S. Pires, N.d.F.F. Soares, L.H.M. da Silva, N.J. de Andrade, M.F.A. Silveira, A.F. de Carvalho, Polydiacetylene as a biosensor: fundamentals and applications in the food industry, Food Bioprocess Technol. 3 (2) (2010) 172–181, https://doi.org/10.1007/s11947-008-0171-x.
[16] T. Yamashita, N. Ookawa, M. Ishida, H. Kanamori, H. Sasaki, Y. Katayose, H. Yokoyama, A novel open-Type biosensor for the in-situ monitoring of biochemical oxygen demand in an aerobic environment, Sci. Rep. 6 (2016), https://doi.org/10.1038/srep38552.
[17] S. Ershad, S. Kangari, Preparation of a fluconazole potentiometric sensor and its application to pharmaceutical analysis and to drug recovery from biological fluids, Int. J. Electrochem. Sci. 4 (8) (2009) 1100–1108. http://www.electrochemsci.org/papers/vol4/4081100.pdf.
[18] A.L. Suherman, E.E.L. Tanner, S. Kuss, S.V. Sokolov, J. Holter, N.P. Young, R.G. Compton, Voltammetric determination of aluminium(III) at tannic acid capped-gold nanoparticle modified electrodes, Sensor. Actuator. B Chem. 265 (2018) 682–690, https://doi.org/10.1016/j.snb.2018.03.098.
[19] R. Ahmad, O.S. Wolfbeis, Y.B. Hahn, H.N. Alshareef, L. Torsi, K.N. Salama, Deposition of nanomaterials: a crucial step in biosensor fabrication, Mat. Today Commun. 17 (2018) 289–321, https://doi.org/10.1016/j.mtcomm.2018.09.024.

[20] V.N. Morozov, T.Y. Morozova, Electrospray deposition as a method to fabricate functionally active protein films, Anal. Chem. 71 (7) (1999b) 1415–1420, https://doi.org/10.1021/ac9808775.
[21] O. Wilhelm, L. Mädler, S.E. Pratsinis, Electrospray evaporation and deposition, J. Aerosol Sci. 34 (7) (2003) 815–836, https://doi.org/10.1016/S0021-8502(03)00034-X.
[22] S. Kavadiya, P. Biswas, Electrospray deposition of biomolecules: applications, challenges, and recommendations, J. Aerosol Sci. 125 (2018) 182–207, https://doi.org/10.1016/j.jaerosci.2018.04.009.
[23] J. Xie, A. Rezvanpour, C.H. Wang, J. Hua, Electric field controlled electrospray deposition for precise particle pattern and cell pattern formation, AIChE J. 56 (10) (2010) 2607–2621, https://doi.org/10.1002/aic.12198.
[24] V.N. Morozov, T.Y. Morozova, Electrospray deposition as a method for mass fabrication of mono- and multicomponent microarrays of biological and biologically active substances, Anal. Chem. 71 (15) (1999a) 3110–3117, https://doi.org/10.1021/ac981412h.
[25] J.G. Lee, H.J. Cho, N. Huh, C. Ko, W.C. Lee, Y.H. Jang, B.S. Lee, I.S. Kang, J.W. Choi, Electrohydrodynamic (EHD) dispensing of nanoliter DNA droplets for microarrays, Biosens. Bioelectron. 21 (12) (2006) 2240–2247, https://doi.org/10.1016/j.bios.2005.11.015.
[26] B. Lee, A. Tajima, J. Kim, Y. Yamagata, T. Nagamune, Fabrication of protein microarrays using the electrospray deposition (ESD) method: application of microfluidic chips in immunoassay, Biotechnol. Bioproc. Eng. 15 (1) (2010) 145–151, https://doi.org/10.1007/s12257-009-3033-0.
[27] N.V. Avseenko, T.Y. Morozova, F.I. Ataullakhanov, V.N. Morozov, Immunoassay with multicomponent protein microarrays fabricated by electrospray deposition, Anal. Chem. 74 (5) (2002) 927–933, https://doi.org/10.1021/ac010970k.
[28] N.V. Avseenko, T.Y. Morozova, F.I. Ataullakhanov, V.N. Morozov, Immobilization of proteins in immunochemical microarrays fabricated by electrospray deposition, Anal. Chem. 73 (24) (2001) 6047–6052, https://doi.org/10.1021/ac010460q.
[29] S.S. Groves, M.J. Turell, C.L. Bailey, V.N. Morozov, Rapid active assay for the detection of antibodies to West Nile virus in chickens, Am. J. Trop. Med. Hyg. 78 (1) (2008) 63–69, https://doi.org/10.4269/ajtmh.2008.78.63.
[30] V.N. Morozov, A.A. Nikolaev, Y.M. Shlyapnikov, A.Y. Mikheev, E.A. Shlyapnikova, T.R. Bagdasaryan, I.A. Burmistrova, T.G. Smirnova, I.Y. Andrievskaya, E.E. Larionova, I.Y. Nikitina, I.V. Lyadova, Non-invasive approach to diagnosis of pulmonary tuberculosis using microdroplets collected from exhaled air, J. Breath Res. 12 (3) (2018), https://doi.org/10.1088/1752-7163/aab3f2.
[31] Y.M. Shlyapnikov, V.N. Morozov, Titration of trace amounts of immunoglobulins in a microarray-based assay with magnetic labels, Anal. Chim. Acta 966 (2017) 47–53, https://doi.org/10.1016/j.aca.2017.02.037.
[32] R. Moerman, J. Frank, J.C.M. Marijnissen, T.G.M. Schalkhammer, G.W.K. Van Dedem, Miniaturized electrospraying as a technique for the production of microarrays of reproducible micrometer-sized protein spots, Anal. Chem. 73 (10) (2001) 2183–2189, https://doi.org/10.1021/ac001041g.
[33] R. Moerman, G.W.K. Van Dedem, A coverslip method for controlled parallel sample introduction into arrays of (sub)nanoliter wells for quantitative analysis, Anal. Chem. 75 (16) (2003) 4132–4138, https://doi.org/10.1021/ac020432n.
[34] P. Bhatnagar, Multiplexed electrospray deposition for protein microarray with micromachined silicon device, Appl. Phys. Lett. 91 (1) (2007), https://doi.org/10.1063/1.2754642.

[35] S. You, K. Han, H. Kim, H. Lee, C.G. Woo, C. Jeong, W. Nam, M. Choi, High-resolution, parallel patterning of nanoparticles via an ion-induced focusing mask, Small 6 (19) (2010) 2146–2152, https://doi.org/10.1002/smll.201000892.
[36] I. Uematsu, H. Matsumoto, K. Morota, M. Minagawa, A. Tanioka, Y. Yamagata, K. Inoue, Surface morphology and biological activity of protein thin films produced by electrospray deposition, J. Colloid Interface Sci. 269 (2) (2004) 336–340, https://doi.org/10.1016/j.jcis.2003.08.069.
[37] S.V. Martyn, H.K. Heywood, P. Rockett, M.D. Paine, M.J. Wang, P.J. Dobson, S.J. Sheard, D.A. Lee, J.P.W. Stark, Electrospray deposited fibronectin retains the ability to promote cell adhesion, J. Biomed. Mater. Res. B Appl. Biomater. (2011) 110–118, https://doi.org/10.1002/jbm.b.31745.
[38] W.C. Yan, J. Xie, C.H. Wang, Electrical field guided electrospray deposition for production of gradient particle patterns, ACS Appl. Mater. Interfaces 10 (22) (2018) 18499–18506, https://doi.org/10.1021/acsami.8b02914.
[39] K. Kim, B.U. Lee, G.B. Hwang, J.H. Lee, S. Kim, Drop-on-demand patterning of bacterial cells using pulsed jet electrospraying, Anal. Chem. 82 (5) (2010) 2109–2112, https://doi.org/10.1021/ac9027966.
[40] E.S. Chong, G.B. Hwang, K. Kim, I.S. Lee, S.H. Han, H.J. Kim, H. Jung, S.J. Kim, H. Il Jung, B. Uk Lee, Viable bacterial cell patterning using a pulsed jet electrospray system, J. Microbiol. Biotechnol. 25 (3) (2014) 381–385, https://doi.org/10.4014/jmb.1401.01012.
[41] S.B. Jeong, E.s. Chong, K.J. Heo, G.W. Lee, H.J. Kim, B.U. Lee, Electrospray patterning of yeast cells for applications in alcoholic fermentation, Sci. Rep. 9 (1) (2019), https://doi.org/10.1038/s41598-019-55225-4.
[42] S.J. Lee, S.M. Park, S.J. Han, D.S. Kim, Electrolyte solution-assisted electrospray deposition for direct coating and patterning of polymeric nanoparticles on non-conductive surfaces, Chem. Eng. J. 379 (2020), https://doi.org/10.1016/j.cej.2019.122318.
[43] R. Moerman, J. Frank, J.C.M. Marijnissen, G.H. van Dedem, Picoliter dispensing in wells of a micro-array by means of electrospraying, J. Aerosol Sci. 30 (1) (1999) S551–S552, https://doi.org/10.1016/S0021-8502(99)80287-0.
[44] M.C. Castrovilli, P. Bolognesi, J. Chiarinelli, L. Avaldi, A. Cartoni, P. Calandra, E. Tempesta, M.T. Giardi, A. Antonacci, F. Arduini, V. Scognamiglio, Electrospray deposition as a smart technique for laccase immobilisation on carbon black-nanomodified screen-printed electrodes, Biosens. Bioelectron. 163 (2020), https://doi.org/10.1016/j.bios.2020.112299.
[45] B. Lee, N. Kamiya, S. Machida, Y. Yamagata, K. Horie, T. Nagamune, Fabrication of a protein film by electrospray deposition method and investigation of photochemical properties by persistent spectral hole burning, Biomaterials 24 (12) (2003) 2045–2051, https://doi.org/10.1016/S0142-9612(02)00637-3.
[46] V.N. Morozov, S. Groves, M.J. Turell, C. Bailey, Three minutes-long electrophoretically assisted zeptomolar microfluidic immunoassay with magnetic-beads detection, J. Am. Chem. Soc. 129 (42) (2007) 12628–12629, https://doi.org/10.1021/ja075069m.
[47] H.S. Kim, D.Y. Lee, J.H. Park, J.H. Kim, J.H. Hwang, H.I. Jung, Optimization of electrohydrodynamic writing technique to print collagen, Exp. Tech. 31 (4) (2007) 15–19, https://doi.org/10.1111/j.1747-1567.2007.00154.x.
[48] M.D. Paine, M.S. Alexander, K.L. Smith, M. Wang, J.P.W. Stark, Controlled electrospray pulsation for deposition of femtoliter fluid droplets onto surfaces, J. Aerosol Sci. 38 (3) (2007) 315–324, https://doi.org/10.1016/j.jaerosci.2006.12.004.
[49] T. Kuilla, S. Bhadra, D. Yao, N.H. Kim, S. Bose, J.H. Lee, Recent advances in graphene based polymer composites, Prog. Polym. Sci. 35 (11) (2010) 1350–1375, https://doi.org/10.1016/j.progpolymsci.2010.07.005.

[50] K.J. Cash, H.A. Clark, Nanosensors and nanomaterials for monitoring glucose in diabetes, Trends Mol. Med. 16 (12) (2010) 584–593, https://doi.org/10.1016/j.molmed.2010.08.002.
[51] D. Liu, M.M. Rahman, C. Ge, J. Kim, J.J. Lee, Highly stable and conductive PEDOT:PSS/graphene nanocomposites for biosensor applications in aqueous medium, New J. Chem. 41 (24) (2017) 15458–15465, https://doi.org/10.1039/c7nj03330c.
[52] N. Ruecha, R. Rangkupan, N. Rodthongkum, O. Chailapakul, Novel paper-based cholesterol biosensor using graphene/polyvinylpyrrolidone/polyaniline nanocomposite, Biosens. Bioelectron. 52 (2014) 13–19, https://doi.org/10.1016/j.bios.2013.08.018.
[53] N. Ruecha, N. Rodthongkum, D.M. Cate, J. Volckens, O. Chailapakul, C.S. Henry, Sensitive electrochemical sensor using a graphene-polyaniline nanocomposite for simultaneous detection of Zn(II), Cd(II), and Pb(II), Anal. Chim. Acta 874 (2015) 40–48, https://doi.org/10.1016/j.aca.2015.02.064.
[54] O.J. Yoon, C.H. Kim, I.Y. Sohn, N.E. Lee, Toxicity analysis of graphene nanoflakes by cell-based electrochemical sensing using an electrode modified with nanocomposite of graphene and Nafion, Sensor. Actuator. B Chem. 188 (2013) 454–461, https://doi.org/10.1016/j.snb.2013.07.039.
[55] V. Penmatsa, T. Kim, M. Beidaghi, H. Kawarada, L. Gu, Z. Wang, C. Wang, Three-dimensional graphene nanosheet encrusted carbon micropillar arrays for electrochemical sensing, Nanoscale 4 (12) (2012) 3673–3678, https://doi.org/10.1039/c2nr30161j.
[56] W. Li, J. Lin, X. Wang, J. Jiang, S. Guo, G. Zheng, Electrospray deposition of ZnO thin films and its application to gas sensors, Micromachines 9 (2) (2018), https://doi.org/10.3390/mi9020066.
[57] A. Ali, K. Ali, K.R. Kwon, M.T. Hyun, K.H. Choi, Electrohydrodynamic atomization approach to graphene/zinc oxide film fabrication for application in electronic devices, J. Mater. Sci. Mater. Electron. 25 (2) (2014) 1097–1104, https://doi.org/10.1007/s10854-013-1693-1.
[58] C.T. Pan, Y.C. Chen, C.C. Hsieh, C.H. Lin, C.Y. Su, C.K. Yen, Z.H. Liu, W.C. Wang, Ultrasonic sensing device with ZnO piezoelectric nanorods by selectively electrospraying method, Sens. Actuators, A 216 (2014) 318–327, https://doi.org/10.1016/j.sna.2014.05.024.
[59] K. Chen, G. Lu, J. Chang, S. Mao, K. Yu, S. Cui, J. Chen, Hg(II) ion detection using thermally reduced graphene oxide decorated with functionalized gold nanoparticles, Anal. Chem. 84 (9) (2012) 4057–4062, https://doi.org/10.1021/ac3000336.
[60] S. Mao, G. Lu, K. Yu, Z. Bo, J. Chen, Specific protein detection using thermally reduced graphene oxide sheet decorated with gold nanoparticle-antibody conjugates, Adv. Mater. 22 (32) (2010) 3521–3526, https://doi.org/10.1002/adma.201000520.
[61] J. Chen, S. Mao, G. Lu, K. Yu, Protein viability on Au nanoparticles during an electrospray and electrostatic-force-directed assembly process, J. Nanomater. 2010 (2010) 6, https://doi.org/10.1155/2010/196393. Article ID 196393.
[62] S. Afsahi, M.B. Lerner, J.M. Goldstein, J. Lee, X. Tang, D.A. Bagarozzi, D. Pan, L. Locascio, A. Walker, F. Barron, B.R. Goldsmith, Novel graphene-based biosensor for early detection of Zika virus infection, Biosens. Bioelectron. 100 (2018) 85–88, https://doi.org/10.1016/j.bios.2017.08.051.
[63] T. Soundappan, K. Haddad, S. Kavadiya, R. Raliya, P. Biswas, Crumpled graphene oxide decorated sno2 nanocolumns for the electrochemical detection of free chlorine, Appl. Nanosci. 7 (8) (2017) 645–653, https://doi.org/10.1007/s13204-017-0603-x.

[64] S. Mao, G. Lu, K. Yu, J. Chen, Specific biosensing using carbon nanotubes functionalized with gold nanoparticle-antibody conjugates, Carbon 48 (2) (2010) 479–486, https://doi.org/10.1016/j.carbon.2009.09.065.

[65] U. Farook, E. Stride, M.J. Edirisinghe, Preparation of suspensions of phospholipid-coated microbubbles by coaxial electrohydrodynamic atomization, J. R. Soc. Interface 5 (32) (2009) 271–277, https://doi.org/10.1098/rsif.2008.0225.

[66] S. Mahalingam, M.B.J. Meinders, M. Edirisinghe, Formation, stability, and mechanical properties of bovine serum albumin stabilized air bubbles produced using coaxial electrohydrodynamic atomization, Langmuir 30 (23) (2014) 6694–6703, https://doi.org/10.1021/la5011715.

[67] W.C. Yan, Q.W. Chua, X.J. Ong, V.K. Sharma, Y.W. Tong, C.H. Wang, Fabrication of ultrasound-responsive microbubbles via coaxial electrohydrodynamic atomization for triggered release of tPA, J. Colloid Interface Sci. 501 (2017) 282–293, https://doi.org/10.1016/j.jcis.2017.04.073.

[68] F. Foroutan, J.V. Jokerst, S.S. Gambhir, O. Vermesh, H.W. Kim, J.C. Knowles, Sol-gel synthesis and electrospraying of biodegradable (P2O5)55-(CaO)30-(Na2O) 15glass nanospheres as a transient contrast agent for ultrasound stem cell imaging, ACS Nano 9 (2) (2015) 1868–1877, https://doi.org/10.1021/nn506789y.

[69] C. Zhang, Z.C. Yao, Q. Ding, J.J. Choi, Z. Ahmad, M.W. Chang, J.S. Li, Tri-needle coaxial electrospray engineering of magnetic polymer yolk-shell particles possessing dual-imaging modality, multiagent compartments, and trigger release potential, ACS Appl. Mater. Interfaces 9 (25) (2017) 21485–21495, https://doi.org/10.1021/acsami.7b05580.

[70] M. Rasekh, Z. Ahmad, R. Cross, J. Hernández-Gil, J.D.E.T. Wilton-Ely, P.W. Miller, Facile preparation of drug-loaded tristearin encapsulated superparamagnetic iron oxide nanoparticles using coaxial electrospray processing, Mol. Pharm. 14 (6) (2017) 2010–2023, https://doi.org/10.1021/acs.molpharmaceut.7b00109.

[71] A.R. Faramarzi, J. Barzin, H. Mobedi, Producing PLGA fine particles containing high magnetite nanoparticles by using the electrospray technique, J. Polym. Res. 24 (1) (2016), https://doi.org/10.1007/s10965-016-1177-0.

[72] Q. Du, L. Li, Y. Liu, J. Zeng, J. Li, C. Zheng, G. Zhou, X. Yang, Fabrication of inherently radiopaque BaSO4@BaAlg microspheres by a one-step electrospraying method for embolization, J. Mater. Chem. B 6 (21) (2018) 3522–3530, https://doi.org/10.1039/c8tb00542g.

[73] J. Zeng, L. Li, H. Zhang, J. Li, L. Liu, G. Zhou, Q. Du, C. Zheng, X. Yang, Radiopaque and uniform alginate microspheres loaded with tantalum nanoparticles for real-time imaging during transcatheter arterial embolization, Theranostics 8 (17) (2018) 4591–4600, https://doi.org/10.7150/thno.27379.

[74] A.S. Reddy, B.A. Lakshmi, S. Kim, J. Kim, Synthesis and characterization of acetyl curcumin-loaded core/shell liposome nanoparticles via an electrospray process for drug delivery, and theranostic applications, Eur. J. Pharm. Biopharm. 142 (2019) 518–530, https://doi.org/10.1016/j.ejpb.2019.07.024.

[75] Y. Wu, L. Li, Y. Mao, L.J. Lee, Static micromixer-coaxial electrospray synthesis of theranostic lipoplexes, ACS Nano 6 (3) (2012) 2245–2252, https://doi.org/10.1021/nn204300s.

[76] F. Wang, H. Wang, A. Ali, Y. Zhang, X. Cui, Y. Liu, In-situ one-step electrospray fabrication of polyvinylidene fluoride encapsulated CsPbBr3 spheres with high stability and cell imaging application, Inorg. Chem. Commun. 106 (2019) 99–103, https://doi.org/10.1016/j.inoche.2019.05.032.

[77] C.W. Jung, G. Jalani, J. Ko, J. Choo, D.W. Lim, Synthesis, characterization, and directional binding of anisotropic biohybrid microparticles for multiplexed

biosensing, Macromol. Rapid Commun. 35 (1) (2014) 56–65, https://doi.org/10.1002/marc.201300652.
[78] H. Jang, E.Y. Hwang, Y. Kim, J. Choo, J. Jeong, D.W. Lim, Surface-enhanced Raman scattering and fluorescence-based dual nanoprobes for multiplexed detection of bacterial pathogens, J. Biomed. Nanotechnol. 12 (10) (2016) 1938–1951, https://doi.org/10.1166/jbn.2016.2309.
[79] X. Ju, X. Wang, Z. Liu, R. Xie, W. Wang, L. Chu, Red-blood-cell-shaped chitosan microparticles prepared by electrospraying, Particuology 30 (2017) 151–157, https://doi.org/10.1016/j.partic.2016.05.011.
[80] S.M. Janib, A.S. Moses, J.A. MacKay, Imaging and drug delivery using theranostic nanoparticles, Adv. Drug Deliv. Rev. 62 (11) (2010) 1052–1063, https://doi.org/10.1016/j.addr.2010.08.004.
[81] X. Luo, A. Morrin, A.J. Killard, M.R. Smyth, Application of nanoparticles in electrochemical sensors and biosensors, Electroanalysis 18 (4) (2006) 319–326, https://doi.org/10.1002/elan.200503415.
[82] J. Wischhusen, F. Padilla, Ultrasound molecular imaging with targeted microbubbles for cancer diagnostics: from bench to bedside, IRBM 40 (1) (2019) 3–9, https://doi.org/10.1016/j.irbm.2018.10.007.
[83] K. Pancholi, E. Stride, M. Edirisinghe, Generation of microbubbles for diagnostic and therapeutic applications using a novel device, J. Drug Target. 16 (6) (2008) 494–501, https://doi.org/10.1080/10611860802184884.
[84] Y. Li, J. Li, H.B. Zhang, Y.S. Su, Microbubble suspensions prepared via electrohydrodynamic jetting process, in: BioMedical Engineering and Informatics: New Development and the Future - Proceedings of the 1st International Conference on BioMedical Engineering and Informatics, BMEI 2008, vol. 2, 2008, pp. 445–449, https://doi.org/10.1109/BMEI.2008.200.
[85] W.C. Yan, X.J. Ong, K.T. Pun, D.Y. Tan, V.K. Sharma, Y.W. Tong, C.H. Wang, Preparation of tPA-loaded microbubbles as potential theranostic agents: a novel one-step method via coaxial electrohydrodynamic atomization technique, Chem. Eng. J. 307 (2017) 168–180, https://doi.org/10.1016/j.cej.2016.08.081.
[86] H.B. Na, I.C. Song, T. Hyeon, Inorganic nanoparticles for MRI contrast agents, Adv. Mater. 21 (21) (2009) 2133–2148, https://doi.org/10.1002/adma.200802366.
[87] K. Hayashi, K. Ono, H. Suzuki, M. Sawada, M. Moriya, W. Sakamoto, T. Yogo, Electrosprayed synthesis of red-blood-cell-like particles with dual modality for magnetic resonance and fluorescence imaging, Small 6 (21) (2010) 2384–2391, https://doi.org/10.1002/smll.201000399.
[88] T. Ahuja, A. Ghosh, S. Mondal, P. Basuri, S.K. Jenifer, P. Srikrishnarka, J.S. Mohanty, S. Bose, T. Pradeep, Ambient electrospray deposition Raman spectroscopy (AESD RS) using soft landed preformed silver nanoparticles for rapid and sensitive analysis, Analyst 144 (24) (2019) 7412–7420, https://doi.org/10.1039/c9an01700c.
[89] A. Li, Z. Baird, S. Bag, D. Sarkar, A. Prabhath, T. Pradeep, Cooks, Using ambient ion beams to write nanostructured patterns for surface enhanced Raman spectroscopy, Angew. Chem. Int. Ed. 53 (46) (2014) 12528–12531, https://doi.org/10.1002/anie.201406660.
[90] P.M. Bulemo, H.J. Cho, D.H. Kim, I.D. Kim, Facile synthesis of Pt-functionalized meso/macroporous SnO_2 hollow spheres through in situ templating with SiO_2 for H_2S sensors, ACS Appl. Mater. Interfaces 10 (21) (2018) 18183–18191, https://doi.org/10.1021/acsami.8b00901.
[91] F.L. Zhou, H.H. Wu, D.J. McHugh, I. Wimpenny, X. Zhang, J.E. Gough, P.L. Hubbard Cristinacce, G.J.M. Parker, Co-electrospraying of tumour cell

mimicking hollow polymeric microspheres for diffusion magnetic resonance imaging, Mater. Sci. Eng. C 101 (2019) 217–227, https://doi.org/10.1016/j.msec.2019.03.062.

[92] H.L. Aaltonen, J.K. Jakobsson, S. Diaz, S. Zackrisson, E. Piitulainen, J. Löndahl, P. Wollmer, Deposition of inhaled nanoparticles is reduced in subjects with COPD and correlates with the extent of emphysema: proof of concept for a novel diagnostic technique, Clin. Physiol. Funct. Imag. 38 (6) (2018) 1008–1014, https://doi.org/10.1111/cpf.12517.

[93] K. Higashi, K. Uchida, A. Hotta, K. Hishida, N. Miki, Micropatterning of silica nanoparticles by electrospray deposition through a stencil mask, J. Lab. Autom. 19 (1) (2014) 75–81, https://doi.org/10.1177/2211068213495205.

[94] C.W. Chiu, P.H. Lin, Core/shell Ag@silicate nanoplatelets and poly(vinyl alcohol) spherical nanohybrids fabricated by coaxial electrospraying as highly sensitive SERS substrates, RSC Adv. 6 (71) (2016) 67204–67211, https://doi.org/10.1039/c6ra06584h.

[95] T. Matsuura, T. Maruyama, Hollow phosphorylcholine polymer vesicles prepared by a coaxial electrospray technique, Colloid Polym. Sci. 295 (7) (2017) 1251–1256, https://doi.org/10.1007/s00396-017-4110-0.

[96] S. Mishra, K. Ranjith, K.K. Khadija, P.C. Ramamurthy, Fabrication of hollow microspheres using single step electrospraying process, J. Res. Updates Polym. Sci. 3 (2014) 108–113, https://doi.org/10.6000/1929-5995.2014.03.02.5.

[97] J. Lee, J. Jang, D. Akin, C.A. Savran, R. Bashir, Real-time detection of airborne viruses on a mass-sensitive device, Appl. Phys. Lett. 93 (1) (2008), https://doi.org/10.1063/1.2956679.

[98] H.L. Aaltonen, S.S. Kindvall, J.K. Jakobsson, J. Löndahl, L.E. Olsson, S. Diaz, S. Zackrisson, P. Wollmer, Airspace Dimension Assessment with nanoparticles reflects lung density as quantified by MRI, Int. J. Nanomed. 13 (2018) 2989–2995, https://doi.org/10.2147/IJN.S160331.

[99] L.T. De Jonge, J. Ju, S.C.G. Leeuwenburgh, Y. Yamagata, T. Higuchi, J.G.C. Wolke, K. Inoue, J.A. Jansen, A comparative study of two advanced spraying techniques for the deposition of biologically active enzyme coatings onto bone-substituting implants, Thin Solid Films 518 (19) (2010) 5615–5621, https://doi.org/10.1016/j.tsf.2010.04.066.

[100] J.W. Kim, Y. Yamagata, M. Takasaki, B.H. Lee, H. Ohmori, T. Higuchi, A device for fabricating protein chips by using a surface acoustic wave atomizer and electrostatic deposition, Sensor. Actuator. B Chem. 107 (2) (2005) 535–545, https://doi.org/10.1016/j.snb.2004.11.012.

[101] K.H. Choi, H.B. Kim, K. Ali, M. Sajid, G.U. Siddiqui, D.E. Chang, H.C. Kim, J.B. Ko, H.W. Dang, Y.H. Doh, Hybrid surface acoustic wave- electrohydrodynamic atomization (SAW-EHDA) for the development of functional thin films, Sci. Rep. 5 (2015), https://doi.org/10.1038/srep15178.

[102] G.U. Siddiqui, M. Sajid, J. Ali, S.W. Kim, Y.H. Doh, K.H. Choi, Wide range highly sensitive relative humidity sensor based on series combination of MoS_2 and PEDOT: PSS sensors array, Sensor. Actuator. B Chem. 266 (2018) 354–363, https://doi.org/10.1016/j.snb.2018.03.134.

[103] J. Jiang, G. Zheng, P. Zhu, J. Liu, Y. Liu, X. Wang, W. Li, S. Guo, Controlling of electrospray deposition for micropatterns, Micromachines 9 (2) (2018), https://doi.org/10.3390/mi9020072.

[104] W. Li, G. Zheng, L. Xu, X. Wang, Fabrication of micro-patterns via near-field electrospray, AIP Adv. 6 (11) (2016), https://doi.org/10.1063/1.4967200.

[105] M. Parhizkar, P.J.T. Reardon, J.C. Knowles, R.J. Browning, E. Stride, R.B. Pedley, T. Grego, M. Edirisinghe, Performance of novel high throughput multi electrospray

systems for forming of polymeric micro/nanoparticles, Mater. Des. 126 (2017) 73–84, https://doi.org/10.1016/j.matdes.2017.04.029.

[106] D. Olvera-Trejo, L.F. Velásquez-García, Additively manufactured MEMS multiplexed coaxial electrospray sources for high-throughput, uniform generation of core-shell microparticles, Lab Chip 16 (21) (2016) 4121–4132, https://doi.org/10.1039/c6lc00729e.

[107] R. Moerman, J. Knoll, C. Apetrei, L.R. Van Den Doel, G.W.K. Van Dedem, Quantitative analysis in nanoliter wells by prefilling of wells using electrospray deposition followed by sample introduction with a coverslip method, Anal. Chem. 77 (2005) 225–231, https://doi.org/10.1021/ac0400515.

PART THREE

Trends in electrospinning and electrospraying

CHAPTER ELEVEN

Trending approaches in electrospinning and electrospraying for biomedical applications

Poornima Dubey[1,a], Ishita Matai[2,3,a], Deepa Garg[2,3,a], Alok Kumar[4], Vinita Takiar[1,5]

[1]Department of Radiation Oncology, University of Cincinnati College of Medicine Cincinnati, Cincinnati, OH, United States
[2]Central Scientific Instruments Organization (CSIR-CSIO), Chandigarh, Punjab, India
[3]Academy of Scientific and Innovative Research, CSIR-CSIO, Chandigarh, Punjab, India
[4]Department of Immunology and Genomic Medicine, Graduate School of Medicine, Kyoto University, Yoshida Campus, Yoshida Konoe-cho, Kyoto, Japan
[5]Cincinnati Department of Veterans Affairs (VA) Medical Center, Cincinnati, OH, United States

11.1 Introduction

Currently, different techniques are available for nanomaterial fabrication, such as electrohydrodynamic (EHD), self-assembly, phase separation, template synthesis, mechanical drawing, etc. Among these, EHD process has emerged to be one of the most reliable, versatile, user-friendly, cost-effective, and point-of-care detection in comparison to others [1,2]. EHD techniques utilize electrostatically charged melts of the substrate to fabricate nano- or microranged fibers, particles, or beads, applicable to medical purposes. *Electrospinning and electrospraying* present two complementary technologies derived from the EHD process and have been extensively explored for fabrication of nanofibers (NFs) and nanoparticles (NPs), respectively [1]. The main difference at preparation stage among them remains the polymer viscosity, hence the concentration of the polymer solution under similar set of conditions. The polymeric solution, with decreased solution concentration, destabilizes the jet leads to bead NFs to particles [1,3]. Typically, NF diameter ranges from nanometers, i.e., less than 1 to 1000 nm [4]. It allows for precise control over the porous microstructure,

[a] Equal contribution.

Biomedical Applications of Electrospinning and Electrospraying
ISBN: 978-0-12-822476-2
https://doi.org/10.1016/B978-0-12-822476-2.00008-X

along with high surface area-to-volume ratio leading to higher biomolecule encapsulation and retention, with capability for processing diverse range of substrates [1]. On the contrary, electrospraying is a liquid atomization process which uses electrical forces to fabricate particles. In comparison to other particles, electrosprayed particles/droplets are highly stable and do not aggregate due to their self-dispersive nature. Similar to electrospun NFs, electrosprayed particles can also be used for implant coatings, drug delivery, and diagnosis [3,5]. Since decades, considerable efforts have been made in the synthesis of nanomaterials to provide a specific and ultrasensitive diagnostic tool for several diseases, including cancer, malaria, diabetes, etc.

However, the potential of their combinatorial approach in the field of tissue engineering, drug delivery, bioimaging, and diagnosis is relatively less explored. Majority of the polymers employed include synthetic such as polystyrene, poly(vinyl chloride), poly ε-caprolactone (PCL), polylactide (PLA), poly(lactide-co-glycolide) (PLGA), and polyglycolide and natural such as collagen, chitosan, gelatin, alginate, and silk fibroin [3,6]. Similarly, a wide variety of biomolecules can be encapsulated or surface functionalized, such as growth factors, nano-/microparticles, protein, nucleic acid, etc.

11.2 Trending approaches in electrospinning and electrospraying for disease diagnosis

Recent advancement in the fabrication of electrospun NFs and electrosprayed particles showed promising alternatives for early diagnosis and monitoring of a disease. An increase in the surface area-to-volume ratio increases the contact area between the actual sensing apparatus and the target cell/molecules, which influences the specificity, selectivity, and limit of detection (LOD) of the NF sensor [7]. Various formulations of electrospun NFs and their potential use in biosensing are recorded in Table 11.1.

11.2.1 Cancer

Cancer, the second leading cause of death in the world, is one of the biggest threats to human health. Alone in 2018, approximately 18.1 million new cases were registered, and 9.6 million lost their lives to cancer and millions more are at a huge risk [8]. Early diagnosis of cancer has been observed to play a significant role in the successful treatment, and therefore improves the survival rate of patients. The overexpression of specific protein biomarkers by cancer cells provides the opportunity to develop strategies for early diagnosis. Some of

Table 11.1 Application of electrospun nanofibers in disease diagnostics.

Base material	Additive component	Further treatment	Type of sensing	Key features	Ref.
ZnO nanofibers	Multiwalled carbon nanotubes	Calcination	Carcinoma antigen-125 (ovarian cancer)	LOD: 0.00113 Um/L Sensitivity: 90.14 μA/(U/mL)/cm^2 Detection range: 0.001Um/L−1 kUm/L	[11]
Carbon nanofibers	Bimetallic MCo (M = Cu, Fe, Ni, and Mn) nanoparticles	Thermal treatment	Glucose (diabetes)	LOD: 1.0 μM Sensitivity: 507 μA m/M cm^2 Detection range: 0.02−11 mM	[23]
PEI-PLGA nanofibers	Hyaluronic acid	Integration in a microfluidic chamber	CD44+ Carcinoma (cancer)	Capable of capturing HeLa cells at low density (20 cells per mL)	[16]
ZnO nanofibers	Carbon nanotubes	Integration in a microfluidic chamber	Histidine-rich protein II (HRPII) (malaria)	LOD: 7.5 fg/mL Sensitivity: 1.19 mA/g/mL/cm^2 Detection range: 10 fg/mL−100 μg/mL	[28]

these biomarkers include carcinoma antigen-125 (ovarian cancer), CD44 (leukemia, breast, ovarian cancer), AFP (liver cancer), BRCA1/BRCA2 (breast/ovarian cancer), and CEA (colorectal cancer) [9,10].

In this direction, electrospinning and electrospraying techniques have been widely explored to detect specific biomarkers. For instance, *Paul* et al. developed a label-free, electrochemical biosensor to achieve ultrasensitive detection of carcinoma antigen-125 with the help of differential pulse voltammetry. The immunosensor platform employed electrospinning technique to fabricate zinc oxide (ZnO) nanowires embedded with multiwalled carbon nanotubes (MWCNTs). This cost-effective and stable biosensor demonstrated good sensitivity (90.14 μA/(U/mL)/cm^2), low detection limit (0.00113 U/mL), and a broad detection range (0.001 U/mL − 1 kU/mL) [11]. Apart from protein-based detectors, gas biosensors based on volatile organic compounds such as toluene and aromatic amines are widely known [12].

In addition, circulating tumor cells are also considered an important biomarker for the early diagnosis of metastatic cancer. These cells often shed from the primary tissue into the bloodstream and reach vasculature or lymphatics, thereby resulting in metastasis [13]. Isolation and capture of such cells from blood is expected to slow down and/or prevent cancer metastasis. To this end, numerous studies have been conducted for capturing cells specific to breast cancer, melanoma, colorectal cancer, and prostate cancer [14,15]. To achieve higher detection sensitivity and selectivity, EHD techniques have been integrated with microfluidic diagnostic systems. *Xu* et al. proposed a facile approach to selectively capture CD44+ cancer cells of various origins (HeLa, KB, A549, and MCF-7 cells). They conjugated hyaluronic acid (HA) with polyethyleneimine (PEI)-functionalized PLGA electrospun NFs, which were then integrated into a microfluidic platform [16].

Often, higher than normal levels of expression of alkaline phosphatase (ALP) in serum have been associated with malignant tumor. Therefore, developing sensitive biosensors capable of detecting ALP concentration seems to benefit early diagnosis of cancer [17]. To achieve this, ALP activity in human serum has been monitored by an NF-based ratiometric assay by *Zhao* et al. First, fluorescein (a fluorescent dye) was covalently immobilized onto polyethylene terephthalate (PET) electrospun fibers, and bisquaternary ammonium salt of tetraphenylethene (TPE-2N+) was adsorbed via electrostatic interactions. If ALP is absent, phosphorylated fluorescein forms a complex with TPE-2N+, resulting in blue color fluorescence (471 nm) due to TPE. However, the presence of ALP leads to hydrolysis of phosphoesters, as a result TPE-2N+ slips away. This results in restoration of green color fluorescein emission (514 nm). Finally, the nanosensor showed excellent LOD of 0−80 mU/mL, and the obtained results were in good agreement with the ELISA results [17].

To meet the high energy demands required for metabolism, cancer cells consume glucose, metabolize it, and excrete large amount of lactate. This leads to localized pH changes in cancer cells, which can be detected by diagnostic tools [18]. *Shaibani* et al. fabricated an addressable potentiometric sensor (LAPS) integrated with pH-sensitive hydrogel NFs, produced using electrospinning. NF-LAPS showed changes in cancer cell acidification by continuous measuring and monitoring the pH changes as a response to therapeutic treatment. This method widens our knowledge on the metabolic process involved in cancer progression, and their possible response to anticancer therapies [19].

11.2.2 Diabetes

Diabetes mellitus has become a global pandemic, with higher prevalence in low- and middle-income countries. According to a report by the World Health Organization, more than 422 million people are suffering from this serious illness, while more than 318 million are at a risk of developing in the near future. It is estimated to be seventh leading cause of death in the upcoming times [20]. To minimize the health risks associated with diabetes, continuous monitoring of blood glucose levels is crucial.

Electrospun NFs play a vital role in developing biosensors for rapid and accurate detection of glucose, and are categorized into enzyme- and nonenzyme-based sensors. However, the activity and stability of the enzyme-based biosensors is limited due to variable environment conditions (pH, temperature, humidity), shifting the complete focus to nonenzymatic biosensors [2,21]. *Zheng* et al. fabricated nonenzymatic biosensor by modifying electrospun cupric oxide NFs (Ag/CuO NFs) with silver (Ag) NP. It was then employed for the detection of glucose using cyclic voltammetry (CV) and chronoamperometry, and exhibited a high sensitivity of 1347 $\mu A/mM\ cm^2$ and an LOD of 51.7 nM. Finally, the similar and reproducible results were obtained after employing the similar strategy on fresh blood samples [22].

In a similar study by *Li* et al., electrocatalytic oxidation and glucose detection efficiency of the different bimetallic MCo (M = Cu, Fe, Ni, and Mn) NPs distributed in electrospun carbon nanofibers (CFs) were investigated using CV and chronoamperometry. All the materials except MnCo—CF formed 3D network films, primarily responsible for the activity of the materials due to high surface area and increased number of active sites. The results revealed good stability and reproducibility of biosensor, with highest performance shown by CuCo—CF, followed by FeCo—CF, NiCo—CF, and MnCo—CF. Moreover, CuCo—CF exhibited a high sensitivity of 507 $\mu A/mM\ cm^2$, low response time of 2 s, and excellent linear response ranging from 0.02 to 11 mM. These results were found to be in accordance with the real blood samples [23].

11.2.3 Malaria

Vector-borne diseases, especially malaria, are of the serious health complications, occurring globally. Nearly 228 million cases of malarial infection were reported in 2018, and 0.18% of them proved to be fatal [24]. Today, several methods for malarial diagnosis are available, including microscopy, polymerase chain reaction, flow cytometry, molecular diagnostic techniques, automated blood cell analyzers, and immune-based rapid diagnostic kits. However, they are expensive, time consuming, and require highly skilled technicians [25]. These limitations of the conventional methods have drawn the attention toward the diagnosis based on nanomaterials, such as NFs and NPs.

In an attempt to improve the LOD, *Brince* et al. fabricated an electrochemical immunoassay-based biosensor for detection of histidine-rich protein-2 (HRPII) antigen, specific to malarial infection. Herein, copper (Cu)-doped ZnO NFs were produced using electrospinning and functionalized with mercaptopropylphosphonic acid. The prepared nanobiosensor showed a good sensitivity of 28.5 KΩ/(gm/mL)/cm^2 and excellent LOD of 6.8 ag/mL [26]. However, the use of additional modification of electrode surface has become a hindrance in the development of an inexpensive, light-weight, and flexible point-of-care diagnosis.

In this view, functionalization of ZnO with a more suitable conductive material could be considered. Therefore, *Brince* et al. replaced Cu with MWCNTs and fabricated a flexible and label-free chemiresistive-based nanobiosensor. Similar to the previous study, MWCNT−ZnO NFs were also synthesized using electrospinning and calcination. After depositing the MWCNT−ZnO NFs between the source and drain electrodes, which were patterned on a flexible and thin film of PET, HRPII-specific antibodies were directly conjugated with the functional groups on ZnO NFs. Finally, the developed nanobiosensor revealed LOD of 0.97 fg/mL, resistivity of 8.29 kΩ/g mL, and detection range of 10 fg/mL−10 ng/mL, thereby promising a better diagnostic approach [27].

Lately, fabrication of microfluidic integrated biosensor has been documented for detecting HRPII (Fig. 11.1). The fabrication and integration of the prefunctionalized sensing platform in the microfluidic channels was done by tune transfer approach, which is much simpler than the traditional methods. Afterward, the sensing platform was integrated with the antibody (AntiHRP11) immobilized CNT−ZnO electrospun NFs. The fabricated biosensor revealed excellent sensitivity of 1.19 mA/g/mL/cm^2 with LOD of 7.5 fg/mL and a wide detection range from 10 fg/mL to 100 μg/mL, for HRPII detection [28].

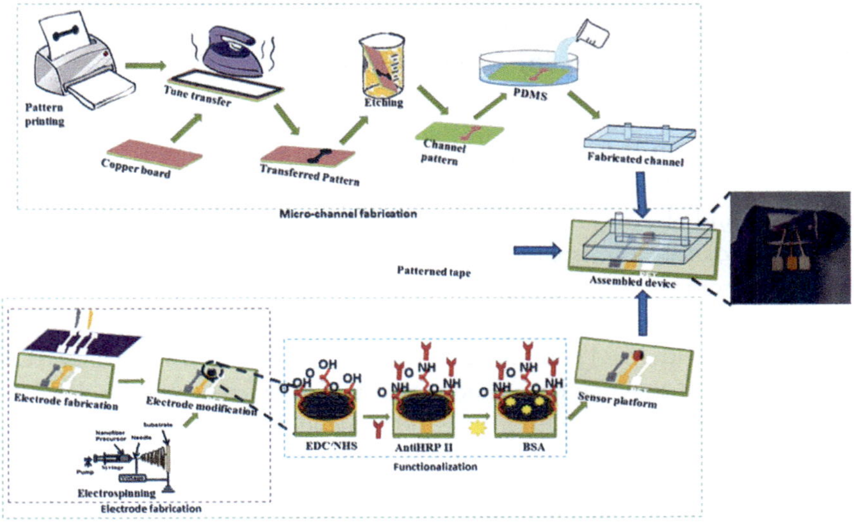

Figure 11.1 Schematic illustration of experimental fabrication and functionalization of the plastic-based biochip for malaria detection. *Reprinted with permission from ref. K. Brince Paul, A.K. Panigrahi, V. Singh, S.G. Singh, Nonlithographic fabrication of plastic-based nanofibers integrated microfluidic biochip for sensitive detection of infectious biomarker, ACS Appl. Mater. Interfaces 9 (2017) 39994–40005. https://doi.org/10.1021/acsami.7b11331, Copyright © 2016, American Chemical Society.*

11.2.4 Other diseases

Mondal et al. fabricated anatase titania NF mat (TiO_2−NF) utilizing PVP as a polymer matrix, to detect esterified cholesterol using electrochemical method. This sensing platform reported excellent catalytic response, with low LOD (0.49 mM), good sensitivity (181.6 μA/mg/dL/cm^2), and very low detection time of 20 s [29].

Electrospun NFs are being used for the detection of some volatile compounds to detect the concentration of breath biomarkers, indicative of a disease. Toward this end, *Choi* et al. reported the synthesis of semiconductor metal oxide−based gas sensors for detection of acetone and hydrogen sulfide (H_2S) in humid air, known as breath markers for diabetes and halitosis. The gas sensor was fabricated by functionalization of stannic acid electrospun NFs with reduced graphene oxide, followed by calcination. LOD as low as 1 ppm for H_2S and 100 ppb for acetone was achieved [30].

In a study, *Marquez* et al. utilized coelectrospinning technique to develop a multifunctional polymeric coaxial NF system with optical oxygen transduction and could detect the concentration of uric acid in serum samples. Moreover, a good correlation between results obtained by them and an external laboratory was reported [31,32].

11.3 Trending approaches in electrospinning and electrospraying for bioimaging

Electrospinning and electrospraying have been widely used to fabricate the NFs modified with imaging agents which allow continuous monitoring of the physiological process. Table 11.2 lists different electrospun NFs and electrosprayed particles applied in bioimaging applications.

Using coaxial electrospinning technique, *Jin* et al. developed a theranostic system to monitor the progression of a disease. A synthetic and biocompatible polymer polyethylene oxide was used as a core polymer for NF synthesis, incorporated with MRI contrast agent (G(III) diethylenetriaminepentaacetate hydrate) and therapeutic drug indomethacin. Finally, the outer shell of the NF core was formed using Eudragit S100 to avoid drug/contrast agent release in the stomach. This core—shell NF system proved to be a good theranostic agent, with sustained release of the drug to colon and excellent contrast properties [33].

A few studies have demonstrated dynamic in vivo monitoring of glucose by introducing implantable biosensors. This is especially beneficial to patients who are prone to frequent fluctuations in glucose level [34]. For instance, *Balaconis* et al. fabricated glucose-sensitive PCL NFs, loaded with boronic acid and alizarin (optical reporter), and showed enhanced response and in vivo residency time in comparison to the spherical nanosensors. In the absence of glucose, a diol group on alizarin binds to boronic acid and exhibits fluorescence. Contrarily, when glucose is present, it competitively binds to the boronic acid and this disturbs its interaction with the alizarin, and as a result, fluorescence is quenched. The fluorescence quenching, therefore, depends on the concentration of glucose. Remarkably, NF sensors could maintain higher residency time, in comparison to spherical nanosensors which diffused away from the injection site within 3 h [34].

Meanwhile, electrospraying has been successfully employed for imaging using techniques, such has ultrasound, magnetic resonance, and fluorescence [35,36]. For example, *Zhang* et al. fabricated polymer-based magnetic polymer yolk—shell particle with both dual-mode (ultrasonic and magnetic) imaging capability, using trineedle coaxial electrospraying. As shown in Fig. 11.2, these particles are of uniform size, and comprise a multicompartment structure. They consist of a polymeric core (with PCL as a matrix), an oily interface layer, and polymeric shell (PCL) embedded with magnetic iron oxide nanoparticles. Briefly, multiple probes/drugs can be encapsulated in the core—shell compartments and their release profiles can be tuned by

Table 11.2 Application of electrospun nanofibers and electrosprayed particles for bioimaging.

Imaging type	Base material	Contrast material	Application	Key features	Ref.
Magnetic resonance imaging (MRI)	Core–shell nanofibers Core: PEO Shell: Eudragit S100	Core: Gd(DTPA)	Delivering drug indomethacin to colon and imaging it simultaneously	Sustained release over 12–29 h Excellent contrast properties	[33]
Dual mode (ultrasonic and MRI)	Yolk-shell particles Core: PCL matrix Shell: PCL matrix	Shell: Magnetic Fe_3O_4 nanoparticles	Developing theranostic agents with dual-mode imaging	Good imaging and coactive delivery	[35]
Fluorescence	PLGA Janus microspheres (dual chamber)	One chamber: Fluorescent drug $TbLa_3(Bim)_{12}$ Second chamber: Magnetic Fe_3O_4 nanoparticles	Monitoring and tracing the delivery of drug benzimidazole (Bim)	High fluorescent intensity	[37]
Desorption electrospray ionization–mass spectrometry imaging (DESI-MS)	–	–	Chemical imaging of small molecules (lipids and other metabolites) in tissue sections	Indicates vital lipids associated with physiological organogenesis	[41]

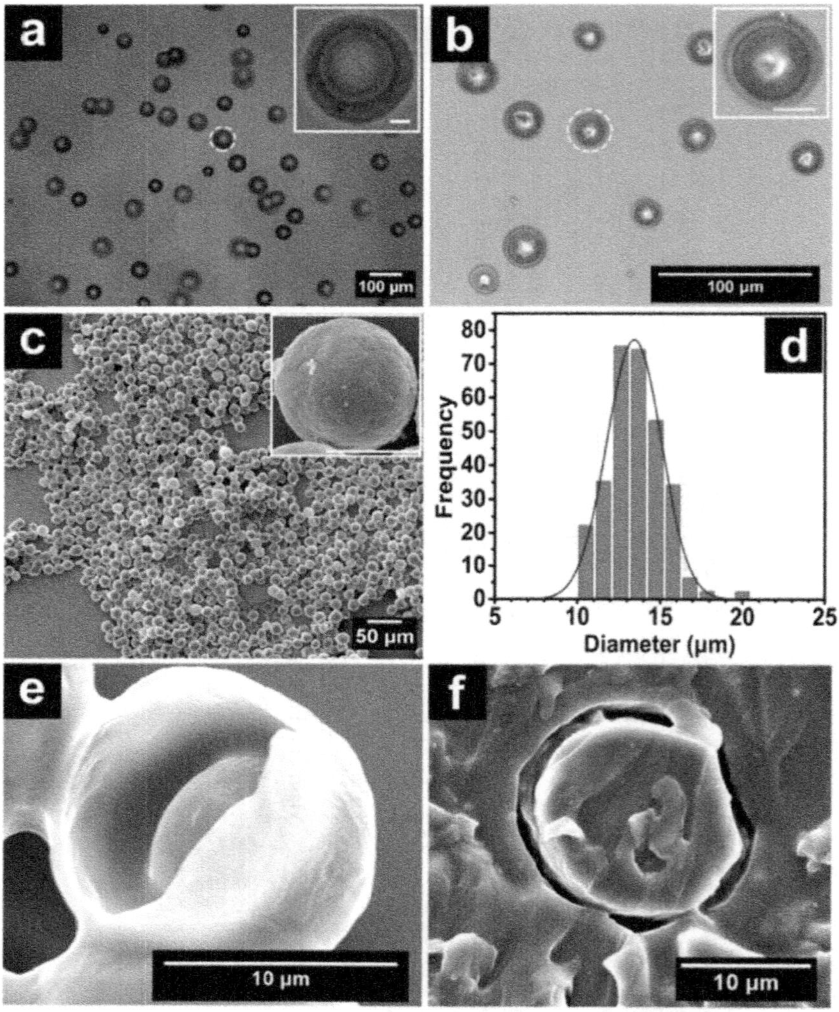

Figure 11.2 Morphological characterization of magnetic polymer yolk–shell particles (YSPs). (a) Optical micrograph, and (b) merged bright field and fluorescence image of YSPs with the interfacing layer labeled with Nile red. (c) Electron micrograph of YSPs (scale bar = 10 μm) and (d) size distribution based on statistical analysis of 300 particles. (e) Electron micrograph of a ruptured microparticle. (f) Cross-sectional electron micrograph of microsphere embedded in epoxy resin. *Reprinted with permission from ref. C. Zhang, Z.C. Yao, Q. Ding, J.J. Choi, Z. Ahmad, M.W. Chang, J.S. Li, Tri-needle coaxial electrospray engineering of magnetic polymer yolk-shell particles possessing dual-imaging modality, multiagent compartments, and trigger release potential, ACS Appl. Mater. Interfaces 9 (2017) 21485–21495. https://doi.org/10.1021/acsami.7b05580, Copyright © 2017, American Chemical Society.*

external auxiliary magnetic field. The electrosprayed particles demonstrated good imaging and coactive delivery [35].

A similar study by *Li* et al. demonstrated the fabrication of a double-chambered drug delivery system and Janus microspheres using double-needle electrospraying. To enhance the fluorescent intensity of the particles, fluorescent and magnetic materials were encapsulated in two chambers, separately. Thus, it was predicted that Janus particles with enhanced fluorescent activity could be potentially used in tracing therapeutic drug delivery [37].

Electrospraying when coupled with mass spectroscopy is commonly known as desorption electrospray ionization mass spectrometry imaging (DESI-MSI), and provides a label-free platform to visualize the distribution of wide variety of metabolites, such as lipids and carbohydrates [38]. This also provides better understanding of cancer biology and development of early diagnostic systems [39].

Hsu et al. reported the utilization of nanospray DESI (nanoDESI) to map and image proteins in tissue samples with minimal invasion. The expression of ubiquitin, β-thymosin, myelin basic protein, and hemoglobin was observed in healthy thymus tissue. The same modality was extended to MYC-induced lymphomas. In contrast to healthy tissue, truncated proteins with spatial heterogeneity were found to be dominant in the area where normal cells were now penetrated by tumor cells. Therefore, this imaging tool is expected to provide in-depth understanding of the cellular process [40].

In recent years, DESI-MS has been explored to study the chemical changes in fetal and embryonic development, and related congenital diseases. *León* et al. reported the DESI-MS-assisted chemical imaging of small molecules (lipids and other metabolites) in tissue sections from a complete swine fetus (gestation period-50 days) and displayed their organ-specific distributions. The chemical information obtained from DES-MS imaging provides an important insight in physiology, and this information, when added complementarily to the already existing anatomical studies, indicates vital lipids associated with physiological organogenesis [41].

Hemalatha et al. illustrated the applicability of electrospun nylon-6 NF mats for detection and imaging via DESI-MS technique. The mats with fibers of diameter ~200 nm were fabricated using needless electrospinning. The prepared NF mats demonstrated rapid detection of analytes in a single drop of dyes (methyl orange), plant extracts (periwinkle flower extract), and inks (Fig. 11.3a–c). These mats were found to be capable of imaging imprinted patterns of diverse materials, including inks and plant parts (leaves,

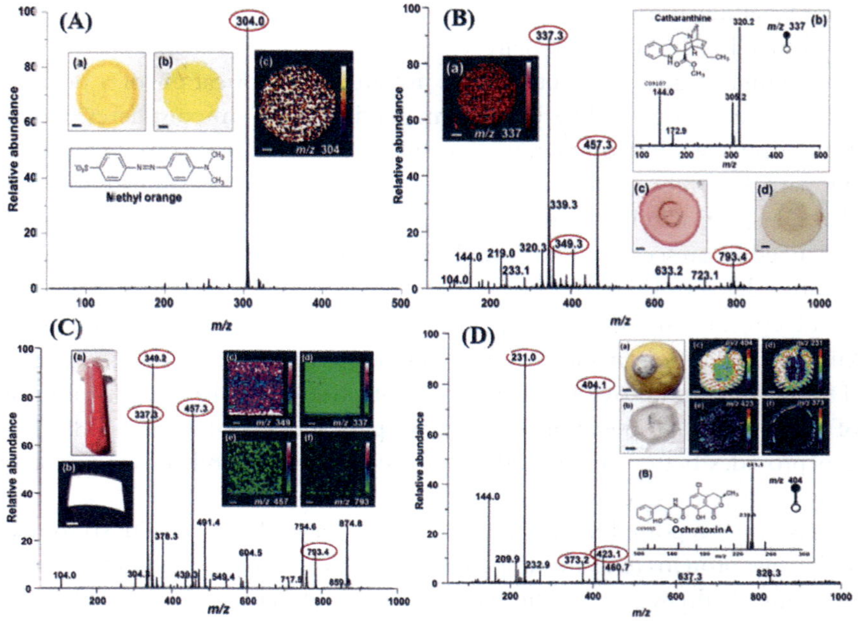

Figure 11.3 (A) DESI-MS spectrum from a single drop of methyl orange (MO) spotted on a nylon nanofiber mat. (a) Images of the corresponding spot of MO on a TLC-plate, revealing the spreading effect, and halo formation on its periphery. (b) Same MO sample when spotted on a nylon nanofiber mat displays uniform spreading. (c) DESI-MS images of characteristic MO peak at m/z 304. (B) DESI-MS spectrum from a single drop of a periwinkle flower extract spotted on a nylon nanofiber mat. (a) DESI-MS image and (b) tandem mass spectrum characteristic of catharanthine at m/z 337. (c) Spreading and (d) fading effects of the flower extract spotted on TLC-plates. Scale bar in all DESI-MS images is 5 mm. (C) DESI-MS spectrum of nylon fiber mat incorporated with periwinkle flower extract. (a) Nylon polymer solution blend with flower extract exhibiting pink color. (b) Optical image of the electrospun nylon fiber mat incorporated with flower extract. (c–f) DESI-MS images of the encircled peaks at m/z 337, 349, 457, and 793. All the compounds showed uniform distribution. Scale bar in all DESI-MS images is 5 mm. (D) (i) DESI-MS spectrum of the fungal-infected region of lemon, swabbed on a nylon nanofiber mat. (a,b) Optical images of (a) infected whole fruit of lemon, and (b) region of fungal infection. (c–f) DESI-MS images of encircled peaks revealing toxic metabolites from fungal species, (ii) tandem mass spectra and structure of Ochratoxin A at m/z 404. *Reprinted with permission from ref. R.G. Hemalatha, M.A. Ganayee, T. Pradeep, Electrospun nanofiber mats as "smart surfaces" for desorption electrospray ionization mass spectrometry (DESI MS)-Based analysis and imprint imaging, Anal. Chem. 88 (2016) 5710–5717. https://doi.org/10.1021/acs.analchem.5b04520, Copyright © 2016, American Chemical Society.*

petals, rhizome slices). Furthermore, the growth of fungal species on fruits such as lemon was imaged on NF mats, and revealed the presence of ochratoxin A, a toxic metabolite secreted by fungus (*Penicillium digitatum*) (Fig. 11.3d) [42]. Altogether, these results signify the efficacy of nylon-6

NF mats to provide a smart surface for detection and imprint imaging of diverse classes of compounds.

11.4 Trending approaches in electrospinning and electrospraying in wound healing and antimicrobial applications

Wound, a status of interrupted anatomical structure of the skin, impairs the function of skins [43]. Wound healing, a biological process, involves the interaction of different cells, growth factors, chemical messengers, and enzymatic cofactors [44]. Wound healing, a dynamic and complex process, requires proper environment that promotes the healing process [45]. Wound healing accomplishes through four phases of hemostasis, inflammation, proliferation, and remodeling. These phases occur in a well-connected cascade and their promotion depends on wound type, pathological conditions of wounds, and the type of dressing material. Depending upon the duration and nature of healing process, wound can be acute (because of accident or surgical injury) or chronic (because of ulcers and burns).

Wound dressings provide proper conditions to rebuild skin. Tissue engineering deals with the use of scaffolds or wound dressings that promote or hasten the formation of new viable tissue. Faster wound healing depends upon the type of wound dressing material. An ideal wound dressing should be biocompatible, sterile, nontoxic, nonallergic, and act as physical barrier to check microbial infection while at the same time must enhance leukocytes migration by providing debridement action. It should also provide a moist environment for controlling the elimination of exudates and water vapor transmission which is a requisite for the fast recovery of wound. Traditional wound dressing simply covers the wound and does not play active role in hastening the healing processes, while nanotechnology-based wound dressings cover many aspects and can be designed to actively involve in hastening healing process by using antibacterials, and by delivering healing-promoting molecules [46]. Scaffolds morphology decides the different aspects of cellular functions at the application site like cell adhesion, proliferation, infiltration, and migration. Different aspects of fiber like porosity, fiber diameter, and surface roughness affect cell adhesion, proliferation, cell migration, and infiltration to the wound area.

Polymeric NFs, because of submicrometric dimension having large area/volume ratio and high porosity, have been considered superior options to be used as scaffolds or wound dressings. Electrohydrodynamic (electrospinning and electrospraying) processes have been widely explored for different biomedical applications. The produced electrospun fibers and electrosprayed particles possess many structural and functional advantages over traditional methods. However, their use in the field of wound dressings with antimicrobial abilities is less explored. Because of the infection, people die from burns and diabetic wounds. As per CDC report, up to 2050, there will be more death because of bacterial infection compared to cancer. This demands the development of antibacterial-based wound dressings to avoid the infection and heal the burns and diabetic wounds. "Nanoparticle dressing," a term being used for incorporating NPs into scaffolds, has gained much more attention.

Many agents have been explored for their use in clinical purposes. Ag and ZnO NPs are the most well studied for their antibacterial properties and have been incorporated with different NFs for the wound dressings. In addition, some redox-active transition metals, for example, Cu, kill the bacteria by producing reactive oxygen species through Fenton's reaction [47]. Other some soft acids, for example, Ag+, Au+, Zn2+, Cu+, and Cu++, form stable covalent bonds with thiol groups of amino acids (especially arginine, histidine, lysine, proline) and proteins and thereby cause oxidation that leads to bacterial death. Ag shows higher affinity for polymeric membranes of bacteria which are highly electronegative in nature. In this section, we will discuss the potential antimicrobial-based applications of electrospinning and electrospraying techniques. Moreover, limitations and future perspectives will also be highlighted.

11.4.1 EHD techniques for wound dressing applications

Electrospinning process provides us an added advantage to produce biomimetic nanofibrous materials from a wide spectrum of natural and synthetic polymers which is nearly impossible with traditional methods. The electrospun nanofibrous materials with morphological features and dimensions allow them to impersonate the extracellular matrix (ECM) which is essential for fostering cell proliferation and attachment with neighbor cells [48].

Natural biopolymers like proteins and polysaccharides, being biocompatible, biodegradable, and able to recreate the natural ECM, are the first choice for polymer selection [49]. Natural fiber—derived proteins like collagen, fibrinogen, and silk fibroin are suitable for electrospun nanofibrous mat preparation since they easily self-assemble into fibrous structures [50]. The natural polysaccharides like chitosan, cellulose, alginate, and glycosaminoglycans and biopolymers like collagen (the major component of ECM), gelatin, chitosan, alginate, and glycosaminoglycans (like HA and chondroitin sulfate) have gained much interest for the selection of polymer because of their peculiar properties.

11.4.2 Nanocomposite scaffolds using metal nanoparticles as antibacterial for the wound dressings

The nanocomposite scaffold requires the biocompatible polymer (discussed in previous section) and the antibacterial NPs. Adding antibacterial NP either directly in the polymer solution or simultaneously electrospraying a NP dispersion generates a composite, NP-embedded or NP-coated polymeric fibers with enhanced and some novel properties. The NPs further enhance the area of contact and increase the surface-dependent properties (like antimicrobial and enzymatic properties) of the nanocomposite fibers.

Metal NPs with antibacterial properties are preferred for the incorporation to prepare nanocomposite fibers. Antibacterial properties of Ag are widespread and are a most common formulation used in different studies [51]. Ag NP gets ionized in the wound fluid and the ionized Ag NP kills the bacteria by binding to tissue protein and bringing structural changes in the bacterial wall. It binds with nucleic acid as well as by denaturing and stops the bacterial replication. We have listed different nanocomposite fibers and mats for wound dressing that used NPs as the antibacterial agent.

Recently, a research group reported the use of plasma-treated electrospun PCL scaffold which was coated with Ag NPs embedded in gelatin. The advantages of this nanocomposite scaffold are that a) thick layer of gelatin on PLC surface has been created using multicoating method and b) gelatin covering on PLC was strengthened by plasma treatment. They tested its antibacterial property using agar diffusion and found it to be effective against gram-positive and gram-negative bacteria as well. The unique property of this nanocomposite scaffold is that because of hydrophilic property of PCL electrospun, it does not cause any damage during dressing removal. Water interaction test was performed to test hydrophilization of PCL fibers [52]. Their work led a way for the application of multicoating technique in optimizing the antibacterial property of a nonadhesive PCL/gelatin/Ag scaffold. In other work, Zhang et al. have shown the beneficial effects of nanocomposite Ag NPs that were doped with collagen—alginate fiber [53]. The biocomposite was found to be effective in killing *Escherichia coli* and *Staphylococcus aureus* in agar diffusion assay. CA—Ag NPs biocomposite possess much higher antimicrobial activity than CA-biocomposite itself, and importantly the antibacterial activity increases with AgNP content linearly.

Chitosan, the natural polysaccharide, has wider applications in tissue engineering and wound healing applications. Some reports suggest chitosan controls inflammatory mediators and thereby helps in faster healing of wounds [54]. Different research groups have shown the nanocomposite of chitosan with other NPs as antimicrobial components in the wound dressing. Abdelrahman et al. have shown the electrospun sheet of chitosan blended with PVA, and incorporated Ag NPs (3142 ppm) have higher antibacterial effects for clearing the microbial load of *E. coli* and hastening the healing of wounds (chitosan—Ag—PVA) [55]. The nanocomposite chitosan—Ag—PVA shows added bactericidal activity since chitosan (polycationic) and Ag (monovalent cationic) have similar mechanism of action by attaching with anionic bacterial membrane. Other groups have used the combination of chitosan with gold [56] and Cu [57] as well.

11.4.3 Nanocomposite scaffolds using metal oxide nanoparticles as antibacterials for the wound dressings

Not only metal NPs but also metal compounds especially oxides of transition metals show antibacterial activity. Most commonly used metal oxide NPs are ZnO and titanium oxide (TiO_2) for the antibacterial compound. Lee et al. have reported the nanocomposite electrospun PVA fibers with TiO_2 NPs and found effectively inhibited *S. aureus* and *Klebsiella pneumoniae* [58]. In a similar work, other research groups also reported the use of TiO_2 (along with small amount of $AgNO_3$) for their antibacterial activity where they have used polymeric electrospun chitosan/PVA blend fibers [59]. They have shown the higher antimicrobial activity of this nanocomposite against *S. aureus* and *E. coli*.

Another antibacterial NPs that attracted the research most is ZnO. Their economical synthesis and antibacterial effectiveness against a broad range of microbes are two important features that keep it in the front line of antibacterial nanostructures. Shalumon et al. have reported the mixed biodegradable and biocompatible fiber sodium alginate/PVA with ZnO as antibacterial for the wound dressing [60]. Sodium alginate being polyelectrolyte increased the electrical conductivity of solution, while alginate promotes the thermal stability. The nanocomposite showed antibacterial effect against *E. coli and S. aureus*. The authors have further shown the nanocomposite to have reduced adhesion which is a beneficial feature for the use as wound dressings. Other research groups have developed electrospun poly(D,L-lactide) fiber and used ZnO NPs (3 wt%) as antibacterial. It is effective against gram-negative *E. coli* and the gram-positive *S. aureus* bacteria. The results suggest ZnO-coated fibrous PLA mats as a potential candidate for applications related to wound dressing materials [61].

11.5 Conclusions and future perspective

Applications of EHD technology comprising electrospinning and electrospraying have widened the possibility of healthcare management. Their astounding properties, including high surface area-to-volume ratio, encapsulation efficiency, and porosity, have proven to be very useful for therapeutics, diagnostics, and for designing nanocomposite scaffolds for tissue engineering applications to name a few. Nevertheless, the polymers and solvents pose risk on safety profile, along with other factors such as quality and uniformity and large-scale production of the products. Interestingly, combination of electrospinning with spraying has shown great promise for designing products such as NF microspheres for improved stem cell viability and proliferation owing to their injectability and biomimetic features. Hence, recent studies done suggest that the combination of electrospun NF with nano-/microparticles offers a new landscape to overcome existing problems of nanoformulations and scaffolding materials and offers improved nanofabricated products and therapeutics for biomedical applications.

References

[1] Z. Chan, Z. Chen, A. Zhang, J. Hu, X. Wang, Z. Yang, Electrospun nanofibers for cancer diagnosis and therapy, Biomater. Sci. 4 (2016) 922–932, https://doi.org/10.1039/c6bm00070c.

[2] P. Prabhu, Nanofibers for medical diagnosis and therapy, in: A. Barhoum, M. Bechelany, A. Makhlouf (Eds.), Handbook of Nanofibers, Springer, Cham, 2019, pp. 831–867, https://doi.org/10.1007/978-3-319-53655-2_48.

[3] R. Sridhar, R. Lakshminarayanan, K. Madhaiyan, V.A. Barathi, K.H.C. Limh, S. Ramakrishna, Electrosprayed nanoparticles and electrospun nanofibers based on natural materials: applications in tissue regeneration, drug delivery and pharmaceuticals, Chem. Soc. Rev. 44 (2015) 790–814, https://doi.org/10.1039/c4cs00226a.

[4] J. Xue, T. Wu, Y. Dai, Y. Xia, Electrospinning and electrospun nanofibers: methods, materials, and applications, Chem. Rev. 119 (2019) 5298–5415, https://doi.org/10.1021/acs.chemrev.8b00593.

[5] D.I. Braghirolli, F. Zamboni, G.A.X. Acasigua, P. Pranke, Association of electrospinning with electrospraying: a strategy to produce 3D scaffolds with incorporated stem cells for use in tissue engineering, Int. J. Nanomed. 10 (2015) 5159–5170, https://doi.org/10.2147/IJN.S84312.

[6] J.D. Schiffman, C.L. Schauer, A review : electrospinning of biopolymer nanofibers and their applications, Polym. Rev. 48 (2008) 317–352, https://doi.org/10.1080/15583720802022182.
[7] J. Horne, L. McLoughlin, B. Bridgers, E.K. Wujcik, Recent developments in nanofiber-based sensors for disease detection, immunosensing, and monitoring, Sens. Actuators Rep. 2 (2020) 100005, https://doi.org/10.1016/j.snr.2020.100005.
[8] Cancer (n.d.). https://www.who.int/health-topics/cancer#tab=tab_1 (Accessed 10 May 2020).
[9] C. Chen, S. Zhao, A. Karnad, J.W. Freeman, The biology and role of CD44 in cancer progression: therapeutic implications, J. Hematol. Oncol. 11 (2018) 1–23, https://doi.org/10.1186/s13045-018-0605-5.
[10] I. Belczacka, A. Latosinska, J. Metzger, D. Marx, A. Vlahou, H. Mischak, M. Frantzi, Proteomics biomarkers for solid tumors: current status and future prospects, Mass Spectrom. Rev. 38 (2019) 49–78, https://doi.org/10.1002/mas.21572.
[11] K.B. Paul, V. Singh, S.R.K. Vanjari, S.G. Singh, One step biofunctionalized electrospun multiwalled carbon nanotubes embedded zinc oxide nanowire interface for highly sensitive detection of carcinoma antigen-125, Biosens. Bioelectron. 88 (2017) 144–152, https://doi.org/10.1016/j.bios.2016.07.114.
[12] Y. Adiguzel, H. Kulah, Breath sensors for lung cancer diagnosis, Biosens. Bioelectron. 65 (2015) 121–138, https://doi.org/10.1016/j.bios.2014.10.023.
[13] Y. Xiao, M. Shen, X. Shi, Design of functional electrospun nanofibers for cancer cell capture applications, J. Mater. Chem. B. 6 (2018) 1420–1432, https://doi.org/10.1039/c7tb03347h.
[14] C.C. Yu, Y.W. Chen, P.Y. Yeh, Y.S. Hsiao, W.T. Lin, C.W. Kuo, D.Y. Chueh, Y.W. You, J.J. Shyue, Y.C. Chang, P. Chen, Random and aligned electrospun PLGA nanofibers embedded in microfluidic chips for cancer cell isolation and integration with air foam technology for cell release, J. Nanobiotechnol. 17 (2019) 1–13, https://doi.org/10.1186/s12951-019-0466-2.
[15] C.C. Yu, B.C. Ho, R.S. Juang, Y.S. Hsiao, R.V.R. Naidu, C.W. Kuo, Y.W. You, J.J. Shyue, J.T. Fang, P. Chen, Poly(3,4-ethylenedioxythiophene)-based nanofiber mats as an organic bioelectronic platform for programming multiple capture/release cycles of circulating tumor cells, ACS Appl. Mater. Interfaces 9 (2017) 30329–30342, https://doi.org/10.1021/acsami.7b07042.
[16] G. Xu, Y. Tan, T. Xu, D. Yin, M. Wang, M. Shen, X. Chen, X. Shi, X. Zhu, Hyaluronic acid-functionalized electrospun PLGA nanofibers embedded in a microfluidic chip for cancer cell capture and culture, Biomater. Sci. 5 (2017) 752–761, https://doi.org/10.1039/c6bm00933f.
[17] L. Zhao, S. Xie, X. Song, J. Wei, Z. Zhang, X. Li, Ratiometric fluorescent response of electrospun fibrous strips for real-time sensing of alkaline phosphatase in serum, Biosens. Bioelectron. 91 (2017) 217–224, https://doi.org/10.1016/j.bios.2016.12.025.
[18] M. Chen, C. Chen, Z. Shen, X. Zhang, Y. Chen, F. Lin, X. Ma, C. Zhuang, Y. Mao, H. Gan, P. Chen, X. Zong, R. Wu, Extracellular pH is a biomarker enabling detection of breast cancer and liver cancer using CEST MRI, Oncotarget 8 (2017) 45759–45767, https://doi.org/10.18632/oncotarget.17404.
[19] P.M. Shaibani, H. Etayash, S. Naicker, K. Kaur, Metabolic study of cancer cells using a pH sensitive hydrogel nano fi ber light addressable potentiometric sensor, ACS Sens. 2 (2016) 151–156, https://doi.org/10.1021/acssensors.6b00632.
[20] Diabetes (n.d.). https://www.who.int/news-room/fact-sheets/detail/diabetes (Accessed 10 May 2020).

[21] M.V. Vellayappan, J.R. Venugopal, S. Ramakrishna, S. Ray, A.F. Ismail, M. Mandal, A. Manikandan, S. Seal, S.K. Jaganathan, Electrospinning applications from diagnosis to treatment of diabetes, RSC Adv. 6 (2016) 83638–83655, https://doi.org/10.1039/c6ra15252j.

[22] B. Zheng, G. Liu, A. Yao, Y. Xiao, J. Du, Y. Guo, D. Xiao, Q. Hu, M.M.F. Choi, A sensitive AgNPs/CuO nanofibers non-enzymatic glucose sensor based on electrospinning technology, Sens. Actuators, B Chem. 195 (2014) 431–438, https://doi.org/10.1016/j.snb.2014.01.046.

[23] M. Li, L. Liu, Y. Xiong, X. Liu, A. Nsabimana, X. Bo, L. Guo, Bimetallic MCo (M = Cu, Fe, Ni, and Mn) nanoparticles doped-carbon nanofibers synthetized by electrospinning for nonenzymatic glucose detection, Sens. Actuators, B Chem. 207 (2015) 614–622, https://doi.org/10.1016/j.snb.2014.10.092.

[24] Malaria (n.d.). https://www.who.int/news-room/fact-sheets/detail/malaria (Accessed 10 May 2020).

[25] K.V. Ragavan, S. Kumar, S. Swaraj, S. Neethirajan, Advances in biosensors and optical assays for diagnosis and detection of malaria, Biosens. Bioelectron. 105 (2018) 188–210, https://doi.org/10.1016/j.bios.2018.01.037.

[26] K. Brince Paul, S. Kumar, S. Tripathy, S.R.K. Vanjari, V. Singh, S.G. Singh, A highly sensitive self assembled monolayer modified copper doped zinc oxide nanofiber interface for detection of Plasmodium falciparum histidine-rich protein-2: targeted towards rapid, early diagnosis of malaria, Biosens. Bioelectron. 80 (2016) 39–46, https://doi.org/10.1016/j.bios.2016.01.036.

[27] B. Paul, A.K. Panigrahi, V. Singh, S.G. Singh, A multi-walled carbon nanotube-zinc oxide nanofiber based flexible chemiresistive biosensor for malaria biomarker detection, Analyst 142 (2017) 2128–2135, https://doi.org/10.1039/c7an00243b.

[28] K. Brince Paul, A.K. Panigrahi, V. Singh, S.G. Singh, Nonlithographic fabrication of plastic-based nanofibers integrated microfluidic biochip for sensitive detection of infectious biomarker, ACS Appl. Mater. Interfaces 9 (2017) 39994–40005, https://doi.org/10.1021/acsami.7b11331.

[29] K. Mondal, M.A. Ali, V.V. Agrawal, B.D. Malhotra, A. Sharma, Highly sensitive biofunctionalized mesoporous electrospun TiO_2 nanofiber based interface for biosensing, ACS Appl. Mater. Interfaces 6 (2014) 2516–2527, https://doi.org/10.1021/am404931f.

[30] I. Kim, Selective detection of acetone and hydrogen sulfide for the diagnosis of diabetes and halitosis using SnO 2 nano fibers functionalized with reduced graphene oxide nanosheets, ACS Appl. Mater. Interfaces 6 (2014) 2588–2597, https://doi.org/10.1021/am405088q.

[31] J.F. Fernandez-sanchez, A multifunctional material based on co-electrospinning for developing biosensors with optical oxygen transduction, Anal. Chim. Acta 1015 (2018) 66–73, https://doi.org/10.1016/j.aca.2018.02.010.

[32] B.M. Serafim, A. Leitolis, S. Crestani, B.H. Marcon, L. Foti, C.L. Petzhold, C. Radtke, M.A. Krieger, C.K. Saul, Electrospinning induced surface activation (EISA) of highly porous PMMA microfiber mats for HIV diagnosis, J. Mater. Chem. B. 4 (2016) 6004–6011, https://doi.org/10.1039/c6tb01435f.

[33] M. Jin, D.G. Yu, C.F.G.C. Geraldes, G.R. Williams, S.W.A. Bligh, Theranostic fibers for simultaneous imaging and drug delivery, Mol. Pharm. 13 (2016) 2457–2465, https://doi.org/10.1021/acs.molpharmaceut.6b00197.

[34] M.K. Balaconis, Y. Luo, H.A. Clark, Glucose-sensitive nanofiber scaffolds with an improved sensing design for physiological conditions, Analyst 140 (2015) 716–723, https://doi.org/10.1039/c4an01775g.

[35] C. Zhang, Z.C. Yao, Q. Ding, J.J. Choi, Z. Ahmad, M.W. Chang, J.S. Li, Tri-needle coaxial electrospray engineering of magnetic polymer yolk-shell particles possessing dual-imaging modality, multiagent compartments, and trigger release potential, ACS Appl. Mater. Interfaces 9 (2017) 21485–21495, https://doi.org/10.1021/acsami.7b05580.
[36] F. Foroutan, J.V. Jokerst, S.S. Gambhir, O. Vermesh, H.W. Kim, J.C. Knowles, Sol-gel synthesis and electrospraying of biodegradable $(P_2O_5)55-(CaO)30-(Na_2O)15$glass nanospheres as a transient contrast agent for ultrasound stem cell imaging, ACS Nano 9 (2015) 1868–1877, https://doi.org/10.1021/nn506789y.
[37] K. Li, P. Li, Z. Jia, B. Qi, J. Xu, D. Kang, M. Liu, Y. Fan, Enhanced fluorescent intensity of magnetic-fluorescent bifunctional PLGA microspheres based on Janus electrospraying for bioapplication, Sci. Rep. 8 (2018) 1–11, https://doi.org/10.1038/s41598-018-34856-z.
[38] A.M. Jeckel, K. Matsumura, K. Nishikawa, Y. Morimoto, R.A. Saporito, T. Grant, D.R. Ifa, Use of whole-body cryosectioning and desorption electrospray ionization mass spectrometry imaging (DESI-MSI) to visualize alkaloid distribution in poison frogs, J. Mass Spectrom. 55 (2020) e4520, https://doi.org/10.1002/jms.4520.
[39] A.M. Porcari, J. Zhang, K.Y. Garza, R.M. Rodrigues-Peres, J.Q. Lin, J.H. Young, R. Tibshirani, C. Nagi, G.R. Paiva, S.A. Carter, L.O. Sarian, M.N. Eberlin, L.S. Eberlin, Multicenter study using desorption-electrospray-ionization-mass-spectrometry imaging for breast-cancer diagnosis, Anal. Chem. 90 (2018) 11324–11332, https://doi.org/10.1021/acs.analchem.8b01961.
[40] C.C. Hsu, P.T. Chou, R.N. Zare, Imaging of proteins in tissue samples using nanospray desorption electrospray ionization mass spectrometry, Anal. Chem. 87 (2015) 11171–11175, https://doi.org/10.1021/acs.analchem.5b03389.
[41] M. León, C.R. Ferreira, L.S. Eberlin, A.K. Jarmusch, V. Pirro, A.C.B. Rodrigues, P.O. Favaron, M.A. Miglino, R.G. Cooks, Metabolites and lipids associated with fetal swine anatomy via desorption electrospray ionization – mass spectrometry imaging, Sci. Rep. 9 (2019) 1–10, https://doi.org/10.1038/s41598-019-43698-2.
[42] R.G. Hemalatha, M.A. Ganayee, T. Pradeep, Electrospun nanofiber mats as "smart surfaces" for desorption electrospray ionization mass spectrometry (DESI MS)-Based analysis and imprint imaging, Anal. Chem. 88 (2016) 5710–5717, https://doi.org/10.1021/acs.analchem.5b04520.
[43] G. Han, R. Ceilley, Chronic wound healing: a review of current management and treatments, Adv. Ther. 34 (2017) 599–610, https://doi.org/10.1007/s12325-017-0478-y.
[44] S. Saghazadeh, C. Rinoldi, M. Schot, S.S. Kashaf, F. Sharifi, E. Jalilian, K. Nuutila, G. Giatsidis, P. Mostafalu, H. Derakhshandeh, K. Yue, W. Swieszkowski, A. Memic, A. Tamayol, A. Khademhosseini, Drug delivery systems and materials for wound healing applications, Adv. Drug Deliv. Rev. 127 (2018) 138–166, https://doi.org/10.1016/j.addr.2018.04.008.
[45] S. Dhivya, V.V. Padma, E. Santhini, Wound dressings - a review, Biomedicine 5 (2015) 24–28, https://doi.org/10.7603/s40681-015-0022-9.
[46] M. Mozafari, Nanotechnology in wound care: one step closer to the clinic, Mol. Ther. 26 (2018) 2085–2086, https://doi.org/10.1016/j.ymthe.2018.08.008.
[47] M.L. Kremer, Promotion of the fenton reaction by Cu^{2+} ions: evidence for intermediates, Int. J. Chem. Kinet. 38 (2006) 725–736, https://doi.org/10.1002/kin.20205.
[48] L.J. Villarreal-Gómez, J.M. Cornejo-Bravo, R. Vera-Graziano, D. Grande, Electrospinning as a powerful technique for biomedical applications: a critically selected survey, J. Biomater. Sci. Polym. Ed. 27 (2016) 157–176, https://doi.org/10.1080/09205063.2015.1116885.

[49] A. Faccendini, B. Vigani, S. Rossi, G. Sandri, M.C. Bonferoni, C.M. Caramella, F. Ferrari, Nanofiber scaffolds as drug delivery systems to bridge spinal cord injury, Pharmaceuticals 10 (2017) 1–30, https://doi.org/10.3390/ph10030063.

[50] E. Mele, Electrospinning of natural polymers for advanced wound care: towards responsive and adaptive dressings, J. Mater. Chem. B. 4 (2016) 4801–4812, https://doi.org/10.1039/C6TB00804F.

[51] M. Rai, A. Yadav, A. Gade, Silver nanoparticles as a new generation of antimicrobials, Biotechnol. Adv. 27 (2009) 76–83, https://doi.org/10.1016/j.biotechadv.2008.09.002.

[52] N. Tra Thanh, M. Ho Hieu, N. Tran Minh Phuong, T. Do Bui Thuan, H. Nguyen Thi Thu, V.P. Thai, T. Do Minh, H. Nguyen Dai, V.T. Vo, H. Nguyen Thi, Optimization and characterization of electrospun polycaprolactone coated with gelatin-silver nanoparticles for wound healing application, Mater. Sci. Eng. C 91 (2018) 318–329, https://doi.org/10.1016/j.msec.2018.05.039.

[53] H. Zhang, M. Peng, T. Cheng, P. Zhao, L. Qiu, J. Zhou, G. Lu, J. Chen, Silver nanoparticles-doped collagen–alginate antimicrobial biocomposite as potential wound dressing, J. Mater. Sci. 53 (2018) 14944–14952, https://doi.org/10.1007/s10853-018-2710-9.

[54] K. Madhumathi, P.T. Sudheesh Kumar, S. Abhilash, V. Sreeja, H. Tamura, K. Manzoor, S.V. Nair, R. Jayakumar, Development of novel chitin/nanosilver composite scaffolds for wound dressing applications, J. Mater. Sci. Mater. Med. 21 (2010) 807–813, https://doi.org/10.1007/s10856-009-3877-z.

[55] A.M. Abdelgawad, S.M. Hudson, O.J. Rojas, Antimicrobial wound dressing nanofiber mats from multicomponent (chitosan/silver-NPs/polyvinyl alcohol) systems, Carbohydr. Polym. 100 (2014) 166–178, https://doi.org/10.1016/j.carbpol.2012.12.043.

[56] A. Regiel-Futyra, M. Kus-Liśkiewicz, V. Sebastian, S. Irusta, M. Arruebo, G. Stochel, A. Kyzioł, Development of noncytotoxic chitosan-gold nanocomposites as efficient antibacterial materials, ACS Appl. Mater. Interfaces 7 (2015) 1087–1099, https://doi.org/10.1021/am508094e.

[57] A. Gopal, V. Kant, A. Gopalakrishnan, S.K. Tandan, D. Kumar, Chitosan-based copper nanocomposite accelerates healing in excision wound model in rats, Eur. J. Pharmacol. 731 (2014) 8–19, https://doi.org/10.1016/j.ejphar.2014.02.033.

[58] K. Lee, S. Lee, Multifunctionality of poly(vinyl alcohol) nanofiber webs containing titanium dioxide, J. Appl. Polym. Sci. 124 (2012) 4038–4046, https://doi.org/10.1002/app.34929.

[59] B. Son, B.-Y. Yeom, S.H. Song, C.-S. Lee, T.S. Hwang, Antibacterial electrospun chitosan/poly(vinyl alcohol) nanofibers containing silver nitrate and titanium dioxide, J. Appl. Polym. Sci. 111 (2009) 2892–2899, https://doi.org/10.1002/app.29233.

[60] K.T. Shalumon, K.H. Anulekha, S.V. Nair, S.V. Nair, K.P. Chennazhi, R. Jayakumar, Sodium alginate/poly(vinyl alcohol)/nano ZnO composite nanofibers for antibacterial wound dressings, Int. J. Biol. Macromol. 49 (2011) 247–254, https://doi.org/10.1016/j.ijbiomac.2011.04.005.

[61] H. Rodríguez-Tobías, G. Morales, A. Ledezma, J. Romero, D. Grande, Novel antibacterial electrospun mats based on poly(D,L-lactide) nanofibers and zinc oxide nanoparticles, J. Mater. Sci. 49 (2014) 8373–8385, https://doi.org/10.1007/s10853-014-8547-y.

Further reading

[1] L. Persano, A. Camposeo, C. Tekmen, D. Pisignano, Industrial upscaling of electrospinning and applications of polymer nanofibers: a review, Macromol. Mater. Eng. 298 (2013) 504–520, https://doi.org/10.1002/mame.201200290.

[2] O. Akampumuza, H. Gao, H. Zhang, D. Wu, X.-H. Qin, Raising nanofiber output: the progress, mechanisms, challenges, and reasons for the pursuit, Macromol. Mater. Eng. 303 (2018) 1700269, https://doi.org/10.1002/mame.201700269.

[3] M. Zamani, M.P. Prabhakaran, S. Ramakrishna, Advances in drug delivery via electrospun and electrosprayed nanomaterials, Int. J. Nanomed. 8 (2013) 2997–3017, https://doi.org/10.2147/IJN.S43575.

[4] S. Chen, S.K. Boda, S.K. Batra, X. Li, J. Xie, Emerging roles of electrospun nanofibers in cancer research, Adv. Healthc. Mater. 7 (2018) 1–20, https://doi.org/10.1002/adhm.201701024.

CHAPTER TWELVE

Combinatorial approaches in electrospinning, electrospraying, and 3D printing for biomedical applications

Jimna Mohamed Ameer*, Roopesh Pai (R)*, Remya Komeri, Vinod Damodaran, P.R. Anil Kumar, Naresh Kasoju
Division of Tissue Culture, Department of Applied Biology, Biomedical Technology Wing, Sree Chitra Tirunal Institute for Medical Sciences and Technology, Thiruvananthapuram, Kerala, India

Abbreviations

3D Three dimensional
EDOT 3,4-ethylene dioxythiophene
HV High voltage
kV Kilovolts
MEW Melt electrospinning writing
NFES Near-field electrospinning
PCL Poly(ε-caprolactone)
PLA Poly(L-lactic acid)
PLGA Poly(lactic-co-glycolic acid)
PVDF Polyvinylidene fluoride

12.1 Introduction

The field of biomedical engineering, particularly tissue engineering, controlled drug delivery, imaging, biosensing, and many other allied themes, has recently seen a surge in research and developmental activities with the introduction of novel materials and fabrication techniques. Electrospinning—a micro-/nanoscale fiber-forming method—has gained much popularity owing to its simplicity, affordability, and versatility [1]. The fibers that resulted out of electrospinning were highly explored in the field of tissue engineering owing to its structural similarity with natural

* These authors contributed equally.

Biomedical Applications of Electrospinning and Electrospraying
ISBN: 978-0-12-822476-2
https://doi.org/10.1016/B978-0-12-822476-2.00011-X

extracellular matrix. These fibrous materials were also highly explored in drug delivery and other allied biomedical fields owing to their high surface-to-volume ratio. However, relatively small pore size and poor mechanical properties and pseudo-3D nature are some of the limitations associated with these materials. On the other hand, electrospraying—a sister technology to electrospinning—has gained extensive attention in the field of drug delivery, imaging, and biosensing [2]. The micro-/nanoparticulate materials produced by electrospraying are much smaller than typical spray-dried particles, and, therefore, offers high surface-to-volume ratio. However, they could not find greater applications in tissue engineering field due to inability to form 3D structures. The latest entry in the field of biomedical engineering, i.e., 3D printing technology, has changed the way the material fabrication is done [3]. However, 3D printed materials are not always desirable owing to poor surface-to-volume ratio when compared to nanomaterials prepared by electrospinning and electrospraying. In this evolving field of material fabrication, recently, electrospinning, electrospraying, and 3D printing techniques have found mutually beneficial partnership with each other in order to develop next generation of materials for potential applications in various themes of biomedical engineering (Fig. 12.1).

In this chapter, we begin with Section 12.2, with a brief background of electrospinning, electrospraying, and 3D printing techniques. This is followed by Section 12.3, which covers a detailed account of various approaches of electrospinning and 3D printing. In particular, we describe various stand-alone electrospinning approaches which form structures

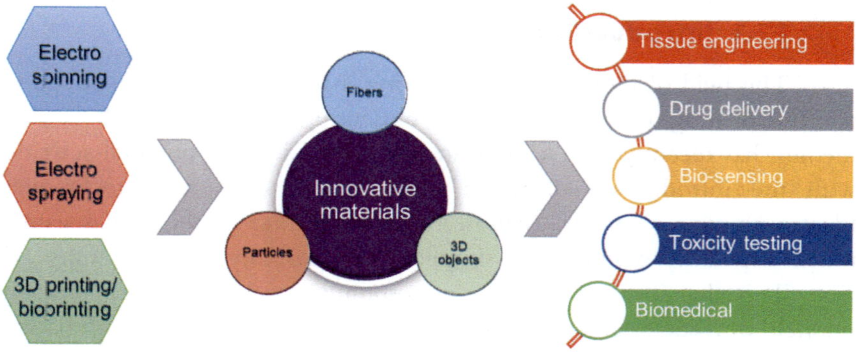

Figure 12.1 Combinatorial approaches and their scope: electrospinning and its sister technology electrospraying are tying up with previously unrelated 3D printing/bioprinting process to develop innovative materials with applications across a range of biomedical fields.

similar to 3D printed materials, followed by interesting approaches involving chopping of electrospun scaffolds into pieces and formulating ink/bioink for 3D printing process, and subsequently, we highlight approaches involving simultaneous use of electrospinning and 3D printing/bioprinting processes that led to materials with innovative structural and functional properties for potential biomedical applications. Next, in Section 12.4, we present details of different combinatorial strategies in electrospraying. In particular, we describe various innovations noted within the basic electrospraying setup in the context of tissue engineering, drug delivery, biosensing, and beyond, followed by combinatorial approaches in electrospraying with electrospinning in order to generate particle impregnated fibrous materials, and subsequently, we describe how electrospraying and 3D printing approaches were cleverly combined in order to generate novel materials for biomedical applications. We conclude this chapter with Section 12.5 highlighting key developments in the field so far and potential opportunities for future.

12.2 Background to electrospinning, electrospraying, and 3D printing

12.2.1 Electrospinning

Electrostatic spinning although much popularized in the field of biomedical engineering in the recent few years, its history dates back to 1600s, when an English physicist Mr. William Gilbert first described the electrostatic phenomena [4]. He discovered that a hemispherical drop of water holding on a dry and flat surface was subjected to electrostatic phenomenon and was evolving into a conical shape drop whenever it was exposed to a rubbed amber object. Subsequently, researchers like Rayleigh, Zeleny, and Formahals studied the phenomenon in detail and developed a working prototype of a modern-day electrospinning unit. In a typical setup (Fig. 12.2), a syringe is loaded with a polymer solution and is passed through the tip of a fine orifice such as a blunt-ended needle. Next, an HV power supply unit connected to the needle would charge the polymer solution and this results in accumulation of electrostatic charge at the tip of the droplet. The charge repulsion dominates the surface tension, causing formation of cone shape droplet and release of polymer solution in the form of a fine jet [5]. This jet travels toward a ground, and in the process loses solvent and transforms into a solid fiber. This micro- to nanoscale fiber-forming method, initially explored in the textile industry, has now ventured into the biomedical engineering field. Several researchers across the globe

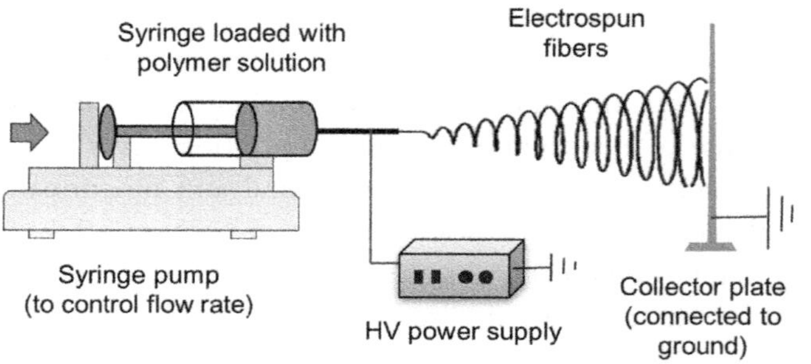

Figure 12.2 Schematic illustration of electrospinning setup and working principle: the setup typically consists of a syringe loaded with polymer solution, blunt-end needle connected to HV power unit, syringe pump controlling flow rate, and a grounded collector plate. When the polymer solution is charged with HV power, the repulsive forces lead to the formation of fine jet that results in the formation of fibers, provided other electrospinning process parameters are optimal.

introduced innovative modifications in the setup to develop a wide variety of structures and thereby expanding the scope of applications in biomedical and applied areas [1,6].

12.2.2 Electrospraying

Electrospraying technique is employed for the generation of micro- and nanoparticulate materials with definite size and shape [7]. In 1952, Vonnegut and Neubauer established the electrospraying by applying HV to generate nano-/microparticles via electrical atomization [8]. They demonstrated that when an electrical charge of 5−10 kV (direct current) was applied to liquids held in small capillaries, a jet of highly electrified droplets was formed which led to formation of particulate matter (Fig. 12.3). In principle, electrospinning and electrospraying can be considered as sister technologies. The difference between these two can be related to the degree of electrostatic interactions within the liquid that were influenced by process parameters. Electrospraying technique has been explored widely in the field of microencapsulation, particularly to entrap, coat, or load substances of various types and characteristics [2]. For instance, electrospray particles loaded with drugs were explored for potential controlled release applications, and electrospray particles loaded with contrast agents were explored in ultrasound imaging. Variously formulated electrospray particles were explored as coatings for biomedical implants. They were also widely used as growth factor carriers in tissue engineering applications. The field still seems evolving as several researchers are coming up with innovative

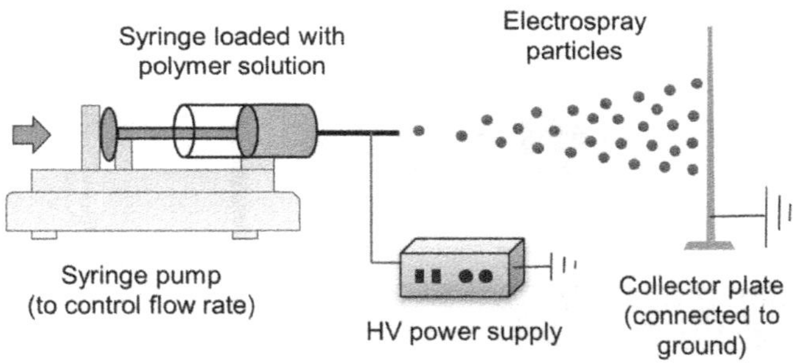

Figure 12.3 Schematic illustration of electrospray setup and working principle: the setup typically is composed of a polymer filled syringe connected to a syringe pump, blunt-end needle connected to HV power supply, and a collector plate connected to ground. Upon applying HV power, the repulsive forces within polymer solution result in the formation of a fine jet that eventually lead to the formation of particles, when other electrospray parameters are also favorable.

modifications in the setup in order to prepare an array of novel materials, including but not limited to hollow particles, porous particles, core—shell particles, multilayered particles, and Janus particles. Further, postfabrication modification to the particles was also reported in order to improve the functional properties and thereby expand its applications in various biomedical and allied fields [9].

12.2.3 3D printing/bioprinting

Three-dimensional printing is an additive manufacturing technique for fabricating solid objects using a digital model. In the 1980s, Charles Hull proposed the concept of stereolithography and develoepd the first commercial 3D printing technology for producing product prototypes in industries [10]. The 3D printing workflow (Fig. 12.4) begins with a 3D model obtained from a digital scanner or generated using designing software. The design file is then translated to a mesh file, in stereolithography (.stl) or object (.obj) file format and put into a slicer software to generate a horizontal layer-by-layer toolpath. The toolpath is saved as a G-code, sent to the 3D printer, and printing starts with the base layer building a series of layers on top according to the design. 3D printing can print virtually any object shape using a wide range of materials, such as metals, ceramics, polymers, even living cells and tissues [11] and comes with advantages such as freedom to produce customized or personalized products, increased cost efficiency, enhanced productivity, and democratization of design across the globe [12]. The conventional method of tissue engineering wherein cells

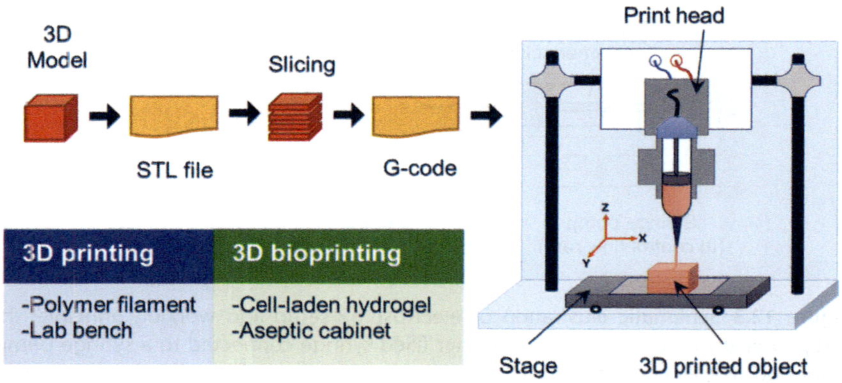

Figure 12.4 Schematic illustration of 3D printing/bioprinting setup and workflow: the setup typically consists of print head and a stage with control over X, Y, and Z movements. In 3D printing a polymer filament is melted to form the scaffold, whereas 3D bioprinting involves cell-laden hydrogel as bioink. Additionally, 3D printing can be done on a lab bench, but 3D bioprinting requires an aseptic cabinet. As for the workflow, typically a computer-generated 3D model is processed and fed into machine using a software to fabricate 3D materials.

are seeded over the premade scaffold restricts the penetration of cells into the structure leading to an engineered tissue with heterogeneous properties [13]. 3D cell printing or bioprinting allows simultaneous deposition of cells, biomaterials, and growth factors, together termed as "bioink," in a layer-by-layer fashion to produce a cell-encapsulated scaffold [14]. Beyond tissue engineering, 3D printing/bioprinting is also finding its applications in various other biomedical engineering fields including but not limited to drug delivery, biosensing, and bioanalytical devices [15—17].

12.3 Combinational approaches in electrospinning

12.3.1 Electrospinning 3D structures

Electrospinning technique has been profoundly known for its ability to produce nonwoven fibrous meshes which are typically thin "two-dimensional" structures [18]. A challenging task is to fabricate a highly ordered 3D object of desired size and shape with intricate structural details. Electrohydrodynamic fibre writing techniques, such as MEW, NFES, and tethered pyro-electrospinning, can potentially address these challenges as they function like the additive manufacturing techniques [19—21]. Brown et al. demonstrated MEW technique wherein an electrified PCL polymer melt was drawn into straight fibers when the collector translated at a speed matching with that of the jet speed [22]. The technique was also adapted to different collector types such as a rotating cylinder to fabricate tubular materials [23] and to explore novel photo-cross-linkable polymer poly(L-lactide-co-ε-caprolactone-co-acryloyl carbonate) to produce high strength structures [24]. The setup was modified by Ristovski et al. to reduce the undesirable charge effects during layer-by-layer stacking of e-spun fibers and thereby fabricated a highly ordered 3D structure comprising 200 layers (2 mm thick) of interwoven PCL fibers [25]. Despite having several advantages, the sole dependence of MEW on low melting thermoplastic substrates narrow down its biomedical applications. Meanwhile, NFES—a modified version of the solution electrospinning technique—was reported by Sun et al. to deposit nanofibers in a direct and continuous manner [26]. In this technique, the electrode-to-collector distance was reduced to few millimeters to utilize the stable liquid jet region for controlled deposition. Later, several studies highlighting the tremendous potential of NFES were reported [27–29]. For example, Luo et al. showed that near-field e-spun fibers could be stacked consistently in a fiber-by-fiber manner to construct a variety of 3D structures using a printing paper as the collector (Fig. 12.5) [30].

12.3.2 3D printing/bioprinting electrospun structures

The growth and development of conventional biomedical engineering applications are being enriched and evolved by new technologies in various cross-disciplinary fields. 3D printing—an additive manufacturing process introduced in late 1980s—is making radical changes in biomedical applications in recent times. Developments in the 3D printing/bioprinting processes have enabled the users to integrate nanotopographical features within the complex 3D structures. For instance, Narayanan et al. described formulation of PLA nanofiber–reinforced bioink made of alginate hydrogel and human adipose–derived stem cells for bioprinting musculoskeletal tissue constructs [31]. Similarly, the addition of aminolyzed PLA microcylinders into gelatin methacryloyl bioink yielded better printability and the bioprinted constructs mimicked the fibrous microenvironment of the cells [32,33]. A similar strategy was used by Chen et al. wherein electrospun matrix derived from a polymer mix of gelatin/PLGA was processed into an ink suitable for 3D printing (Fig. 12.6) [34]. The 3D printed scaffolds exhibited water-induced shape memory, fibrous surface morphology, and achieved satisfactory cartilage regeneration in vivo when seeded with chondrocytes. Of late, another study conducted by the same group showed that

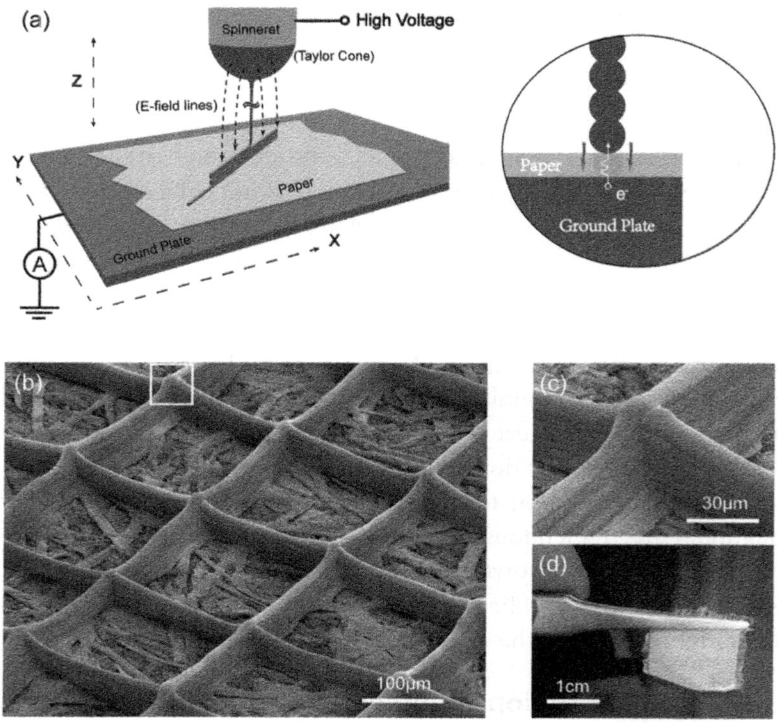

Figure 12.5 Fabrication of 3D objects by near-field electrospinning: 3D structured objects composed of PVDF fibers were prepared by direct-write electrospinning approach; (a) setup, (b) scanning electron microscope image of a 10-layer 3D structure, (c) magnified image of crossover area, and (d) a gross scale picture of the material. *Reproduced with permission from G. Luo, K.S. Teh, Y. Liu, X. Zang, Z. Wen, L. Lin, Direct-write, self-aligned electrospinning on paper for controllable fabrication of three-dimensional structures. ACS Appl. Mater. Interfaces 7(50) (2015) 27765–27770. https://doi.org/10.1021/acsami.5b08909; ©2015 American Chemical Society.*

the 3D printed scaffold derived from fiber-reinforced decellularized matrix-based bioink served both the need for good mechanical stability and biocompatibility [35]. The 3D printing/bioprinting technology has revolutionized the field of biomedical engineering in many ways. This relatively new technology is still evolving and is finding interesting relationship with electrospinning technology resulting in the formation of novel materials and systems, we believe this interesting combination will evolve in the days to come and expand the horizons of electrospinning applications in biomedical engineering, including but not limited to tissue engineering, drug delivery, bionics, biosensing, toxicological testing, wearable devices, etc.

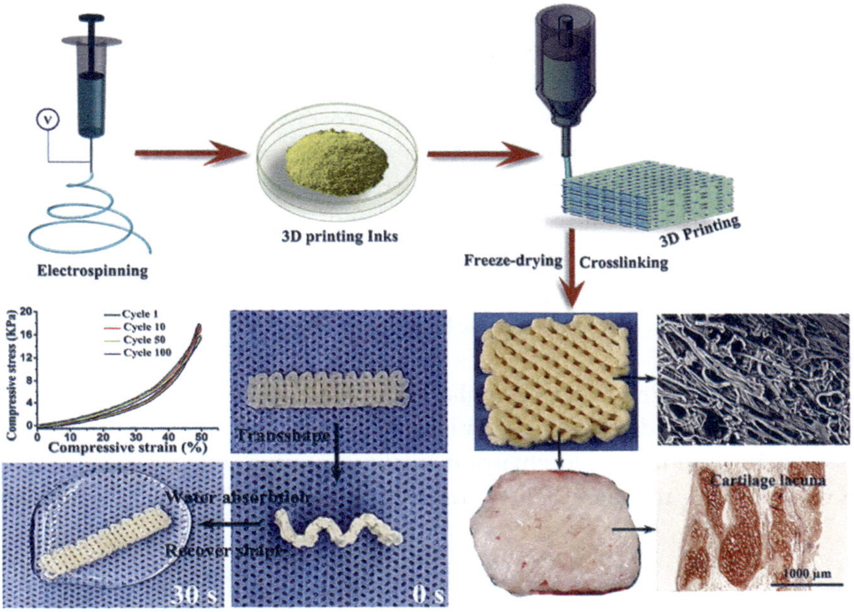

Figure 12.6 3D printing/bioprinting electrospun structures: Gelatin PLGA electrospun fibers were processed into 3D printed objects and subsequently evaluated for its potential application in cartilage tissue engineering. *https://doi.org/10.1021/acsbiomaterials.6b00196. Reproduced from Chen et al. 2019 [32]; © 2019 The Authors. Published by Elsevier Ltd.*

12.3.3 Simultaneous electrospinning and 3D printing

Owing to the individual limitations of electrospinning and 3D printing technique in fabricating complex 3D structures with nano- to microscale features, a hybrid process methodology has been explored recently for developing products with a wide range of biomedical applications [35–37]. For example, Pensa et al. introduced a combinatorial approach, in which a PCL mesh was 3D printed over the electrospun PCL/gelatin matrix to enhance the strength and stiffness [38]. The reinforced scaffolds showed good biocompatibility when used as membrane cover for bone graft particles in rat calvarial defect model. In contrast to the above method, Spackman et al. used a novel 3D printing platform to stamp electrospun nylon mat over inkjet printed UV curable polymer matrix to enhance the elastic modulus and tensile strength of soft composites [39]. Meanwhile, a facile method was developed to decorate 3D printed PCL scaffolds with electrospun nanofiber segments of PLGA–collagen–gelatin and bioactive peptide molecules for bone regeneration application [40]. Similarly, a hybrid scaffold, exhibiting a controlled drug release kinetics, was fabricated by combining melt plotted PCL microfibers with the electrospun PEO/rhodamine fibers [41]. The utility of concurrent processes was also reflected in the fabrication of implantable tissue grafts with regenerative capabilities. For instance, a small diameter triple-layered vascular graft, fabricated by combining 3D printing and electrospinning, favored endothelialization and tissue integration in vivo [42]. Similarly, transplantation of a two-layered tracheal graft composed of a cell-loaded mesoscale fibrous matrix formed ciliated columnar epithelium in rabbit tracheal defect model (Fig. 12.7) [43].

Beyond tissue engineering applications, conductive 3D electrospun mats were also explored for its inexpensive applications in portable and wearable devices for healthcare and environmental monitoring systems. For instance, Kweon et al. revealed a new route toward the fabrication of highly

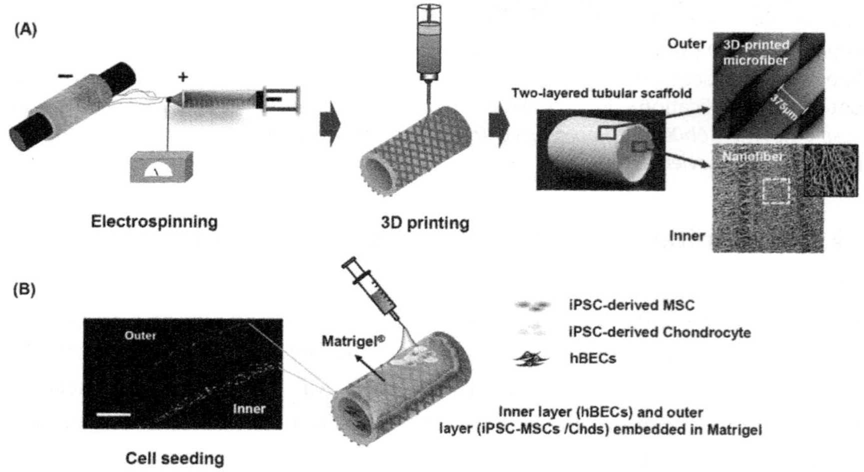

Figure 12.7 Combinatorial electrospinning and 3D printing approach: Electrospun PCL tubular scaffold was reinforced by 3D printed PCL strands and subsequently cultured with iPSC-derived chondrocytes and bronchial epithelial cells in order to bioengineer trachea. (a) electrospun PCL nanofibrous tube covered with 3D-printed PCL strands and the corresponding surface morphologies, (b) Cells in different layers were detected by PKH-26 staining (red color; iPSC-chds) and DAPI (blue color; hBECs) staining (scale bar = 200 μm). *Reproduced from I.G. Kim, S.A. Park, S-H. Lee, J.S. Choi, H. Cho, S.J. Lee, Y-W. Kwon, S.K. Kwon, Transplantation of a 3D-printed tracheal graft combined with iPS cell-derived MSCs and chondrocytes. Sci. Rep. 10(1) (2020) 4326. https://doi.org/10.1038/s41598-020-61405-4; ©2020 The Authors. Published by Springer Nature.*

conductive PVDF-co-hexafluoropropylene/poly (EDOT) mats for its potent applications in piezoresistive-type pressure sensors [44]. Typically, PVDF-HFP fibers were electrospun directly onto inkjet printed poly(EDOT): PSS/PET substrates for the formation of flexible electrode, followed by vapor deposition polymerization EDOT that led poly(EDOT) shell and spherical bumps formation on the surface of a PVDF-co-hexafluoropropylene fiber. Kozior et al. demonstrated another combinatorial approach involving 3D printed PLA matrix and electrospun polyacrylonitrile matrix for fabrication of mechanically stable 3D composites for filtration applications [45]. Extending the application of 3D printed and electrospun composite materials further, Wei et al. described a new method to record extracellular electrical signals through microelectrode arrays integrated into bionic engineered cardiac tissue on a composite material [46]. This bionic heart model was functionally evaluated by administrating isoprenaline. This particular example clearly provides a solution to develop cutting edge in vitro models that could be explored for efficient understanding of mechanisms of drug therapy on cardiovascular disease and beyond. The above-mentioned examples and approaches are only to give an idea about the various possibilities in the field of electrospinning. Given the versatility of both electrospinning as well as 3D printing technologies, quite a few innovations in the field of materials science and engineering with potential for various biomedical applications are yet to come in near future.

12.4 Combinational approaches in electrospraying

12.4.1 Innovations in electrospraying

Electrospraying method is reliable than conventional emulsion method for micro-/nanoparticle generation and ensures narrow size distribution of particles with spherical, porous, core—shell, or hollow shapes. Micro-/nanoparticles are used as injectable suspension or embedded on scaffolds having immense application as carrier of various bioactive cargoes, such as cells, genes, drugs, enzymes, or growth factors. For instance, e-sprayed drug-loaded PLGA microparticles are well adapted for localized anticancer therapy, especially, to deliver the lipophilic drugs like Paclitaxel [47] or Cisplatin [48], which otherwise have serious systemic side effects on intravenous application. Coaxial electrospraying technique was envisaged in fabrication of monodisperse microbubbles as contrasting agents for ultrasound imaging [49] and to design drug carriers for theranostic applications [50].

The higher surface area-to-volume ratio of e-sprayed particles is well adapted for tissue engineering and for ex vivo expansion of cells such as mesenchymal stem cells [51]. Additionally, the encapsulation of live cells within e-sprayed particles was achieved through the concept of bioelectrospraying. There were apprehensions about the effect of heat or HV on encapsulated cells; however, several investigations on this subject revealed that the cells remain viable and functional at lower voltages (<10 kV) but exhibit deteriorating alterations at higher voltages (>10 kV) [52,53]. Further, the electrical charge in electrospraying process was also well-explored in gene therapy applications. For instance, Lee et al. demonstrated that when 3T3 fibroblast cell suspension is e-sprayed with green fluorescence protein gene complex, the resultant encapsulated cells were transfected with the given gene through electroporation during electrospray process [54].

12.4.2 Electrospraying and electrospinning

Electrospray particles as such have made significant impact in various biomedical applications, including but not limited to tissue engineering, drug delivery, and biosensing. Nevertheless, researchers have constantly come with clever modalities by combining electrospraying with its sister technology, i.e., electrospinning in order to develop a new set of materials with multitude of applications. For instance, simultaneous bioelectrospraying and electrospinning can ensure better cell distribution for uniform tissue formation throughout the scaffold. To this end, Weidenbacher et al. have reported similar attempt in which skeletal myoblast cells mixed in gelatin were sprayed over e-spun PVDF-co-hexafluoropropylene scaffolds for vascular/muscle reconstruction (Fig. 12.8) [55]. In an exciting approach, Boda et al. homogenized e-spun fibrous scaffolds that were e-sprayed to form nanofibrous microspheres with high surface-to-volume ratio which led to higher cell carrying efficiency when compared to solid microspheres [56]. It is anticipated that such nanofibrous particles could be suitable for irregular defect management compared to solid microspheres. To tackle the issue of low pore size in e-spun scaffolds, Wang et al. employed the combinatorial approach to introduce desirable porosity to the silk fibroin—based e-spun scaffolds by electrospraying sacrificial poly(-ethylene oxide) microparticles of different diameter [57]. In order to create a gradient fibrous and particulate structure, Wu et al. explored a hybrid process including electrospinning of PCL and electrospraying of hydroxyapatite for potential tendon—bone interface tissue engineering [58].

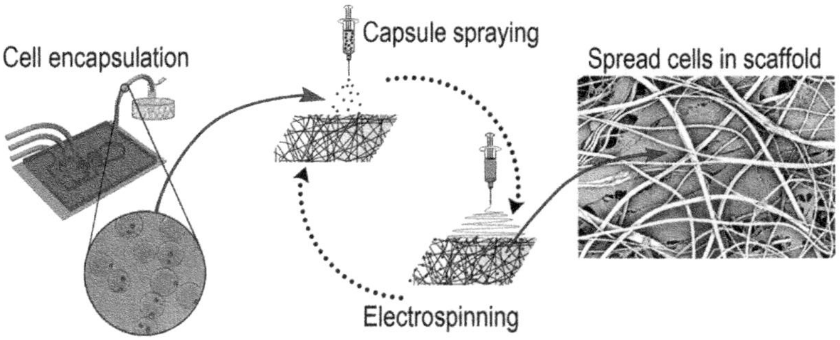

Figure 12.8 Combinatorial electrospraying and electrospinning approach: microfluidic cell encapsulation of murine skeletal myoblast cell line (C2C12) in gelatin followed by electrospraying onto PVDF electrospun fibrous matrix offered control over spatial distribution and infiltration of cells throughout the scaffolds. *Reproduced with permission from L. Weidenbacher, A. Abrishamkar, M. Rottmar, A.G. Guex, K. Maniura-Weber, A.J. deMello, S.J. Ferguson, R.M. Rossi, G. Fortunato, Electrospraying of microfluidic encapsulated cells for the fabrication of cell-laden electrospun hybrid tissue constructs. Acta Biomater. 64 (2017) 137–147. https://doi.org/10.1016/j.actbio.2017.10.012; ©2017Acta Materialia Inc, published by Elsevier Ltd.*

The combinational approach of electrospray with electrospinning was well-explored in tissue engineering; however, this was not yet fully explored in drug delivery, biosensing, and other biomedical applications.

12.4.3 Electrospraying and 3D printing

Recently, with the advent of additive manufacturing technologies, or otherwise called 3D printing, several innovative combinatorial approaches have been described in the literature. Although electrospinning was well-explored with 3D printing, its counterpart electrospraying was yet to be explored with 3D printing to its full extent. There were only a couple of examples in this regard. First by Olvera-Trejo and Velásquez-García who described preparation of core–shell particles with up to 25 coaxial electrospray emitters following 3D printing approach. The clever adaptation of an array of miniaturized coaxial electrospray emitters as the 3D printing platform not only allowed precise control over particle size distribution but also allowed enhancement in the throughput [59]. The second example involved facile combination of electrospraying with 3D printing technology in the field of tissue engineering. Xu et al. e-sprayed human bone marrow–derived MSC-laden alginate–gelatin solution into microspheres and collected in $CaCl_2$ bath (Fig. 12.9). Subsequently, the cell-laden particles

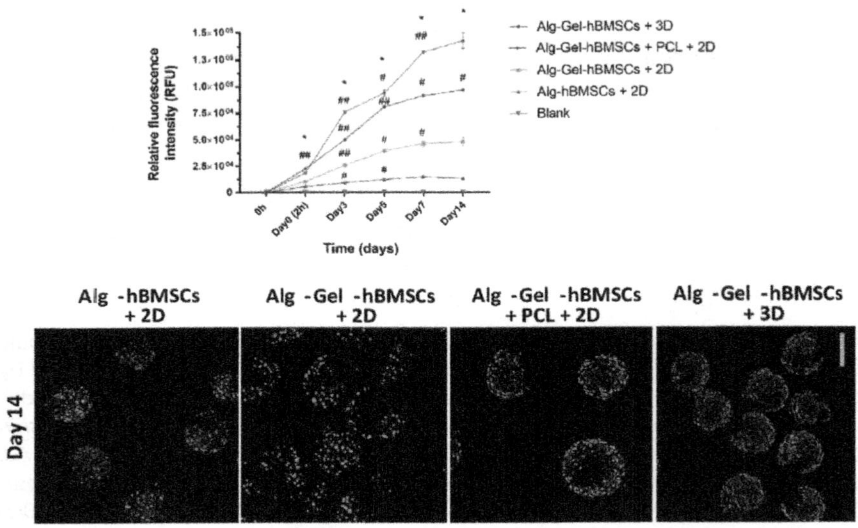

Figure 12.9 Combinational electrospraying and electrospinning approach: hBMSCs embedded in alginate (Alg) and gelatin (Gel) containing electrosprayed microsprayed when cultured on 3D printed PCL scaffold in dynamic conditions exhibited superior cell response. *Y. Xu, J. Peng, G. Richards, S. Lu, D. Eglin, Optimization of electrospray fabrication of stem cell-embedded alginate-gelatin microspheres and their assembly in 3D-printed poly(ε-caprolactone) scaffold for cartilage tissue engineering. J. Orthop. Trans. 18 (2019) 128–141. https://doi.org/10.1016/j.jot.2019.05.003; © 2019 The Authors, published by Elsevier (Singapore) Pvt Ltd on behalf of Chinese Speaking Orthopedic Society.*

were loaded into a 3D printed PCL scaffolds for potential cartilage tissue engineering applications. It was said that the hybrid approach was selected to compensate the limitations of each technique by the other to improve the complexity of engineered tissue construct toward the natural counterpart. Further, we envisage greater attention to this combinatorial approach since it would enable controlled spatial deposition of particles containing cells, growth factors, imaging molecules, or biosensing agents, in the form of complex 3D printed constructs of desired size, shape, and functional requirement and thereby further expand its applications in tissue engineering, drug delivery, imaging, biosensing, and beyond [60].

12.5 Summary and future prospects

Dating back to early 1900s, electrospinning has evolved and received significant attention in the field of materials and manufacturing engineering.

A simple process involving electrostatic pull of a charged polymer toward a grounded or oppositely charged collector resulted in the formation of fibers. Several modifications in the setup were reported in order to generate novel fibrous materials with a control over fiber size and controlled deposition. Apart from simplicity and versatility of the technique, researchers across various fields were attracted because of high surface-to-volume ratio offered by the electrospun fibers. These fibers were variously explored in tissue engineering, drug delivery, biosensing, and other biomedical fields. Its sister technology, electrospraying—a particle forming process—has also attracted the attention of many biomedical engineers owing its simplicity, versatility, and striking features of the resultant micro-/nanoparticles. Lately, 3D printing/bioprinting technology—an additive manufacturing process—is revolutionizing the biomedical field. This discrete technology has found an interesting relationship with electrospinning and electrospraying technologies and has resulted in a new set of materials with a magnitude of applications in tissue engineering, drug delivery, imaging, biosensing, etc. However, based on the amount of available literature, we can say that the combinatorial approaches involving electrospinning/electrospraying and 3D printing/bioprinting are in its infancy stage. Yet, in view of paramount demand for new materials across various disciplines of biomedical engineering, and keeping in view of the potential of these technologies, we envisage great spark in the combinatorial approaches in the days to come.

Acknowledgments

Authors acknowledge Department of Science and Technology, Government of India, and Sree Chitra Tirunal Institute for Medical Sciences and Technology (An Institution of National Importance), Thiruvananthapuram, for funding projects based on electrospinning and 3D printing (TDF-P6219, TRC-P8141, and TRC-P8137).

References

[1] J. Xue, T. Wu, Y. Dai, Y. Xia, Electrospinning and electrospun nanofibers: methods, materials, and applications, Chem. Rev. 119 (2019) 5298–5415, https://doi.org/10.1021/acs.chemrev.8b00593.

[2] J. Wang, J.A. Jansen, F. Yang, Electrospraying: possibilities and challenges of engineering carriers for biomedical applications - a mini review, Front. Chem. 7 (2019), 258, https://doi.org/10.3389/fchem.2019.00258.

[3] J. Chang, J. He, M. Mao, W. Zhou, Q. Lei, X. Li, D. Li, C.K. Chua, X. Zhao, Advanced material strategies for next-generation additive manufacturing, Materials 11 (2018), 166, https://doi.org/10.3390/ma11010166.

[4] N. Tucker, J.J. Stanger, M.P. Staiger, H. Razzaq, K. Hofman, The history of the science and technology of electrospinning from 1600 to 1995, J. Eng. Fibers Fabr. 7 (2012) 63–73, https://doi.org/10.1177/155892501200702S10.

[5] A.L. Yarin, S. Koombhongse, D.H. Reneker, Taylor cone and jetting from liquid droplets in electrospinning of nanofibers, J. Appl. Phys. 90 (2001) 4836–4846, https://doi.org/10.1063/1.1408260.

[6] J.M. Ameer, P.R. Anil Kumar, N. Kasoju, Strategies to tune electrospun scaffold porosity for effective cell response in tissue engineering, J. Funct. Biomater. 10 (2019), 30, https://doi.org/10.3390/jfb10030030.

[7] N. Bock, M.A. Woodruff, D.W. Hutmacher, T.R. Dargaville, Electrospraying, a reproducible method for production of polymeric microspheres for biomedical applications, Polymers 3 (2011) 131–149, https://doi.org/10.3390/polym3010131.

[8] A. Alehosseini, B. Ghorani, M. Sarabi-Jamab, N. Tucker, Principles of electrospraying: a new approach in protection of bioactive compounds in foods, Crit. Rev. Food Sci. Nutr. 58 (2018) 2346–2363, https://doi.org/10.1080/10408398.2017.1323723.

[9] H. Lee, S. An, S. Kim, B. Jeon, M. Kim, I.S. Kim, Readily functionalizable and stabilizable polymeric particles with controlled size and morphology by electrospray, Sci. Rep. 8 (2018), 15725, https://doi.org/10.1038/s41598-018-34124-0.

[10] C.W. Hull, Apparatus for Production of Three-Dimensional Objects by Stereolithography, vol. 4575330, 1986.

[11] A. Haleem, M. Javaid, 3D printed medical parts with different materials using additive manufacturing, Clin. Epidemiol. Glob. Health 8 (2020) 215–223, https://doi.org/10.1016/j.cegh.2019.08.002.

[12] C. Lee Ventola, Medical applications for 3D printing: current and projected uses, P T 39 (2014) 704–711. http://www.ptcommunity.com/system/files/pdf/ptj3910704.pdf.

[13] B.P. Chan, K.W. Leong, Scaffolding in tissue engineering: general approaches and tissue-specific considerations, Eur. Spine J. 17 (2008) 467–479, https://doi.org/10.1007/s00586-008-0745-3.

[14] J. Groll, J.A. Burdick, D.-W. Cho, B. Derby, M. Gelinsky, S.C. Heilshorn, T. Jüngst, J. Malda, V.A. Mironov, K. Nakayama, A. Ovsianikov, W. Sun, S. Takeuchi, J.J. Yoo, T.B.F. Woodfield, A definition of bioinks and their distinction from biomaterial inks, Biofabrication 11 (2018), 013001, https://doi.org/10.1088/1758-5090/aaec52.

[15] G.W. Bishop, J.E. Satterwhite-Warden, K. Kadimisetty, J.F. Rusling, 3D-printed bioanalytical devices, Nanotechnology 27 (2016), 284002, https://doi.org/10.1088/0957-4484/27/28/284002.

[16] S. Kotta, A. Nair, N. Alsabeelah, 3D printing technology in drug delivery: recent progress and application, Curr. Pharm. Des. 24 (2018) 5039–5048, https://doi.org/10.2174/1381612825666181206123828.

[17] M. Sharafeldin, A. Jones, J.F. Rusling, 3D-printed biosensor arrays for medical diagnostics, Micromachines 9 (2018), 394, https://doi.org/10.3390/mi9080394.

[18] I. Jun, H.-S. Han, J.R. Edwards, H. Jeon, Electrospun fibrous scaffolds for tissue engineering: viewpoints on architecture and fabrication, Int. J. Mol. Sci. 19 (2018), 745, https://doi.org/10.3390/ijms19030745.

[19] E.L. Gill, X. Li, M.A. Birch, Y.Y.S. Huang, Multi-length scale bioprinting towards simulating microenvironmental cues, Bio-Des. Manuf. 1 (2018) 77–88, https://doi.org/10.1007/s42242-018-0014-1.

[20] Y. Jin, Q. Gao, C. Xie, G. Li, J. Du, J. Fu, Y. He, Fabrication of heterogeneous scaffolds using melt electrospinning writing: design and optimization, Mater. Des. 185 (2020), 108274, https://doi.org/10.1016/j.matdes.2019.108274.
[21] C. Sara, N. Giuseppe, V. Veronica, F. Pietro, Layered 3D printing by tethered pyro-electrospinning, Adv. Polym. Technol. 2020 (2020), 1252960, https://doi.org/10.1155/2020/1252960.
[22] T.D. Brown, P.D. Dalton, D.W. Hutmacher, Direct writing by way of melt electrospinning, Adv. Mater. 23 (2011) 5651−5657, https://doi.org/10.1002/adma.201103482.
[23] T.D. Brown, A. Slotosch, L. Thibaudeau, A. Taubenberger, D. Loessner, C. Vaquette, P.D. Dalton, D.W. Hutmacher, Design and fabrication of tubular scaffolds via direct writing in a melt electrospinning mode, Biointerphases 7 (2012) 1−16, https://doi.org/10.1007/s13758-011-0013-7.
[24] F. Chen, G. Hochleitner, T. Woodfield, J. Groll, P.D. Dalton, B.G. Amsden, Additive manufacturing of a photo-cross-linkable polymer via direct melt electrospinning writing for producing high strength structures, Biomacromolecules 17 (2016) 208−214, https://doi.org/10.1021/acs.biomac.5b01316.
[25] N. Ristovski, N. Bock, S. Liao, S.K. Powell, J. Ren, G.T.S. Kirby, K.A. Blackwood, M.A. Woodruff, Improved fabrication of melt electrospun tissue engineering scaffolds using direct writing and advanced electric field control, Biointerphases 10 (2015), 011006, https://doi.org/10.1116/1.4914380.
[26] D. Sun, C. Chang, S. Li, L. Lin, Near-field electrospinning, Nano Lett. 6 (2006) 839−842, https://doi.org/10.1021/nl0602701.
[27] P. Fattahi, J.T. Dover, J.L. Brown, 3D near-field electrospinning of biomaterial microfibers with potential for blended microfiber-cell-loaded gel composite structures, Adv. Healthcare Mater. 6 (2017), 1700456, https://doi.org/10.1002/adhm.201700456.
[28] E.L. Gill, S. Willis, M. Gerigk, P. Cohen, D. Zhang, X. Li, Y.Y.S. Huang, Fabrication of designable and suspended microfibers via low-voltage 3D micropatterning, ACS Appl. Mater. Interfaces 11 (2019) 19679−19690, https://doi.org/10.1021/acsami.9b01258.
[29] B. Kong, Y. Chen, R. Liu, X. Liu, C. Liu, Z. Shao, L. Xiong, X. Liu, W. Sun, S. Mi, Fiber reinforced GelMA hydrogel to induce the regeneration of corneal stroma, Nat. Commun. 11 (2020), 1435, https://doi.org/10.1038/s41467-020-14887-9.
[30] G. Luo, K.S. Teh, Y. Liu, X. Zang, Z. Wen, L. Lin, Direct-write, self-aligned electrospinning on paper for controllable fabrication of three-dimensional structures, ACS Appl. Mater. Interfaces 7 (2015) 27765−27770, https://doi.org/10.1021/acsami.5b08909.
[31] L.K. Narayanan, P. Huebner, M.B. Fisher, J.T. Spang, B. Starly, R.A. Shirwaiker, 3D-bioprinting of polylactic acid (PLA) nanofiber-alginate hydrogel bioink containing human adipose-derived stem cells, ACS Biomater. Sci. Eng. 2 (2016) 1732−1742, https://doi.org/10.1021/acsbiomaterials.6b00196.
[32] W. Chen, Y. Xu, Y. Liu, Z. Wang, Y. Li, G. Jiang, X. Mo, G. Zhou, Three-dimensional printed electrospun fiber-based scaffold for cartilage regeneration, Mater. Des. 179 (2019), 107886, https://doi.org/10.1016/j.matdes.2019.107886.
[33] J. Lee, C.H. Park, C.S. Kim, Microcylinder-laden gelatin-based bioink engineered for 3D bioprinting, Mater. Lett. 233 (2018) 24−27, https://doi.org/10.1016/j.matlet.2018.08.138.
[34] W. Chen, Y. Xu, Y. Li, L. Jia, X. Mo, G. Jiang, G. Zhou, 3D printing electrospinning fiber-reinforced decellularized extracellular matrix for cartilage regeneration, Chem. Eng. J. 382 (2020), 122986, https://doi.org/10.1016/j.cej.2019.122986.

[35] I. Rajzer, A. Kurowska, A. Jabłoński, S. Jatteau, M. Śliwka, M. Ziąbka, E. Menaszek, Layered gelatin/PLLA scaffolds fabricated by electrospinning and 3D printing- for nasal cartilages and subchondral bone reconstruction, Mater. Des. 155 (2018) 297–306, https://doi.org/10.1016/j.matdes.2018.06.012.
[36] S. Naghieh, E. Foroozmehr, M. Badrossamay, M. Kharaziha, Combinational processing of 3D printing and electrospinning of hierarchical poly(lactic acid)/gelatin-forsterite scaffolds as a biocomposite: mechanical and biological assessment, Mater. Des. 133 (2017) 128–135, https://doi.org/10.1016/j.matdes.2017.07.051.
[37] S.H. Park, T.G. Kim, H.C. Kim, D.Y. Yang, T.G. Park, Development of dual scale scaffolds via direct polymer melt deposition and electrospinning for applications in tissue regeneration, Acta Biomater. 4 (2008) 1198–1207, https://doi.org/10.1016/j.actbio.2008.03.019.
[38] N.W. Pensa, A.S. Curry, P.P. Bonvallet, N.F. Bellis, K.M. Rettig, M.S. Reddy, A.W. Eberhardt, S.L. Bellis, 3D printed mesh reinforcements enhance the mechanical properties of electrospun scaffolds, Biomater. Res. 23 (1) (2019), 22, https://doi.org/10.1186/s40824-019-0171-0.
[39] C.C. Spackman, C.R. Frank, K.C. Picha, J. Samuel, 3D printing of fiber-reinforced soft composites: process study and material characterization, J. Manuf. Process. 23 (2016) 296–305, https://doi.org/10.1016/j.jmapro.2016.04.006.
[40] R. Li, A. McCarthy, Y.S. Zhang, J. Xie, Decorating 3D printed scaffolds with electrospun nanofiber segments for tissue engineering, Adv. Biosyst. 3 (2019), 1900137, https://doi.org/10.1002/adbi.201900137.
[41] H. Yoon, G. Kim, A three-dimensional polycaprolactone scaffold combined with a drug delivery system consisting of electrospun nanofibers, J. Pharm. Sci. 100 (2011) 424–430, https://doi.org/10.1002/jps.22310.
[42] K. Huang, X. Gao, J. Wang, H. Chen, C. Tong, Y. Tan, Z. Tan, Triple-layer vascular grafts fabricated by combined e-jet 3D printing and electrospinning, Ann. Biomed. Eng. 46 (2018) 1254–1266, https://doi.org/10.1007/s10439-018-2065-z.
[43] I.G. Kim, S.A. Park, S.-H. Lee, J.S. Choi, H. Cho, S.J. Lee, Y.-W. Kwon, S.K. Kwon, Transplantation of a 3D-printed tracheal graft combined with iPS cell-derived MSCs and chondrocytes, Sci. Rep. 10 (2020), 4326, https://doi.org/10.1038/s41598-020-61405-4.
[44] O.Y. Kweon, S.J. Lee, J.H. Oh, Wearable high-performance pressure sensors based on three-dimensional electrospun conductive nanofibers, NPG Asia Mater. 10 (2018) 540–551, https://doi.org/10.1038/s41427-018-0041-6.
[45] T. Kozior, A. Mamun, M. Trabelsi, M. Wortmann, S. Lilia, A. Ehrmann, Electrospinning on 3D printed polymers for mechanically stabilized filter composites, Polymers 11 (2019), 2034, https://doi.org/10.3390/polym11122034.
[46] X. Wei, Q. Gao, C. Xie, C. Gu, T. Liang, H. Wan, L. Zhuang, Y. He, P. Wang, Extracellular recordings of bionic engineered cardiac tissue based on a porous scaffold and microelectrode arrays, Anal. Methods 11 (2019) 5872–5879, https://doi.org/10.1039/c9ay01888c.
[47] S.H. Ranganath, I. Kee, W.B. Krantz, P.K.H. Chow, C.H. Wang, Hydrogel matrix entrapping PLGA-paclitaxel microspheres: drug delivery with near zero-order release and implantability advantages for malignant brain tumour chemotherapy, Pharm. Res. 26 (2009) 2101–2114, https://doi.org/10.1007/s11095-009-9922-2.
[48] M. Parhizkar, P.J.T. Reardon, J.C. Knowles, R.J. Browning, E. Stride, P.R. Barbara, A.H. Harker, M. Edirisinghe, Electrohydrodynamic encapsulation of cisplatin in poly (lactic-co-glycolic acid) nanoparticles for controlled drug delivery, Nanomed. Nanotechnol. Biol. Med. 12 (2016) 1919–1929, https://doi.org/10.1016/j.nano.2016.05.005.

[49] Q. Wen, S. Wan, Z. Liu, S. Xu, H. Wang, B. Yang, Ultrasound contrast agents and ultrasound molecular imaging, J. Nanosci. Nanotechnol. 14 (2014) 190–209, https://doi.org/10.1166/jnn.2014.9114.
[50] M. Rasekh, Z. Ahmad, R. Cross, J. Hernández-Gil, J.D.E.T. Wilton-Ely, P.W. Miller, Facile preparation of drug-loaded tristearin encapsulated superparamagnetic iron oxide nanoparticles using coaxial electrospray processing, Mol. Pharm. 14 (2017) 2010–2023, https://doi.org/10.1021/acs.molpharmaceut.7b00109.
[51] C.Y. Chui, A. Odeleye, L. Nguyen, N. Kasoju, E. Soliman, H. Ye, Electrosprayed genipin cross-linked alginate–chitosan microcarriers for ex vivo expansion of mesenchymal stem cells, J. Biomed. Mater. Res. A 107 (2019) 122–133, https://doi.org/10.1002/jbm.a.36539.
[52] Y. Liu, Y. Zhang, T. Zhang, X. Wang, M. Qu, A. Tan, M. Bogari, M. Zhu, L. Lin, Q. Hu, Analysis of multiple types of human cells subsequent to bioprinting with electrospraying technology, Biomed. Rep. 5 (2016) 723–730, https://doi.org/10.3892/br.2016.790.
[53] S. Sahoo, W.C. Lee, J.C. Goh, S.L. Toh, Bio-electrospraying: A potentially safe technique for delivering progenitor cells, Biotechnol. Bioeng. 106 (2010) 690–698, https://doi.org/10.1002/bit.22734.
[54] J.H. Chung, H. Seonwoo, P. Garg, K.J. Jang, S. Pandey, H.B. Kim, S.B. Park, J.B. Ku, J.H. Kim, K.T. Lim, Development of a bio-electrospray system for cell and non-viral gene delivery, RSC Adv. 8 (2018) 6452–6459, https://doi.org/10.1039/c7ra12477e.
[55] L. Weidenbacher, A. Abrishamkar, M. Rottmar, A.G. Guex, K. Maniura-Weber, A.J. deMello, S.J. Ferguson, R.M. Rossi, G. Fortunato, Electrospraying of microfluidic encapsulated cells for the fabrication of cell-laden electrospun hybrid tissue constructs, Acta Biomater. 64 (2017) 137–147, https://doi.org/10.1016/j.actbio.2017.10.012.
[56] S.K. Boda, S. Chen, K. Chu, H.J. Kim, J. Xie, Electrospraying electrospun nanofiber segments into injectable microspheres for potential cell delivery, ACS Appl. Mater. Interfaces 10 (2018) 25069–25079, https://doi.org/10.1021/acsami.8b06386.
[57] K. Wang, M. Xu, M. Zhu, H. Su, H. Wang, D. Kong, L. Wang, Creation of macropores in electrospun silk fibroin scaffolds using sacrificial PEO-microparticles to enhance cellular infiltration, J. Biomed. Mater. Res. A 101 (2013) 3474–3481, https://doi.org/10.1002/jbm.a.34656.
[58] Y. Wu, J. Fuh, Y. San Wong, J. Sun, A hybrid electrospinning and electrospraying 3D printing for tissue engineered scaffolds, Rapid Prototyp. J. 23 (2017) 1011–1019, https://doi.org/10.1108/RPJ-08-2015-0111.
[59] D. Olvera-Trejo, L.F. Velásquez-García, Additively manufactured MEMS multiplexed coaxial electrospray sources for high-throughput, uniform generation of core-shell microparticles, Lab Chip 16 (2016) 4121–4132, https://doi.org/10.1039/c6lc00729e.
[60] Y. Xu, J. Peng, G. Richards, S. Lu, D. Eglin, Optimization of electrospray fabrication of stem cell-embedded alginate-gelatin microspheres and their assembly in 3D-printed poly(ε-caprolactone) scaffold for cartilage tissue engineering, J. Orthop. Trans. 18 (2019) 128–141, https://doi.org/10.1016/j.jot.2019.05.003.

CHAPTER THIRTEEN

Electrospinning and electrospraying in biomedical engineering: retrospect and prospects

Naresh Kasoju[1], Hua Ye[2], Zhanfeng Cui[2], Seeram Ramakrishna[3]
[1]Division of Tissue Culture, Department of Applied Biology, Biomedical Technology Wing, Sree Chitra Tirunal Institute for Medical Sciences and Technology, Thiruvananthapuram, Kerala, India
[2]Institute of Biomedical Engineering, Department of Engineering Science, University of Oxford, Oxford, United Kingdom
[3]Center for Nanotechnology and Sustainability, Department of Mechanical Engineering, National University of Singapore, Singapore, Republic of Singapore

13.1 Introduction

The nanomaterials are favored in many fields, including biomedical, for their high surface-to-volume ratio and unique functional properties. To this end, several groups explored various strategies to prepare nanostructures. However, electrostatic spinning/spraying, introduced in 1900s and ignored for many years, has recently emerged as the hot favorite strategy for fabricating nanomaterials [1−3]. Typically, electrospinning/spraying consists of (a) a syringe loaded with polymer solution, connected to a syringe pump, (b) a high-voltage power supply connected to a spinneret, and (c) a grounded collector (Fig. 13.1). When a sufficiently high voltage is applied, the electrostatic repulsion within the polymer solution at the tip of spinneret causes the droplet to stretch and accelerate towards the collector. Meanwhile, the solvent evaporates and thereby forms solid nanomaterials [4,5]. Depending on the process parameters, one can produce either nanofibers or nanoparticles. This simple, cost-effective, and versatile setup was highly experimented in recent times, as evident from the publication trends (Fig. 13.1).

Over the time, these two sister technologies were highly explored with several other disciplines to develop next-generation biomaterials with unique features. In this chapter, we present highlights of scientific developments in electrospinning and electrospraying, followed by applications of

Biomedical Applications of Electrospinning and Electrospraying
ISBN: 978-0-12-822476-2
https://doi.org/10.1016/B978-0-12-822476-2.00015-7

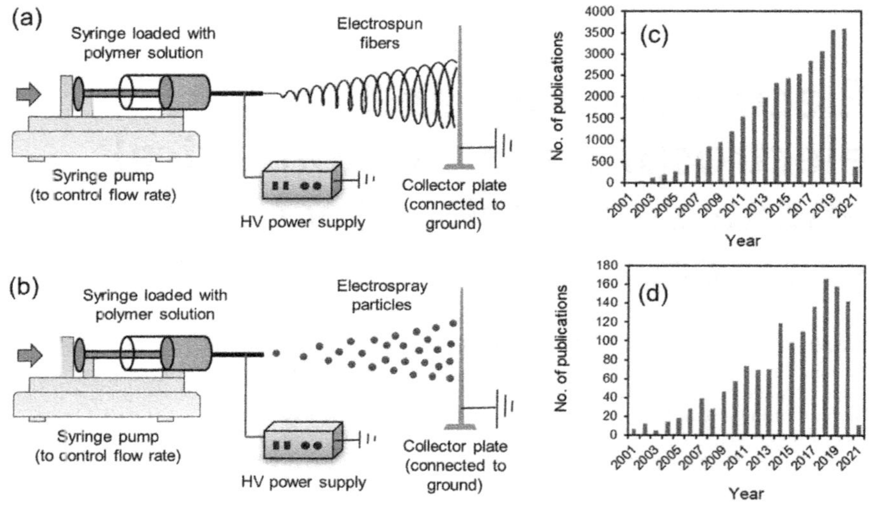

Figure 13.1 Schematic of setups and corresponding publication trends of electrospinning (a, c) and electrospraying (b, d) *Source: Web of science.*

electrospinning and electrospraying materials in biomedical field, and developments in the electrospinning and electrospraying units. Here, we begin with Section 13.2. focusing on technological advances in electrospinning and electrospraying, including cross-disciplinary systems. The following Section 13.3. deals with applications of electrospinning and electrospraying materials in biomedical field, in particular tissue engineering, drug delivery, biosensing, bioimaging, and diagnostics. In Section 13.4, we highlight about the developments in the electrospinning and electrospraying units, including lab-scale, large-scale, and point-of-care devices. In Section 13.5, we highlight the transformation of e-spun/e-spray materials into intelligent human—machine interface systems, including smart wearable sensors and neuroprosthetics. Lastly, in Section 13.6, we summarize the overall developments and highlight future prospects in the field of electrospinning and electrospraying.

13.2 Trends in advanced and combinatorial approaches

Electrospinning/spraying is quite comparable to other spinning/spraying techniques where a tensile force leads to the formation of a fiber/particle. In conventional spinning/spraying techniques mechanical forces initiate the jet, whereas in electrospinning/spraying, the electrical forces initiate the jet. As presented in Fig. 13.1, the setup is quite simple consisting of an HV power supply unit, a syringe loaded with polymer solution, and a grounded collector. However, there are more than 20 parameters that would influence the spinning/spraying process, including system properties (nozzle diameter, nozzle to collector distance, voltage applied, collecting mode viz. static or dynamic, collector type viz. plain or patterned, syringe pump speed, etc.), solution properties (type, molecular weight, and concentration of polymer, boiling point and conductivity of solvent, viscosity of the solution, etc.), and ambient properties (temperature, humidity, and air velocity) (refer to Chapters 1 and 6 of this book for further reading on fundamental principles). Overall simplicity of the setup and the multitude of influencing factors collectively offers the user to manipulate the setup and/or process so as to create nanomaterials with a variety of morphologies and other physicochemical properties.

When we look at the setup and the operating principle, it is quite evident that there are three major stages of fiber or particle production where one can manipulate to achieve versatility in the resultant product features: first—jet formation, second—jet elongation, and third—jet collection (Fig. 13.2). In terms of jet formation, typically, there are two types of electrospinning/spraying setups viz. nozzle-based versus nozzle-free setups. Both these setups were variously experimented to develop innovative ways of jet formation. To name a few, in case of nozzle-based setup, multinozzle system was

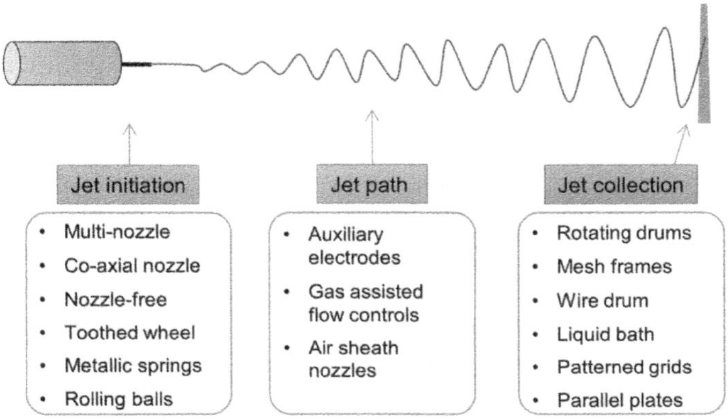

Figure 13.2 Schematic flow chart showing three key aspects of e-spin/e-spray process, i.e., jet formation, jet path control, and jet collection and examples of various innovations thereof.

evolved to increase the throughput of the product. These systems could have either multiple number of conventional syringes or a specialized head unit with multiple orifices, including coaxial [6,7]. Similarly, in case of nozzle-free systems, a wide variety of innovations were seen in the way the jet was formed. These include elements that would aid in jet formation viz. air bubbles, magnetic flakes, metallic springs, toothed wheel, rolling balls, etc. [8]. In terms of second aspect, i.e., the jet elongation, auxiliary electrodes, sheath gas, etc., were used to control the jet path so as to improve the productivity as well as uniformity of the nanofibers [9,10]. As for the third aspect, i.e., the jet collection, apart from the typical static versus rotating drum collectors, a variety of innovative collectors viz. patterned grids, liquid bath, parallel plates, wire drum, etc., were reported in order to generate interesting product forms such as patterned fibers, yarns, capsules, etc. [11,12]. For further reading, refer to Chapter 2 of this book for innovations in electrospinning by Davoodi et al. and to Chapter 7 of this book for advances in electrospraying technology by Yu et al.

Besides alterations in the conventional setups, several curios innovations were also reported combining the two electrohydrodynamic techniques, i.e., electrospinning, that produces nanoscale fibers, with its sister technology electrospraying, that offers nanoscale particles. Given the fact that both these technologies follow same principle and similar setup but different products, several researchers used these two in various combinations to generate products with complimenting properties. In the nozzle-based setups, electrospinning and electrospraying spinnerets were explored in sequential manner to develop nanofiber—nanoparticle assembly in layer-by-layer manner or in concurrent manner to develop nanoparticle-impregnated nanofibrous materials [13—15]. These innovations were also seen in case of the nozzle-free systems as well, wherein needleless electrospinning was used along with needleless electrospraying setup to produce hybrid nanomaterials [16]. In any case, typical setups result in the random organization of nanofiber—nanoparticle assemblies; however, innovations were also reported on the controlled patterning of nanofiber—nanoparticle assemblies by electrostatic template-assisted deposition of electrosprayed particles on electrospun nanofibers [17]. The nanoparticle impregnated nanofibrous materials were explored in various biomedical applications including drug delivery, tissue engineering, cancer research, etc. For further reading, refer to Chapter 11 of this book focusing on innovations in electrospinning-co-electrospraying technologies.

With latest developments in the field of materials engineering and manufacturing technologies, quite a few innovative concepts are emerging, such as 3D printing/bioprinting, microfluidics, etc. These developments were closely observed by the researchers in the field of electrospinning/spraying, and eventually, the electrohydrodynamic technologies have evolved by including elements from other technologies such as 3D printing/bioprinting and microfluidics (Fig. 13.3). For instance, electrospinning/spraying system has reshaped itself from high-voltage to low-voltage system, far-field to near-field system, solution to melt system, and traditional deposition to direct writing system in order to develop next-generation electrospun/spray biomaterials [18–21]. Further, combinatorial approaches of electrospinning/spraying with 3D printing/bioprinting and microfluidics are being reported in recent times [22]. Particularly, 3D printing/bioprinting is being used both in concurrent or sequential manner with electrospinning/spraying to generate next-generation biomaterials, wherein the 3D printed construct gives shape fidelity and required mechanical strength, and the electrospun/spray component offers high surface-to-volume ratio for enhanced functionality in drug delivery, tissue engineering, or other biomedical applications. For further reading, refer to Chapter 12 of this book for innovations in electrospinning with 3D printing/bioprinting and for innovations in electrospraying with 3D printing/bioprinting, respectively.

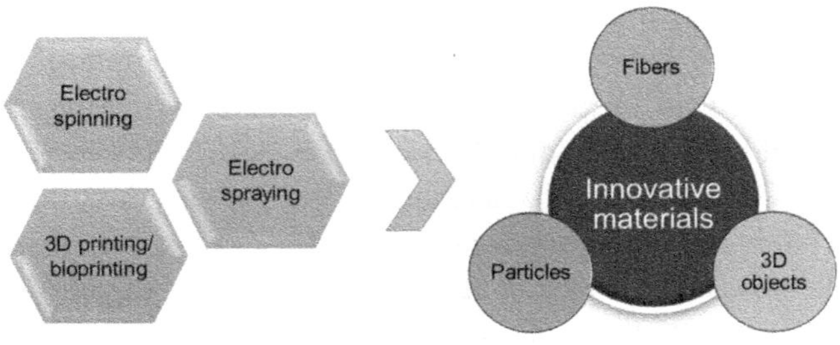

Figure 13.3 Schematic illustration depicting the combinatorial approaches in electrospinning, electrospraying, and 3D printing/bioprinting toward development of innovative materials.

13.3 Trends in applications across various biomedical fields

Tissue engineering is the major application focus for e-spun/e-spray materials [23–25]. Tissue engineering aims to develop artificial human tissues, where-in the biomaterial-based scaffold is the core element of the process. While methods such as phase separation were conventionally explored to make porous scaffolds [26–28], the e-spinning technique came out as a favorite scaffold fabricating approach owing to the high surface-to-volume ratio and high porosity of the resultant scaffold [29]. Similarly, the e-spray materials have also become a favorite scaffolding material, particularly for bottom-up approaches, ex vivo stem cell expansion, and cell encapsulation through bioelectrospraying [30,31]. The e-spun/e-spray materials have evolved from being a mere space filling materials to bioactive and smart scaffolds in the context of tissue engineering and regenerative medicine [32,33]. At the same time, several investigations are shedding light on the process—property—function relationship studies and how the e-spun/e-spray material properties influence the cell response [34–36]. With extensive R&D over the last few years and inputs from various other disciplines such as 3D printing, microfluidics, etc., several innovative materials and medical devices are under development for potential applications in tissue engineering field. In Chapter 3 of this book, Aggarwal and Sah described the use of e-spun articles as scaffolding material for engineering hard, soft, and specialized tissues. Similarly, in Chapter 8 of this book, Dubey et al. elaborated various applications of electrospraying in tissue engineering and beyond.

Another major field of e-spun/e-spray material applications is drug delivery [37,38]. Typically, the systemic administration of drugs in their pristine form could suffer from drawbacks such as poor solubility in the physiological fluids, insufficient bioavailability at the site of action, fluctuations in drug concentration, and inconsistency in the drug stability or shelf life, which collectively could result in the ineffectiveness of the drug and/or adverse reaction side effects. To this end, the pristine drug was formulated or made into the form of a device in order to achieve control on delivery rate over a sustained period of time and thereby enhance the safety, efficacy, and performance of the drug. Over the last few decades, an array of polymeric micro/nanostructures prepared by various methods have been explored as drug-delivery systems. Among them, the e-spun/e-spray materials were extensively investigated as drug-delivery systems to incorporate several therapeutic agents. One of the attractive feature of e-spin/e-spray technology was that it offers control over several process parameters, versatility over material choice, and tunability over shape, size, and morphology of the e-spun/e-spray products. A variety of polymers such as polycaprolactone, polylactic acid, collagen, silk fibroin, and composites were explored to encapsulate drugs such as paclitaxel, curcumin, etc., by e-spinning/e-spraying. For further reading, refer to Chapters 4 and 9 of this book for state-of-the-art applications of e-spun and e-spray materials as drug delivery systems in biomedical field, respectively.

The ongoing COVID-19 pandemic has made everyone realize the need for efficient and quick sensing and diagnostic systems. Biosensing and diagnostics is one key subarea in the biomedical field and the versatile e-spun/e-spray materials could very well be explored in this field too [39]. The high surface-to-volume ratio and porosity of the e-spun nanofibers or the e-spray nanoparticles means that there would be excellent scope for ligand and analyte interaction, and this means ultrafast and efficient sensing [40]. An array of e-spun materials was used for sensing applications by combining or functionalizing inert polymeric systems with other materials or building blocks with optical, electrical, chemical, or other stimuli-responsive properties. In Chapter 5 of this book, Wei presented state-of-the-art review on e-spun materials composed of zero-, one-, and two-dimensional materials for subsequent applications in colorimetric, fluorescent, luminescence, electrochemical, and other biosensing field. Similar to e-spun materials, its sister products, the e-spray materials were being explored in biosensing mainly because of the simple yet versatile nature of the setup, and the fact that the e-spray materials loaded with active sensing elements could be mass produced with ease and accuracy. In Chapter 10 of this book, Nguyen and Yang described up-to-date review on the use of e-spray materials as biosensing systems and beyond.

Besides, the e-spun/e-spray materials are being explored in a wide variety of specialized biomedical applications (Fig. 13.4). For instance, Jin et al. 2010 demonstrated the "photocurrent therapy" by using e-spun materials [41]. Here, the authors reported the preparation of electrospun poly(3-hexylthiophene)/polycaprolactone nanofibers and their subsequent application as photo/electro-sensitive scaffolds for skin regeneration in presence of applied photocurrent. Medical imaging, such as magnetic resonance imaging (MRI), is another interesting area where the e-spun/e-spray materials are being explored. Lately, Jin et al. 2016 have reported e-spun core—shell polymeric materials loaded with gadolinium (III) complex to the porcine colon and thereby proved that such contrast-enhancing agent—loaded e-spun

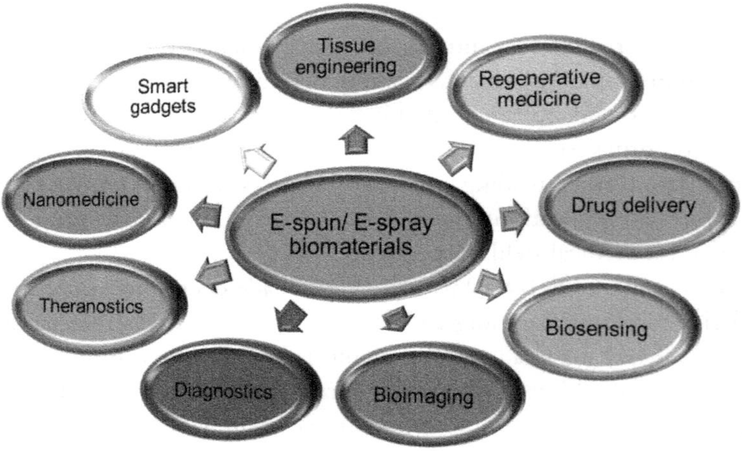

Figure 13.4 Schematic illustration showing electrospinning and electrospraying applications across multiple biomedical fields.

materials could be explored for effective medical imaging of colonic or other abnormalities [42]. Theranostics is yet another exciting avenue for e-spun/e-spray materials in the recent years. Jin et al. 2016 first reported the use of e-spun core—shell materials loaded with the MRI contrast agent gadolinium (III) complex and indomethacin as a model drug for image-guided drug delivery [43]. Similarly, Ramachandran et al. 2017 reported e-spun—based theranostic nanoimplant for prolonged and localized treatment of recurrent glioma [44].

13.4 Trends in setups from lab-scale to industrial as well as point-of-care devices

Any science and/or engineering principles could be considered successful when it becomes a technology, and any technology could be considered successful when it moves from bench to bedside, especially in the biomedical field. The electrospinning and electrospraying technologies are fascinating nanomaterial fabrication processes that gained tremendous attention in the research and product development activities. While its high surface-to-volume ratio was much appreciated, many speculated that its relatively poor yield and assembling various components into a single portable unit could impede this technology in transforming from laboratory bench to commercial scale and to bedside. However, detailed investigations into the electrospinning and electrospraying process engineering and more importantly the passionate efforts of many electrohydrodynamic enthusiasts led to several innovations and development of commercial as well as point-of-care electrospinning and electrospraying devices.

Setting up an electrospinning/spraying setup in the laboratory was once initiated as a do-it-yourself activity by purchasing several components individually and assembling it together to make it work with bit of trial and error. While such systems were accepted for R&D activities, they often lack control over many process parameters and also contain safety risks. However, several commercial entities across the globe have realized the potential of this process, worked on the basic setups and started to offer a ready-to-install basic system, with control over many, if not all, process parameters and with maximum safety features. As detailed in previous Section 13.2, the basic unit of electrospinning/spraying has been variously modified so as to develop next-generation biomaterials. These laboratory-scale R&D activities were also picked up by the electrospinning/spraying companies and successfully upgraded their systems from time to time to offer versatile and evolving features of the technology to their customers. These include a variety of specialized components such as coaxial spinnerets, collectors, and other accessories that aid in jet formation, jet elongation, or jet collection. Further, commercial setups of advanced versions of electrospinning/spraying such as multijet systems, direct-write systems, melt electrospinning system, etc., have also been introduced into the market [45]. For further reading, refer to Chapter 14 of this book detailing practical aspects of setting up e-spin/e-spray units.

Moving on, these setups have evolved from typical R&D activities to large-scale production in factories for the real biomedical applications in clinics. Both nozzle-based and nozzle-free systems were upgraded to yield high-throughput fiber/particle production; however, looking at the reports and product portfolio in the market, perhaps the nozzle-free systems are more profitable. These nozzle-free systems, otherwise called as free surface electrospinning systems, are mostly focused on achieving more number of jets formed with less free feed volume. Nanospider electrospinning systems from Elmarco, Czech Republic, stands out among all as the most successful commercial scale nozzle-free system [46]. Besides, Molanr and Nagy introduced "corona electrospinning" which includes a novel metal electrode having sharp edge as the spinneret [47]. Further high-throughput systems were reported by Wei et al. [48], Wu et al. [49], Shao et al. [50], Wei et al. [51], etc. The field is still active and reports are continuously emerging on this aspect. Recently, Kara et al. reported shear-aided electrospinning as a nozzle-free process for high-throughput nanomaterial fabrication [52]. Apart from conventional single component nanomaterial producing setups, drug-loaded and multicomponent nanomaterial producing high-throughput setups have also evolved successfully. For instance, Krogstad and Woodrow reported successful manufacturing scale-up of electrospun poly(vinyl alcohol) nanofibrous matrices loaded with tenofovir for potential applications in the vaginal drug delivery [53]. Similarly, Jiang and Qin reported a modified nozzle-free electrospinning setup for massive production of core—shell nanofibers [54]. Further, advanced systems such as those based on melt electrospinning are also emerging; recently, Koenig et al. reported a new prototype melt electrospinning with 600 nozzles (Fig. 13.5) [45].

COVID-19, the ongoing corona virus pandemic, has taught us the importance of "rapid" action, in terms of testing or treating. For any technology to be available to the patients at a "rapid" pace, it is important to make it available at the point of care. The electrospinning/spraying technologies have evolved over the last few years and developed into point-of-care systems. For instance, Mouthuy et al. reported a small, battery-operated electrospinning/spraying apparatus with a microcontroller to regulate voltage and feed rate (Fig. 13.6). Using this portable machine, the authors demonstrated

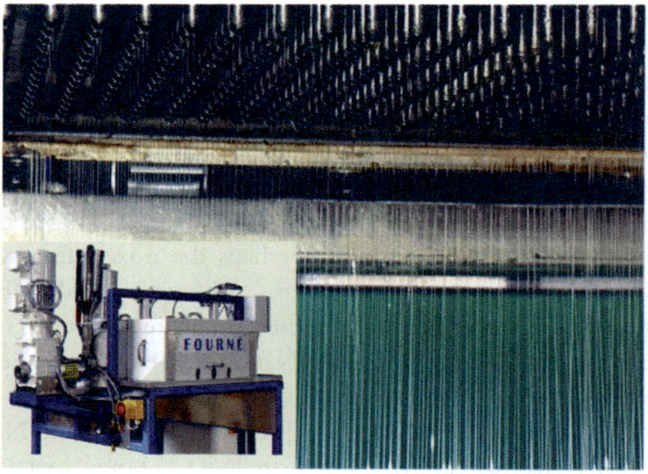

Figure 13.5 The 600-nozzle melt-electrospinning prototype developed at the AMIBM. *Reproduced from K. Koenig, K. Beukenberg, F. Langensiepen, G. Seide, A new prototype melt-electrospinning device for the production of biobased thermoplastic sub-microfibers and nanofibers, Biomater. Res. 23 (2019) 10. https://doi.org/10.1186/s40824-019-0159-9. Copyright © 2019, The Author(s). Publisher Springer Nature.*

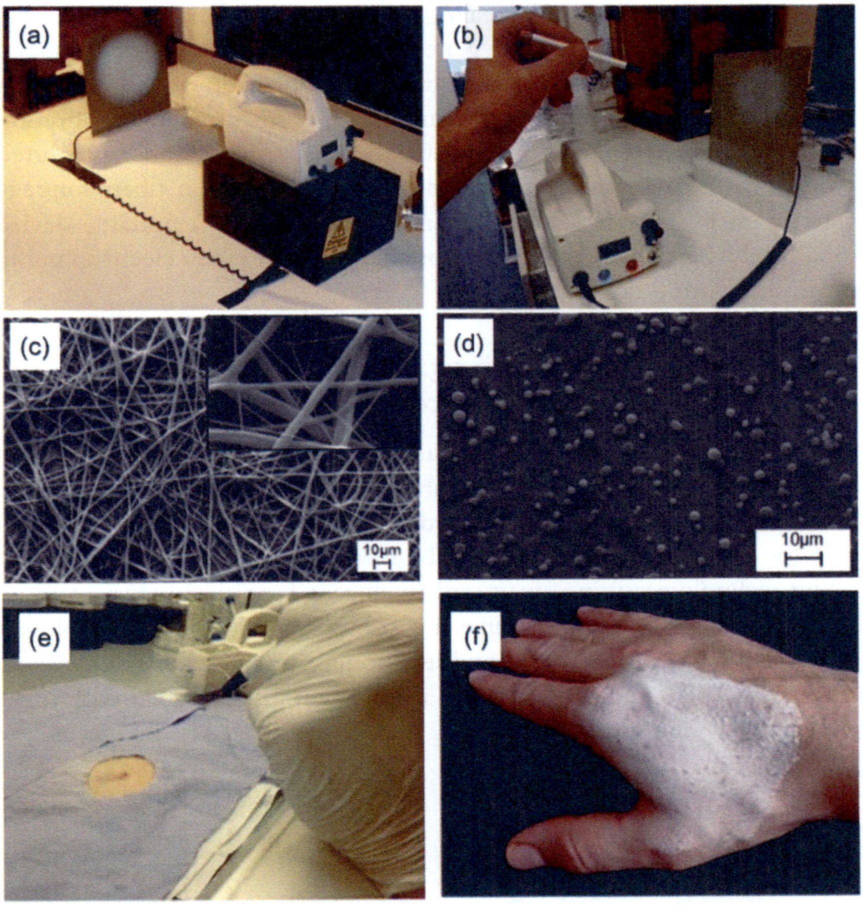

Figure 13.6 A portable electrospinning/electrospraying device in action ((a) stand-alone device, (b) device with a pen extension, (c) SEM image of e-spun fibers, (d) SEM image e-spray particles, (e) portable device electrospinning fibers onto porcine wound site, and (f) portable device–derived e-spun patch on a healthy human volunteer). *Reproduced from P.-A. Mouthuy, L. Groszkowski, H. Ye, Performances of a portable electrospinning apparatus, Biotechnol. Lett. 37 (2015) 1107–1116. https://doi.org/10.1007/s10529-014-1760-6. Copyright © 2015, The Author(s). Publisher: Springer Nature.*

successful spinning as well spraying of a variety of polymer solutions directly onto the skin surface [55,56]. Subsequently, Xu et al. developed a similar battery-operated portable handheld electrospinning apparatus [57]. In the following years, Haik et al. demonstrated the feasibility of a handheld electrospinning device for the application of nanofibrous wound dressings at various stages of wound healing [58]. Similarly, Brako et al. 2018 reported a portable device for generation of silver nanoparticle—doped cellulose acetate nanofibers for advanced wound dressing [59] Revia et al. reported a portable system for nanofiber synthesis and its application for cosmetic treatment of alopecia [60], and Fuenteslópez and Ye reported production of polycaprolactone and gelatine electrospun fibers impregnated with hyaluronic acid—chitosan nanoparticles by a portable device [61]. Lately, Zhao et al. reported a portable device for melt electrospinning for in situ wound dressing [62].

13.5 Transformation of E-spin/E-spray materials into human—machine interface systems

Smart materials, intelligent systems, human—machine interface systems, bionics, wearable sensors, flexible electronics, big data, and internet of things are some of the buzzing words these days. An emerging application field for e-spun/e-spray materials in biomedical engineering include interfacing technologies using smart and intelligent biomaterials for real-time sensing, including internet of things (Fig. 13.7) [63—65]. These technologies are upcoming in both invasive and less/noninvasive devices. For instance, Zhang et al. reported fabrication of alginate nanofibers loaded with silver nanoparticles and demonstrated its use as smart fabrics for accurately

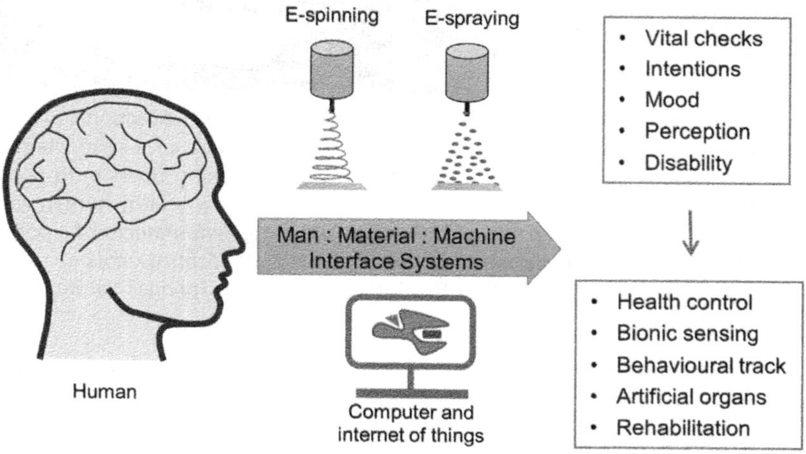

Figure 13.7 An illustrative flow chart of human—machine or more specifically man-material—machine interface systems, including e-spun/e-spray materials, in transforming human health monitoring, diagnosis, and rehabilitation in the days to come.

monitoring human's rate and depth of respiration during exercise and emotion changes [66]. The authors claimed that it could be a low-cost approach for tracking respiration and for avoiding sleep apnea. Similarly, Ma et al. reported highly oriented electrospun poly[(vinylidenefluoride-co-trifluoroethylene] materials with piezoelectric property and high mechanical endurance and showed that these materials can be twisted and woven into daily outfit for body motion sensing, including monitor body gestures such as elbow bending angle, swinging arm direction, etc. [67]. Similar reports on e-spun/e-spray smart systems for health monitoring, diagnosis, and rehabilitation are very recently reviewed by Ghosh et al. and are thus not covered here to avoid duplication [68].

Other existing biomedical applications such as bionics are on the rise for e-spun/e-spray materials [69]. Here, the e-spun/e-spray materials are being used individually and by integrating with other smart systems. One particular area of focus to mention here is the neuroprosthetics, which are interfaced with several other tissues in the body to regain the lost functions [70]. For instance, Dirk et al. reported electrospun-based conductive and porous scaffolds as potential neural interface materials, wherein the conductivity of the material was tuned by manipulating the multiwalled carbon nanotubes content [71]. These systems are also converted into multifunctional bioelectrodes in neuroscience, such as those reported by Reddy et al., wherein bionanotube/poly(3,4-ethylenedioxythiophene) nanohybrid was explored as an electrode for dopamine sensor and neural interfacing [72]. Similarly, Chen et al. reported the fabrication of poly(3,4-ethylenedioxythiophene)-carbon nanotube composite for neural interfacing [73]. In this context, the cell–material interaction studies are extensively being investigated both for reparative and regenerative purposes [74–78].

13.6 Summary and future prospects

Initially reported in the early 1900s, ignored for many years thereafter, then rejuvenated in the recent past, the electrospinning/spraying technologies have seen ups and downs in their life time. Currently, these technologies are enjoying the best of their time by attracting attention from scientists of various backgrounds who are looking for materials with submicron scale features. Innovative research and developmental activities are ongoing in the field focusing on various aspects of these technologies viz. improvisations in the setup, transformation of fibers/particles into medical devices, and expanding the scope of applications in biomedical field. On the other hand, developments on setups that would scale up the production and regulatory activities that are required to streamline successful translation of e-spun/e-spray devices from bench to bedside are also going on in full swing (refer to Chapter 15 of this book for further reading). Cherry on the cake aspect would be the fact that e-spin/e-spray technologies are finding interesting relationships with other technologies such as 3D printing, and this means several exciting innovations are in the pipeline particularly as smart and intelligent human−machine interface systems. Overall, the current trends in the field of electrospinning/spraying technologies are highly exciting and we envisage greater scope of these technologies in biomedical field in the days to come.

Acknowledgment

NK thanks Sree Chitra Tirunal Institute for Medical Sciences and Technology, Thiruvananthapuram, for Technology Development Fund (P6219).

References

[1] S. Ramakrishna, K. Fujihara, W.-E. Teo, T. Yong, Z. Ma, R. Ramaseshan, Electrospun nanofibers: solving global issues, Mater. Today 9 (2006) 40−50, https://doi.org/10.1016/S1369-7021(06)71389-X.

[2] Z. Ma, M. Kotaki, R. Inai, S. Ramakrishna, Potential of nanofiber matrix as tissue-engineering scaffolds, Tissue Eng. 11 (2005) 101−109, https://doi.org/10.1089/ten.2005.11.101.

[3] S.-H. Tan, R. Inai, M. Kotaki, S. Ramakrishna, Systematic parameter study for ultra-fine fiber fabrication via electrospinning process, Polymer 46 (2005) 6128−6134, https://doi.org/10.1016/j.polymer.2005.05.068.

[4] P.-A. Mouthuy, Y. El-Sherbini, Z. Cui, H. Ye, Layering PLGA-based electrospun membranes and cell sheets for engineering cartilage-bone transition: electrospinning and cell sheet engineering, J. Tissue Eng. Regen. Med. 10 (2016) E263−E274, https://doi.org/10.1002/term.1765.

[5] E. Soliman, F. Bianchi, J.N. Sleigh, J.H. George, M.Z. Cader, Z. Cui, H. Ye, Engineered method for directional growth of muscle sheets on electrospun fibers: engineered method for directional growth, J. Biomed. Mater. Res. 106 (2018) 1165−1176, https://doi.org/10.1002/jbm.a.36312.

[6] Y. Zheng, H. Cao, Z. Zhou, X. Mei, L. Yu, X. Chen, G. He, Y. Zhao, D. Wu, D. Sun, Concentrated multi-nozzle electrospinning, Fibers Polym. 20 (2019) 1180−1186, https://doi.org/10.1007/s12221-019-8984-y.

[7] Y. Zhang, Z. Cheng, Z. Han, S. Zhao, X. Zhao, L. Kang, Stable multi-jet electrospinning with high throughput using the bead structure nozzle, RSC Adv. 8 (2018) 6069−6074, https://doi.org/10.1039/C7RA13125A.

[8] A. Ahmad, U. Ali, A. Nazir, A. Shahzad, Z. Khaliq, M.B. Qadir, M.A. Khan, S. Ali, M. Aamir Hassan, S. Abid, R. Tahir, B. Mushtaq, Toothed wheel needleless electrospinning: a versatile way to fabricate uniform and finer nanomembrane, J. Mater. Sci. 54 (2019) 13834−13847, https://doi.org/10.1007/s10853-019-03875-0.

[9] G. Zheng, J. Jiang, D. Chen, J. Liu, Y. Liu, J. Zheng, X. Wang, W. Li, Multinozzle high efficiency electrospinning with the constraint of sheath gas, J. Appl. Polym. Sci. 136 (2019) 47574, https://doi.org/10.1002/app.47574.
[10] G. Zheng, J. Jiang, X. Wang, W. Li, J. Liu, G. Fu, L. Lin, Nanofiber membranes by multi-jet electrospinning arranged as arc-array with sheath gas for electrodialysis applications, Mater. Des. 189 (2020) 108504, https://doi.org/10.1016/j.matdes.2020.108504.
[11] A.Y. Nuryantini, M.M. Munir, M.P. Ekaputra, T. Suciati, Khairurrijal, electrospinning of poly(vinyl alcohol)/chitosan via multi-nozzle spinneret and drum collector, AMR 896 (2014) 41–44, https://doi.org/10.4028/www.scientific.net/AMR.896.41.
[12] N. Kasoju, J. George, H. Ye, Z. Cui, Sacrificial core-based electrospinning: a facile and versatile approach to fabricate devices for potential cell and tissue encapsulation applications, Nanomaterials 8 (2018) 863, https://doi.org/10.3390/nano8100863.
[13] K.M. Sajesh, K. Kiran, S.V. Nair, R. Jayakumar, Sequential layer-by-layer electrospinning of nano SrCO3/PRP loaded PHBV fibrous scaffold for bone tissue engineering, Compos. B Eng. 99 (2016) 445–452, https://doi.org/10.1016/j.compositesb.2016.06.026.
[14] W. Li, X. Li, W. Li, T. Wang, X. Li, S. Pan, H. Deng, Nanofibrous mats layer-by-layer assembled via electrospun cellulose acetate and electrosprayed chitosan for cell culture, Eur. Polym. J. 48 (2012) 1846–1853, https://doi.org/10.1016/j.eurpolymj.2012.08.001.
[15] H. Rodríguez-Tobías, G. Morales, D. Grande, Electrospinning and electrospraying techniques for designing antimicrobial polymeric biocomposite mats, in: M.M. Rahman, A.M. Asiri (Eds.), Nanofiber Research - Reaching New Heights, InTech, 2016, https://doi.org/10.5772/63470.
[16] A. Shaid, L. Wang, R. Padhye, A. Jadhav, Needleless electrospinning and electrospraying of mixture of polymer and aerogel particles on textile, Adv. Mater. Sci. Eng. 2018 (2018) 1–7, https://doi.org/10.1155/2018/1781930.
[17] S. Nedjari, A. Hébraud, S. Eap, S. Siegwald, C. Mélart, N. Benkirane-Jessel, G. Schlatter, Electrostatic template-assisted deposition of microparticles on electrospun nanofibers: towards microstructured functional biochips for screening applications, RSC Adv. 5 (2015) 83600–83607, https://doi.org/10.1039/C5RA15931H.
[18] D. Sun, C. Chang, S. Li, L. Lin, Near-field electrospinning, Nano Lett. 6 (2006) 839–842, https://doi.org/10.1021/nl0602701.
[19] X. Li, Z. Li, L. Wang, G. Ma, F. Meng, R.H. Pritchard, E.L. Gill, Y. Liu, Y.Y.S. Huang, Low-voltage continuous electrospinning patterning, ACS Appl. Mater. Interfaces 8 (2016) 32120–32131, https://doi.org/10.1021/acsami.6b07797.
[20] R. Nayak, R. Padhye, L. Arnold, Melt-electrospinning of nanofibers, in: Electrospun Nanofibers, Elsevier, 2017, pp. 11–40, https://doi.org/10.1016/B978-0-08-100907-9.00002-7.
[21] H. Chen, A. de B.F.B. Malheiro, C. van Blitterswijk, C. Mota, P.A. Wieringa, L. Moroni, Direct writing electrospinning of scaffolds with multidimensional fiber architecture for hierarchical tissue engineering, ACS Appl. Mater. Interfaces 9 (2017) 38187–38200, https://doi.org/10.1021/acsami.7b07151.
[22] S.M. Giannitelli, M. Costantini, F. Basoli, M. Trombetta, A. Rainer, Electrospinning and microfluidics, in: Electrofluidodynamic Technologies (EFDTs) for Biomaterials and Medical Devices, Elsevier, 2018, pp. 139–155, https://doi.org/10.1016/B978-0-08-101745-6.00008-6.
[23] M. Rahmati, D.K. Mills, A.M. Urbanska, M.R. Saeb, J.R. Venugopal, S. Ramakrishna, M. Mozafari, Electrospinning for tissue engineering applications, Prog. Mater. Sci. (2020) 100721, https://doi.org/10.1016/j.pmatsci.2020.100721.

[24] A. Bigham, F. Foroughi, E. Rezvani Ghomi, M. Rafienia, R.E. Neisiany, S. Ramakrishna, The journey of multifunctional bone scaffolds fabricated from traditional toward modern techniques, Bio-Des. Manuf. 3 (2020) 281–306, https://doi.org/10.1007/s42242-020-00094-4.
[25] M. Goswami, P. Rekhi, M. Debnath, S. Ramakrishna, Microbial polyhydroxyalkanoates granules: an approach targeting biopolymer for medical applications and developing bone scaffolds, Molecules 26 (2021) 860, https://doi.org/10.3390/molecules26040860.
[26] N. Kasoju, D. Kubies, M.M. Kumorek, J. Kříž, E. Fábryová, L. Machová, J. Kovářová, F. Rypáček, Dip TIPS as a facile and versatile method for fabrication of polymer foams with controlled shape, size and pore architecture for bioengineering applications, PloS One 9 (2014) e108792, https://doi.org/10.1371/journal.pone.0108792.
[27] N. Kasoju, D. Kubies, T. Sedlačík, O. Janoušková, J. Koubková, M.M. Kumorek, F. Rypáček, Polymer scaffolds with no skin-effect for tissue engineering applications fabricated by thermally induced phase separation, Biomed. Mater. 11 (2016) 015002, https://doi.org/10.1088/1748-6041/11/1/015002.
[28] N. Kasoju, D. Kubies, E. Fábryová, J. Kříž, M.M. Kumorek, E. Sticová, F. Rypáček, In vivo vascularization of anisotropic channeled porous polylactide-based capsules for islet transplantation: the effects of scaffold architecture and implantation site, Physiol. Res. 64 (2015) S75–S84, https://doi.org/10.33549/physiolres.933138.
[29] N. Kasoju, U. Bora, Silk fibroin based biomimetic artificial extracellular matrix for hepatic tissue engineering applications, Biomed. Mater. 7 (2012) 045004, https://doi.org/10.1088/1748-6041/7/4/045004.
[30] C.-Y. Chui, A. Odeleye, L. Nguyen, N. Kasoju, E. Soliman, H. Ye, Electrosprayed genipin cross-linked alginate–chitosan microcarriers for ex vivo expansion of mesenchymal stem cells, J. Biomed. Mater. Res. 107 (2019) 122–133, https://doi.org/10.1002/jbm.a.36539.
[31] M.C. Lee, H. Seonwoo, P. Garg, K.J. Jang, S. Pandey, H.B. Kim, S.B. Park, J.B. Ku, J.H. Kim, K.T. Lim, J.H. Chung, Development of a bio-electrospray system for cell and non-viral gene delivery, RSC Adv. 8 (2018) 6452–6459, https://doi.org/10.1039/C7RA12477E.
[32] A. Alehosseini, B. Ghorani, M. Sarabi-Jamab, N. Tucker, Principles of electrospraying: a new approach in protection of bioactive compounds in foods, Crit. Rev. Food Sci. Nutr. 58 (2018) 2346–2363, https://doi.org/10.1080/10408398.2017.1323723.
[33] I. Otsuka, C.J. Barrett, Electrospinning of photo-responsive Azo-Cellulose: towards smart fibrous materials, Cellulose 26 (2019) 6903–6915, https://doi.org/10.1007/s10570-019-02585-9.
[34] Q. Li, B. Zhang, N. Kasoju, J. Ma, A. Yang, Z. Cui, H. Wang, H. Ye, Differential and interactive effects of substrate topography and chemistry on human mesenchymal stem cell gene expression, IJMS 19 (2018) 2344, https://doi.org/10.3390/ijms19082344.
[35] B. Zhang, N. Kasoju, Q. Li, J. Ma, A. Yang, Z. Cui, H. Wang, H. Ye, Effect of substrate topography and chemistry on human mesenchymal stem cell markers: a transcriptome study, IJSC 12 (2019) 84–94, https://doi.org/10.15283/ijsc18102.
[36] B. Zhang, N. Kasoju, Q. Li, E. Soliman, A. Yang, Z. Cui, J. Ma, H. Wang, H. Ye, Culture surfaces induce hypoxia-regulated genes in human mesenchymal stromal cells, Biomed. Mater. 14 (2019) 035012, https://doi.org/10.1088/1748-605X/ab0e61.
[37] M. Farokhi, F. Mottaghitalab, R.L. Reis, S. Ramakrishna, S.C. Kundu, Functionalized silk fibroin nanofibers as drug carriers: advantages and challenges, J. Contr. Release 321 (2020) 324–347, https://doi.org/10.1016/j.jconrel.2020.02.022.
[38] S. Mohammadi, S. Ramakrishna, S. Laurent, M.A. Shokrgozar, D. Semnani, D. Sadeghi, S. Bonakdar, M. Akbari, Fabrication of nanofibrous PVA/Alginate-Sulfate

substrates for growth factor delivery: fabrication of nanofibrous PVA/Alginate-Sulfate substrates for growth factor delivery, J. Biomed. Mater. Res. 107 (2019) 403–413, https://doi.org/10.1002/jbm.a.36552.

[39] N. Xin, D. Wei, Y. Zhu, M. Yang, S. Ramakrishna, O. Lee, H. Luo, H. Fan, Upconversion nanomaterials: a platform for biosensing, theranostic and photoregulation, Mater. Today Chem. 17 (2020) 100329, https://doi.org/10.1016/j.mtchem.2020.100329.

[40] C. Wolf, M. Tscherner, S. Köstler, Ultra-fast opto-chemical sensors by using electrospun nanofibers as sensing layers, Sensor. Actuator. B Chem. 209 (2015) 1064–1069, https://doi.org/10.1016/j.snb.2014.11.070.

[41] G. Jin, M.P. Prabhakaran, S. Liao, S. Ramakrishna, Photosensitive materials and potential of photocurrent mediated tissue regeneration, J. Photochem. Photobiol. B Biol. 102 (2011) 93–101, https://doi.org/10.1016/j.jphotobiol.2010.09.010.

[42] M. Jin, D.-G. Yu, X. Wang, C.F.G.C. Geraldes, G.R. Williams, S.W.A. Bligh, Electrospun contrast-agent-loaded fibers for colon-targeted MRI, Adv. Healthcare Mater. 5 (2016) 977–985, https://doi.org/10.1002/adhm.201500872.

[43] M. Jin, D.-G. Yu, C.F.G.C. Geraldes, G.R. Williams, S.W.A. Bligh, Theranostic fibers for simultaneous imaging and drug delivery, Mol. Pharm. 13 (2016) 2457–2465, https://doi.org/10.1021/acs.molpharmaceut.6b00197.

[44] R. Ramachandran, V.R. Junnuthula, G.S. Gowd, A. Ashokan, J. Thomas, R. Peethambaran, A. Thomas, A.K.K. Unni, D. Panikar, S.V. Nair, M. Koyakutty, Theranostic 3-Dimensional nano brain-implant for prolonged and localized treatment of recurrent glioma, Sci. Rep. 7 (2017) 43271, https://doi.org/10.1038/srep43271.

[45] K. Koenig, K. Beukenberg, F. Langensiepen, G. Seide, A new prototype melt-electrospinning device for the production of biobased thermoplastic sub-microfibers and nanofibers, Biomater. Res. 23 (2019) 10, https://doi.org/10.1186/s40824-019-0159-9.

[46] M.H. El-Newehy, S.S. Al-Deyab, E.-R. Kenawy, A. Abdel-Megeed, Nanospider technology for the production of nylon-6 nanofibers for biomedical applications, J. Nanomater. 2011 (2011) 1–8, https://doi.org/10.1155/2011/626589.

[47] K. Molnar, Z.K. Nagy, Corona-electrospinning: needleless method for high-throughput continuous nanofiber production, Eur. Polym. J. 74 (2016) 279–286, https://doi.org/10.1016/j.eurpolymj.2015.11.028.

[48] L. Wei, H. Yu, L. Jia, X. Qin, High-throughput nanofiber produced by needleless electrospinning using a metal dish as the spinneret, Textil. Res. J. 88 (2018) 80–88, https://doi.org/10.1177/0040517516677232.

[49] D. Wu, Z. Xiao, K.S. Teh, Z. Han, G. Luo, C. Shi, D. Sun, J. Zhao, L. Lin, High-throughput rod-induced electrospinning, J. Phys. D Appl. Phys. 49 (2016) 365302, https://doi.org/10.1088/0022-3727/49/36/365302.

[50] Z. Shao, L. Yu, L. Xu, M. Wang, High-throughput fabrication of quality nanofibers using a modified free surface electrospinning, Nanoscale Res. Lett. 12 (2017) 470, https://doi.org/10.1186/s11671-017-2240-4.

[51] L. Wei, R. Sun, C. Liu, J. Xiong, X. Qin, Mass production of nanofibers from needleless electrospinning by a novel annular spinneret, Mater. Des. 179 (2019) 107885, https://doi.org/10.1016/j.matdes.2019.107885.

[52] Y. Kara, H. He, K. Molnár, Shear-aided high-throughput electrospinning: a needleless method with enhanced jet formation, J. Appl. Polym. Sci. 137 (2020) 49104, https://doi.org/10.1002/app.49104.

[53] E.A. Krogstad, K.A. Woodrow, Manufacturing scale-up of electrospun poly(vinyl alcohol) fibers containing tenofovir for vaginal drug delivery, Int. J. Pharm. 475 (2014) 282–291, https://doi.org/10.1016/j.ijpharm.2014.08.039.

[54] G. Jiang, X. Qin, An improved free surface electrospinning for high throughput manufacturing of core—shell nanofibers, Mater. Lett. 128 (2014) 259—262, https://doi.org/10.1016/j.matlet.2014.04.074.

[55] P.-A. Mouthuy, L. Groszkowski, H. Ye, Performances of a portable electrospinning apparatus, Biotechnol. Lett. 37 (2015) 1107—1116, https://doi.org/10.1007/s10529-014-1760-6.

[56] C.-Y. Chui, P.-A. Mouthuy, H. Ye, Direct electrospinning of poly(vinyl butyral) onto human dermal fibroblasts using a portable device, Biotechnol. Lett. 40 (2018) 737—744, https://doi.org/10.1007/s10529-018-2522-7.

[57] S.-C. Xu, C.-C. Qin, M. Yu, R.-H. Dong, X. Yan, H. Zhao, W.-P. Han, H.-D. Zhang, Y.-Z. Long, A battery-operated portable handheld electrospinning apparatus, Nanoscale 7 (2015) 12351—12355, https://doi.org/10.1039/C5NR02922H.

[58] J. Haik, R. Kornhaber, B. Blal, M. Harats, The feasibility of a handheld electrospinning device for the application of nanofibrous wound dressings, Adv. Wound Care 6 (2017) 166—174, https://doi.org/10.1089/wound.2016.0722.

[59] F. Brako, C. Luo, D.Q.M. Craig, M. Edirisinghe, An inexpensive, portable device for point-of-need generation of silver-nanoparticle doped cellulose acetate nanofibers for advanced wound dressing, Macromol. Mater. Eng. 303 (2018) 1700586, https://doi.org/10.1002/mame.201700586.

[60] Revia, Z. Wagner, A portable electrospinner for nanofiber synthesis and its application for cosmetic treatment of alopecia, Nanomaterials 9 (2019) 1317, https://doi.org/10.3390/nano9091317.

[61] C.V. Fuenteslópez, H. Ye, Electrospun fibres with hyaluronic acid-chitosan nanoparticles produced by a portable device, Nanomaterials 10 (2020), https://doi.org/10.3390/nano10102016, 2016.

[62] Y.-T. Zhao, J. Zhang, Y. Gao, X.-F. Liu, J.-J. Liu, X.-X. Wang, H.-F. Xiang, Y.-Z. Long, Self-powered portable melt electrospinning for in situ wound dressing, J. Nanobiotechnol. 18 (2020) 111, https://doi.org/10.1186/s12951-020-00671-w.

[63] W.A.D.M. Jayathilaka, K. Qi, Y. Qin, A. Chinnappan, W. Serrano-García, C. Baskar, H. Wang, J. He, S. Cui, S.W. Thomas, S. Ramakrishna, Significance of nanomaterials in wearables: a review on wearable actuators and sensors, Adv. Mater. 31 (2019) 1805921, https://doi.org/10.1002/adma.201805921.

[64] O.Y. Kweon, S.J. Lee, J.H. Oh, Wearable high-performance pressure sensors based on three-dimensional electrospun conductive nanofibers, NPG Asia Mater. 10 (2018) 540—551, https://doi.org/10.1038/s41427-018-0041-6.

[65] T. Yang, L. Zhan, C.Z. Huang, Recent insights into functionalized electrospun nanofibrous films for chemo-/bio-sensors, Trac. Trends Anal. Chem. 124 (2020) 115813, https://doi.org/10.1016/j.trac.2020.115813.

[56] J. Zhang, X.-X. Wang, B. Zhang, S. Ramakrishna, M. Yu, J.-W. Ma, Y.-Z. Long, In situ assembly of well-dispersed Ag nanoparticles throughout electrospun alginate nanofibers for monitoring human breath—smart fabrics, ACS Appl. Mater. Interfaces 10 (2018) 19863—19870, https://doi.org/10.1021/acsami.8b01718.

[67] S. Ma, T. Ye, T. Zhang, Z. Wang, K. Li, M. Chen, J. Zhang, Z. Wang, S. Ramakrishna, L. Wei, Highly oriented electrospun P(VDF-TrFE) fibers via mechanical stretching for wearable motion sensing, Adv. Mater. Technol. 3 (2018) 1800033, https://doi.org/10.1002/admt.201800033.

[68] R. Ghosh, K.Y. Pin, V.S. Reddy, W.A.D.M. Jayathilaka, D. Ji, W. Serrano-García, S.K. Bhargava, S. Ramakrishna, A. Chinnappan, Micro/nanofiber-based noninvasive devices for health monitoring diagnosis and rehabilitation, Appl. Phys. Rev. 7 (2020) 041309, https://doi.org/10.1063/5.0010766.

[69] K. Zhang, X. Wang, D. Jing, Y. Yang, M. Zhu, Bionic electrospun ultrafine fibrous poly(L-lactic acid) scaffolds with a multi-scale structure, Biomed. Mater. 4 (2009) 035004, https://doi.org/10.1088/1748-6041/4/3/035004.
[70] R.M. Rothschild, Neuroengineering tools/applications for bidirectional interfaces, brain—computer interfaces, and neuroprosthetic implants — a review of recent progress, Front. Neuroeng. 3 (2010) 112, https://doi.org/10.3389/fneng.2010.00112.
[71] S.M. Dirk, K.N. Cicotte, E.L. Hedberg-Dirk, S. Buerger, P.P. Lin, G. Reece, Conductive electrospun and micro-Stereolithographically produced porous scaffolds as potential neural interface materials, MRS Proc. 1418 (2012), https://doi.org/10.1557/opl.2012.102 mrsf11-1418-mm05-05.
[72] S. Reddy, Q. Xiao, H. Liu, C. Li, S. Chen, C. Wang, K. Chiu, N. Chen, Y. Tu, S. Ramakrishna, L. He, Bionanotube/Poly(3,4-ethylenedioxythiophene) nanohybrid as an electrode for the neural interface and dopamine sensor, ACS Appl. Mater. Interfaces 11 (2019) 18254—18267, https://doi.org/10.1021/acsami.9b04862.
[73] N. Chen, B. Luo, A.C. Patil, J. Wang, G.G.L. Gammad, Z. Yi, X. Liu, S.-C. Yen, S. Ramakrishna, N.V. Thakor, Nanotunnels within poly(3,4-ethylenedioxythiophene)-carbon nanotube composite for highly sensitive neural interfacing, ACS Nano 14 (2020) 8059—8073, https://doi.org/10.1021/acsnano.0c00672.
[74] S. Politi, F. Carotenuto, A. Rinaldi, P. Di Nardo, V. Manzari, M.C. Albertini, R. Araneo, S. Ramakrishna, L. Teodori, Smart ECM-based electrospun biomaterials for skeletal muscle regeneration, Nanomaterials 10 (2020) 1781, https://doi.org/10.3390/nano10091781.
[75] E. Soliman, F. Bianchi, J.N. Sleigh, J.H. George, M.Z. Cader, Z. Cui, H. Ye, Aligned electrospun fibers for neural patterning, Biotechnol. Lett. 40 (2018) 601—607, https://doi.org/10.1007/s10529-017-2494-z.
[76] N. Ghane, S. Khalili, S. Nouri Khorasani, R. Esmaeely Neisiany, O. Das, S. Ramakrishna, Regeneration of the peripheral nerve via multifunctional electrospun scaffolds, J. Biomed. Mater. Res. 109A (n.d.) 437—452. https://doi.org/10.1002/jbm.a.37092.
[77] R. Zhu, Z. Sun, C. Li, S. Ramakrishna, K. Chiu, L. He, Electrical stimulation affects neural stem cell fate and function in vitro, Exp. Neurol. 319 (2019) 112963, https://doi.org/10.1016/j.expneurol.2019.112963.
[78] H. Liu, X. Xu, Y. Tu, K. Chen, L. Song, J. Zhai, S. Chen, L. Rong, L. Zhou, W. Wu, K.-F. So, S. Ramakrishna, L. He, Engineering microenvironment for endogenous neural regeneration after spinal cord injury by reassembling extracellular matrix, ACS Appl. Mater. Interfaces 12 (2020) 17207—17219, https://doi.org/10.1021/acsami.9b19638.

PART FOUR

Laboratory to clinical translational aspects in electrospinning and electrospraying

CHAPTER FOURTEEN

Electrospinning and electrospraying instrumentation: critical insights, practical considerations and commercial landscape

Ellen Byrne
Business Development at Spraybase (Biofabrication Division of Avectas), MaynoothWorks, Maynooth, Co. Kildare, Ireland

Abbreviations

MEW Melt electrowriting
MSDS Material safety data sheet
PCL Polycaprolactone
PPE Personal protective equipment
PVP Polyvinyl pyrrolidone

14.1 Introduction

The versatile nature of electrospinning and electrospraying has led to an increased popularity of the technologies in recent years, a portion of which can be attributed to significant, ever-evolving improvements that have been made to the equipment and apparatus design [1,2]. The hardware is low cost and simplistic, which allows a basic hardware setup to be applied for both electrohydrodynamic processes, the main differentiation between the technologies instead relies considerably on the solution properties and composition. As the number of commercial providers increase, the fundamental setup of both technologies remains the same; a needle/emitter connected to a reservoir, i.e., syringe containing the desired solution, a method of fluidic control, i.e., syringe pump, a power supply, and a grounded collector [3,4]. The flexible nature of the technologies encourages involvement from end users spanning a wide range of backgrounds and experiences and contributes to the growth of the literature concerning the area of both electrospinning and electrospraying. Most critically, the popular

Biomedical Applications of Electrospinning and Electrospraying
ISBN: 978-0-12-822476-2
https://doi.org/10.1016/B978-0-12-822476-2.00012-1

techniques have also garnered the interest of researchers within the biomedical space, due to the ability of the fibrous scaffold to act as a temporary, functional environment for cells in tissue engineering and regenerative medicine applications, as encapsulation of poorly soluble therapeutic drugs for sustained delivery applications, as carriers for enzymes and other reactants for biocatalysis or biosensing applications, and beyond [5]. The principles of which are widely applied to a number of applications including but not limited to vascular, bone, and skin grafts [6–8]. This chapter will examine the practical preparation steps required for employing these technologies within a laboratory environment. The apparatus design, including the various components and the impact that they have on the end product output, will be reviewed in detail. The final perspective will examine the competitive landscape and availability of lab scale equipment.

14.2 Preparatory considerations for setting up a lab unit

14.2.1 Facilities and utilities requirements

There are several forethoughts necessary in advance of using or purchasing electrospinning or electrospraying equipment, regardless if the end user opts for a commercial or homemade system. The first of which is the available facilities and most importantly adequate bench space. The setup and installation of a lab scale instrument is often a straightforward operation due to the compact nature of the device. In most cases the term "lab scale" is intended to describe a bench top unit; often interchangeable or recognized as Entry Level, Research, Basic, Starter, or Bench Top. However, in some instances "lab scale" may also incorporate an integrated fume hood. Consideration must be adhered to with respect to equipment dimensions. For example, two commercial providers who market their products as "lab scale" vary immensely in footprint, dimensions provided on their respective websites are as follows: Product 1: 1050 mm × 960 mm × 890 mm, whereas Product 2: 560 mm × 520 mm × 500 mm. Product 1 is almost double the size; therefore, in the research of the different offerings, reviewing the footprint in line with the space available to host the equipment is essential. Additional space may also be required for the clearance of cables and wires and to allow ventilation around the hardware. It is also advisable to have a separate materials preparation area to minimize the likelihood of liquid spills damaging the equipment. Consideration must be given to the exact location of the equipment within the lab environment and its proximity to other equipment and facilities that will be used during the experimental process such as chemical storage and waste, such as a flammable cabinet which may be essential to host the toxic or flammable solvents. If a fume hood is required to host the apparatus, review if an existing hood can be repurposed for the equipment or alternatively that a new fume hood entirely is required and the space is available in the lab to accommodate the equipment. The fume hood size must be relative to the equipment that it will hold. Ref. [9] have recommended a fume hood interior should be at least twice the size of the equipment to host and its ancillary components.

Access to utilities is a crucial factor to operate the equipment. Mains power supply and most likely, in the case of electrospraying, a compressed air source is necessary to operate the equipment. In practical terms, the geographic origin of the equipment and its intended location of use must be considered. Also ensure the electrical input, i.e., voltage, frequency, current, and amperage, is appropriate for local use, i.e., 110VAC for USA and 240VAC for EU. Furthermore, the preparation for the installation of the hardware should take into account the availability of access points or plugs to run the equipment and the various supporting components, i.e., multiple power supplies will each require an individual power source. A compressed air supply line (air or N_2) is in most cases offered as standard across academic and industry labs, although this is suitable for use, it is recommended to attach a regulator to the airline to avoid damage to the electrospinning or electrospraying equipment. Should this resource not be available within the working space, cylinders of compressed air are also acceptable, again ensuring they are connected to a regulator and comply with the local safety directives.

As the commercial equipment designs continue to evolve and become more sophisticated, they often include a PC Software Interface which may be incorporated or independent and as a result require the use of a laptop or computer. It is important to ensure the operating system and specification of the device is compatible with the software supplied by the hardware provider and further to this that the correct serial port and associated cables are available. Technical specifications supplied with the equipment of choice will clarify this.

The final consideration for the practical preparation is the availability and access to personal protective equipment to reduce the danger of exposure to solvents or harmful materials, or potential injury from an electric shock. Industry recommendations include protective footwear, a grounding mat, and grounding wrist band to minimize any impact of a stray electrical discharge. However, the likelihood of injury is highly dependent on the competence of the end user and safety standard of the equipment. With respect to standard lab practices and additional protection from harmful solvents, goggles, a lab coat, and gloves which are of an appropriate resistance and quality standard are recommended. It is advised to consult locally with the institution or facility regarding any specific health and safety guidelines in place for additional protective measures.

14.2.2 Health and safety aspects

Electrospinning and electrospraying attracts the attention of multiple safety perspectives given that high voltage is applied in the presence of flammable solvents along with other electrical, fluidic, and potentially laser and optical considerations that must be adhered to. Safety directives within Europe have been established and revised on multiple occasions to govern this process and most recently updated in 2015 [10,11]. It is advisable to complete a risk assessment and seek approval, if applicable locally, prior to engaging in any experimental activity. Evaluation of all potential hazards, the level of risk, and preventive controls must be noted. A selection of potential risks related to electrospinning and electrospraying has been identified in Table 14.1. When transitioning from electrospraying to electrospinning, solvent selection is pivotal and, furthermore, the solution concentration [12]. To this effect a material safety data sheet (MSDS) is supplied for each solvent and polymer that will be used. The details captured within this MSDS will advise the correct handling, storage, transport, and disposal details. Further to this the safe storage of potentially dangerous materials is also a requirement. Access to a flammable cabinet is necessary in the instance flammable solvents are used in the experimental process, or alternatively toxic solvents are stored in a well-ventilated cabinet. A competent individual must have the adequate skill set to deal with hazards deftly and efficiently, such as spills and the correct waste management in the event an incident arises.

14.2.3 Environmental factors

Electrospinning and electrospraying are reliant on a combination of parameters, they are frequently grouped into the following categories [5,13]:

- Polymer solutions properties, both rheological and chemical
- Processing conditions, which are generally influenced by the hardware, e.g., voltage and flow rate
- Environmental or ambient parameters such as temperature and humidity

Table 14.1 Sample of potential risks from electrospinning and electrospraying.

Potential risk	Level of risk	Mitigation action
Use of compressed air supply—risk of explosion, leak, etc.	High	Do not exceed the prescribed maximum input pressure as designated by the vendor.
Use of high voltage—overload, short circuit, arcing; resulting in fire or electrocution	High	Advise the end user that there is no serviceable parts, do not manipulate or interfere with internal components. Use all safety mitigation features, e.g., safety covers.
Use of harmful solvents (see hazard symbols)—flammable, explosive, toxic, harmful/irritant, corrosive	High	Wear appropriate recommended personal protective equipment. Complete MSDS and ensure end user is familiar with the potential hazards of each material.
Sharps injury from needles	Medium	Do not manually blunt surgical needles, invest in needles which are already blunt and fit for purpose to avoid injury.
Mechanical injury from the syringe pump	Low	Consider using third-party software to control syringe pump movement mechanisms. Be conscious and aware of moving parts.
Moving/installing the equipment	Low	Manual handling approach for safe lifting. Get assistance if applicable.

An important criterion to help determine commercial viability, principally within the biomedical field, is ensuring the fibers or particles are generated with reproducible characteristics. However, as noted there are several interdependent variables that influence reproducibility, each material specific. With respect to preparation, temperature and humidity can have a major impact on reproducibility, depending on the location of the equipment in a laboratory setting. Experimental work is conducted at the ambient temperature and humidity; therefore, it is suggested to place the device in a well-ventilated space and not in direct sunlight. Both temperature and humidity are highly variable factors and contingent on time of day, time of year, and geographic location. There is little investigation into the use of ambient parameters compared to the other two categories, typically due to the additional instrumentation required. An elevated temperature can accelerate the solvent evaporation during the electrospinning or electrospraying process, having detrimental effects on the fiber or the particle formation, on the contrary an increase in relative humidity results in a decreased evaporation, highlighting that even a small variation can cause significant change to the structures formed [13,14]. Due to the volatile influence of both temperature and humidity, it is recommended to consider the addition of a climatic controlled chamber to the equipment setup. This will establish a more consistent environment to generate reproducible fibers and particles. As demonstrated in Fig. 14.1, temperatures tested for each electrosprayed polymer were at 20, 30, and 40°C; with humidity altered at each temperature time point at 30%, 40%, and 50% humidity. The surface morphology is shown to be altered from indented to smooth, through the presence of increased humidity at all three temperature sets. Alternatively, if this is not possible due to budget limitations or lack of justification with respect to the materials choice, it is advised to monitor and record the ambient parameters via a digital thermometer and hygrometer.

The SEM micrographs reported in Fig. 14.1 are an example to illustrate the impact of temperature and humidity on particle size, morphology, and polydispersity of particles generated from the electrospray of PVP (polyvinylpyrrolidone) dissolved in ethanol. Without delving too deep into the interplay of a specific solvent system with temperature and humidity which is not the scope of this chapter, it is possible to notice how the secondary morphology of the particles changes from indented spheres to smooth spheres as the humidity increases.

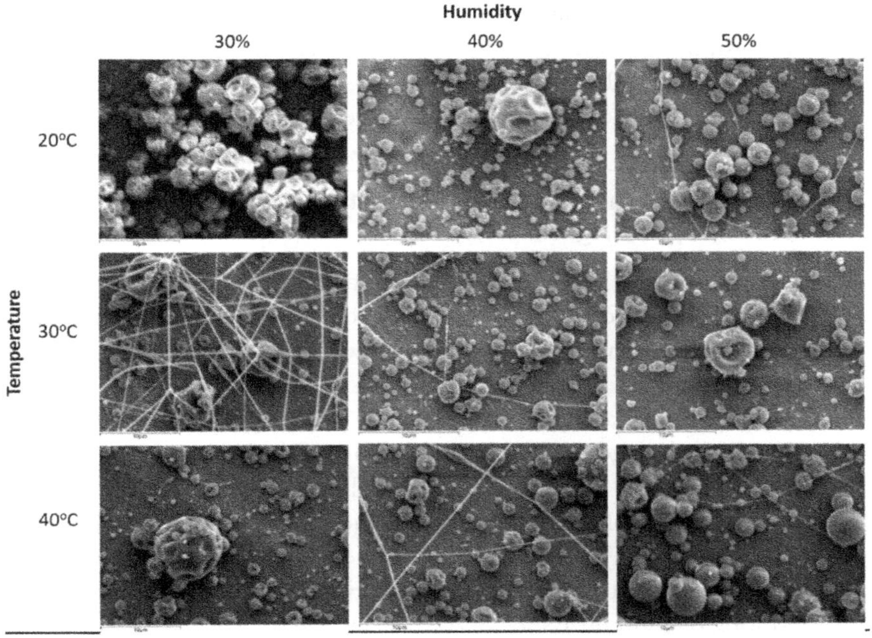

Figure 14.1 SEM images of Electrosprayed Particles of PVP in EtOH within a climate control chamber at temperature sets 20, 30, and 40°C with humidity at each temperature set tested at 30%, 40%, and 50% respectively.

14.2.4 The end user competency

Although electrospinning and electrospraying are recognized as well-established techniques, it is evident that there are a compelling number of interplaying factors which require a strong technical competence. This is even more so critical whereby the end user intends to build a homemade system. Notwithstanding this, not all end users may possess the expertise to do so; therefore, the global availability of "plug and play" commercial systems alleviates the requirement of building a homemade system for those who do not have the skill set or interest in doing so. This can be directly influenced by the timeline available to the end user, often pending submissions deadlines of research grants and dissertations do not allow the time for designing and building a homemade system. Challenges are not limited to one's expertise but also reliant on multiple suppliers with respect to lead times and stock availability. An appreciation for the technology and the chosen materials and awareness of the potential associated risks are also necessary. An understanding of the materials is recommended for a straightforward and successful experimental process, making a materials science or polymer chemistry background extremely beneficial.

14.3 Hardware for typical electrospinning and electrospraying

With respect to vertical vs horizontal design considerations, there are favorable arguments for each arrangement for both vertical and horizontal experimental setups, however they are not without their challenges. A primary disadvantage of a vertical setup is large droplets falling on to the substrate or collector as a result of an unstable or unoptimized experimental setup causing damage to the sample [15]. If a horizontal or reverse (bottom-up) design is chosen, this in turn allows only the smaller particles to deposit on the collector as the larger heavier droplets are eliminated due to gravity [15]. A further design consideration is the build materials choice, all components must tolerate the harsh conditions of toxic solvents. Furthermore, one should avoid conductive surfaces so materials are primarily attracted to collector.

Electrospinning and electrospraying equipment share the same essential features; a high-voltage power supply, a vessel to hold the solution, i.e., syringe, a syringe pump to control the flow, and a grounded collector [3,4]. As previously noted there are three main categories of parameters, polymer, processing, and environmental, which influence the desired dimensions and morphology of the structures. In this section, the processing parameters will be reviewed with respect to the hardware components and demonstrated in Fig. 14.2.

14.3.1 High-voltage power supply

It has been concluded that applied voltage is one of the most compelling factors influencing fiber or particle morphology [16,17]. It is also one of the main determining factors for generating either fibers or particles (Fig. 14.3). When using a lower applied voltage, the surface tension of the solution is not overcome, resulting in a spray of droplets, the output of successful electrospraying, or the anthesis, the by-product of the process, beads. As the voltage increases, the surface tension and viscoelastic forces allow the formation of stable charged jet which results in fibers, i.e., electrospinning [18]. There are many high-voltage power supplies available on the

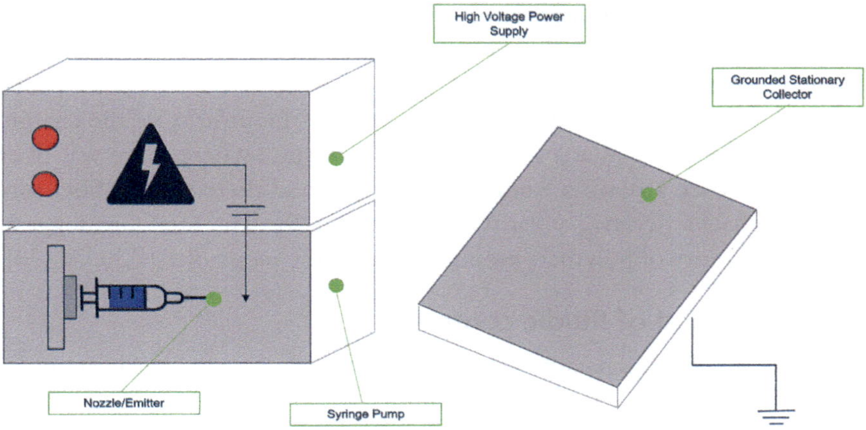

Figure 14.2 Schematic illustration of electrospinning setup. The key components of a typical setup include a polymer solution–loaded syringe with a blunt-ended needle, a syringe pump, a high-voltage power supply connected to the needle, and a grounded metallic collector.

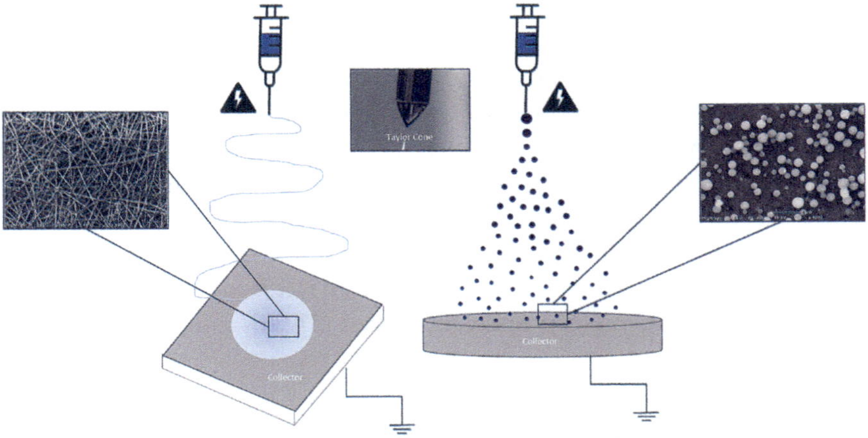

Figure 14.3 Schematic illustration of fibers and particles generated from, respectively, electrospinning and electrospraying, common feature of Taylor cone highlighted at emitter tip.

market with a portion designed specifically with electrospinning and electrospraying in mind. Not only is the voltage range important but also the polarity of the terminals (positive or negative) and connections employed with it. For example, a homemade system may use a power supply with a range of up to +60 kV with crocodile connection clips which is inefficient in comparison to a commercial power supply purposefully designed with a gold-push pin connection. The former may require higher voltages to compensate for loss of power during the process. However, the processability of the material/solution is also influenced by the polarity of the charge. Tong and colleague Wang discuss specific examples where there was fiber formation when a positive voltage was applied and there was no fiber formation when a negative polarity was applied [19]. The literature suggests that the majority of polymers produce fibers in the range of 10–30 kV [20].

14.3.2 Method of fluidic control

An additional process parameter that is determined using the hardware is the flow rate or feed rate whereby a minimum feed solution is required to obtain fibers [21]. This has a direct influence on the size, shape, and porosity of the fibers [1]. The traditional method to control the flow rate in electrospinning is a syringe pump, a device which is often automated and controlled by third-party software provider such as Syringe Pump Pro (https://syringepumppro.com/). Although a syringe pump is also suitable for generating particles, its peristaltic nature often lends itself to variable particle distribution, the result of which can be beading. When the feed rate is not constant and the fiber generation does not occur, the defects that arise as a result are commonly recognized as beading (Fig. 14.4). This is generally not observed when using a pneumatically driven fluid system due to the continuous feed flow and superior control over the flow rate. The importance of controlling the feed rate is recognized in the jet velocity and transfer rate of the solution which in turn impacts the ability of the solvent to evaporate, if this balance is not achieved and the feed rate is too low, it will inhibit the electrospinning or electrospraying process [21,22]. If the feed rate is too

(a) (b) (c)

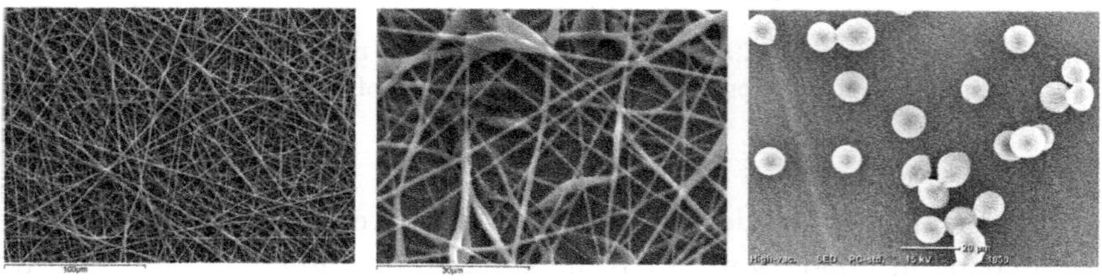

Figure 14.4 (L–R) Fibers, Beading. Particles (PCL). (L–R) (a) fibers—a good example of fiber formation using a syringe pump. (b) Beading—result of a lack of accurate fluidic control, (c) particles—a good example of particles generated using a pressure over fluid method of fluidic control. All samples are PCL.

high, a Taylor cone will be unable to form and the impact of this is having dripping of the solvent on to the collector, which will damage the sample collected prior to the dripping. An alternative less common method is needle-free electrospinning whereby fibers are generated directly from on open liquid surface such as a water bath [23]. This method has demonstrated positive indications toward the scaling and mass production of fibers due the multiple jets formed during the process [24].

14.3.3 Syringes and spinnerets

The vessel containing the polymer solution, i.e., syringe component, is attached either directly or with a tube feed to a nozzle, which is flat ended or blunt and often interchangeable for the emitter, needle, or spinneret [15]. A single nozzle configuration is the most common [1]. High-quality connections minimize dead volume and ensure the material is easily transferred from the syringe source to the targeted collector. The gauge size of the emitter and internal diameter of the tubing directly influence the morphology of the end structure. Materials that possess a higher viscosity and are intended to fabricate fibers require a larger internal diameter tubing and lower emitter gauge (e.g., 12–18 gauge) to successfully create fibers. Axlarger gauge emitter (e.g., 22–30 gauge) and smaller internal diameter tubing are most suitable for generating particles from materials with a lower viscosity. The primary function of the tubing is to regulate flow rate and is chosen based on the viscosity of the materials. Variations of the emitter include coaxial arrangements which use two concentric needles with different diameters, two materials or polymers (either the same or different) are then fed into the emitter and a compound droplet is formed followed by a compound jet used in the formation of nanocomposite particles or fibers [5,15,25]. Modifications of this include a hollow core and up to three or four concentric layers identified as triaxial and tetraxial, respectively. The material that is most often used for the emitters is stainless steel as it is a relatively good conductor. The emitter is supported by a Z-axis, which can be interpreted as a retort stand. This simple yet important component is critical for controlling the emitter to collector distance and dictating the whipping time for the jet, i.e., deposition time and the evaporation rate. A greater distance increases the opportunity for solvent to evaporate and decreases the fiber wetness [26–28]. On the other hand, an increased emitter to collector distance can potentially cause fiber splitting due to prolonged exposure to the electric field [29]. Ref. [1] have speculated that the emitter to collector distance is one of the contributing factors that distinguishes electrospinning from electrospraying. Electrospinning requires a larger separation distance typically in the range of 10–20 cm [20], this distance allows the fiber to stretch thin and enter in to the "whipping" phase which allows the solvents to evaporate. Electrospraying has a much smaller separation distance from emitter to collector, generally in the range of 2–6 cm, as the jet escapes its accelerates toward the collector allowing the solvent to evaporate as the droplet repeatedly splits in to atomized particles as they dry.

14.3.4 Collectors

Collectors for electrospinning and electrospraying can vary massively with respect to sophistication, functionality, and complexity which directly influence the morphological features and architecture of the end product. For example, random deposition of fibers is achieved using a flat plate collector, while aligned fiber deposition can be obtained using a parallel plate collector, as shown in (Fig. 14.5). Commercially the most common collectors are stationary or a rotating drum; however, there are many variations of both which vary in the size of the collector, the yield of end product, the fiber orientation, and the particle deposition [1] (Fig. 14.6, Table 14.2). In order to increase the potential difference, the end user preference may charge the collector with a negative or positive voltage, which can be the case in relation to homemade systems where the connections are weaker. On one end of the scale a sheet of aluminum foil will suffice, more advanced collectors can include additional control over fiber diameter by implementing the use

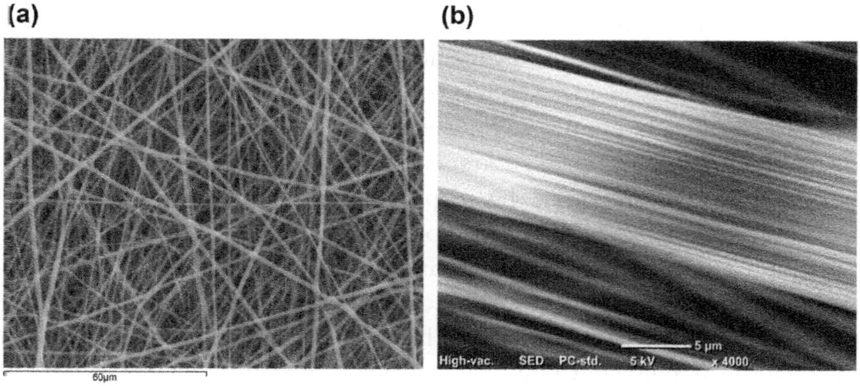

Figure 14.5 Possible geometries of fibers generated from electrospinning using the (a) flat plate—random (b) parallel plates—aligned.

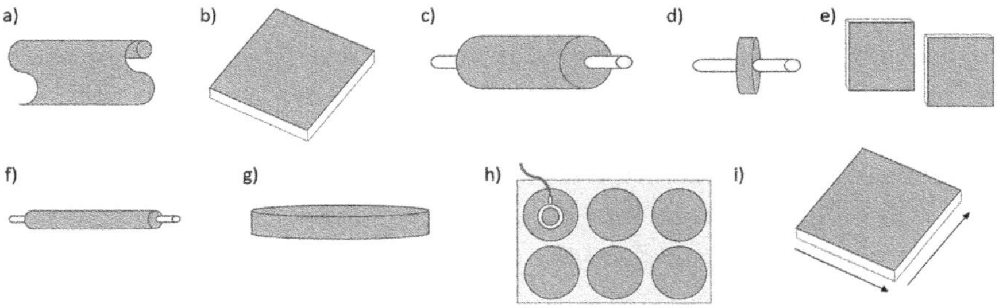

Figure 14.6 Schematics representing the various collectors for generating different geometries - a) Aluminum Foil, b) Flat Metallic Plate Stationary, c) Rotating Drum, d) Disk Collector, e) Parallel Plates, f) Rotating Mandrel, g) Dish Collector, h) Ring Electrode, i) Moving Stage.

Table 14.2 Types of collectors.

	Collector	Fiber orientation/ Particle distribution	Electrospinning	Electrospraying
(a)	Aluminum oil	Random/non-woven	✔	✔
(b)	Flat metallic plate	Random/non-woven	✔	✔
(c)	Rotating drum	Aligned	✔	
(d)	Disk collector	Aligned	✔	
(e)	Parallel plates	Aligned	✔	
(f)	Rotating mandrel	Tubular (random)	✔	
(g)	Dish collector	Monolayer		✔
(h)	Ring electrode	Monolayer		✔
(i)	Moving stage	Controlled/pattern	✔	✔

of rotational and translational speed [25,28]. An advantage of having the option of various collector options which are easily interchangeable is allowing multiple projects to coexist simultaneously without any major interference to your setup. The most common type of collectors are summarized in Table 14.2.

14.3.5 Ancillary components

In homemade systems, the most common electrical connector item identified is crocodile clips (or alligator wire) which lack efficiency and are also a cause for concern with respect to safety. Crocodile clips generally encourage the end user to operate at higher applied voltage than what would be necessary in a commercial system. Furthermore, there is a potential risk to short circuit if the clip contacts two terminals at the same time.

Furthermore, there are a number of ancillary components which can enhance the electrospinning or electrospraying process, an exhaust hood if a fume hood is not available, a camera to record the process in real time, a laptop or computer if needed to run third-party software, and finally an air compressor. Not all of these products are essential for the experiments and will only need to be introduced depending on specific circumstances the equipment being used and the competency level of the end user.

14.4 Modified versions of electrospinning and electrospraying setups

14.4.1 Melt electrowriting setup

Melt electrowriting (MEW) is described by Ref. [30] as "a high-resolution AM method with the capability to produce fibers in the micro- and nanometer range." The electrohydrodynamic process has increasingly gained momentum in recent years, evident through the large number of journal articles, a surge which has been attributed to the controllable diameters and excellent uniformity that can be more challenging for solution electrospinning to achieve. In MEW, the electric potential difference is applied to a polymer melt rather than to a polymer solution. Solution and melt electrospinning share many of the same basic components including high voltage, a nozzle, and collector area. However, there are several distinct characteristics dividing the two methods which relate to fiber formation, compatible materials, and drug loading [31]. MEW is often referred to as a "green technology" due to the lack of toxic solvents required; furthermore, the temperamental nature of solution electrospinning favors the MEW process as a suitable superior alternative to standard electrospinning for applications in the biomedical and tissue engineering domain. Not requiring solvent is a significant advantage when generating implantable scaffolds for biomedical applications as there is no risk of residual solvent. MEW is employed to generate reproducible 3D scaffolds with a defined structure, examples are depicted in Fig. 14.7. The scaffolds are designed to replicate the desirable features of the extracellular matrix to enhance both cell growth and function, successful applications include cardiac tissue, skeletal muscle, and skin [32–35]. Despite a large portion of MEW research originating in academic groups from homemade melt electrospinning systems, this is a more complex route for end users to pursue. Moreover, the

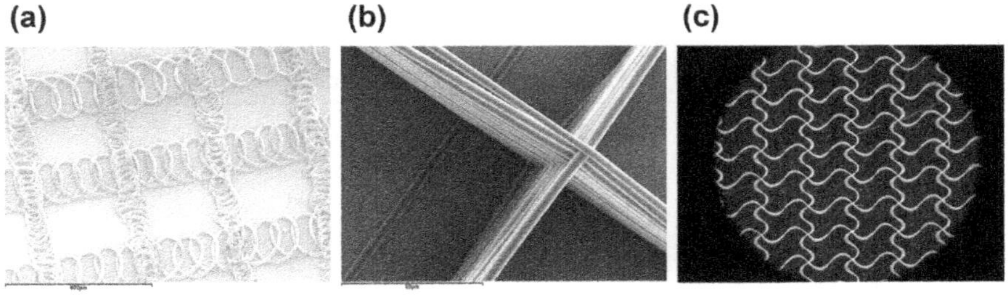

Figure 14.7 Various melt electrospinning scaffolds, (a) slow speed—curly fibers, (b) layers of junction, (c) auxetic scaffold.

availability of commercial systems is increasing with up to as many as six different companies globally offering both dedicated and modular MEW options [36].

14.4.2 Near-field electrospinning setup

As the name suggests, the primary differences between low-voltage near-field electrospinning approach and solution electrospinning is the emitter to collector distance which can be as low as 8 mm in comparison to 10–20 cm and the working voltage which is generally less than 3 kV in comparison to 10–30 kV [20]. Although this approach is not as popular, it does cite multiple novel functional advantages over standard electrospinning including the ability to print [37] or deposit living bacteria and to create single fiber suspensions [38]. An in-depth dive into near-field electrospinning transcends the aim of this chapter but the research advances; future prospects and insight on process parameters concerning this emerging technology were discussed in a recent review by He and colleagues [39].

14.4.3 Combinatorial setups

Due to the shared commonalities in hardware for both electrospinning and electrospraying, many commercial providers offer modular equipment capable of producing both fibers and particles with minimal change to the setup (Table 14.3). Differentiations can occur with respect to the collectors, emitter, and tubing dimensions and method of fluidic control. Although many of the items are interchangeable between the technologies and are generally application dependent, the solution parameters will far outweigh that of the hardware.

In recent years, combinatorial setups which previously focused on 3D printing or bioprinting are now also offering the option of electrospinning

Table 14.3 Commercial providers of lab scale equipment.

Company/Website	Country	Electrospinning lab scale	Electrospraying lab scale
Contipro/4SPIN https://www.4spin.info/	Czech Republic	✔	
ElMarco https://www.elmarco.com/	Czech Republic	✔	
Epsin NanoTech https://www.espinnanotech.com/	India	✔	
FNM Co. http://en.fnm.ir/	Iran	✔	
Genvolt https://www.genvolt.com/en-IE	India	✔	
Holmarc https://www.holmarc.com/	India	✔	
IME Medical Electrospinning https://www.ime-electrospinning.com/	Netherlands	✔	
Inocure https://inocure.cz/	Czech Republic	✔	
Inovenso https://www.inovenso.com/	Turkey	✔	
Kato Tech https://english.keskato.co.jp/	Japan	✔	
Linarai Nanotech https://www.linarinanotech.com/	Italy	✔	
MECC Co. Ltd. https://www.mecc-nano.com/technology01.html	Japan	✔	
MTI Corp. https://www.mtixtl.com/	USA	✔	
Nadetech Innovations https://nadetech.com/	Spain	✔	
NanoNC http://nanonc.co.kr/wordpress/	Korea	✔	✔
NovaSpider http://novaspider.com/	Spain	✔	
Physics Equipment http://www.phyeqpt.in/	India	✔	
Progene Link Sdn Bhd https://www.progenelink.com/	Malaysia	✔	
SKE Research Equipment https://www.ske.it/	Italy	✔	
Spinbox https://www.spinboxsystems.com/	Spain	✔	✔
Spinbow http://www.spinbow.it/	Italy	✔	

Table 14.3 Commercial providers of lab scale equipment.—cont'd

Company/Website	Country	Electrospinning lab scale	Electrospraying lab scale
Spraybase https://www.spraybase.com/	Ireland	✔	✔
Tong Li Tech https://www.electro-spinning.com/	China	✔	
Ucalery https://www.electro-spinning.com/	China	✔	
Weistron https://www.weistron.com/electrospinning-tech/	USA/China	✔	
Y Flow http://www.yflow.com/	Spain	✔	✔

or MEW due to their increased popularity and versatile nature. Although this can create a positive impact in creating awareness for the technologies and in turn increase the number of end users, the downside of this may be that there is not a sufficient level of knowledge or support available due to an unfamiliarity of the technology from the supplier.

14.5 Equipment maintenance and troubleshooting

To prolong the life span of the hardware, routine cleaning and maintenance is advised. Accessories such as the tubing and nozzles should be cleaned after every use to avoid blockages or degrading of the component quality and replaced periodically. Remaining items should be cleaned regularly or after each time a new material is processed using the equipment. Many of the supporting accessories are generally autoclavable and dishwasher safe, however please consult to supplier recommendations for the best guidance, as they may offer a service or maintenance contract with the equipment. An often occurrence after a long deposition duration is random fiber deposition on the surfaces close by the collector area. To avoid material build up, it is advised to remove and clean these areas post each experiment, this is even more important if moving parts are involved such a motors or translational sliders. Additional common errors encountered while electrospinning and electrospraying are reviewed in Table 14.4 and images in support of this detail as shown in Fig. 14.8.

Table 14.4 Troubleshooting. Common errors encountered while electrospinning and electrospraying and troubleshooting to solve the issue.

Issue	Potential cause	Suggestions to resolve
Taylor cone is not forming	Voltage has not been turned on. Voltage setting is not appropriate for your sample. Grounding is not connected. Wear and tear in your connections.	Ensure the power supply is connected to the mains power supply. Ensure mains switches are connected and increasing as expected. Ensure grounding is connected. Ensure the equipment is fit for purpose.
High voltage will not increase	Wear and tear in your connections. Safety interlock not engaged.	Ensure the equipment is fit for purpose. If there is safety cover that is interlocked, ensure it is engaged.
No material emerges from the nozzle	Tubing is blocked. Spinneret is blocked. Tubing or spinneret are not connected correctly. There is an air leak in the system (pressure over fluid only).	Remove tubing and ensure it is free from debris, clean as recommended. Remove spinneret and ensure it is free from debris, and clean as recommended. Ensure tubing and spinneret are setup as per company recommendation.
Sample is landing on sites other than the collector	Grounding is not connected. Grounding point of contact is worm, loose, or dirty. The hardware has not been cleaned correctly. Collector area is insulated, and material is no longer attracted. Distance is too large.	Ensure grounding is connected. Remove all stray fiber or particles that have built up on surfaces other than the collector with a damp cloth, ensure equipment is in a clean condition.
Polymer solidifying at the emitter tip	Solvent is too volatile.	Review solution parameters.

Table 14.4 Troubleshooting. Common errors encountered while electrospinning and electrospraying and troubleshooting to solve the issue.—cont'd

Issue	Potential cause	Suggestions to resolve
Dripping of material from the nozzle	The flow rate is too high, too much sample at the nozzle tip. Tubing diameter is too large. Voltage setting is not appropriate for your sample. Emitter to collector distance is too large.	Decrease the flow rate. Decrease the tubing diameter size. Increase the voltage. Decrease the emitter to collector distance.
The jet has multiple streams instead of a single stream	Voltage is too high, Taylor cone has formed multiple jets.	Decrease the voltage to avoid different fiber sizes being deposited.

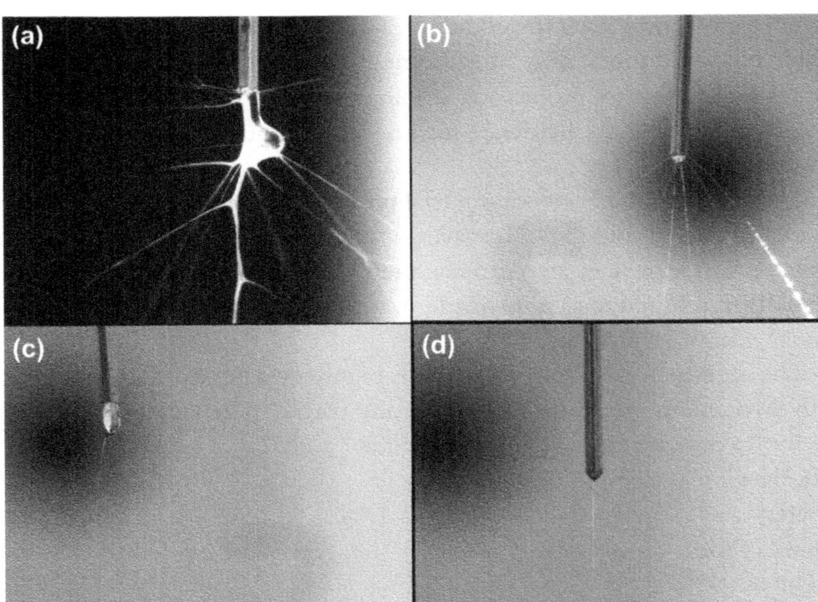

Figure 14.8 L–R, (a) polymer solidifying at the emitter tip, (b) multijet forming from voltage being too high, (c) dripping at the emitter tip, flow rate needs to be reduced, (d) a good example of Taylor cone.

14.6 Competitive landscape

The availability of lab scale setups has expanded in recent years, with a growing interest in the technologies encouraging increased competition among suppliers, with many companies marketing systems dedicated to electrospinning only and others promoting the availability of combination electrospinning and electrospraying systems [40]. The market potential for nanofiber products is expected to grow to $4.3 billion by 2023, with the dominant portion of the lab scale apparatus associated with the academic market [41]. There are dedicated companies who specialize in laboratory and industrial scale hardware and others whose primary focus is the commercialization of electrospun and electrosprayed products [40]. However, there is now a movement toward a "one-stop shop" business model that can capture the end-to-end process, one vendor that can offer both lab scale and industrial scale equipment for the various stages of the research and validation process, further evolving through to GMP facilities for product commercialization. The key considerations sought after by the standard academic customer are generally

- Value for money with the addition of academic discounts
- Flexibility and modularity of equipment with the potential to upgrade or change hardware as projects or funding demands
- Size/footprint of the hardware for ease of installation with limited bench space available

There are a number of commercial providers of lab scale apparatus, they are identified in Table 14.3. However, a large portion of electrospinning and electrospraying devices are manufactured or assembled by the researchers themselves, referred to as homemade systems, although opting for this route is not without its challenges.

The argument of build versus buy is highly evident within the industry, with favorable motions for both opposing parties. The factors which offer the most contradicting viewpoints include

- Budget
- Safety
- Ease of use
- Timelines
- External support
- Literature justification

Although opting to build a system can save money in the short term, further investment will be required to improve the system in time with respect to safety and efficiency. This can be the after-effect of opting for poor quality components, which in turn can be detrimental to the process resulting in inconsistencies or a lack of reproducibility, a common occurrence for homemade systems where production is rarely consistent. Although a commercial system is more costly to begin with and require a larger initial investment, savings will be recognized later when the apparatus allows for reproducible experimental work and minimal waste of precious or expensive materials.

The safety of the equipment is referred to in Section 14.2; however, its importance must not be underestimated explicitly with respect to homemade or self-assembled equipment. It is the expectation that commercial providers' equipment is compliant with national safety regulations, i.e., CE Certification if in Europe. This enforces confidence and trust in the commercial provider that the system is fit for purpose and will not cause harm to the end user if used as specified and the system has not been compromised in any way. It is critical that end users do not interfere with any safety features of the system which may preclude the system from performing as specified. Particular guidance and attention should be adhered to any supporting documentation supplied with a commercial system. The correct use and maintenance of the provided cables and power cords is essential to the appropriate functioning of the system. A homemade system unfortunately cannot offer this type of reassurance; furthermore, homemade systems are often used without any additional protective measures for the safety of the end user, e.g., safety cover with interlock, therefore it is not surprising that there are reported cases of fire damage to labs where homemade systems are involved. Regardless if the system is self-developed or commercial, the simplistic nature of the technology should follow through to the functionality of the equipment. The ability to adjust basic parameters such as voltage and pressure must be present.

Factors such as project deadlines and lack of expertise do not allow for carefully developed and rigorously tested equipment. Reliance on multiple suppliers and their stock levels, access to the compatible components, and lengthy timelines are the primary sources of build delays. Purchasing a commercial system is generally a straightforward process with one contact point who can guide the end user through the full equipment purchase process eliminating the unknown factors. Warranty, although a less critical however an important level of assurance, is generally offered as standard with all commercial kits, this can offer the purchaser peace of mind when budgets are limited and funds are not available for repairs in the early stages. Further to this, external support and guidance, both technical and practical, is available which is not the case for a homemade system. If an end user experiences an issue, the commercial provider will have the expertise to troubleshoot and share solutions much more efficiently in comparison to issues with a homemade system.

Further aids are available in the format of literature justification, Electrospinning and electrospraying companies are willing to share published work, posters, case studies, and blog posts relating to their internal scientific teams and end users if publicly available, as a testament to the functionality and versatility of their equipment. Customer publications can in turn act as a readymade library of application notes for new users across a variety of applications and a collection of different materials and polymers combinations.

14.7 Conclusion and outlook

In conclusion, although electrospinning and electrospraying technologies are widely recognized for their operational simplicity and low-cost nature, they are not without their challenges in the initial establishment and equipment setup stages. There are several practical considerations with respect to facilities and utilities prior to completing any experimental work. This is further supported by the health and safety particulars, environmental factors, and the competency of the end user. The end user preference, in addition to the time and budget available to them, is the most significant determining factor while opting between a commercial system and a homemade system. The global availability of lab scale devices in recent years has contributed significantly to the growth of literature and popularity of the techniques. This is encouraged by the development and advances of the technologies and their prevalence within the biomedical industry, predominantly tissue engineering and regenerative medicine. The potential applications of fibers and particles have been largely demonstrated in the literature and looking forward large-scale production is highly desirable for biomedical applications. However, Ref. [1] have highlighted a number of potential issues relating to scale including "low output per spinneret, clogging of the spinneret tip, inter-jet interface, recovery of vaporized solvents involved in the process, and fiber alignment over a large area." More attention is required in optimizing the hardware and process to achieve a higher yield without blocking the emitter, potential avenues to overcome this issue include a multi needle approach. Lab scale equipment is a definitive starting point for research and development into the potential of nano- and mircoparticles and fibers for biomedical applications. Scale-up and mass production of electrospinning has been demonstrated [24,42]; therefore, the commercial potential exists, however optimization of the process at a lab scale level is a critical step before industrial options can be explored. Furthermore, the applications within the biomedical engineering industry which would have been previously limited to tissue engineering and regenerative medicine have expanded beyond these domains in drug delivery and cell encapsulation in recent years. Looking forward, this is eagerly supported and encouraged through the availability of process development guidance where GMP facilities are available to manufacture clinical and commercial end products.

References

[1] R.S. Bhattarai, R.D. Bachu, S.H.S. Boddu, S. Bhaduri, Biomedical applications of electrospun nanofibers: drug and nanoparticle delivery, Pharmaceutics 11 (1) (2019), https://doi.org/10.3390/pharmaceutics11010005.

[2] A. Haider, S. Haider, I.K. Kang, A comprehensive review summarizing the effect of electrospinning parameters and potential applications of nanofibers in biomedical and biotechnology, Arab. J. Chem. 11 (8) (2018) 1165–1188, https://doi.org/10.1016/j.arabjc.2015.11.015.

[3] S.A. Park, K. Park, H. Yoon, J.G. Son, T. Min, G.H. Kim, Apparatus for preparing electrospun nanofibers: designing an electrospinning process for nanofiber fabrication, Polym. Int. 56 (11) (2007) 1361–1366, https://doi.org/10.1002/pi.2345.

[4] J. Wang, J.A. Jansen, F. Yang, Electrospraying: possibilities and challenges of engineering carriers for biomedical applications - a mini review, Front. Chem. 7 (2019), https://doi.org/10.3389/fchem.2019.00258.

[5] A.P. Kishan, E.M. Cosgriff-Hernandez, Recent advancements in electrospinning design for tissue engineering applications: a review, J. Biomed. Mater. Res. A 105 (10) (2017) 2892–2905, https://doi.org/10.1002/jbm.a.36124.

[6] H. Ahn, Y.M. Ju, H. Takahashi, D.F. Williams, J.J. Yoo, S.J. Lee, T. Okano, A. Atala, Engineered small diameter vascular grafts by combining cell sheet engineering and electrospinning technology, Acta Biomater. 16 (1) (2015) 14–22, https://doi.org/10.1016/j.actbio.2015.01.030.

[7] H. Nie, W.S. Beng, Y.C. Fu, C.H. Wang, Three-dimensional fibrous PLGA/HAp composite scaffold for BMP-2 delivery, Biotechnol. Bioeng. 99 (1) (2008) 223–234, https://doi.org/10.1002/bit.21517.

[8] D. Steffens, M. Lersch, A. Rosa, C. Scher, T. Crestani, M.G. Morais, J.A.V. Costa, P. Pranke, A new biomaterial of nanofibers with the microalga spirulina as scaffolds to cultivate with stem cells for use in tissue engineering, J. Biomed. Nanotechnol. 9 (4) (2013) 710–718, https://doi.org/10.1166/jbn.2013.1571.

[9] R.J. McCarthy, K.P. Giapis, An adaptable device for scalable electrospinning of low- and high-viscosity solutions, Instruments 37 (2019), https://doi.org/10.3390/instruments3030037.

[10] C.J. Luo, S.D. Stoyanov, E. Stride, E. Pelan, M. Edirisinghe, Electrospinning versus fibre production methods: from specifics to technological convergence, Chem. Soc. Rev. 4708 (2012), https://doi.org/10.1039/c2cs35083a.

[11] National Standards Authority of Ireland, Stationary Electrostatic Application Equipment for Ignitable Flock Material - Safety Requirements, 2015. https://infostore.saiglobal.com/en-us/Standards/I-S-EN-50223-2015-859960_SAIG_NSAI_NSAI_2045866/.
[12] C.J. Luo, M. Nangrejo, M. Edirisinghe, A novel method of selecting solvents for polymer electrospinning, Polymer 51 (7) (2010) 1654–1662, https://doi.org/10.1016/j.polymer.2010.01.031.
[13] O. Hardick, B. Stevens, D.G. Bracewell, Nanofibre fabrication in a temperature and humidity controlled environment for improved fibre consistency, J. Mater. Sci. 46 (11) (2011) 3890–3898, https://doi.org/10.1007/s10853-011-5310-5.
[14] G.Z. Yang, H.P. Li, J.H. Yang, J. Wan, D.G. Yu, Influence of working temperature on the formation of electrospun polymer nanofibers, Nanoscale Res. Lett. 12 (1) (2017), https://doi.org/10.1186/s11671-016-1824-8.
[15] A. Jaworek, A.T. Sobczyk, A. Krupa, Electrospray application to powder production and surface coating, J. Aerosol Sci. 125 (2018) 57–92, https://doi.org/10.1016/j.jaerosci.2018.04.006.
[16] O.S. Yördem, M. Papila, Y.Z. Menceloğlu, Effects of electrospinning parameters on polyacrylonitrile nanofiber diameter: an investigation by response surface methodology, Mater. Des. 29 (1) (2008) 34–44, https://doi.org/10.1016/j.matdes.2006.12.013.
[17] M. Ziabari, V. Mottaghitalab, A.K. Haghi, A new approach for optimization of electrospun nanofiber formation process, Kor. J. Chem. Eng. 27 (1) (2010) 340–354, https://doi.org/10.1007/s11814-009-0309-1.
[18] J. Lasprilla-Botero, M. Álvarez-Láinez, J.M. Lagaron, The influence of electrospinning parameters and solvent selection on the morphology and diameter of polyimide nanofibers, Mater. Today Commun. 14 (2018) 1–9, https://doi.org/10.1016/j.mtcomm.2017.12.003.
[19] H.-W. Tong, M. Wang, Electrospinning of fibrous polymer scaffolds using positive voltage or negative voltage: a comparative study, Biomed. Mater. 5 (5) (2010) 054110, https://doi.org/10.1088/1748-6041/5/5/054110.
[20] Z. Jie, L. Yun-Ze, S. Bin, Z. Zhi-Hua, S. Feng, Z. Hong-Di, Z. Zhi-Ming, H. Jia-Yin, Polymer nanofibers prepared by low-voltage near-field electrospinning, Chin. Phys. Soc. IOP Publ. 21 (4) (2012).
[21] N. Okutan, P. Terzi, F. Altay, Affecting parameters on electrospinning process and characterization of electrospun gelatin nanofibers, Food Hydrocolloids 39 (2014) 19–26, https://doi.org/10.1016/j.foodhyd.2013.12.022.
[22] A. Andrady, Science and Technology of Polymer Nanofibers, John Wiley & Sons, Ltd, 2008.
[23] G. Yan, H. Niu, T. Lin, Needle-less electrospinning, in: Electrospinning: Nanofabrication and Applications, Elsevier, 2018, pp. 219–247, https://doi.org/10.1016/B978-0-323-51270-1.00007-8.
[24] L. Wei, R. Sun, C. Liu, J. Xiong, X. Qin, Mass production of nanofibers from needleless electrospinning by a novel annular spinneret, Mater. Des. 179 (2019), https://doi.org/10.1016/j.matdes.2019.107885.
[25] G.R. Mitchell, Electrospinning: Principles, Practice and Possibilities, 2015. https://books.google.ie/books?hl=en&lr=&id=znMoDwAAQBAJ&oi=fnd&pg=PP1&dq=electrospinning+hardware&ots=UdRAE3pyjI&sig=ZpoEYQ_gL3G4j40AiHqa3AgUT5g&redir_esc=y#v=onepage&q=electrospinning hardware&f=false.
[26] C.J. Buchko, L.C. Chen, Y. Shen, D.C. Martin, Processing and microstructural characterization of porous biocompatible protein polymer thin films, Polymer 40 (26) (1999) 7397–7407, https://doi.org/10.1016/S0032-3861(98)00866-0.

[27] J.S. Lee, K.H. Choi, H.D. Ghim, S.S. Kim, D.H. Chun, H.Y. Kim, W.S. Lyoo, Role of molecular weight of atactic poly(vinyl alcohol) (PVA) in the structure and properties of PVA nanofabric prepared by electrospinning, J. Appl. Polym. Sci. 93 (4) (2004) 1638−1646, https://doi.org/10.1002/app.20602.
[28] M. Mirjalili, S. Zohoori, Review for application of electrospinning and electrospun nanofibers technology in textile industry, J. Nanostructure Chem. (2016) 207−213, https://doi.org/10.1007/s40097-016-0189-y.
[29] X.Y. Yuan, Y.Y. Zhang, C. Dong, J. Sheng, Morphology of ultrafine polysulfone fibers prepared by electrospinning, Polym. Int. 53 (11) (2004) 1704−1710, https://doi.org/10.1002/pi.1538.
[30] J.C. Kade, P.D. Dalton, Polymers for melt electrowriting, Adv. Healthc. Mater. (2020) 2001232.
[31] H. Lian, Z. Meng, Melt electrospinning vs. solution electrospinning: a comparative study of drug-loaded poly (ε-caprolactone) fibres, Mater. Sci. Eng. C 74 (2017) 117−123, https://doi.org/10.1016/j.msec.2017.02.024.
[32] B.L. Farrugia, T.D. Brown, Z. Upton, D.W. Hutmacher, P.D. Dalton, T.R. Dargaville, Dermal fibroblast infiltration of poly(ε-caprolactone) scaffolds fabricated by melt electrospinning in a direct writing mode, Biofabrication 5 (2) (2013), https://doi.org/10.1088/1758-5082/5/2/025001.
[33] D. Olvera, M. Sohrabi Molina, G. Hendy, M.G. Monaghan, Electroconductive melt electrowritten patches matching the mechanical anisotropy of human myocardium, Adv. Funct. Mater. (2020), https://doi.org/10.1002/adfm.201909880.
[34] U. Tamer, E. Kny, Electrospun materials for tissue engineering and biomedical applications: research, design and commercialization, in: Electrospun Materials for Tissue Engineering and Biomedical Applications: Research, Design and Commercialization, Elsevier Inc, 2017, pp. 1−428. http://www.sciencedirect.com/science/book/9780081010228.
[35] Y. Zhang, Z. Zhang, Y. Wang, Y. Su, M. Chen, 3D myotube guidance on hierarchically organized anisotropic and conductive fibers for skeletal muscle tissue engineering, Mater. Sci. Eng. C 116 (2020), https://doi.org/10.1016/j.msec.2020.111070.
[36] T.M. Robinson, D.W. Hutmacher, P.D. Dalton, The next frontier in melt electrospinning: taming the jet, Adv. Funct. Mater. 29 (44) (2019), https://doi.org/10.1002/adfm.201904664.
[37] C. Chang, V.H. Tran, J. Wang, Y.-K. Fuh, L. Lin, Direct-write piezoelectric polymeric nanogenerator with high energy conversion efficiency, Nano Lett. 10 (2) (2010) 726−731.
[38] Xia Li, et al., Low-voltage continuous electrospinning patterning, ACS Appl. Mater. Interfaces 8 (47) (2016), https://doi.org/10.1021/acsami.6b07797.
[39] X.-X. He, J. Zheng, G.-F. Yu, M. You, M. Yu, X. Ning, Y.-Z. Long, Near-field electrospinning: progress and applications, J. Phys. Chem. 121 (16) (2017) 8663−8678.
[40] L. Persano, A. Camposeo, C. Tekmen, D. Pisignano, Industrial upscaling of electrospinning and applications of polymer nanofibers: a review, Macromol. Mater. Eng. 298 (5) (2013) 504−520, https://doi.org/10.1002/mame.201200290.
[41] BCC Publishing, Global Nanofiber Market Trends, Applications & Size Report, BCC Publishing, 2019. https://www.bccresearch.com/market-research/nanotechnology/global-markets-and-technologies-for-nanofibers.html.
[42] P. Vass, E. Szabó, A. Domokos, E. Hirsch, D. Galata, B. Farkas, B. Démuth, S.K. Andersen, T. Vigh, G. Verreck, G. Marosi, Z.K. Nagy, Scale-up of electrospinning technology: applications in the pharmaceutical industry, Wiley Interdiscip. Rev. Nanomed. Nanobiotechnol. 12 (4) (2020), https://doi.org/10.1002/wnan.1611.

CHAPTER FIFTEEN

Translational path for electrospun and electrosprayed medical devices from bench to bedside

Hayley L. Morris, Joana A. Martins, Antonina A. Lach, Andrew J. Carr, Pierre–Alexis Mouthuy
Botnar Research Centre, University of Oxford, Oxford, United Kingdom

15.1 Introduction

The development of electrospinning/spun or electrospraying/sprayed (grouped under the acronym "ES" in this chapter) products for biomedical applications can be a daunting prospect even when utilizing well-characterized materials and manufacturing methods. The novelty of ES materials and the small scale of ES fibers and beads—which are often exploited with the intent to induce a specific cell response in tissues and organs—mean that they present significant challenges in their translational journey from bench to bedside. Many promising novel concepts fail to bridge the translational gap between biomedical research and clinical use, thus never benefitting the intended patient population. Numerous challenges are faced at the early stages of the translational pathway, including the need to secure significant funding for translational activities, recruit necessary expertise into the project team, develop scalable and clean manufacturing processes, identify and collect all sufficient preclinical data, document all activities in an evolving regulatory landscape, perform clinical trials (likely required for most implantable ES devices) and obtain regulatory compliance [1–3].

Within this chapter, we aim to explore some salient aspects in the development pathway of ES products designed for medical applications. A broad overview of this pathway is shown in Fig. 15.1. It should be noted that the primary focus of this chapter is on the translation process within the European Union (EU), in which the process of CE marking is the route to market. We will also mainly concentrate on Class III ES medical devices, i.e., those typically intended for implantation. ES products combined with

Biomedical Applications of Electrospinning and Electrospraying
ISBN: 978-0-12-822476-2
https://doi.org/10.1016/B978-0-12-822476-2.00014-5

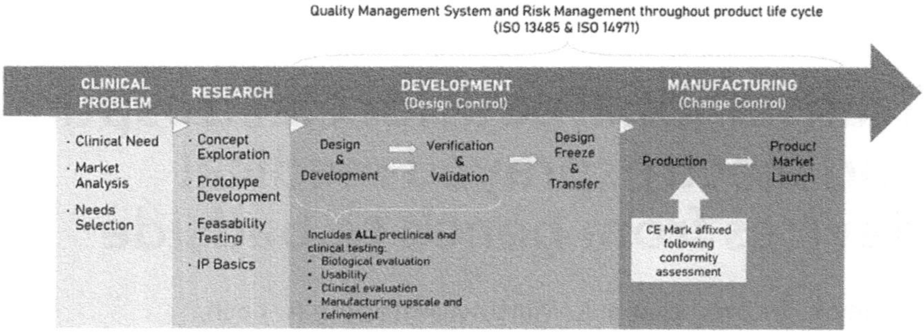

Figure 15.1 Generic translation process in Europe, showing the key activities required to steer a new ES product from bench to bedside via the CE marking route.

drugs and cells are excluded from the scope, although all the topics discussed here are relevant for those strategies. Detailing the entire translational journey of an ES product is not practical within the scope of this chapter. As such, the authors have focused on introducing the current EU medical device regulatory structure and device classifications, followed by summarizing the key activities required to steer the product from a research position through to a saleable CE marked device available to the end user or patient. These activities include design control, risk management, quality control, manufacturing, and upscale. Finally, we will provide examples of ES devices that have undergone or are undergoing clinical trials and that have received approval for commercialization.

15.2 ES device regulation and device classifications

15.2.1 The regulatory framework: ES products as medical devices

The first step in the development of a new ES product is to define which form of regulation the design, function, and intended use of the product falls under. This will set the basis for all ongoing regulatory compliance and commercial strategies. Herein, we will focus on ES devices in the context of biomedical applications, the vast majority of which fall under the category of medical devices.

Medical devices are defined broadly as *"any instrument, apparatus, appliance, software, implant, reagent, material or other article intended by the manufacturer to be used, alone or in combination, for human beings"*. A full definition can be found in Article 2 of the *Medical Devices Regulation* 2017/745 (MDR) [4]. It is worth noting that in order to be considered a medical device, the primary mechanism of action must be purely physical in its operation. Therefore, if a combination device is presented (e.g., combining both a chemically mediated and physically mediated response, such as an electrospun mesh or ES beads loaded with bioactive molecules), a robust justification must be made for the physical nature of the device as the primary actor in the device achieving its intended use. It should also be noted that while informal and nonbinding consultation can be sought from the regulators, it is ultimately the manufacturers who are wholly responsible for the selection and justification of the regulatory qualification of their products.

Regulatory frameworks aim to ensure the safety and efficacy of medical devices and facilitate patients' access to devices in the market. At the time of writing, medical devices within the EU are regulated by three directives:

- Council Directive 90/385/EEC on Active Implantable Medical Devices (AIMDD) (1990)
- Council Directive 93/42/EEC on Medical Devices (MDD) (1993)
- Directive 98/79/EC of the European Parliament and of the Council on in vitro Diagnostic Medical Devices (IVDMD)

However, the European regulation surrounding medical devices is undergoing a significant change and two new regulations were introduced in 2017 to modernize the EU legislative framework with an increased focus on patient safety to provide better protection of public health:

- Regulation (EU) 2017/745 (MDR) of the European Parliament and of the Council of April 5, 2017 on medical devices, amending Directive 2001/83/EC, Regulation (EC) No 178/2002 and Regulation (EC) No 1223/2009 and repealing Council Directives 90/385/EEC and 93/42/EEC.
- Regulation (EU) 2017/746 of the European Parliament and of the Council of April 5, 2017 on in vitro diagnostic medical devices and repealing Directive 98/79/EC and Commission Decision 2010/227/EU.

As a sector experiencing rapid and continuous scientific and technological development, the update of these regulations will work to further guarantee safety and innovation following on from the publication of the previous directives, which date back to the early 1990s. The new regulations (MDR) entered into force on May 25, 2017 and will progressively replace the existing medical device directives (MDD) following a transition period which ends in May 2021 for medical devices and May 2022 for in vitro diagnostic medical devices (IVDs).

There is a common perception when first approaching medical device development that the ultimate goal is to seek regulatory "approval", within the EU framework this is not a fully accurate view of the process. To explain this more clearly, it is necessary to investigate the different actors involved in the CE marking process. Principally, the European Commission (EC) is the executive body of the EU and is accountable to the European Parliament. The EC is responsible for the generation of EU medical device legislation and regulation. Downstream from the EC are the Competent Authorities (CA), each EU member state will have its own CA (e.g., ANSM in France, AIFA in Italy). The CA is responsible for the implementation and enforcement of the legislation. Below the CA for each member state sits the Notified Bodies. These are designated by the CA and hold the responsibility for the conformity assessment of medical devices and manufacturing processes against the regulation. The final category contains the manufacturers and authorized representatives. Ultimately, as mentioned above, it is the manufacturer who is responsible for conforming to the regulation and who declares via a written statement (EC Declaration of Conformity) that the product meets the applicable provisions of the regulation.

15.2.2 Classification of ES medical devices

Once it is clear a new ES product meets the definition of a medical device, the next step is to "classify" the device. While classification can sometimes appear to be an arbitrary process, it has wide ranging implications on the regulatory requirements applied to the product and ultimately the route to market. Classification rules for the MDR can be found in Annex VIII "classification rules". Devices are categorized by risk to the end user (Fig. 15.2). Increased risk is reflected in a higher device classification, and risk is calculated based on the device's duration of contact, level of invasiveness, and location of application in the body. Where more than one classification rule may be applied, the highest risk category is selected. This classification system enables the legally binding medical device

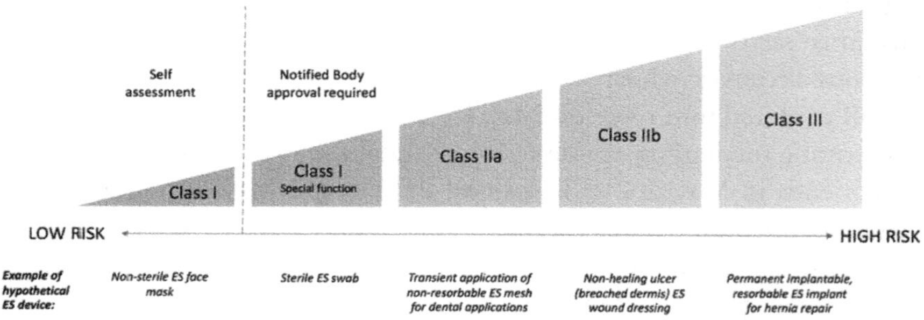

Figure 15.2 Classification of medical devices by risk to the end user.

regulation to apply over a wide range of medical device products from spectacles (Class I) through to deep brain stimulation devices for the treatment of Parkinson's disease (Class III). An example of hypothetical ES device for each category is provided in Fig. 15.2.

In the EU, the conformity assessment procedure will vary with the classification of the device. For Class I devices which are not sterile and do not perform a measuring function, devices can be self-certified by the manufacturer, meaning they are responsible for assessing and certifying that the device is compliant with the relevant regulation. For Class I devices that are sterile or perform a measuring function, these are still largely certified by the manufacturer, however, parts of the technical file relating to sterilization or measurement must be assessed by a Notified Body prior to placing a CE mark on the device.

Any Class II and Class III devices will involve some level of interaction with a Notified Body (NB). For details on the role of Notified Bodies within the structure of the regulatory landscape, the reader is invited to review the EC documentation [5]. The importance of the NB involvement and the level of evidence and control applied to the device increases with increasing classification. On the extreme end, Class III implantable and degradable (absorbable) devices will require a full Notified Body conformity assessment, reviewing the technical documentation and design history of the device, production quality assurance, product verification, product sterility assurance and full review of clinical evaluation. Due to the novelty in processing techniques that ES technologies represent, alongside the likelihood that the polymers utilized are biodegradable (absorbable), most ES medical devices will fall under the Class III umbrella. With this in mind, the following sections cover details of the underpinning activities required to support the development and manufacture of Class III ES devices including design control, technical and regulatory documentation, and quality and risk management.

15.2.3 Note on regulatory processes outside of the EU

The approval process discussed above is relevant to CE marking only. Regions which will only accept CE marked products include 27 EU member states, 4 EFTA countries (Norway/Iceland/Lichtenstein/Switzerland), and Turkey. Other countries are able to accept CE marked products in addition to those approved through other regulatory processes, currently for the MDD. This is orchestrated through mutual recognition agreements and covers territories such as Canada, New Zealand, and Australia. In the

United States, the Centre for Devices and Radiological Health (CDRH) of the United States Food and Drug Administration (USFDA) is responsible for regulating the firms who make, repack, relabel, and/or import medical devices and IVDs, through Federal Food, Drug and Cosmetic Act, particularly following the Code of Federal Regulations (CFR) Title 21, parts 800−1299 [6]. Similar to European Union, the United States classifies the medical devices into Class I, II, and III based on the risk involved, wherein Class II devices require premarket notification 510(k) and Class III devices require premarket approval. In India, a major importer and emerging hub for medical device startups, the medical devices, including IVDs, are regulated through the Medical Device Rules 2017 (gazette notification GSR 78(E), dt. Jan 31, 2017, effective from Jan 01, 2018) as required under the Drugs and Cosmetics Act by the Ministry of Health and Family Welfare, Government of India. The Central Drugs Standard Control Organization (CDCSO) under Directorate General of Health Services is the National Regulatory Authority. Similar to European Union, the CDCSO classifies the medical devices as well as IVDs into Class A, B, C, and D based on the risk involved.

As can be seen from the examples above, similarities and differences exist within the regulation of medical devices throughout the globe, various countries and agencies are involved in a push to streamline the medical device regulations internationally. However, there remain many areas of ambiguity. To this end, a consortium of voluntary medical device regulators from around the world known as the International Medical Device Regulators Forum (IMDRF) (a successor organization of the Global Harmonization Task Force). The IMDRF aims to accelerate international medical device regulatory harmonization and convergence through bringing together regulatory officials and medical device stakeholders from throughout the world. For further information about the regulatory processes outside the European Union, we invite the reader to consult the documentation from the World Health Organization [7] and the IMDRF [8], as well as other existing reviews [9−11].

15.3 Control and development of ES medical devices

15.3.1 Design control

Following on from clarifying the regulatory strategy and classification of the ES medical device, more detailed development activities required to steer the product from research to CE marking can be investigated. Initial activities will be to implement a level of design control, the intent of design control is to accurately document the design and development of the product, covering all aspects ranging from early prototyping and design testing through to establishment of manufacturing and upscale. Design control applies to modifications of existing designs, or changes to processes and becomes crucial once a particular design has been selected as the candidate for translation. Design controls create a transparent and contemporaneous audit trail for future scrutiny by both the CA at the stage of clinical trial submission (if required by the class of the device) and later by a Notified Body for CE marking. It will help to ensure that the new ES device meets the user needs, its intended uses and its targeted clinical requirements.

Fig. 15.3 shows a flow diagram of the application of design control during the design and development of an ES medical device. Design control initiates with an establishment of user needs and the associated regulatory requirements around the proposed device. Having a clear idea of the medical device, what it should do, what problem it will solve and what is required by users, will form the basis of the design and development of the device. User needs are then converted into design inputs. For example, a user need may be identified as "the device must be sterile for implantation and not cause infection". Design inputs falling out from this need may include more specific design criteria based on this need such as "device packaging must maintain sterility for the duration of the shelf life" and "terminal sterilization must be established". The design is then iteratively developed and tested based on the design inputs. This process is termed "verification" and

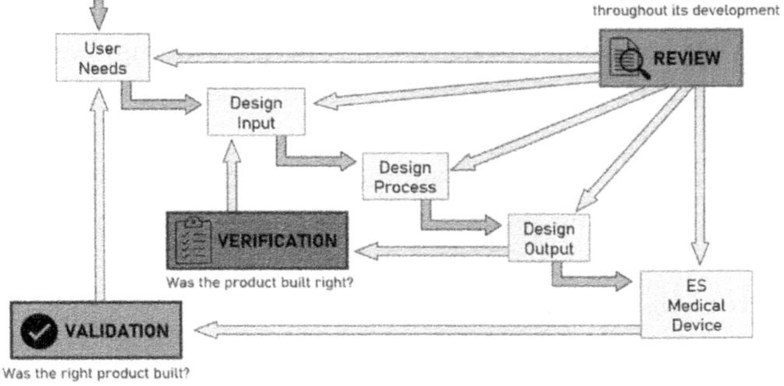

Figure 15.3 The overall design control model applied during the design and development of a medical device. *Adapted from FDA, Design Control Guidance for Medical Device Manufacturers. FDA 21 CFR 820.30 and Sub-clause 4.4 Od ISO 9001, 1997.*

confirms the designed product meets its specifications. Once the design is verified, validation activities can then be performed to confirm the designed device actually meets the clinical and user needs it was designed for.

The following subsections will introduce the technical and regulatory documentation involved in design control as well as the documentation related to risk management and evaluation of biological safety.

15.3.1.1 Technical and regulatory documentation for ES medical devices

For ES medical devices intended to be commercialized in the European Union, the MDR defines requirements for their manufacturing and necessitates the implementation of technical documentation evidencing project activities. This evidence trail must include identification and description of the device, intended use, labeling (with instructions for use), information on the design and manufacture of the device, the risk management file and the verification and validation of the device - proving that it meets the general safety and performance requirements of the MDR. Moreover, the MDR requires appropriate postmarket surveillance planning and implementation, to proactively evaluate the safety of the device longterm. Technical documentation will be reviewed by Notified Bodies—if appropriate for the classification of the device—and may also be the subject of ISO 13485 audits [12]. This is an underpinning standard, guiding manufacturers in the key processes to conform to the requirements of the MDD. Further details on this critical standard can be found in Section 15.3.2.2.

Technical and regulatory documentation is an ongoing process and as the project matures from pure research and development, the project team will begin to require a different structure. Representation will be necessary from different fields involved in device development including technical, quality, clinical, manufacturing, regulatory and commercial interests. At this stage it is often useful to develop a responsibility matrix to define each individual's input on the project. This also aids in the appropriate review and approval of the documentation being produced. Additionally, diversifying the team at this point in development adds critical new perspectives that can inform on all aspects of the design being developed.

As with quality documentation (see later sections), proper procedures for document review, approval and archive should be applied to technical documentation. Collectively this process is termed document control. Following ISO 13485 guidance, key initial documents to be implemented include the following: Design and Development Plan, Design Input Requirements, Biological Evaluation Plan, and Risk Management Plan. At the early stages these documents will be sparsely populated, but as the project and team expand, so will the detail contained within these "live" documents. These ongoing documents can provide critical design information early in the process and reduce expensive and extensive design changes later on [13]. Technical documentation has a high value in capturing iterative studies, tests performed and intellectual property developed. However, it should be noted that applying overly stringent controls to the design too early in the process could lead to additional documentation burden. A balance needs to be struck between accurately recording device development, retaining project know-how and allowing the flexibility and adaptability to change the design, if verification activities produce unforeseen results.

15.3.1.2 Risk management throughout ES medical device life cycle

ISO 14971:2019, *Medical devices. Application of risk management to medical devices* [14], is an international standard which describes the application of risk management to medical devices and defines risk as the combination of the probability of occurrence of harm and the severity of said harm. This standard serves as foundation for ISO 13485, as all quality management system (QMS) processes require a risk-based approach, including purchasing procedures and training. Risk management is a regulatory requirement which incorporates risk assessment from the design, manufacturing, and clinical use of the device. Usability is of particular note in the most current update to the standard. Human factors (and use errors) can represent a high risk to the use of the device in the real world. For example, poorly designed components may make an elegantly designed ES device difficult to implant, leading to poor surgical placement, device complications and failures. By considering human factors within risk management of the ES device under development, there will be reduced need for end user training and user error when the device is used in a clinical setting—leading to more positive clinical outcomes. Early consideration of usability and other risks within the risk management process can mitigate a lot of potential clinical and commercial issues. As exemplified by usability engineering, performing and updating comprehensive risk assessments throughout product life cycle (as an ongoing, repetitive, and systematic process) will assess and mitigate potential harm and risks to the end user, as well as demonstrating monitoring and risk control during a regulatory audit [15].

A risk management plan should be prepared initially and personnel with different expertise should all be involved. Risks, either systematic or random, should be identified at this stage and throughout the process. Then, by assessing the likelihood and severity, manufacturers must identify ways to reduce or mitigate the risks identified [16].

Failure Mode Effect Analysis (FMEA) is a standard technique to assess risk during design development and production. However, FMEAs only evaluate risks relating to failure and do not include risks from normal use. ISO 14971 assesses severity based on harm to the end user, while the FMEA process evaluates severity from a system performance point of view [17]. Therefore, FMEAs in isolation may not be the most appropriate, single tool for risk management. Other techniques such as risk management traceability tables, fault tree analysis, and hazard analysis of critical control point can be used in combination [18]. It is the responsibility of the manufacturer to select and justify the risk management tools utilized on a project.

15.3.1.3 Evaluation of biological safety

Biological evaluation of medical devices is a subsection of the risk management process which specifically considers the biological risks associated with the device. The biological evaluation of medical devices is covered in a series of standards summarized in ISO 10993-1:2018 [19]. ISO 10993 is a series of harmonized and state of the art standards. The scope of topics covered within this series is wide, as they are designed to provide guidance for all the possible iterations of devices permitted under the MDR. This series is composed of many subsections covering biological evaluation testing, from in vitro cytotoxicity [20] through to guidance on in vivo systemic toxicity assessments [21]. Not all parts of ISO 10993 are relevant to the biological evaluation of every device, it is the responsibility of the manufacturer to justify the testing performed for their product by assessing the device characteristics and intended use, being guided by the process outlined in ISO 10993-1. The extent and complexity of testing is determined ultimately through a risk evaluation of the product in development. As such, the level of testing of a non-implantable or Class I device is generally less onerous and less expensive than an implantable, degradable (resorbable) Class III device, due to the more extensive evaluation and testing required to provide robust risk mitigation though testing to evidence biological safety.

When approaching the biological evaluation of ES devices, particular unique challenges present themselves both from production and implantation viewpoints. During production the manufacturer must endeavor to understand and control polymeric raw materials which often display batch to batch variability from suppliers (variation in molecular weight, crystallinity, and impurities). The manufacturer must also document changes in polymer properties with processing steps and sterilization (and how this impacts the final product), record potential residuals and contaminants introduced to the device during processing (high surface area and porous features can add particular complications for ES devices). Finally, storage of final and interim product may also need to be tightly monitored and controlled for degradable devices including the impact of potential shelf life on the device characteristics must be recorded. Focusing on implantation, degradable ES devices require particular attention to be paid to the local tissue effects during implantation including matching of the degradation rate with the local tissue infiltration, and assessment of degradation products (including issues around acidification of the local tissue environment and potential degradation fragments which may fall under the categorization for nanomaterials). The terminal degradation pathway of the device must also be assessed to determine the method of clearance from the body, and assessment of potential systemic toxicity and accumulation of degradation components in the organs of body.

Biological evaluation must be performed within a risk management process to minimize biological risks for patients from the use of ES medical devices. A biological evaluation plan must first be established. When all testing is completed, results must be documented in a biological evaluation report. It is critical to understand that biological evaluation is an ongoing activity that should be assessed whenever the device undergoes design modifications (including processes such as packaging and sterilization) and as new information from postmarket surveillance is received [22].

The biological evaluation process includes the screening and assessment of all raw materials and materials used in the processing and manufacturing of the ES medical device (including transient contact such as storage boxes and cleaning materials). Manufacturers must document that the materials utilized in device processing meet the requirements of device performance, biocompatibility, and clinical suitability according to intended use. It is also required to identify device constituents and manufacturing residues, which can be achieved via chemical characterization following ISO 10993-18 [23].

It should be noted that, while a conservative risk-based approach can be taken in device preclinical testing to assure safety and feasibility wherever possible, residual risks may remain and will need to be justified in a risk—benefit analysis. Postmarket surveillance is critical as follow on from the preclinical risk analysis phase, to ensure that residual risks are monitored and mitigated throughout the commercialization process and beyond. During postmarket surveillance manufacturers must proactively collect data to improve risk management, update design and manufacturing information, detect and report trends and identify needs for corrective and preventative action (CAPA) [22].

15.3.2 Quality management

15.3.2.1 The importance of quality

Given the high regulatory scrutiny involved in the development pathway of ES medical devices, a quality mindset is crucial for successfully translating an ES product to market, as it is for any medical device. Within small companies and startups, commercial interests often favor rapid innovation and a push for early commercialization. In some sectors, these financial drivers can take precedence over the establishment of a reliable and reproducibly manufactured product. Product quality can offer long-term advantages that are key for device success if implemented as a priority from the start, and incorporated at every stage of the medical device development. A quality culture leads to long-term cost reduction, better product functionality, higher speed to market, increased customer trust and improved work environment, despite the associated costs (see Fig. 15.4) [24–28]. In a report from 2013, it was estimated that nonroutine quality events (namely major observations, recalls, and warning letters) costed the medical device industry between $2.5 billion and $5 billion per year on average, including lost sales of new and existing products [25]. Examples of good quality practices include automating data collection, creating a holistic quality improvement program,

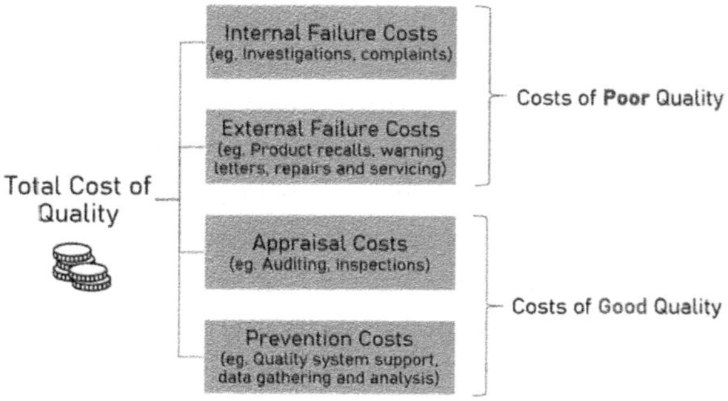

Figure 15.4 Different types of cost associated with poor and good quality. *Adapted from ASQ, Cost of Quality, n.d. Available from: https://asq.org/quality-resources/cost-of-quality.*

improving yield, driving line improvements, and using predictive modeling of parts failure [27]. These practices should consider the diverse challenges of different types of medical devices and manufacturing processes.

15.3.2.2 Implementation of a robust quality management system

A proper Quality Management System (QMS) ensures that all regulatory standards are met, with accurate keeping of records, audit reports, deviations, and CAPA investigations. Additionally, it enforces the correct approval and version control of all documentation, namely standard operating procedures, protocols, reports and batch production records. Using a robust QMS is a demonstration of commitment to quality, and a state of control that are needed to produce high quality products. QMS is closely integrated with design control and risk management as seen in Fig. 15.5.

As for all medical devices, ES medical device manufacturers should follow ISO 13485 [12]. The fulfillment of this standard is mandatory in Canada and Japan. In the European Union, ISO 13485 is not mandatory but it is considered as the de facto standard for medical device development [29]. In United States, the Food and Drug Administration (FDA, a federal agency of the US Department of Health) intends to harmonize its quality system regulation with ISO 13485 but this is yet to be implemented. Certification to this standard (and others) assures both existing and future clients and investors that medical devices are safe and effective. This standard specifies requirements that can be used by medical device companies involved in

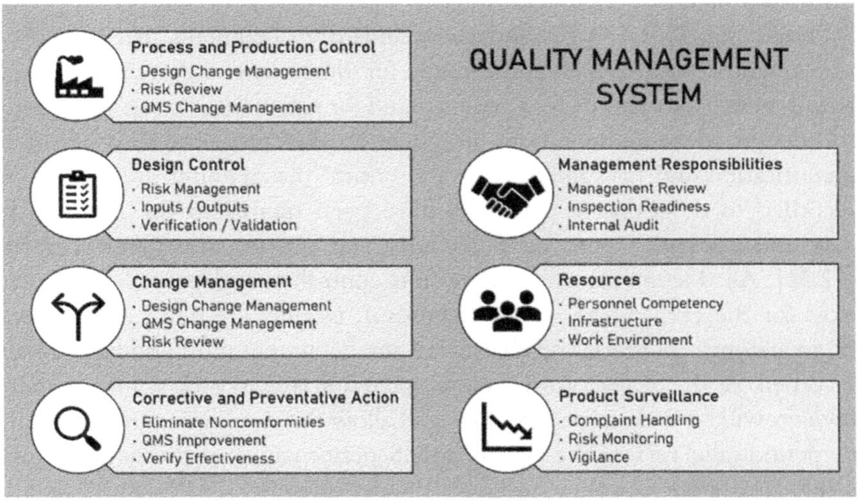
Process and Production Control
· Design Change Management
· Risk Review
· QMS Change Management
QUALITY MANAGEMENT SYSTEM
Design Control
· Risk Management
· Inputs / Outputs
· Verification / Validation
Management Responsibilities
· Management Review
· Inspection Readiness
· Internal Audit
Change Management
· Design Change Management
· QMS Change Management
· Risk Review
Resources
· Personnel Competency
· Infrastructure
· Work Environment
Corrective and Preventative Action
· Eliminate Noncomformities
· QMS Improvement
· Verify Effectiveness
Product Surveillance
· Complaint Handling
· Risk Monitoring
· Vigilance

Figure 15.5 Components of quality management system. *Adapted from [73].*

one or more stages of the life cycle of a medical device. It covers design and development, production, storage, distribution, installation, servicing, and final decommissioning and disposal [12]. ISO 13485 should be used as a complement to the local regulations and requirements, together with all other relevant standards specific for each medical device type. This standard also requires appropriate supplier management, clear roles and responsibilities of all staff (including senior management), personnel training, and contamination control. Finally, the most extensive section covers all the processes that are required to manufacture a medical device from design stages to postmarket surveillance [29].

QMS involves a high level of detail and organization. A robust QMS relies on proper documented procedures, which must be followed in the same way by everyone, ensuring product consistency, and accurate and complete records. It relies on the old adage "if it is not documented, it did not happen." However, it should be noted that a high number of documented procedures do not equate to a better system. The size of QMS is typically dependent on a company size, type, stages, and milestones. For instance, the preclinical and clinical testing stage will involve a more conservative QMS than when the product is commercialized. Documentation must be clear and concise and cover every procedure that is being implemented. However, documentation must not be too restrictive as to impair efficiency and productivity but it also must not give too much flexibility that will allow a low quality product to pass quality controls and reach the market. There must be a balance based on a risk evaluation approach.

Following ISO 13485, there are mandatory documents that should be implemented first, namely procedures for document and record control; requirements for maintenance activities and for risk management; procedures for design, development, and production; also procedures for product identification and traceability. It is also critical that training procedures are recorded to demonstrate personnel have been trained to the most up to date and currently approved procedures and can execute them correctly [12,31]. All documents must be version controlled and procedures should exist for the preparation, review, approval, issuance, retrieval and archival of documents. All preceding changes to any document must also be properly recorded. As the project grows, additional requirements such as management reviews will become necessary. This will allow the developing product team to periodically review the overall QMS performance, addressing resource issues and nonconforming product, discuss ongoing CAPA and schedule and review internal audits.

15.3.2.3 Good documentation practices

Good documentation practices (GDP) and document control help ensure good quality product and traceability and are expected throughout the device life cycle. Good documentation consists of an established system for approval and review of documents, with clear identification of changes and current revision status, correct availability and distribution of documents as required, legible and identifiable documents, identification of documents of external origin, prevention of unintended use and archiving of obsolete documents [32,33]. GDP principles can be found in Fig. 15.6. Records must provide evidence that activities have been performed or results have been achieved. GDP is accomplished during manufacturing by following simple rules that must be highlighted during training, such as using only a ballpoint pen or other pen with indelible ink, following the specified date format, sign and date when required and writing legibly [33]. These main rules ensure better communication and a clear audit trail, ensure traceability, create evidence and protect data integrity. Additionally, it provides compliance to the regulatory system and correct, complete and current information that may be used if required during reviews and CAPA investigations. It must be noted that documentation of any form is only useful if it is accurate. After a product is released and sold to a customer, what remains behind in the organization is the documentation. Therefore, accurate and correct completion of documentation is crucial.

It is important to have critical documents stored safely, physically, and/or electronically, to avoid loss of documentation or loss of access due to floods or fire, software malfunction, or pandemics. Startups and small companies

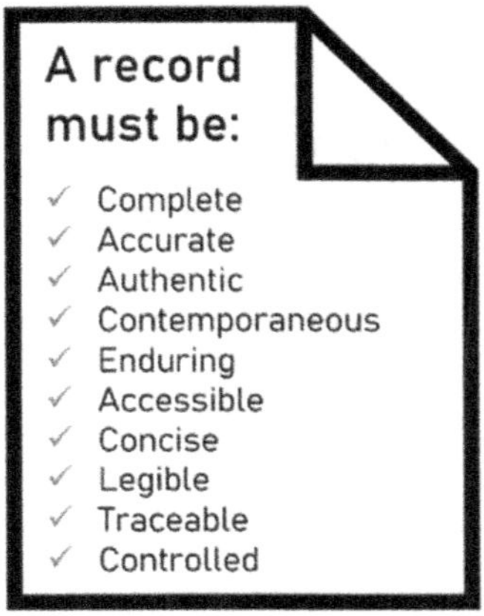
A record must be:
✓ Complete
✓ Accurate
✓ Authentic
✓ Contemporaneous
✓ Enduring
✓ Accessible
✓ Concise
✓ Legible
✓ Traceable
✓ Controlled

Figure 15.6 Good documentation practice principles to ensure data integrity.

usually start with a paper-based QMS, as only a small number of documents are needed, with few personnel. As companies grow, the need for an automated, electronic, cloud-based QMS (also known as eQMS) increases, to aid in document approval, replacement of superseded versions and document access as required in different sites. Additionally, some eQMS help in achieving regulatory requirements. Currently, there are many different options available in the market. The most common include MasterControl Quality Management System, Greenlight Guru Quality Management Software, qmsWrapper, ETQ Reliance, and Qualio [34].

15.3.2.4 The importance of product traceability

ISO 13485 requires documented procedures for product identification and traceability [12]. As a result, each interim and final ES product must have its own unique code. Interim product coding can also be developed to inform about the stage of manufacturing and allow traceability through processes and raw materials. This is particularly beneficial in the event of CAPAs and investigation of nonconforming products.

In the European Union, as defined by the MDR, all medical devices on the market must have a unique device identifier (UDI), stored in a database called EUDAMED [4]. If required, for instance, as part of an ES device adverse incidence investigation, the UDI can be used as a starting point to verify and analyze all the processes and constituents that were involved in the manufacturing of this particular device to identify the root cause of the problem. Good traceability procedures could then inform if the problem could be present only in the specific device or in the whole batch. If the latter, it could lead to a batch recall to prevent further complications and minimize the impact on patient/user safety.

15.4 Manufacturing and upscale

15.4.1 Manufacturing cleanliness

15.4.1.1 Cleanrooms and controlled environments

Cleanrooms and controlled environments are key facilities for manufacturing ES medical devices. They ensure the quality of the products, the safety of end users and also of production employees. They are particularly indispensable for Class II and III ES devices since bacterial, viral or particle contamination can have serious negative implications for patients [35]. With their high surface to volume ratios and microscale features, ES products carry an inherent high risk of catching and entrapping particulate matter including microbes.

Cleanrooms and controlled environments are by definition contained spaces constructed in a manner to control the introduction, generation, and retention of particles and contaminants inside the room. This is achieved by processing the incoming air by means of filtration through HEPA and ULPA filters and control of air pressure cascades, ensuring that any particulates produced are directed out of the manufacturing area [36]. Cleanrooms are widely used in a range of industries from pharmaceutical and food manufacturing to optics, nanotechnology, and aerospace applications [30,36–38]. Due to this wide variety of cleanroom uses, many different types of cleanroom exist. As such, there is no "one size fits all" cleanroom design, it will be specific to the manufacturing requirements of each product. Guidance on the use of cleanrooms specifically for medical device manufacture is outlined in ISO 14644 [39], detailing the expected standards of air quality and contamination control [35]. While a cleanroom's functionality highly depends on its design, the use of a cleanroom does not guarantee a clean and safe product. A raft of underpinning procedures must be in place to ensure the environment is maintained. These include correct equipment placement (to allow adequate airflow), controlled process flow of materials (including raw materials, product, and waste), robust cleaning procedures and adequate training of cleanroom personnel to prevent manufacturing errors and contamination [17].

15.4.1.2 Cleanroom monitoring

Environmental monitoring in the manufacturing area ensures that levels of contamination of an ES product remain low. Microbial and particulate contamination largely derives from operators in the cleanroom. However, other sources such as faulty air exchange systems, machinery with rotating parts and materials releasing particles that are used in the cleanroom, can all contribute to particulate build up. Leaking or broken air filters, inadequate cleaning procedures, or selection of items or materials which facilitate bacterial growth may also allow entry and build-up of microbial contamination in the cleanroom [36,40].

Contamination control should be approached holistically and be documented. ISO 13485 states, that "For sterile medical devices, the organization shall document requirements for control of contamination with microorganisms or particulate matter and maintain the required cleanliness during assembly or packaging processes" [12,41]. Further guidance on microbial contamination and control can be found in ISO 14698-1, *Cleanrooms and associated controlled environments—Biocontamination control,*

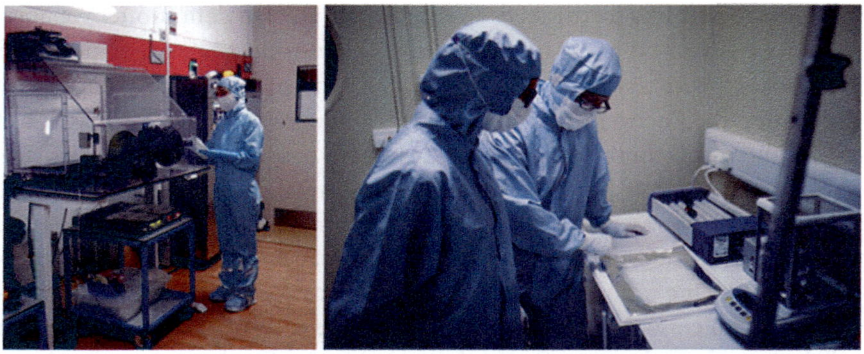

Figure 15.7 Manufacturing staff in cleanroom garments working on ES manufacturing and quality control procedures in a Class 7 cleanroom.

where the methods required for monitoring risk zones and for applying control measures are specified [42]. Evidence of the cleanroom performance is based on measurement of particles per cubic meter, as detailed in ISO 14644-1, *Cleanrooms and associated controlled environments—Part 1: Classification of cleanliness by particle concentration* [72]. While there is no rule on what classification of a cleanroom is required against any product type, due to the broad range of medical devices being produced, cleanrooms Class 7 are commonly used for ES medical device manufacture.

Personnel operating in the cleanroom represent the main source of contamination. To curtail risk of contamination from manufacturing operators, cleanroom gowns are utilized to prevent personnel from releasing particles (e.g., from clothing) and microbial contamination (e.g., from hair/skin flakes). Strict gowning and behavioral procedures are also applied within the cleanroom area, with access to the site being restricted to trained staff only [30]. A thorough cleaning regime (with varying frequency and procedures) must be implemented to minimize microbial and particle build-up on surfaces [43]. Fig. 15.7 shows cleanroom operators working in a Class 7 cleanroom and gives an example of the type of gowning which can be utilized in an ES manufacturing facility.

15.4.1.3 Bioburden

It should be noted that while production of a device can be entirely performed under cleanroom conditions, some level of device microbial contamination will remain. This is known as product bioburden and it specifically refers to the number of viable bacteria (gram positive and gram negative) on or in the product, prior to sterilization. Bioburden should be assessed frequently to build up a picture of the microbial contamination on devices produced over time, allowing the evaluation of routine cleaning and manufacturing procedures in addition to informing the effective sterilization dose.

When assessing bioburden, it is useful to have a basic level of speciation of the colonies found on the device. Gram-negative bacteria typically pose a higher risk to the patient than gram-positive, as the cell membranes are a source of lipopolysaccharides (LPS), also called endotoxins. Endotoxins are released upon cell death, as the bacterial membrane is destroyed (therefore, certain types of sterilization can actually cause an increase in the quantity of endotoxin), but this process also occurs during bacterial growth and division [44]. Endotoxin removal from a device is immensely challenging - due to the heat stability of LPS - endotoxins are not destroyed under regular sterilizing conditions, as a result it is critical to prevent device contamination with gram-negative bacteria during manufacturing [44]. Endotoxins elicit a wide range of cellular responses including pyrogenicity. They can cause symptoms ranging from fever and shivering to hypotension, acute respiratory distress syndrome, disseminated intravascular coagulation and endotoxin shock [44]. Risks from endotoxins must be considered and mitigated as part of device development.

15.4.2 Scale-up considerations

15.4.2.1 Early product and process development steps

Product development typically starts with prototyping. This usually happens in research labs and ES product prototypes are often made using research grade raw materials and reagents. The equipment is of small manufacturing capacity and manufacturing is rather manual, with a high level of product handling being inevitable. Typically a number of samples are made as part of the proof-of-concept (POC) stage to develop the manufacturing methods, characterize the product and define its design parameters [45]. The ES product and its manufacturing process can be defined and established in parallel. It is useful to recognize potential pitfalls of future processes and materials at the earliest stages of the device development. For example, processes such as sterilization can place constraints on the product design [46]. Developing the prototype, working on manufacturing process, and overcoming its challenges often results in Intellectual Property (IP) and know-how being generated. This IP should be retained by properly documenting the development and changes, as well as keeping records of development directions and failed research avenues [47]. Device innovations as well as breakthrough improvement strategies can be patented prior to publication (which is often aimed for in academic research), enabling translation of these concepts to actual products with adequate protections, exclusivities, and necessary profit motives. New strategies leading to product development and future production require reliable IP protection and related essential guarantees for return-on-investment that support the translational process [48].

15.4.2.2 ES product development and design freeze

The successful translation of a product to clinical application often hinges on how thoroughly its early design criteria were developed. For each design iteration, changes in design criteria and their impact of the design inputs should be formally identified and reviewed prior to any high value prototyping or animal testing [49]. The formal process of documenting these design iterations is via a design review meeting. This meeting should include participation from personnel from different aspects of the project including clinical, quality, risk, manufacturing and technical. Following review, the design can be "frozen" allowing for a clear testing strategy on that version of the design. "Design freeze" is a critical point in project timeline that defines the end point of that design iteration, when a technical product description is established and production and testing on that version of the design can commence. A design freeze is a binding decision that defines the whole product, its parts or parameters and allows the continuation of the design based on that decision. It also reduces further potential engineering changes: although these are still permissible, strict change control procedures to be observed to ensure clarity of preclinical testing [50].

An important point to highlight is that while design iterations - and multiple design freezes - are a natural part of the design and verification process, ultimately, the data making up the preclinical evidence package of safety and feasibility need to be performed on the same version of the design which will be implanted into patients (either commercially or for a first in human clinical study). Any changes or upgrades to the manufacturing process, or the materials used, can disrupt the previously established processes or design, which will impact the validity of the preclinical testing already performed on the product and may necessitate repeat testing on the new design. This includes *in-vivo* testing in small and large animal models. This obviously adds extra cost and time to the translation route as well as raising ethical issues around animal use. The design review process facilitates a formal documentation of proposed design changes and investigation of their impact.

Manufacturing capacity should also be taken into consideration at this stage, to ensure a method to allow reproducible and consistent production of the ES medical device is in place. It is strongly advised to establish the manufacturing process in the controlled environment prior to establishing the version of design freeze against which the preclinical testing will be performed. Sufficient upscale of the manufacturing should also be considered, not only to ensure provision of samples for the clinical investigation and early commercialization, but also to demonstrate the upscale potential to meet the long-term demand.

15.4.2.3 Scale up and automation

When scaling up a manufacturing process, numerous aspects should be considered including required equipment capability, equipment robustness and reliability, production rate and yield, constituent parts, materials and quality of the build, level of manual intervention or automation, cleanliness, size and available space, generic or bespoke equipment, equipment and maintenance costs. For highly regulated medical devices (Class III), the cleanliness of operating machinery is a key aspect to be maintained throughout the stages of scale up.

During ES product manufacturing, electrospinning or electrospraying is often the limiting step as it typically has a low production rate. Several high-throughput electrospinning methods and devices have been proposed to overcome this low productivity issue, such as those using multiple nozzles or a liquid-bath approach. However, opting for these methods can cause problems of jet repulsion and reduce the control over the ES jet and ES material deposition [51]. Importantly, this can have a deleterious effect on the ES product quality, which should not be compromised. Besides the ES jetting system, considering the scale up of accessories may also be important, as their scale-up abilities may be limited (e.g. rotating drums). Although various upscaled ES systems and accessories are available in the market, bespoke or semi-bespoke equipment may be needed to ensure suitability to a specific process. An example of an upscale process for the fabrication of continuous filaments is shown in Fig. 15.8.

It is worth considering the introduction of automated processes at early stage of translation as this typically increases production rates, quality, and reliability. Once the project progresses further toward commercialization, further upscale and automation can take place. Process automation should provide time and cost-efficient solutions, while maintaining high quality standards. Low or cost-efficient maintenance is crucial since servicing and calibration must be done regularly to comply with regulatory requirements.

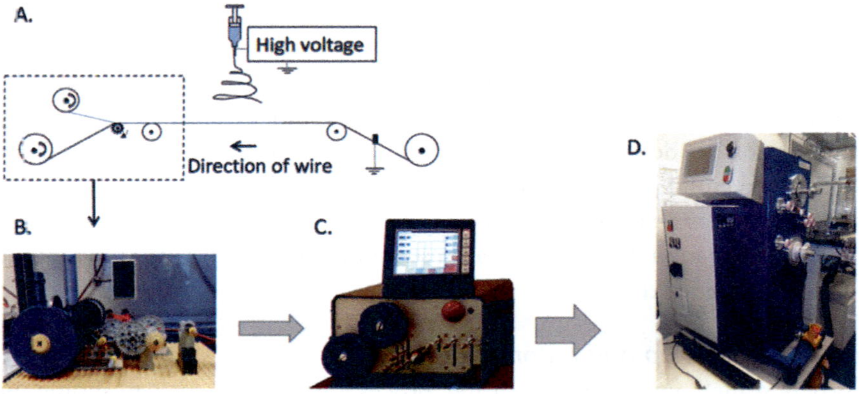

Figure 15.8 Manufacturing upscale of a collection system for producing continuous electrospun filaments during the translation of the process from research to product development. (a) Schematic of the electrospinning process, with the collection system highlighted in the dashed line boundary [52–54]; (b) initial prototype made with LEGO parts, (c) small automated collecting unit, operated via a touchscreen, used in research labs; (d) large collecting unit capable of 24/7 operation, suitable for use in a cleanroom environment.

It should also be noted that the validation of equipment is a part of the process validation required for medical devices, as stated in ISO 13485. Equipment validation covers the installation qualification (functional requirements and how these were met during installation), the operational qualification (key operating parameters, settings, tolerance ranges, and verified operation), and the performance qualification (verified reproducibility and repeatability) [55,56].

15.5 ES devices: clinical trials and commercialization

15.5.1 The importance of preclinical and clinical trials

As mentioned previously, evidencing the biological safety and efficacy of ES medical devices is crucial for their progress to market, especially for Class III medical implants. Following EU regulations, it is highly likely for a Class III device that a rigorously planned clinical trial will be necessary to prove the safety and efficacy of the device. However, these may only be performed after obtaining satisfactory results from preclinical testing. This phase can be a very long and expensive process for Class III devices. Some of the preclinical barriers include lack of accurate preclinical models or the need to do in vivo testing in multiple animal models [3]. Additionally, changes in regulations may result in additional testing that was not planned for financially or temporally. For instance, recent regulatory changes now require that medical implants are assessed throughout the duration and life cycle, thus until an ES device is degraded, removed from the body, or reaches a steady state [57].

Devices often go through different phases of clinical trials, from Phase 1 (exploratory trial or first in man trial, covering safety and feasibility) to Phase 4 (postmarket surveillance studies). For each phase, the number of patients is increased. Ideally (though not a specified regulatory requirement), a new Class III device should be evaluated under a large multicenter randomized clinical trial (Phase 2 and 3), but double blinding can be challenging and not always possible, due to the intended application of the device [3].

15.5.2 Under trial and approved ES medical devices

To identify approved ES devices and those under clinical trials, a search was performed through the FDA databases (510(k), Premarket Approval (PMA) and De Novo), and through ClinicalTrials.gov. Inclusion criteria applied were clinical trials, and studies or case reports where electrospun or ES medical devices represented at least one of independent variables. Exclusion criteria applied were electrospun or ES devices not used on medical applications, non-English language publications, devices not made, at least partly, by electrospinning or electrospraying, reviews and abstract only publications. All searches were performed between May and July 2020.

Our FDA searches revealed that five ES devices were approved for commercialization. Among them, four were approved via the 510(k) route, which is based on substantial equivalence to other devices already on the market, termed predicates (Fig. 15.9). These devices were manufactured by Acera Surgical Inc. and are made of poly(lactic-co-glycolic acid) and polydioxanone. However, substantial equivalence of the first ES device (Cerafix Dura Substitute K153613) was based on material properties, instead of manufacturing methods. This device was in turn used, directly or indirectly, as a predicate or reference device for the other ES products. The fifth device, manufactured by Biotronik Inc., is made of polyurethane for cardiovascular applications and was approved via the PMA route in 2019.

The clinicaltrials.gov search revealed 17 human trials performed with ES devices (Table 15.1), the first being initiated in 2005. Of the 17, 11 of the trials (64.7%) can be classed as wound dressing applications. Wound dressing trials included ulcer treatments (6 trials), surgical incision or excision (2 trials), vitiligo treatment (1 trial), cutaneous leishmaniosis treatment (1 trial), and treatment of split skin graft donor sites (1 trial, using a hand held portable

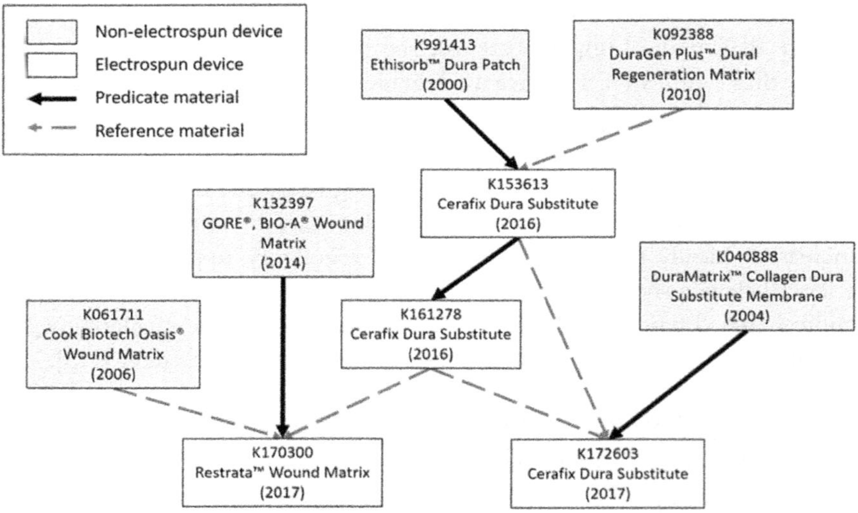

Figure 15.9 Predicate tree of ES devices by Acera Surgical Inc., indicating how ES devices were approved through equivalence to non-ES devices in 2016–17.

point-of-care electrospinning device). Wound dressing applications represent low patient risk and a high clinical incidence which will look positive to a health economics valuation by a potential investor. An aging population and elevated incidence of type II diabetes may also explain the large number of wound dressing trials specifically focused on ulcer treatment. Applications concerned in the remaining six trials included dental applications (3 trials), clotting device for cancellous bone bleeding (1 trial), neurosurgical repair (1 trial) and vascular prosthesis (1 trial). Two trials were terminated before their completion but no reason was specified. Overall, only a low percentage of the trials (17.6%) were for permanent implantable devices. This may be because these type of devices falls under the highest classification (Class III) meaning there is a high level of regulatory burden prior to commencement of the first in man studies, which translates directly to high research and development costs. Also, investment for these devices is more difficult to attract (they are "high-risk, high-reward" products as failure may lead to high patient harm) and this reduces the number of devices translating to clinical use. It is worth noting that the maximum follow-up duration in any of the 17 trials was 1 year, which is relatively short. This may be due to the transient application of the wound dressing devices or perhaps due to the degradable nature of materials used.

Table 15.1 List of ES medical devices that have undergone or are undergoing clinical trials.

ES medical device	Clinical trial Number/ID	Start-end year	Country	Trial phase	Number of patients	Maximum follow-up time
Transdermal patch	NCT00428727	2005–11	Colombia	3	100	90 days
Transdermal patch	NCT00317629	2006–09	Colombia	3	178	10 months
Taliderm	NCT00686296	2008–11	United States	NA	56	2–3 weeks
Taliderm	NCT00720239	2008–10	United States	1	50	20 weeks
Taliderm	NCT02237287	2011–12	Switzerland	1	24	Up to 1 year
ReDura Onlay	NCT02129114	2014–15	China	NA	132 (aim)	6 months
Vascular prostheses (PCL/gelatin/PLGA/Nylon)	NCT02255188	2014–15	Russia	-	120	1 day
EktoTherix tissue repair	NCT02409628	2015–17	United Kingdom	NA	12	3 months
SurgiClot	NCT02509208	2015–16	Norway/United Kingdom	NA	30	6 weeks
Bilayer: silk fibroin—decellularized amniotic	IRCT2016071328903N1	2016–Unknown	Iran	2	20	60 days
Hand held ES device	NCT02680106	2016–17	Israel	NA	40	21 days
Restrata wound matrix	NCT03312595	2017–18	United States	NA	30	14 weeks
Rivelin patch	NCT03592342	2018–ongoing	Several	2	240 (aim)	4 weeks
Rivelin patch	NCT03686800	2018–18	Denmark	NA	12	2 days
TAP nanofibers	NCT03690960	2018–2020 (estimated dates)	Egypt	NA	30 (aim)	2–3 weeks
Biodegradable dressing	IRCT20130812014333N133	2020–ongoing	Iran	2–3	130 (aim)	6 months
Restrata wound matrix	NCT04405050	2020–22 (estimated dates)	United States	4	146 (aim)	12 weeks

It should be highlighted that these observations were only based on the trials which were found through our search criteria. As mentioned above, ES devices can be passed through an equivalence route and be commercialized without a clinical study.

Searches over four research databases (Embase, MEDLINE, Scopus, and Web of Science) revealed 14 publications on ES devices being used in a clinical setting, covering interventional or observational (retrospective) studies [58–71]. The primary function of ES devices was treatment for 13 publications, with only one publication assessing usability. Five publications evaluated AVflo (Nicast Ltd.) - a polycarbonate-urethane and silicone vascular graft - and found no systemic or local reactions to the graft and with similar patency rates as other devices [58,59,65,68,69]. Two publications assessed Restrata Wound Matrix (Acera Surgical Ltd.) for treatment of chronic wounds. Results indicate marked improvement in wound quality and significant reduction in local inflammation, with 85% complete wound closure at 12 weeks [62,70]. Other commercial ES devices found in these publications include Cerafix Dura Substitute (Acera Surgical Ltd.) [66] and SurgiClot (St. Teresa Medical) [71]. Overall, these publications showed that ES devices performed well in their intended applications.

15.5.3 Commercialized ES medical devices

From the information available, we found 28 companies that either commercialize ES products and/or provide ES services and equipment. These are distributed over 12 countries, with United States having the highest number (Fig. 15.10). Among these companies, 46% claim that they are certified to either ISO 13485 or CE marking or that they have FDA

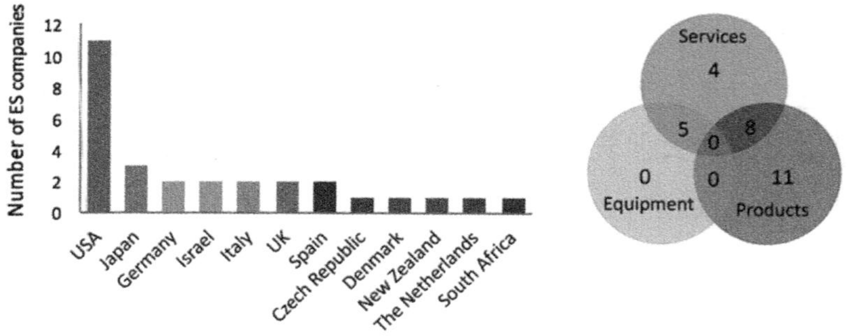

Figure 15.10 Companies that commercialize ES medical devices and/or provide ES medical device services and equipment. Left: Number per country, right: distribution of activities.

approval/clearance. For the remaining companies, it was not possible to find evidence of any certification. It is possible ES companies were not identified, since it was sometimes challenging to identify if a product involved ES technologies due to IP restrictions.

Overall, this indicates that, 30 years after the emergence of ES materials in biomedical research, commercialization of ES devices is still a niche field with opportunities for new companies worldwide. The small number of companies reflects the important preclinical, clinical, commercial and regulatory barriers that companies encounter when trying to translate ES medical devices.

15.6 Summary and way forward

Translating ES products from bench to bedside can represent a challenging prospect for the development of products with novel functions and applications. Adaptation from a scientific and investigative approach to one with the strict requirements and procedures required for regulatory evidence is an exacting shift of working practices.

There continues to be much debate in the regulatory environment in the attempt to balance commercial success and device safety. This, combined with new technological developments (drug eluting ES devices, combinational ES devices, *etc.*), means that the regulatory landscape is constantly evolving. While the regulatory and ISO guidance can provide requirements and test methods, it is generally in the format of an overall framework rather than a fully prescriptive list of what testing is required. It is ultimately the responsibility of the manufacturer to assess, develop and justify the exact regulatory strategy and preclinical testing plan applied to the product. The EU regulatory process is driven by a relative risk versus benefit approach, with an emphasis on risk reduction throughout the translational journey. It will certainly be of benefit to a prospective ES device manufacturer to adopt this mindset early in development. With this in mind, it is highly desirable to initiate the ES product design based on a clear clinical focus, as this will help to strengthen the market and health economics case for later device investment and commercialization. In addition, this strategy assists with the design of the biological safety and efficacy evaluation plan of the device, by focusing on the clinical performance requirements and working backward many of the critical testing parameters will become clear. Close contact with other device developers and regulatory experts is critical at these early stages of design and development.

With an increasing number of ES devices undergoing translation, the methods behind implementing quality, design control, and risk management from a preliminary development stage are becoming increasingly important. Setting these structures in place early will add to the quality and consistency of the final product as well as paving the way for the eventual conformity assessment leading to CE marking and commercial approval. Similarly, it is key to be able to demonstrate manufacturing feasibility in a clean environment (cleanroom) and capacity for scale up early on in ES device development. This ensures that there will be minimal design changes when upscaling. It is also critically important in calculating the cost of goods based on raw materials, manufacturing capacity and processing time. Moreover, having a well-established and documented manufacturing process will allow for clear design modifications, which may be required based on the outcomes of the verification activities being performed. This also facilitates a system for a straightforward gap analysis of the manufacturing process when moving to a clean environment and when undergoing upscale.

Even when utilizing clinically well-characterized polymers, the novel character of ES devices imparts greater challenges in this journey. The submicron features of ES devices, along with manufacturing procedures unfamiliar to the wider medical device regulatory network, make evidencing preclinical safety challenging. However, it is necessary to face those challenges in order to safely bring ES devices to a stage where they can be useful to patients. While several devices have already managed to reach the clinics and commercialization, their numbers and use remain limited. A long-term evaluation of the safety and efficacy of the ES devices, with a clear demonstration of their advantages over conventional processing techniques or products, will hopefully contribute to the successful translation of more devices in the future.

Acknowledgments

The authors gratefully acknowledge the contributions of Anne Jury and Dr. Jo Proffitt in reviewing in this chapter. This work was supported by the National Institute for Health Research (NIHR), the Wellcome Trust, the Norman Collisson Foundation (NCF), and Versus Arthritis (VA). The views expressed in this chapter are those of the authors and not necessarily those of the NIHR, Wellcome, NCF, or VA.

References

[1] D. Clark, G. Dean, S. Bolton, B. Beeson, Bench to bedside: the technology adoption pathway in healthcare, Health Technol. 10 (2) (2020) 537–545.

[2] H.-D. Volk, M.M. Stevens, D.J. Mooney, D.W. Grainger, G.N. Duda, Key elements for nourishing the translational research environment, Sci. Transl. Med. 7 (282) (2015), 282cm2-cm2.

[3] E.T. Stace, S.G. Dakin, P.-A. Mouthuy, A.J. Carr, Translating regenerative biomaterials into clinical practice, J. Cell. Physiol. 231 (1) (2016) 36–49.
[4] Regulation (EU) 2017/745 of the European Parliament and of the Council - of 5 April 2017 - on Medical Devices, 2017.
[5] Notified bodies: European Commission, n.d. Available from: https://ec.europa.eu/growth/single-market/goods/building-blocks/notified-bodies_en.
[6] FDA. CFR Title 21 - Food and Drugs: Parts 800 to 1299, n.d. Available from: https://www.accessdata.fda.gov/scripts/cdrh/cfdocs/cfcfr/CFRSearch.cfm?CFRPartFrom=800&CFRPartTo=1299.
[7] World Health O. Medical Device Regulations: Global Overview and Guiding Principles, World Health Organization, Geneva, 2003.
[8] IMDRF. International Medical Device Regulators Forum, 2021. Available from: http://www.imdrf.org/.
[9] S. Lamph, Regulation of medical devices outside the European Union, J. R. Soc. Med. 105 (Suppl. 1) (2012) S12–S21.
[10] G.A. Van Norman, Drugs and devices: comparison of European and U.S. Approval processes, JACC (J. Am. Coll. Cardiol.): Basic Transl. Sci. 1 (5) (2016) 399–412.
[11] FDA, Design Control Guidance for Medical Device Manufacturers. FDA 21 CFR 820.30 and Sub-clause 4.4 Od ISO 9001, 1997.
[12] BS EN ISO 13485, Medical Devices — Quality Management Systems — Requirements for Regulatory Purposes 2016, 2016.
[13] E.C. Honour, Understanding the value of systems engineering, INCOSE Int. Symp. 14 (1) (2004) 1207–1222.
[14] BS EN ISO 14971, 2019 Medical Devices — Application of Risk Management to Medical Devices, 2019.
[15] J. Speer, What You Need to Know for an Effective Risk Assessment, 2020.
[16] M. Leimbeck, Risk Management in the New Regulatory Environment - Patient-Centered Risk Management Programs for Medical Device Companies, 2018.
[17] Class 2 - 3 Medical Device Cleanrooms: Production Automation Corporation, n.d. Available from: https://blog.gotopac.com/2018/12/20/cleanroom-design-medical-device-class/.
[18] E. Bills, An Exclusive Look at the New ISO 14971:2019 and ISO TR 24971:2020, 2020.
[19] BS EN ISO 10993-1:2018, Biological Evaluation of Medical Devices – Part 1: Evaluation and Testing within a Risk Management Process, 2018.
[20] BS EN ISO 10993-5:2009, Biological Evaluation of Medical Devices – Part 5:Tests for In Vitro Cytotoxicity, 2009.
[21] BS EN ISO 10993-11:2018, Biological Evaluation of Medical Devices – Part 11:Tests for Systemic Toxicity, 2018.
[22] A. Pétiard, ISO 10993-1 and Biocompatibility – Conducting a Biological Evaluation of a Medical Device, 2017.
[23] BS EN ISO 10993-19:2020, Biological Evaluation of Medical Devices – Part 18: Chemical Characterization of Medical Device Materials within a Risk Management Process, 2020.
[24] ASQ, Cost of Quality, n.d. Available from: https://asq.org/quality-resources/cost-of-quality.
[25] T. Fuhr, K. George, J. Pai, The Business Case for Medical Device Quality, 2013.
[26] Etq, The Rise of Quality as a Strategic Business Initiative Research into the State of Quality Management, 2020.
[27] T. Fuhr, E. Makarova, S. Silverman, V. Telpis, Capturing the Value of Good Quality in Medical Devices, 2017.
[28] Medical Device QMS, What It Is, Where It's Required, and Key Regulations to Know: Oriel Stat a Matrix, n.d. Available from: https://www.orielstat.com/blog/medical-device-qms-overview/.

[29] P. White, Understanding ISO 13485:2016 - A Brief, yet Comprehensive, Overview, 2017.
[30] C. Moissl-Eichinger, A.K. Auerbach, A.J. Probst, A. Mahnert, L. Tom, Y. Piceno, et al., Quo vadis? Microbial profiling revealed strong effects of cleanroom maintenance and routes of contamination in indoor environments, Sci. Rep. 5 (2015) 9156.
[31] Checklist of Mandatory Documentation Required by ISO 13485:2016, 2017.
[32] V. Sachdeva, Good Documentation and Quality Management Principles, n.d.
[33] T. Sandle, Good documentation practices, J. Validation Technol. 20(3) (n.d.).
[34] The Best eQMS for Medical Devices, 2020.
[35] How Medical Device Manufacturers Use Cleanrooms to Keep Products Safe for Patients: NS Medical Devices, 2020. Available from: https://www.nsmedicaldevices.com/analysis/medical-device-cleanrooms/.
[36] D.A. Newcombe, M.T. La Duc, P. Vaishampayan, K. Venkateswaran, Impact of assembly, testing and launch operations on the airborne bacterial diversity within a spacecraft assembly facility clean-room, Int. J. Astrobiol. 7 (3−4) (2008) 223−236.
[37] Cleanroom Services Industry: Advanced Cleanroom Microclean, n.d. Available from: https://advancedcleanroom.com/industries/.
[38] Industries That Use Cleanrooms: Specialty Optical Systems, Inc., n.d. Available from: https://www.soscleanroom.com/blog/industries-that-use-cleanrooms/.
[39] BS EN ISO 14644, 2015 Cleanrooms and Associated Controlled Environments. Classification of Air Cleanliness by Particle Concentration, 2015.
[40] T. Sandle, A review of cleanroom microflora: types, trends, and patterns, J. Pharmaceut. Sci. Technol. 65 (4) (2011).
[41] Maetrics, White Paper: Contamination Control of Medical Device Cleanrooms, 2015.
[42] ISO 14698-1 Cleanrooms and Associated Controlled Environments — Biocontamination Control, 2003.
[43] GMP Annex: Clean Air and Containment, 2015.
[44] M.B. Gorbet, M.V. Sefton, Endotoxin: the uninvited guest, Biomaterials 26 (34) (2005) 6811−6817.
[45] O.V. Bitkina, H.K. Kim, J. Park, Usability and user experience of medical devices: an overview of the current state, analysis methodologies, and future challenges, Int. J. Ind. Ergon. 76 (2020) 102932.
[46] K. Alexander, P. Clarkson, Good design practice for medical devices and equipment, Part II: design for validation, J. Med. Eng. Technol. 24 (2) (2000) 53−62.
[47] J.E. Lincoln, Medical device development under design control, J. Validation Technol. 16 (1) (2010) 43.
[48] D.W. Grainger, H.C. van der Mei, P.C. Jutte, J.J. van den Dungen, M.J. Schultz, B.F. van der Laan, et al., Critical factors in the translation of improved antimicrobial strategies for medical implants and devices, Biomaterials 34 (37) (2013) 9237−9243.
[49] H. Charkhkar, B.P. Christie, G.J. Pinault, D.J. Tyler, R.J. Triolo, A translational framework for peripheral nerve stimulating electrodes: reviewing the journey from concept to clinic, J. Neurosci. Methods 328 (2019) 108414.
[50] The role of design freeze in product development, in: T. Eger, C. Eckert, P.J. Clarkson (Eds.), DS 35: Proceedings ICED 05, the 15th International Conference on Engineering Design, Melbourne, Australia, 15-1808 2005, 2005.
[51] H.S. SalehHudin, E.N. Mohamad, W.N.L. Mahadi, A. Muhammad Afifi, Multiple-jet electrospinning methods for nanofiber processing: a review, Mater. Manuf. Process. 33 (5) (2018) 479−498.
[52] P.A. Mouthuy, N. Zargar, O. Hakimi, E. Lostis, A. Carr, Fabrication of continuous electrospun filaments with potential for use as medical fibres, Biofabrication 7 (2) (2015) 025006.

[53] R.E. Abhari, A.J. Carr, P.-A. Mouthuy, 15 - Multifilament electrospun scaffolds for soft tissue reconstruction, in: V. Guarino, L. Ambrosio (Eds.), Electrofluidodynamic Technologies (EFDTs) for Biomaterials and Medical Devices, Woodhead Publishing, 2018, pp. 295–328.
[54] A.A. Lach, H.L. Morris, J.A. Martins, E.T. Stace, A.J. Carr, P.-A. Mouthuy, Pyridine as an additive to improve the deposition of continuous electrospun filaments, PLoS One 14 (4) (2019) e0214419.
[55] J.E. Lincoln, Medical device product verification and validation, J. Validation Technol. 16 (2) (2010) 58.
[56] K.B. Ahir, K.D. Singh, S.P. Yadav, H.S. Patel, C.B. Poyahari, Overview of validation and basic concepts of process validation, Scholars Acad. J. Pharm. 3 (2014) 178–190.
[57] E.T. Stace, P.A. Mouthuy, A.J. Carr, H.C. Ye, Biomaterials: Electrospinning. Comprehensive Biotechnology, Elsevier, 2019.
[58] M. Ferraresso, S. Bertoli, P. Nobili, E.M. Bortolani, Early experience with a newly developed electrospun polycarbonate-urethane vascular graft for hemodialysis access, J. Vasc. Access 14 (3) (2013) 252–256.
[59] S. Yilmaz, Early experience with a novel self-sealing nanofabric vascular graft for early hemodialysis access, Vascular 24 (4) (2016) 421–424.
[60] S. Li, H. Xiao, L. Yang, L. Hua, Z. Qiu, X. Hu, et al., Electrospun P(LLA-CL) nanoscale fibrinogen patch vs porcine small intestine submucosa graft repair of inguinal hernia in adults: a randomized, single-blind, controlled, multicenter, noninferiority trial, J. Am. Coll. Surg. 229 (6) (2019) 541–551.e1.
[61] M. Arenbergerova, P. Arenberger, M. Bednar, P. Kubat, J. Mosinger, Light-activated nanofibre textiles exert antibacterial effects in the setting of chronic wound healing, Exp. Dermatol. 21 (8) (2012) 619–624.
[62] M.J. Regulski, M.R. MacEwan, Implantable nanomedical scaffold facilitates healing of chronic lower extremity wounds, Wounds Compend. Clin. Res. & Pract. 30 (8) (2018) E77–e80.
[63] N.D. Laborde, J. Leslie, E. Krogstad, N. Morar, P. Mutero, J. Etima, et al., Perceptions of the "Fabric" - an exploratory study of a novel multi-purpose technology among women in Sub Saharan Africa, PLoS One 13 (10) (2018) e0204821.
[64] X. Wu, Y. Wang, C. Zhu, X. Tong, M. Yang, L. Yang, et al., Preclinical animal study and human clinical trial data of co-electrospun poly(L-lactide-co-caprolactone) and fibrinogen mesh for anterior pelvic floor reconstruction, Int. J. Nanomed. 11 (2016) 389–397.
[65] S.M. Wijeyaratne, L. Kannangara, Safety and efficacy of electrospun polycarbonate-urethane vascular graft for early hemodialysis access: first clinical results in man, J. Vasc. Access 12 (1) (2011) 28–35.
[66] P. Schmalz, C. Griessenauer, C.S. Ogilvy, A.J. Thomas, Use of an absorbable synthetic polymer dural substitute for repair of dural defects: a technical note, Cureus 10 (1) (2018) e2127-e.
[67] P. López-Jaramillo, M.Y. Rincón, R.G. García, S.Y. Silva, E. Smith, P. Kampeerapappun, et al., A controlled, randomized-blinded clinical trial to assess the efficacy of a nitric oxide releasing patch in the treatment of cutaneous leishmaniasis by Leishmania (V.) panamensis, Am. J. Trop. Med. Hyg. 83 (1) (2010) 97–101.
[68] C. Karatepe, L. Aitinay, T.D. Yetim, C. Dagli, S. Dursun, A novel electrospun nano-fabric graft allows early cannulation access and reduces exposure to central venous catheters, J. Vasc. Access 14 (3) (2013) 273–280.
[69] M. Ferraresso, E.M. Bortolani, G. Amnon, A two-year experience with a rapid access, self-sealing, polycarbonate urethane nanofiber vascular access graft for hemodialysis, J. Vasc. Access 17 (3) (2016) 210–214.

[70] M.J. Regulski, M.R. MacEwan, Clinical evaluation of a novel nanofiber wound matrix for the treatment of chronic wounds, in: A. Academics (Ed.), Wound Care, Tissue Repair and Regenerative Medicine & Breast Cancer Management and Therapy, 2018.
[71] B. Balain, N. Craig, K. Gnanalingham, S. Madan, H. Sharma, G. Wynne-Jones, et al., Safety and efficacy of a novel fibrin dressing on bleeding cancellous bone, J. Clin. Exp. Ophthalmol. 4 (50) (2018).
[72] ISO 14644-1, Cleanrooms and Associated Controlled Environments-Part 1: Classification of Air Cleanliness by Particle Concentration (2015).
[73] Medical Device QMS, What It Is, Where It's Required, and Key Regulations to Know: Oriel Stat a Matrix (2021). https://www.orielstat.com/blog/medical-device-qms-overview/. (Accessed 5 March 2021).

Index

Note: 'Page numbers followed by "f" indicate figures and "t" indicate tables.'

D

E

F

R

S

U

V

W

X

Y

Z

CPI Antony Rowe
Eastbourne, UK
February 18, 2023